ASSISTING IN

SEVENTH EDITION

LONG-TERM CARE

ASSISTING IN
LONG-TERM CARE

SEVENTH EDITION

LEANN MILLER • MARY JO MIRLENBRINK GERLACH

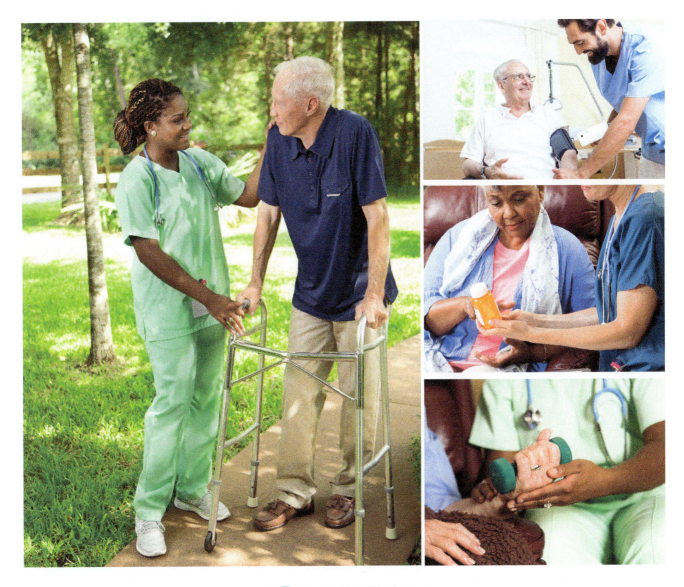

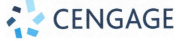

CENGAGE

Australia • Brazil • Mexico • Singapore • Spain • United Kingdom • United States

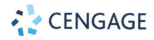

Assisting in Long-Term Care, Seventh Edition
Leann Miller, Mary Jo Mirlenbrink

SVP, GM Skills & Global Product Management:
Jonathan Lau

Product Director: Matthew Seeley

Product Team Manager: Stephen Smith

Associate Product Manager: Lauren Whalen

Product Assistant: Jessica Molesky

Executive Director, Content Design:
Marah Bellegarde

Director, Learning Design: Juliet Steiner

Learning Designer: Deborah Bordeaux

Vice President, Marketing Services:
Jennifer Ann Baker

Marketing Director: Sean Chamberland

Marketing Manager: Jonathan Sheehan

Senior Director, Content Delivery: Wendy Troeger

Senior Content Manager: Thomas Heffernan

Digital Delivery Lead: Derek Allison

Managing Art Director: Jack Pendleton

Senior Designer: Angela Sheehan

Cover Images: iStockPhoto.com/fstop123,
iStockPhoto.com/kzenon

Library of Congress Control Number: 2018965083

ISBN: 978-1-337-62507-4

Cengage
20 Channel Center Street
Boston, MA 02210
USA

Cengage is a leading provider of customized learning solutions with employees residing in nearly 40 different countries and sales in more than 125 countries around the world. Find your local representative at **www.cengage.com.**

Cengage products are represented in Canada by Nelson Education, Ltd.

To learn more about Cengage platforms and services, register or access your online learning solution, or purchase materials for your course, visit **www.cengage.com.**

Notice to the Reader
Publisher does not warrant or guarantee any of the products described herein or perform any independent analysis in connection with any of the product information contained herein. Publisher does not assume, and expressly disclaims, any obligation to obtain and include information other than that provided to it by the manufacturer. The reader is expressly warned to consider and adopt all safety precautions that might be indicated by the activities described herein and to avoid all potential hazards. By following the instructions contained herein, the reader willingly assumes all risks in connection with such instructions. The publisher makes no representations or warranties of any kind, including but not limited to, the warranties of fitness for particular purpose or merchantability, nor are any such representations implied with respect to the material set forth herein, and the publisher takes no responsibility with respect to such material. The publisher shall not be liable for any special, consequential, or exemplary damages resulting, in whole or part, from the readers' use of, or reliance upon, this material.

Printed in the United States of America
Print Number: 01   Print Year: 2018

DEDICATION

This edition is dedicated to the residents and families we serve, and to the skilled and caring individuals who provide this honorable service.

CONTENTS

4 Characteristics of the Long-Term Care Resident | 241

5 Meeting the Residents' Basic Needs | 289

6 Special Nursing Assistant Activities | 431

7 Introduction to Restorative Care | 491

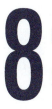

Residents with Specific Disorders | 575

9 Residents with Special Needs | 681

10 Employment | 769

LIST OF PROCEDURES

PREFACE

INTRODUCTION

Assisting in Long-Term Care, Seventh Edition provides the nursing assistant student and the instructor with the necessary tools to guide learning in preparation for a career as a Certified Nursing Assistant. This seventh edition builds on the long-respected foundation of *Assisting in Long-Term Care* and has been updated to ensure information is current and accurate. Hundreds of vibrant photographs illustrate nursing assistant skills and to reflect contemporary nursing assistant practice. With clear, straightforward writing and numerous features to support learning, this text proudly has helped individuals realize their goal of becoming a professional Certified Nursing Assistants since its first edition was published in 1988. Like the profession this text supports, much has changed since that first edition, but the commitment to excellence in client care remains steadfast.

CONCEPTUAL APPROACH

Because of the rising cost of health care, emphasis has been placed on reducing the length of time that individuals spend in an acute care facility. Short- and long-term rehabilitation is taking place in the long-term care facility, as well as in the home. The need for qualified nursing assistants continues to expand as the older adult populations continue to grow. The role of the nursing assistant in the long-term care setting has evolved from an untrained worker to that of an educated provider of care. The nursing assistant role is one of the most important in the para-professional, interdisciplinary team. Nursing assistants spend more time caring for the resident each day. Hence, the nursing assistant must be acutely aware of the needs of the resident and be able to identify and communicate any changes in the resident's condition that may determine a need to alter and adapt the plan of care. This text weighs these professional shifts carefully and endeavors to give nursing assisting students the skills, knowledge, and confidence needed to provide compete care.

One of the unique aspects of nursing assisting is that there is no standardized curriculum. To provide consistency, the National Council of State Boards of Nursing, Inc. established the Nurse Aide Competency and Evaluation Program to provide guidelines for evaluating the nursing assistant program. These guidelines have been incorporated into the OBRA requirements. This is essential content. It incorporates the federal and state core curriculum requirements in the absence of a standardized curriculum. Readers will see that these OBRA requirements are consistently highlighted throughout this text with an easy to identify icon.

ORGANIZATION

The seventh edition has taken the textbook a step further to assure the student understands the information covered. This is done by workbook style activities throughout each lesson. These activities provide the learner with the opportunity to test their understanding of many of the topics in each lesson. As a former teacher, the author is well aware of the rigors that faculty face in developing and revising course outlines. Throughout the revision process we were careful not to change what worked, but to instead make it better. But, at the same time, the content has been updated and expanded within the Lessons to include the elements that are required by the Omnibus Budget Reconciliation Act of 1987 (OBRA). The basic content meets the needs of the individual states that certify the nursing assistant programs. An invaluable tool during the nursing assistant education process, this book will continue to serve as a valuable reference after having achieved the objective of becoming a Certified Nursing Assistant. The general outline of the text is as follows:

The text contains 10 Sections and 35 Lessons. Section 1 has been expanded to discuss Medicare Reporting Regulations as well as the new Minimum Data Set (MDS3.0), highlighting the importance of quality care. To retain federal and state certification, long-term care facilities are routinely visited by a team of surveyors to determine compliance with federal regulations for Medicare and Medicaid program requirement. In an attempt to demystify the survey, deficiency categories are discussed so that the nursing assistant is fully aware of the importance of quality care and the criteria that surveyors use to measure that level of care.

Effective communication skills are pivotal to ensuring that care is provided in a safe and thorough manner. The nursing assistant primarily communicates with the resident and the nursing team. Knowledge of the make-up of the interdisciplinary team, however, is important, as is the understanding of the chain of command. This is discussed in Section 2. In addition, as we enter the twenty-first century, the impact of technological changes becomes even more apparent. The computer is increasingly being utilized to record resident data, and discussion of this is provided in Section 2 as well.

Because the nursing assistant spends the greatest amount of time with the resident it is helpful to the nurse to have a precise and thorough assessment of the resident's condition. Accurate assessment of pain levels is expanded in Section 2. The PAINAD scale has been included to assist the nursing assistant to more effectively communicate the resident with advanced dementia's needs.

Protecting resident rights is a vital component of the care of the resident. A thorough understanding is absolutely essential; this content is discussed in detail in Section 3. Resident Rights are outlined in the OBRA regulations as essential components of care. To help ensure that Resident Rights are implemented, the Ombudsman Program was instituted and continues to be an essential component of care. Discussion of this topic has been expanded.

Also in Section 3, emergency care has been expanded to include discussion of the impact of power outages, natural disasters, such as flood and tornados, as well as the threat of bioterrorism on residents and staff of the long-term care facility. The nursing assistant role is discussed to allay some of the apprehension that could be associated with such occurrences.

Finally, Section 3 covers principles of hand hygiene. *Clostridium difficile* infections are becoming more prevalent in health care facilities. An expanded discussion helps the student understand why this and other microorganisms, such as methicillin-resistant *Staphylococcus aureus* (MRSA) as well as community-based MRSA create significant problems in long-term care facilities.

Section 4 discusses the characteristics of the long-term care resident. The in-depth content enables the nursing assistant to understand the complexity and varied characteristics of those persons who are the resident population for whom they are providing care.

The nursing assistant is the primary provider of care for the long-term care resident. Understanding of the principles involved in the care of a resident is essential. Sections 5 and 6 discuss ways to meet the basic needs as well as any specialized needs the resident may have.

In order to prevent further decline in the resident, addressing nutritional needs is vitally important. The newest revision of the *2010 Dietary Guidelines for Americans* is discussed and *MyPlate* directives are presented. The Guidelines help the nursing assistant follow acceptable patterns of lifestyle in their own lives as well as in the resident's.

Section 7 deals with restorative and rehabilitative care. Many residents of long-term care facilities are admitted with a variety of conditions and health problems. The aim of rehabilitative and restorative care is to, at a minimum, help the resident to maintain or increase their current abilities and health status. Several assessment tools are discussed including the MDS3.0 and the CATs. Nursing assistants are vital members of the team to ensure that residents are fulfilling their potential. An in-depth discussion is provided.

Since nursing assistants and orderlies are among the groups most at risk for musculoskeletal injury, the "No Lift" policy is explained. Awareness of this policy can help to reduce the number and incidence of musculoskeletal injuries and occurrences. This policy affects the resident as well as the nursing assistant.

Many persons who become residents of long-term care facilities suffer from a variety of chronic diseases. Section 8 uses the systems approach to discuss the various conditions that might be present in the population. Each system includes an introduction to the anatomy and physiology as well a discussion and update of the various conditions, so the nursing assistant is able to understand the rationale for the care they provide. Increased emphasis is place on the nervous system.

Rosa's Law, which was passed in 2010, has clarified the definition of "intellectual disability" and use of the older term "mental retardation". Section 9 provides a discussion of this topic along with an in-depth presentation on Alzheimer's and other dementias. Primarily because of the age of the population to which the nursing assistant is providing care, death and dying becomes an essential part of living. The nursing assistant is provided with information to help guide them through this process. Some nursing assistants will choose to work in subacute units. Additional skills that are required are presented to meet those needs.

Section 10 discusses employment opportunities for the nursing assistant. Some persons will choose to work in the arena of home health; this lesson outlines some of the duties that are required. Additional certification, however, will be needed in order to be employed. Emphasis is placed on safety measures for the caregiver as well as the client. Suggestions for seeking, applying, and accepting a position as a nursing assistant are provided. The nursing assistant is a valuable member of the team providing care in a variety of long-term care facilities. It is important to present the best image to the prospective employer.

FEATURES

- Contains over 100 Procedures.
- Case Study at the beginning of each lesson personalizes lesson content with a scenario about a patient or certified nursing assistant, which is followed up by critical thinking questions at the end of each lesson.
- On the Job boxes feature important "real world" insights into the job and the health care industry.
- Building Cultural Awareness boxes throughout the text highlight important information related to meeting the needs of a culturally diverse resident population.
- Each lesson closes with a Lesson Synthesis, which serves as a review of chapter content with matching, multiple choice, true/false, and critical thinking questions.
- A key term list with pronunciations and a comprehensive end of book glossary support learning and mastery of new terminology.
- OBRA icon located throughout the text identifies federally mandated content for the nursing assistant training program.

NEW TO THIS EDITION

Over 200 exercises added to the text to check and enhance learner understanding of all major topics.

- MSDS updates to reflect OSHA changes to SDS.
- Expanded discussion of the Ombudsman Program in Section 3.
- Updated information on emergency care now includes discussion of the impact of power outages, natural disasters, and the threat of bioterrorism on residents and staff of the long-term care facility.
- Thoroughly revised and updated nutrition information includes the newest revision of the *2010 Dietary Guidelines for Americans* and *MyPlate* directives.
- Discussion of the PAINAD scale is now included to help the nursing assistant more effectively communicate the resident's needs related to pain management.
- Coverage of Rosa's Law clarifies the definition of intellectual disabilities and use of the older term *mental retardation*, in addition to more detailed discussion of Alzheimer's and other dementias.

TEACHING AND LEARNING PACKAGE TO ACCOMPANY THE SEVENTH EDITION

A complete teaching and learning package has been created for this text to aid instructors and students as they cover material.

MINDTAP

MindTap is a personalized teaching experience with relevant assignments that guide students to analyze, apply, and improve thinking, allowing you to measure skills and outcomes with ease.

- MindTap features a complete integrated course combining additional quizzing and assignments, and application activities along with the enhanced ebook to further facilitate learning.
- Personalized Teaching: Becomes yours with a Learning Path that is built with key student objectives. Control what students see and when they see it. Use it as-is or match to your syllabus exactly–hide, rearrange, add and create your own content.

- Guide Students: A unique learning path of relevant readings and activities that move students up the learning taxonomy from basic knowledge and comprehension to analysis and application.
- Promote Better Outcomes: Empower instructors and motivate students with analytics and reports that provide a snapshot of class progress, time in course, engagement and completion rates.

SPEND LESS TIME PLANNING AND MORE TIME TEACHING!

With Cengage's Instructor Resources to Accompany *Assisting in Long-Term Care*, preparing for class and evaluating students has never been easier! As an instructor, you will find this tool offers invaluable assistance by giving you access to all of your resources—anywhere and at any time.

Features:

- Each chapter in the **Instructor's Manual** provides (1) an overview of the content of the chapter; (2) instructional objectives; (3) key terms; (4) instructor and student resources; and (5) a chapter lesson plan and Overview
- The **Computerized Testbank** in **Cognero®** makes generating tests and quizzes a snap. With over 500 questions you can create customized assessments for your students with the click of a button. Add your own unique questions and print answers for easy class preparation. All questions have been thoroughly updated to reflect content updates made to the seventh edition.
- Customizable instructor support slide presentations in **PowerPoint®** format focus on key points for each chapter and have been fully updated to correlate to the content updates made to the seventh edition.

ABOUT THE AUTHORS

LEANN MILLER

Leann Miller is a consultant with more than two decades of teaching experience in health care settings. Her consulting practice with long-term and sub-acute facilities focuses on helping clients meet regulatory and clinical compliance requirements. Formerly a health sciences instructor at Kirkwood Community College, she has served as a Clinical Instructor in the Nurse Aide Program and nurse educator in the 75-hour Certified Nursing Assistant Program.

MARY JO MIRLENBRINK GERLACH

Mary Jo Mirlenbrink Gerlach, RN, MSN Ed, began her career in nursing began when she became a nursing assistant in high school. She graduated from the College of Mount Saint Joseph with a BSN and received her MSN Ed from Indiana University. Ms. Mary Jo Mirlenbrink Gerlach has had a long career in nursing education and consulting, and recently retired as Assistant Professor of Adult Nursing from Georgia Health Sciences University College of Nursing, Athens (formerly the Medical College of Georgia School of Nursing). She has received a number of awards for her outstanding teaching, including the Distinguished Alumni Nurse Leader Award from the College of Mount Saint Joseph.

Gerontology and long-term care have been Ms. Mary Jo Mirlenbrink Gerlach's areas of interest for a number of years, and she has served as nurse consultant to several long-term care facilities. She has been involved in curriculum development and instruction for nursing assistant training, and has participated in continuing education programs in both nursing and long-term care settings.

Ms. Mary Jo Mirlenbrink Gerlach also coauthored *Nutrition in Clinical Nursing* for Cengage Learning. In addition, she has written in the areas of Pharmacology and Adult Nursing, and has juried articles in professional journals of gerontology. She was a contributor to the first edition and contributor and co-editor for the second edition of *Adult Nursing: Acute and Community Care*. She also developed the review and study guides for both editions. Ms. Mary Jo Mirlenbrink Gerlach contributed selected chapters to *Clinical Medical-Surgical Nursing: A Decision-making Reference*, *Essentials of Clinical Pharmacology* (Third Edition), and served as the editor for *Concepts and Activities in Nursing Pharmacology*.

BARBARA R. HEGNER

Barbara Robinson Hegner, RN, MSN, was a graduate of a three-year diploma nursing program where direct and total care was the focus. She earned a BSN at Boston College and an MS in nursing from Boston University, with a minor in biologic sciences. She was Professor Emeritus of Nursing and Life Sciences at Long Beach City College, Long Beach (CA).

Throughout her professional career, she had a deep interest in both hospital-based and long-term care nursing.

Ms. Hegner believed that ensuring the rights and well-being of residents in long-term care requires the care of competent, caring nursing assistants under the supervision of professional nurses. The nursing assistants who provide this care should be thoroughly trained and consistently encouraged, evaluated, and given the opportunity for continued learning. Providing the tools to prepare these health care providers in the most effective and efficient way is the goal of *Assisting in Long-Term Care*, Fifth Edition. Barbara R. Hegner also authored *Nursing Assistant: A Nursing Process Approach*, Ninth Edition, for Cengage Learning.

REVIEWERS

This revision was aided by a dedicated group of instructors who reviewed content at various stages of the revision process. For their valuable suggestions and insights we would like to thank:

Dawn Howard, RN, BSN, NHA, CCM
Director of Education
Family Life Enrichment Centers, Inc
High Shoals, Georgia

Georgette Howard, RN, MSN
Nursing Assistant Program Coordinator
Glendale Community College
Glendale, Arizona

Betty Rivers, RN
Assistant Program Coordinator
Health Education Programs Corporate & Continuing Education Division
Forsyth Technical Community College
Winston-Salem, North Carolina

Linda Romano, BSN, RN
Health Science Education Teacher/Nurse Aide Program
Newburgh Enlarged City School District, Newburgh, NY 12550

Cindy Scott, RN, BSN
Director of Nursing
The MethWick Community
Cedar Rapids, Iowa

Vicki Jo Sodermark, RN, MSN
Faculty, Long Term CNA Program
Metropolitan Community College
Omaha, Nebraska

HOW TO USE THIS BOOK

PROCEDURE BEGINNING AND PROCEDURE COMPLETION ACTIONS

The listing of beginning procedure actions gives the essential steps to be performed before beginning any direct resident care procedure. These steps assure the rights of the resident and the safety of the resident and you, the nursing assistant. The procedure completion actions are performed at the end of each procedure to ensure that the resident is comfortable and safe, the resident's environment is clean, all equipment used is cleaned or discarded according to facility policy, and the proper documentation is completed.

TABLE OF CONTENTS

The table of contents lists, for each lesson, the lesson title, major topic headings, general guidelines for specific areas of care or topics of importance to the nursing assistant, and resident care procedures.

LESSON OPENING PAGE

The **Case Study** presents a common resident care situation and in the **Clinical Focus** asks you to think about ways to address the situation as the lesson content is studied. The **Objectives** help you know what is expected of you as you read the text. Your success in achieving each objective is measured by your completion of the unit end reviews.

BUILDING CULTURAL AWARENESS

These brief examples are designed to help you become aware of the differences between people from different groups. They help you recognize that people react differently to health and sickness and that their reactions are determined largely by the culture of which they are a part. The text suggests that if you observe, listen and learn, and accept people as they are, you will provide a high level of caring service.

PROCEDURES

The text contains 111 clinical procedures that provide step-by-step directions for a specific aspect of care. Each procedure reminds you to perform the beginning procedure actions. A list of equipment and supplies needed for the procedure follows. Any notes or cautions about performing the precaution are given. The steps take you carefully through the procedure, emphasizing at all times the need to work safely and to protect the resident's dignity. At the end, you are reminded of the procedure completion actions (refer to the inside back cover to refresh your memory of these actions).

Three icons may be used with the procedures:

OBRA to indicate an essential procedure required for certification

Gloves to indicate the need to observe Standard Precautions and wear personal protective equipment

OBRA

GUIDELINES

The guidelines included in each lesson highlight important points that you need to remember for specific situations or types of care. They are presented in an easy to use format that you can refer to repeatedly until you know the actions you must take when confronted with the situation.

LESSON SYNTHESIS: PUTTING IT ALL TOGETHER

At the end of each lesson, you are asked to return to the situation presented in the **Case Study** at the beginning of the lesson. Based upon what you have learned from the lesson, you are to answer a series of questions related to the resident or nursing assistant discussed. This exercise helps you to integrate what you have learned and apply it to a common clinical situation.

1

The Long-Term Care Setting

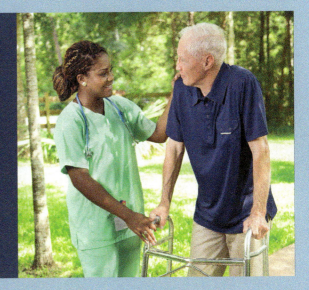

LESSON 1
THE LONG-TERM CARE FACILITY

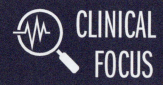

CLINICAL FOCUS

Think about the different types of agencies and facilities available to provide care and services to people with health needs. Consider how the services are paid for and regulated and how people may move from one agency or facility as their health needs change.

OBJECTIVES

After studying this lesson, you should be able to:

• Define and spell vocabulary words and terms.

• Describe community facilities that offer health care services.

• Explain the differences in services offered by health care facilities.

• List names applied to types of long-term care facilities.

• Describe the functional areas and equipment related to a long-term care facility.

• Describe state and federal licensing standards and regulations.

• Identify ways HIPAA laws affect care of the resident in a long-term care facility.

• State the importance of OBRA regulations to nursing assistant certification.

• Identify the role Medicare plays in helping to finance the care of long-term care residents.

• Explain the importance of records related to regulation and reimbursements.

• Describe the survey process, stating the assistants' responsibilities and the consequences of an unsatisfactory survey.

VOCABULARY

assignment (ah-SIGHN-ment)
certification (sir-tih-fih-KAY-shun)

client (KLIGH-ent)
communal (kum-MYOU-nul)

CASE STUDY

Rudolph McCarver is recovering from a stroke. He is 79 years old and is eligible for Medicare. Although he no longer needs the services of an acute care hospital, he will still require weeks of rehabilitation in long-term care before he can return to his home.

compliance (kom-PLY-ans)
confidential (kon-fih-DEN-shul)
decline (dih-KLINE)
deficiencies (dee-FISH-en-seez)
geriatric (jer-ee-AT-rick)
holistic (hoh-LISS-tik)
Kardex (KAR-dex)
licensure (LIE-sen-shur)
long-term care facility (lawng turm kair fah-SILL-ih-tee)
Medicaid (MEH-dih-kaid)
Medicare (MEH-dih-kare)
nurses' station (nur-ses STAY-shun)
OBRA (OH-brah)

patient (PAY-shent)
policy book (POL-ah-see book)
procedure book (proh-SEE-jur book)
rehabilitation (ree-hah-BILL-ih-tay-shun)
resident (REZ-ih-dent)
resident unit (REZ-ih-dent YOU-nit)
restoration (reh-stor-AY-shun)
skilled nursing facility (skilled NUR-sing fah-SILL-ih-tee)
Skilled care (sub-ah-KYOOT kair)
survey (SIR-vay)
surveyor (sir-VAY-er)
terminal (TER-mih-nul)

Nursing assistants make valuable contributions in providing health care. Nursing assistants are trained to care for people who are ill or need help in caring for themselves. The care given is always under the guidance and supervision of licensed health care providers such as nurses or physicians.

COMMUNITY HEALTH CARE FACILITIES

The health needs of the nation are met in various community settings (Figure 1-1). Although trained nursing assistants may work in any type of agency or facility, they find their greatest opportunity for employment in agencies or facilities that provide:

- Life care communities
- Assisted living facilities
- Health and personal care for people in their homes
- Hospice care for the terminally ill
- Care for the developmentally disabled
- Health services in acute care hospitals
- Extended (long-term) care

- Subacute care services
- Skilled care facilities

Each care setting provides basic care in addition to special services to meet individual needs. Figure 1-2 compares some of the characteristics of three care settings where nursing assistants are employed.

Home health care, assisted living facilities, hospices, and homes for the developmentally disabled offer similar services:

- They are conducted in a homelike setting.
- They stress supportive psychosocial services.
- They provide for physical needs.
- They assist clients to maintain and achieve the maximum level of personal control and functioning.

Home Health Care

Home health services provide for the health and daily living activity needs of people who are ill or have disabilities when family members cannot provide the necessary care in the home.

Acute care hospitals	Assisted living facilities
Facilities for the mentally ill	Community health centers
Physicians' offices	Subacute care facilities
Clinics of various kinds	Life care communities
Hospices for the terminally ill	Adult day care facilities
Facilities for the developmentally disabled	Group homes
Facilities for long-term care	Adult foster care
Rehabilitation facilities	

Figure 1-1 Different types of health care facilities are needed to meet the nation's health needs.

Facility	Care Recipient	Length of Stay	Characteristics/Service	Nursing Assistant Participation
Acute care	Patient	Few days to weeks	Cure-oriented; frequent physician visits; high-level skilled nursing; high-technology equipment; multiple support services; multiple support departments; multiple personnel; may be specialized according to patient needs; care of acutely ill persons; limited term.	Employed by the hospital; may or may not require certificate; gives basic care under direct supervision; assists professionals in more complex care; carries out special techniques under supervision and for which they have been specially educated; contributes to nursing care plan or clinical pathway through observing and reporting.
Long-term care	Resident	Weeks, months, years	Subacute care; restoration, maintenance-oriented; assistance with activities of daily living; rehabilitative techniques; less complex equipment; stress on social and psychological needs; fewer physician visits; professional nursing supervision; long-term care of chronically ill, infirm, and developmentally disabled; pediatric and in some cases psychiatric services.	Requires certification; encourages self-care when possible; provides complete personal care for those who are unable to help themselves; participates in rehabilitative efforts; contributes to nursing care plan through observing and reporting.
Home health care	Client	Intermittent, may have periodic hospital stays	Some procedures may be assigned and monitored by the RN. Other procedures may be *delegated* (assigned to another care provider) and supervised periodically.	Employed by the agency; time spent with a client may range from 1 hour to a full 8-hour shift; may visit several clients in 1 day for 1–3 hours each; must interact with family members to provide required services to client; offers emotional support to family; carries out basic care under indirect supervision; promotes self-care and rehabilitation; contributes to the nursing care plan by observing, reporting, and documenting; keeps records related to reimbursements.

Figure 1-2 Comparison of the health care provided in different health care settings.

⊘N THE JOB

Although many health care services are available, people are not always able to access the services necessary to meet their health needs. This is a critical problem in health care delivery.

The care needed is assessed and planned by the nurse along with other health care specialists. The nursing assistant, who works for the home health care agency, carries out the care in the person's home. Additional preparation and certification are required for working in home health care. The person who receives the care is called a client. The home care nursing assistant is supervised by professionals but usually works alone with clients. The client is assisted in performing activities of daily living (ADL) and needed personal and basic nursing care is given. The nursing assistant reports directly to the supervising nurse and is involved in the planning, implementation, and documentation of care. The private home care provider (PHCP) is a specially prepared nursing assistant who gives care to clients in their own homes under the direction of a registered nurse (RN). The PHCP may assist with personal care, household and housekeeping tasks, and preparation and serving of meals, as well as provide transportation for appointments, shopping, or other social activities.

Hospice and Palliative Care

Hospice is a concept of care, providing supportive care (relief of symptoms) rather than cure of a disease. Personal, individualized care can be provided in a variety of settings: in the person's own home, a personal care home, an assisted living facility or a "home-like" private hospice facility (Figure 1-3), a long-term care facility, or a hospital setting. A more detailed explanation can be found in Lesson 32.

Care for the Developmentally Disabled

Services for the developmentally disabled are designed to assist in the care and training of persons whose mental and physical limitations affect self-care (Figure 1-4).

Many developmentally disabled clients live in a long-term care facility. Some clients live at home but spend time daily in the facility for care and training, such as in ADL. The nursing assistant who works with this group of clients also needs basic nursing and interpersonal skills.

Acute Care Hospitals

People receiving care in an acute care hospital are called patients. These people are usually seriously ill or injured, or they have some special health need. They require a high level of skilled professional care. Nursing assistants, sometimes called patient care assistants or patient care technicians in the acute care setting, provide basic care and are supervised as they perform special technical skills that they have been taught. Patients stay in hospitals for a limited time and

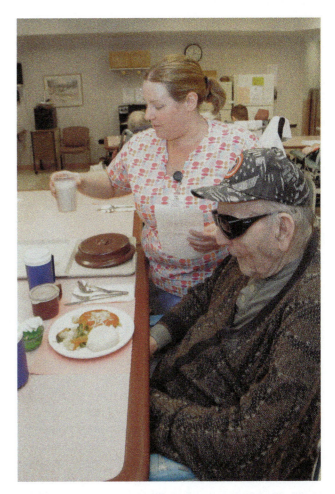

Figure 1-4 People with developmental disabilities have a limited ability to care for themselves.

may then be transferred to long-term care facilities or home as their conditions change.

Because patients in an acute care facility need closer attention and more care, the nursing assistant is assigned to care for a specific number of people at a time and is always under the direct supervision of a professional health provider. The nursing assistant working in an acute care facility needs basic nursing skills and interpersonal relationship skills and may be trained by the facility in special technical skills.

Physicians' Offices/Clinics

People visit physicians' offices for acute short-term care and referrals. Nursing assistants may assist the professional staff by receiving patients and performing basic procedures such as measuring temperature, pulse, respiration, and blood pressure. Nursing assistants may be asked to measure and weigh patients and to record and report the information. Selected nursing assistants are trained to do other special procedures under the direct supervision of the physician or nurse.

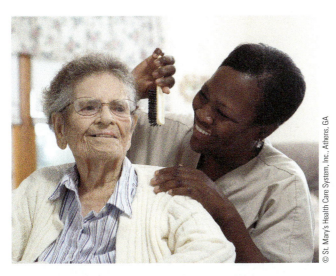

© St. Mary's Health Care System, Inc., Athens, GA

Figure 1-3 Hospice care assists people with a limited life span.

Facilities for the Mentally Ill

Patients are admitted to facilities for mental illness to receive care and therapy. Some patients may stay for a short time, whereas others are admitted for long periods. The trend today is to move patients out of institutions as soon as possible and into community-based outpatient programs. Nursing assistants employed by the facility perform basic care skills and make a major contribution to the nursing care plan through careful observation and reporting of the patients' behavior and response to care.

Rehabilitation Facilities

Patients may visit rehabilitation facilities as an outpatient for a period of weeks or months, or they may spend a period of time in a long-term care facility recuperating from a stroke or hip fracture and receiving intensive therapy. These types of settings are also known as Post Acute Facilities. The focus of care is based on evaluating, maintaining, and restoring the patient's or resident's mobility and independence in carrying out ADL. This level of therapy is more intensive than that received in a nursing home. Nursing assistants work with RNs and therapists (physical, occupational, and speech) in positioning persons, using adaptive equipment, and providing emotional support and encouragement. Some facilities utilize restorative nursing assistants who have taken additional training in rehabilitative nursing after their basic CNA program. Restorative aides help the residents with a Functional Maintenance Plan (FMP) to prevent additional physical decline.

Community Health Centers

These centers may also be referred to as public health nursing clinics. Care is provided on a regular outpatient basis. Nurses in the centers provide health teaching and monitor chronic conditions such as diabetes and high blood pressure (hypertension). They also offer weight control counseling and focus on overall wellness, including activities and lifestyles. The centers may provide reproductive health services, breast and cervical cancer screening, immunizations, well baby clinics, and AIDS testing and counseling. Nursing assistants provide basic skills such as measuring and weighing clients and taking vital signs. They may also help with examinations and care for equipment and records. Some metropolitan areas have nonprofit community-based clinics for the medically underserved. These clinics provide free and low-cost health care services.

Long-Term Care Facilities

The person cared for in a **long-term care facility** is called a **resident**. The facility becomes home for the resident for an extended period, which may be for weeks or months as the resident is restored to better health. In some cases, the facility may become the resident's permanent home.

People are discharged from an acute care facility because they no longer need the specialized care

---

❓ EXERCISE 1-1

COMPLETION
Select the correct term(s) from the following list to complete each statement.

seriously	mental	resident
care	patients	semi-independent
client	physical	technical
injured	supportive	training

1. The person receiving care at home is called a(an) _____.
2. The nursing assistant working in home care works in a(an) _____ manner.
3. Hospice care provides _____ care rather than cure of a disease.
4. Developmentally disabled persons are those whose _____ and _____ impairments limit self-care.
5. Some developmentally disabled clients live at home but spend time in a care facility for _____ and _____.
6. People being cared for in acute care hospitals are called _____.
7. People being cared for in acute care facilities are usually _____ ill, _____, or have some special health need.
8. Nursing assistants working in acute care may be trained in special _____ skills.
9. The person being cared for in a long-term care facility is called a(an) _____.

Complete the following statement by providing brief answers.

1. Five community facilities that offer health care services are:

    a. _____

    b. _____

    c. _____

    d. _____

    e. _____

provided there. However, they may still require skilled care and not be ready to return home. Often they are admitted to the **skilled care** unit in a hospital or in a long-term care facility. Here, they receive short-term nursing care until they are ready to go home.

The different types of long-term care facilities employ many nursing assistants who play a vital role in the success of the care given. Nursing assistants who work in long-term care must be certified. This text is designed to help students become successful certified nursing assistants.

TYPES OF LONG-TERM CARE FACILITIES

Several different names are applied to long-term care (LTC) facilities. Some of the names you will hear include:

- Nursing home
- Nursing facility (NF)
- Skilled nursing facility
- Rehabilitation care center
- Assisted living facility
- Alzheimer's care center

People who need long-term care are those who:

- Need to regain the ability to care for themselves (restoration or rehabilitation)
- Cannot, because of illness or disability, care for themselves and have no one else to provide such care
- Are older and frail and need continuous nursing care (geriatric care)

All long-term care facilities provide housing, protection, and assistance as needed to meet individual needs (Figure 1-5). Some also provide skilled nursing care. Placement in a specific long-term care facility is determined by the level of care and type of services needed (Figure 1-6). Some of the service is supported by governmental funds such as Medicare and Medicaid.

In an attempt to make nursing homes and long-term care facilities more "home-like," the Centers for Medicare and Medicaid Services issued new guidelines

All long-term care facilities provide:

Holistic care

Physical care

Emotional care

Dementia care

Help with activities of daily living (ADLs)

Restorative care

Safety and security

Opportunities for social interaction

Spiritual/religious activities

Figure 1-5 Health care facility functions.

in 2009, which provide surveyors detailed information for assessing facility compliance with OBRA regulations (discussed later in this Lesson) that deal with issues related to the physical environment, health and safety matters, and resident rights.

The Eden Alternative concept is one way to deinstitutionalize facility environments. The Eden Alternative philosophy, with a focus on anything "living," incorporates the use of plants and animals and encourages regular visits by children. It has been documented that this philosophy helps to eliminate loneliness, helplessness, and boredom that may frequent residents in long-term care facilities.

The Skilled Nursing Facility

In order to qualify for federal funding such as Medicare or Medicaid, a facility must guarantee that the bed is certified for skilled care. The number of certified beds within a facility may vary. Some facilities certify all the available beds as skilled, whereas others may certify only a percentage of the beds as skilled. Persons who require restorative care on a less intensive level and who are not utilizing any federal funding source can reside in a skilled care facility in one of the noncertified beds.

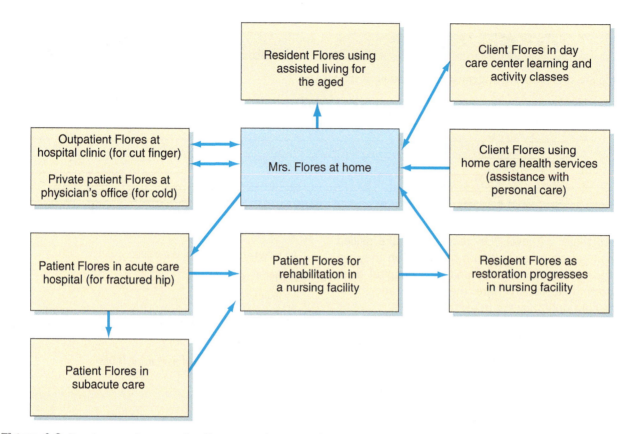

Figure 1-6 People move from one health care service to another as their needs household model and integrate resident centered care/culture change.

The **skilled nursing facility** (SNF) offers professional nursing care to chronically ill or disabled persons and those who are recovering but do not require the high-cost services of an acute hospital setting. Many of these people are older; some are in the **terminal** (last) stage of life. They have many needs and require the services of many skilled professionals. Highly trained team members provide this specialized care. Physicians, professional nurses, and pharmacy services are readily available. Other support personnel and specialists, such as physical, occupational, and speech therapists, are available as required.

Skilled nursing facilities provide many of the services offered in the acute hospital setting. The care is aimed at maintenance and **restoration (rehabilitation)** (Figure 1-7). Maintenance is aimed at preventing further loss and limitations.

Restoration or rehabilitation is the process of assisting residents to do as much as they can, as well as they can, for as long as they can for themselves. Residents of any age who are admitted primarily for rehabilitation usually stay about 1 to 3 months before they are discharged. The cost of care in such an SNF is higher than for some other types of extended care because

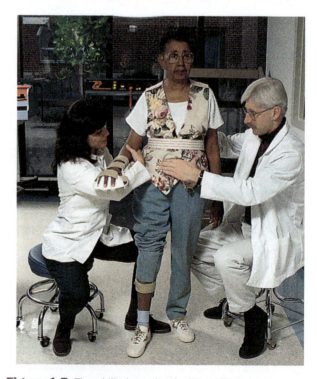

Figure 1-7 The skilled nursing facility (SNF) provides technical nursing care and emphasizes rehabilitation.

? EXERCISE 1-3

Complete the following statement by providing brief answers.

1. Four common services offered by home health care, assisted living facilities, hospices, and homes for the developmentally disabled include:

   a. _____

   b. _____

   c. _____

   d. _____

more services are available. As soon as appropriate, residents are transferred, usually to a less expensive care setting such as a nursing facility or to their homes.

Assisted Living Facility

Residents in this type of facility may not require constant care but may need help with ADLs such as meals, bathing, dressing, housekeeping, as well as assistance with medication administration. Assisted Living Facilities are known as "a hotel with medical services." The person also may experience confusion or memory problems. Assisted living facilities bridge the gap between independent living and nursing home care. Residents are predominantly private pay clients. If the resident was a veteran or the spouse of a veteran, some monetary support may be available through the Veterans' Administration.

Personal Care Homes

Residents of personal care homes do not have an illness or disability that requires chronic care; but need an environment that offers protective care. The size of the facility tends to range in size from 2 to 12 or more residents. Facilities that advertise to provide personal care services are licensed in their respective state to provide *only* this type of care.

Retirement Communities

Continuing care retirement communities (CCRC), also known as life care communities, offer a complete range of housing and care to meet the current and future needs of residents. These communities offer the opportunity for independent living, assisted living, and long-term care. A resident may move in and out of the various levels of care as individual needs dictate. There is usually an entrance fee and a monthly maintenance fee, and with that, a provision for care for the rest of their life.

Livable Communities aka Villages

Another relatively new concept that has been evolving across the United States in recent years is that of the livable or lifelong communities, frequently referred to as "villages." Studies and surveys have shown that the majority of older adults would prefer to "age in place," that is, to live in their own homes for as long as possible.

In response to these findings, local communities have become aware of the needs of its senior citizens and are developing areas where an older person can remain at home and stay socially connected to the community as their physical needs may change. Emphasis is placed on transportation, home repair, modifications, social connections, and health support services. Membership fees offer support services for older adults, both healthy and disabled in all income brackets. Most of the services are provided by "vetted" volunteers and a number of service providers who offer members a discount. The older adult who wishes to participate is one who does not require long-term care. Membership in the "village" helps one obtain services through a trusted source with the goal of preventing preinstitutionalization. This type of service is less expensive than living in a retirement community or residing in a long-term care facility. Increasing emphasis will be placed on the role of home health services in this type of system.

FUNCTIONAL AREAS IN A LONG-TERM CARE FACILITY

Facilities vary to some degree in physical layout, but certain elements are common to all.

The Resident Room

The resident's room may be called a **resident unit**. An adjustable bed, bedside stand, overbed table, chair, wastebasket, privacy curtain, and a storage area (closet) are provided for each person (Figure 1-8).

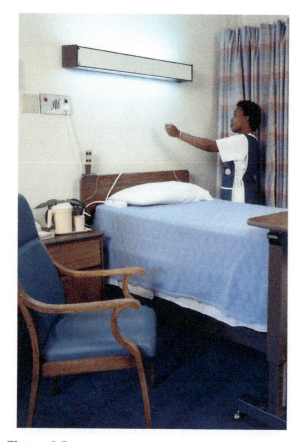

Figure 1-8 Standard furniture provided in a resident unit.

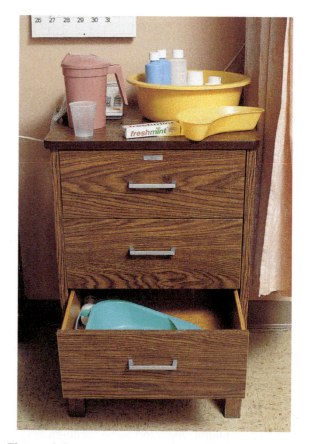

Figure 1-9 Clean and soiled items must be kept separate in the drawers (or shelves) of the bedside stand.

Resident rooms may be designed for occupancy by a single individual, but they usually accommodate two persons. In some instances, several residents share a single room.

Many facilities encourage residents who will be making the facility their home to bring personal articles as space permits. A familiar chest of drawers, a lamp, or bedside table may replace some of the facility's equipment to add a sense of familiarity and security for the resident. Personal mementos such as pictures or religious articles are important to residents and are kept at the bedside or displayed.

The Bed

The bed is usually adjustable for height. It can be raised during care (eliminating bending for the caregiver) and lowered so that residents can get into or out of bed safely. Some beds are lowered to 8 to 10 inches from the ground to prevent risk of falls. The head and bottom of the bed can also be raised or lowered for resident comfort.

Each bed can be equipped with side rails. Side rails should be securely in place if they are ordered for a specific resident. Not all residents need the side rails up. Many facilities remove side rails completely so they do not act as restraints.

Some beds are electric; others are adjusted by hand with a crank. The assistant should be thoroughly familiar with the bed controls before attempting to operate them.

Personal Equipment

The bedside stand in each unit is equipped with articles for the resident's personal care and use. Many of the articles are purchased by the resident or the resident's family. These articles should not be shared with other residents.

All items in the bedside stand should be clearly marked with the resident's name.

The contents of the bedside table should be arranged so that "clean" items are stored separately from those items that are considered "dirty," such as the bedpan or urinal (Figure 1-9). Clean items include:

- Washbasin or bath pan
- Kidney-shaped emesis basin
- Soap dish
- Comb and hairbrush
- Toothbrush, toothpaste, denture cup
- Personal items, such as lotion, makeup, or shaving cream

Call Lights

Each unit has a signaling device, such as a call light (Figure 1-10). Call lights may be attached to the wall or may be part of a more complex panel attached to the side rail of the bed. The panel may also control a radio, television, or telephone. Call lights are also located in the bathroom and shower area. The shower and bathroom lights blink differently and have a different sound, indicating the need for immediate attention. When a resident needs help and uses the call signal, a light over the door of the resident's room and at the nurses' station comes on, showing the room number of the resident who called (Figure 1-11). The call light should

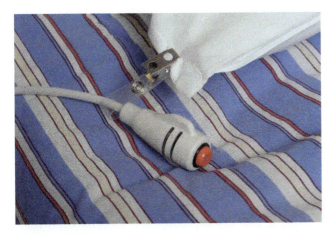

Figure 1-10 Each resident unit has a way for the resident to signal for assistance.

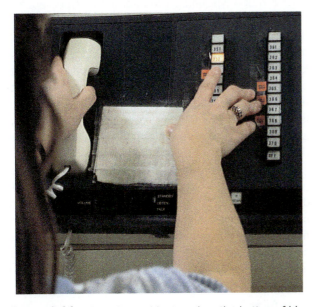

Figure 1-11 When the resident pushes the button of his or her signaling device, a light shows at the communications center at the nurses' station and over the door of the resident's room to indicate which resident is calling for assistance.

always be within reach of the resident. It is important that the staff answer the resident's call light promptly, within 15 minutes or less if possible.

An overbed table, which is adjustable in height, may be placed over the bed, providing a place to serve meals or hold equipment during care. Each unit has a closet for storing the resident's personal articles.

Dining Room

Residents who are able are encouraged to eat in a communal (group) setting, so each facility has a common dining room. This helps to provide social stimulation and may encourage better food intake.

Dining rooms sometimes are used for activities and socialization at times other than meals.

Lounges, Activity Areas, and Gardens

Because talking with others, watching television, and playing cards are enjoyable activities for those whose physical needs are limited, a television set, playing cards, and other games may be available in the facility's lounges. These areas also provide a place for visiting with family and friends outside the resident's own room. Many facilities also have outdoor areas that are suitable for a variety of activities. All of these areas are safe and handicapped accessible so the resident does not have to be confined indoors. Group exercises, singing, and parties that celebrate a special occasion, such as a resident's birthday or a holiday, are also usually held in the lounge or dining room.

Nurses' Station

Every facility has an area where records of care are kept. This area is called the nurses' station. Part of the nurses' station is set aside for the control and dispensing of medications; unauthorized persons are not permitted in this area. Authorized persons include the physician, the pharmacist, the registered nurse, the licensed vocational/practical nurse (LVN or LPN), and, in some states, the certified medication aide (CMA). This part of the nurses' station is kept locked when unattended.

Medications are delivered to residents by the medication nurse using a medicine cart. Medication carts must always be locked when unattended to prevent unauthorized persons from taking anything from the cart.

Reports of residents' needs and care are usually given within the nurses' station. This is confidential (private, personal) information and should not be discussed within hearing of the residents or guests. This information should never be discussed outside the facility. Nursing assistants use this area to report and record their observations and the care given. Directions and **assignments** (list of duties) are received at the nurses' station.

Records

Important records are found in the nurses' station including the:

- Procedure book
- Policy book
- Resident's chart
- Kardex or resident profile
- Assignment sheet
- Care plans
- Fire and safety manual
- Medication and treatment books
- Disaster plan
- Material Safety Data Sheets
- Infection control manual

The **procedure book** explains how care is to be given. The **policy book** (Figure 1-12) outlines the rules for the facility and explains what will be done for the residents.

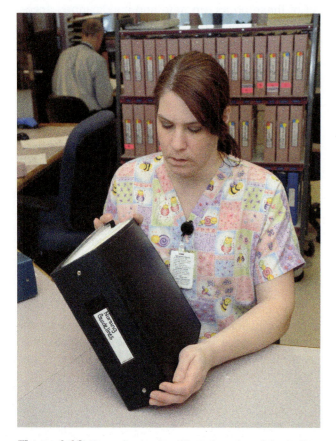

Figure 1-12 The policy book outlines the rules of the facility.

The resident's chart contains a record of the care given and the progress reported, as well as information about the resident. The resident profile or **Kardex** contains information about the specific daily care to be given to a particular resident. The information on the Kardex reflects a plan called the interdisciplinary care plan that has been developed for each resident. The assignment sheet lists the specific assignments and duties for the staff for the shift. The fire and safety manual outlines procedures to follow if a fire or accident occurs in the facility. Also kept at each nurses station is a crash cart for medical emergencies.

Computers

Computers are used in health care facilities to:

- Maintain records such as care plans, nursing assessments, physicians' orders, and required reports to state and federal agencies
- Inventory supplies
- Record medications and treatments
- Schedule appointments
- Set work schedules. Transmission of medical information to government

If your facility uses computers to process information, you may be asked to use one. You will be trained to use the computer and then be supervised until you can operate it properly.

Computers have a central processing unit, a drive, a display screen, and a keyboard. The keyboard is like the keyboard of a typewriter. The information typed appears on the screen. Information can be stored in the drive of the computer or on disks. A disk has a menu that lists the files of information on the disk. Once information is entered and named, the file name can be selected on the menu and opened. The information can then be reviewed and revised as needed. For privacy reasons, it is important for the CNA, or anyone using the computer system to enter or review information related to the resident, to "lock out" of the system when finished.

Computers provide ready access to essential information that can be used to make medical and nursing decisions (Figure 1-13). Because documentation by the certified nursing assistant is crucial to patient care and financial reimbursement, many facilities install kiosks, or computers on the wall in each service area, so that documentation can be completed as patient care is given.

Fax Machines

Fax machines allow you to send information from printed sheets over telephone lines to other locations. These locations may be within the same building or

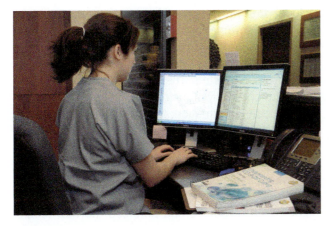

Figure 1-13 Computers provide immediate access to resident information.

city, across the United States, or in another country. The sending and receiving of information by fax machines can be accomplished in a few minutes. To operate the fax machine, you dial a telephone number that prepares a machine at the other end to receive and print the message. The fax machine is frequently used to send physicians' orders and laboratory test results until the permanent document can be attached to the chart.

Areas for Specific Rehabilitation

To make it easier to work with residents, facilities have special areas devoted to the rehabilitation process.

- In the physical therapy department, physical therapists and physical therapy aides focus on exercises to strengthen the residents' larger muscles for ambulation and transfer. Residents are also taught to use prostheses (artificial limbs), canes, walkers, or crutches to increase their mobility and independence.

- In the occupational therapy department, occupational therapists and occupational therapy aides focus on improving the flexibility of the smaller muscles of the residents' hands and arms and focus on specific tasks to aid with ADLs. This is especially helpful when a resident has arthritis and for rehabilitation after a stroke.

- In the speech therapy department, residents are evaluated for speech and swallowing problems. Speech therapists assist residents to improve their written and oral communication abilities, as well as recommending the proper diet to minimize potential choking issues.

- In the respiratory therapy department, residents are helped to make the most efficient use of

their breathing capacity. For example, they may be taught respiratory exercises to clear the airway and how to do pursed-lip breathing.

Kitchen

Meals are prepared and food is stored in the kitchen. The kitchen area should only be accessible to food service personnel. Meals are then delivered to residents in the dining room or, when necessary, in their rooms.

Both regular and special diets are prepared for residents in this area and then delivered in special carts.

Each wing of a facility may be equipped with a small kitchen area equipped with a refrigerator that is used for storage of milk, juice, and snacks for exclusive use of the residents. No medications, specimens, or employee snacks should be kept in these refrigerators. Food must be labeled and dated. The temperature in the refrigerator must be monitored and should not be more than 40°F. A temperature log must be kept daily and posted at each refrigerator.

Laundry

Some facilities have laundries that wash and dry residents' personal clothes (Figure 1-14). Basic linens needed in resident care may be commercially laundered and delivered to the facility, and soiled laundry and clothing may be picked up for cleaning. Some facilities may handle all laundry needs on the premises. In some instances, the family may choose to launder the resident's clothes and return them to the facility. Soiled clothing should be put into a specially marked container and never stored with the resident's clean clothing. Gloves are required when handling soiled linen of any kind. Clothing must be marked with the resident's name in an inconspicuous place.

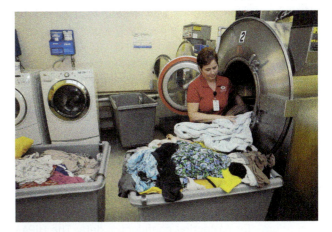

Figure 1-14 When the facility launders resident's personal clothing, individual items must be labeled with the resident's name to avoid mix-ups.

MULTIPLE CHOICE
Select the one best answer.

1. A machine used to keep records and schedule appointments in health facilities is the
   (A) fax machine
   (B) telephone
   (C) intercom
   (D) computer

2. What is considered an appropriate response time for answering a call light?
   (A) 5 to 10 minutes
   (B) 10 to 20 minutes
   (C) 30 minutes
   (D) Whenever you can get there

Standards and Regulations

All facilities must adhere to standards that are set by official public agencies. These standards govern the:

- Qualifications of the caregivers
- Care that is given
- Safety of the facility
- Sanitary conditions
- Quality of food

HEALTH INSURANCE PORTABILITY AND ACCOUNTABILITY ACT

The Health Insurance Portability and Accountability Act (HIPAA), a law that protects confidential resident/patient medical records and other health information, took effect in 2003. These standards were developed by the Department of Health and Human Services (HHS) to provide persons with access to their individual medical records and allow them more control over how this information is used.

Many health care providers are affected by this law. This group includes physician, nurses, pharmacies, hospitals, clinics, and nursing homes. In addition, health insurance companies, health maintenance organizations (HMOs), most employer group health plans, as well as government programs that pay for health care, such as Medicare and Medicaid, must comply with the law.

HIPAA rules ask providers to analyze how and where resident information is used and to develop procedures for protecting confidential data. The HIPAA policies and procedures for each agency are individualized to that agency. The information that is protected includes that which is contained in the medical record as well as conversations a person has with health care providers that deal with care or treatment. Billing information and any data stored in an agency's computer system are protected. The law also outlines requirements for physically storing and transmitting any confidential health information. National uniform standards regulate the transmission of data in any form, whether by letter, fax, or computer.

For certain violations of the law, by individuals or agencies, penalties of a monetary fine as well as imprisonment may be imposed. The HHS Office for Civil Rights (OCR) oversees and enforces the new federal privacy regulations.[1]

OBRA LEGISLATION

In 1987, the first OBRA (Omnibus Budget Reconciliation Act) was passed. This legislation established training and evaluation standards for nursing assistants working in such facilities. A new OBRA is passed each year. This legislation requires all nursing assistants to complete an evaluation program (written and skills testing) and be entered into a state registry before they can work in long-term care.

OBRA also requires the:

- promotion of resident independence
- elimination of restraints
- promotion of improved quality of life, care, health, and safety for all residents

OBRA legislation focuses on all aspects of the resident's social, mental, physical, emotional, and spiritual life. Facilities and nursing assistants must follow the OBRA rules and regulations to be in compliance (accord) with the law.

Nursing Assistant Certification Under the Omnibus Budget Reconciliation Act

Nursing assistants must be certified within 120 days by the state before they can work in long-term care. State regulations for the training and certification of nursing assistants are guided by the OBRA. Since October 1, 1990, all persons working as nursing assistants must complete a competency evaluation program or approved course.

[1]U.S. Department of Health and Human Services. (2003, April). *Fact Sheet: Protecting the privacy of patient's health information.* Retrieved May 20, 2011, from Health and Human Services online via: http:www.hhs.gov/news/facts/privacy.html.

The National Nurse Aide Assessment Program

The National Nurse Aide Assessment Program (NNAAP) is an examination made up of two parts: a written (or oral) examination and a skills examination. These examinations test the aide's ability to safely perform entry-level job skills and demonstrate the related knowledge and ability to support such care. Both parts of the examination must be passed for the aide to be certified and to become listed in the nurse aide registry. Some states may require that certification be renewed every 2 years unless one has worked as a CNA in the past 24 months.

Areas of testing include:

- Physical care skills, including ADL, basic nursing skills, and restorative services
- Psychosocial care skills, including meeting emotional, mental health, and spiritual needs
- Role of the nurse aide, including communication, residents' rights, ethical behavior, and being a member of the health care team
- Role of the nurse aide in following infection control guidelines
- Role of the nurse aide in maintaining safety of resident at all times

Nursing assistants who are not certified have three opportunities to meet the requirements for certification. In some states, a new training and competency evaluation program must be completed by nursing assistants who previously finished such a program but have not performed nursing-related services for pay for a continuous 24-month period. Certified nursing assistants must complete at least 12 hours of continuing education per year. In some states, the continuing education requirement is 24 hours per year.

The OBRA regulations are important because they:

- Give nursing assistants recognition through certification and listing on the state registry
- Help define the scope of nursing assistant practice
- Ensure better uniformity of care by nursing assistants
- Promote educational standards for nursing assistants

Be sure you are familiar with any specific state regulations or legislation that relate to your job as a nursing assistant.

FINANCING IN LONG-TERM CARE

Long-term care is paid for in several ways, such as through:

- Private sources—residents pay the costs out of their own funds
- Prepaid insurance—residents pay premiums to insurance companies that, in turn, pay providers for care
- Preferred provider organization (PPO)—members are given a list of providers from which to choose a primary care provider
- Health maintenance organization (HMO)
- Charitable organizations and community agencies
- Medicare
- Medicaid

Not all facilities accept Medicare payment, but those that do must follow Medicare rules and regulations to receive reimbursement.

Medicaid

Medicaid (Title XIX) is a state and federally funded program designed to provide health care for eligible low-income individuals. Federal money is issued to the states, which then determine how to distribute the money to health care facilities. Facilities must be approved (certified) to participate in the program. Not all facilities choose to participate.

Medicare

The Medicare program is federally funded and is under the administration of the Centers for Medicare and Medicaid Services. Facilities must be approved to participate in the program. Medicare is divided into four parts: A, B, C, and D.

Part A

Also known as hospital insurance, helps pay for some of the cost of care in acute settings and in skilled nursing facilities. It may also cover some of the costs related to home health care and hospice care. There is no monthly premium; the taxes people pay while they are working help cover the cost of Part A Medicare.

Part B

Medicare beneficiaries may pay an additional premium monthly, which makes them eligible for additional services, such as some diagnostic tests, splints, braces, prosthetics, therapy evaluation, limited rehabilitation services, and other outpatient care. These services must be considered medically necessary in order to be covered by Part B.

Part C

Medicare Part C, also known as Medicare Advantage plans (MA Plans), combine Medicare parts A and B to cover all medically needed services for persons who require a larger amount of services. It can be a lower cost alternative to Parts A and B. Part C coverage is administered by approved private insurance companies under contracts with Medicare. Prescription drug coverage under Medicare Part C is usually included in this plan. It is important to determine the plan's rules since there are wide variations among insurance companies. Persons who require extensive amounts of health care services receive these specialized services through approved network providers.

Part D

The Medicare Prescription, Drug, Improvement, and Modernization Act of 2003 created prescription drug benefits that were added to Medicare in 2006. The new program is voluntary and will offer a variety of choices for prescription drug coverage.

Medicare Reporting Regulations. To be in compliance and receive reimbursement, specific reports must be submitted to show that the facility is assisting the resident to function at the highest possible level. The government developed a Resident Assessment Instrument (RAI) to help with the assessment and reporting process. The nursing care plan that is developed guides the resident's care using the data from the RAI.

Resident Assessment Instrument. The RAI has been in use since the early 1990s. The information that was gathered for the RAI was sent electronically to the state. The state then transmitted the information to the federal government. Medicare and Medicaid payments were made to the facility based on the residents' conditions and needs as identified on the RAI (Figure 1-15).

The information is also used to track resident progress within the facility (advances as well as declines). If the residents show a pattern of too many declines, an unannounced survey may be triggered.

The RAI components include:

- The Minimum Data Set (MDS3.0)
- Care Area Assessment (CAA): 20 Care Areas identified
- RAI Utilization Guidelines

The RAI is used to:

- Set payment to the facility
- Identify resident problems, needs, and risks
- Develop a care plan that maintains or improves the resident's condition
- Coordinate facility staff to better meet resident needs

Minimum Data Set (MDS3.0). Since the origin of the MDS, the uses have expanded. The primary purpose is a screening and assessment tool to identify resident problems (clinical and functional) on an individualized basis that provides common definitions and coding categories that help to standardize communication between caregivers and between agencies. Data collected from the assessment is used for the Medicare reimbursement system as well as state Medicaid reimbursement. It is also an important tool to monitor the quality of care that is provided. Quality Indicators (QI) and Quality Measures (QM) were developed by researchers to assist survey teams in identifying potential care problems in a facility, to provide caregivers with quality improvement activities, and to provide information to consumers. Consumer information includes characteristics of a facility, the staffing patterns, and the quality of the care. Facilities are given a star rating, based on the QI and QM scores. Scores range from 1 to 5 and the higher the score, the better the facility, overall.

The changes in the MDS3.0, which were implemented in 2010, were redesigned to improve the reliability and usefulness of the data obtained. The assessment information is derived from multiple sources. Mandatory sources include the **resident** and direct care staff *on all shifts*. In addition, the resident's medical record, physician, family members, and any other appropriate sources are used. All data are then transmitted, within 14 days of the care plan completion date, to the national system. This system offers the staff an opportunity to improve the quality of care for the residents.

Care Assessment Areas (CAAs). There are 20 CAA problem areas that cover the majority of problems that may affect facility residents and may be *triggered* by the MDS3.0 responses. These problem areas are referred to as Care Area Triggers (CATs). All CATs must be thoroughly assessed; this information then helps the staff to develop *individualized* care plans for the residents. CATs were called Resident Assessment Protocols (RAPs) in the MDS2.0 version. For example, the resident may have an actual condition, such as weight loss, with the potential for complications or an infection that could cause his or her health to worsen. The resident may be a candidate for a restorative program.

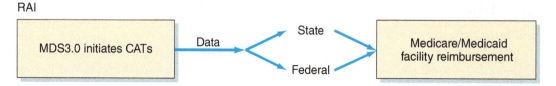

Figure 1-15 Reimbursement for resident care services in long-term care.

? EXERCISE 1-5

MATCHING

Match the term on the right with the definition on the left.

Definition	Term
1. _____ contains information about residents' daily care	a. client
2. _____ private	b. confidential
3. _____ federal legislation that guides state regulations for the training and certification of nursing assistants	c. procedure book
4. _____ outline of rules governing the facility	d. Kardex
5. _____ accordance with the law	e. policy book
6. _____ reviews and evaluates various aspects of a health care facility	f. OBRA
7. _____ home care recipient	g. compliance
8. _____ explains how care is to be given	h. survey
9. _____ law designed to give control over how health information is used	i. HIPAA

Reporting Times. To be in compliance and receive reimbursement, reports (MDS3.0 and CATs) must be completed and submitted on time (Figure 1-16). OBRA requires that an RAI be completed within 14 days of admission of a new resident. With the implementation of the new Rules of Participation in 2016-2018, care plans must be initiated within 48 hours of admission. All disciplines are to be made aware of the basic needs of the resident identified on these care plans. Care plans may change if the MDS3.0 assessment changes. These care plans are reassessed quarterly, or upon a significant condition change.

THE COMPLAINT SURVEY, ANNUAL AND EXTENDED

All health care facilities must be licensed by the state to provide care. The license is awarded by the agency that regulates care. In most states this is the Department of Public Health or the Department of Inspections and Appeals.

Facilities that receive Medicare funds participate in a certification process. One survey is usually done for both licensure and certification. All health care facilities undergo surveys on a regular basis. Facilities also may seek accreditation by The Joint Commission Long-term Care Accrediting Program, which is a voluntary program that can be used to demonstrate the positive quality of care provided.

A team of health care professionals (surveyors) is responsible for conducting the survey. The team determines whether the facility is following all state and federal regulations and whether the facility is in compliance (doing what it is supposed to do). Every day has the potential for a survey. Facilities should be ready at all times. Surveys are always unannounced and a certain percentage are conducted on Saturdays and Sundays. In addition to the *annual visit*, a facility may be surveyed as the result of a complaint. A follow-up survey visit will then occur to determine whether the deficiency has been corrected. All survey information must be made available in a public place within the facility and is posted online for consumers to read.

Purpose

The purpose of the survey is to:

- Review the quality of life for the residents
- Review the quality of care given to residents
- Review cleanliness and sanitation of the environment
- Review food preparation, quality, and service

Report	RAI	MDS3.0	Short Version MDS3.0	New MDS3.0*
Due	Within 14 days of resident admission	Days 5–14 30–60 90	Quarterly	Annually and when significant changes in resident's condition occur

*A new MDS3.0 is necessary if resident shows decline or improvement in two or more ADLs

Figure 1-16 Required reporting periods.

- Evaluate facility safety
- Determine areas of deficient care
- Review policies and procedures

Survey Process

Surveyors make judgments about a facility by:

- Gathering information before the visit using past surveys and MDSs
- Identifying:
  - areas of concern
  - special features of the facility, such as Alzheimer's units
  - residents and families to interview
  - contacting the facility ombudsman to learn about reported complaints
- During the survey:
  - Making observations related to:
  - how care is provided
  - cleanliness and safety issues
  - privacy, dignity, and implementing resident rights
- Interviewing:
  - staff members
  - residents and their families
- Reviewing:
  - medical records and care plans
  - facility manuals and records
  - budgets and finances
  - state requirements related to: licensing and/or registry listing for employees
- Touring the facility (signs are posted around the facility indicating that a survey is in progress)

Nursing Assistant Responsibilities During a Survey

During a survey there is always a higher level of tension and anxiety among caregivers. You give your best level of care if you *always* use good work habits and:

- Be calm and confident
- Know the residents you care for
- Know and follow the care plan for each resident in your care
- Cooperate with the surveyors
- Keep all work areas clean and tidy
- Perform each procedure as outlined in the facility procedure manual
- Know the policies that affect you in your facility
- Know how to operate all equipment properly
- Respect the residents' rights
- Report for duty where and when assigned and carry out your normally assigned tasks

- Attend inservice education programs and cooperate in presurvey audits conducted by the quality assurance committee of the facility
- Answer surveyor questions honestly
- If the surveyor asks you a question you cannot answer, you might say "I do not know the answer, but I will find out for you." Be sure you know where to find the requested information. Do not give excuses such as:
  - "I don't usually work on this floor."
  - "No one ever told me that."
  - "I'm new here."
- Do not try to outsmart a surveyor. Answer only the questions they ask you.

Survey Completion

The findings of the survey are important and are discussed with the facility administration during an exit conference. If **deficiencies** (Figure 1-17) are found, the facility is usually given 10 days to prepare a plan to correct them. Up to 60 days are allowed for the facility to correct the deficiencies.

Serious deficiencies can result in:

- Fines of up to $10,000 per day until all deficiencies are corrected
- A stop on payment for Medicare and Medicaid
- Loss of certification
- A 2-year loss of approval to hold a CNA class in the facility
- Loss of licensure to operate as a long-term care facility
- Loss of your job

Nursing assistants are important to the success of the survey!

Inadequate Quality of Care:
Accident hazards, urinary incontinence and urinary tract infections, failure to prevent and treat pressure ulcers, unwarranted use of physical and chemical restraints, failure to provide the highest level of care for the residents

Resident Assessment:
Lack of comprehensive care plans, failure to meet professional standards for employees, services provided by unqualified personnel

Quality of Life:
Failure to provide a safe, clean, comfortable, homelike environment; failure to respect Resident Rights and dignity

Figure 1-17 Survey deficiency categories.

? EXERCISE 1-6

MULTIPLE CHOICE

Select the one best answer.

1. The National Nurse Aide Assessment Program
   (A) tests physical care skills only in an oral exam
   (B) does not test the aide's ability to perform entry-level job skills
   (C) must be passed for an aide to be certified
   (D) does not address the aide's understanding of ethical behavior

2. Nursing assistants who are not certified have
   (A) one opportunity to meet certification requirements
   (B) a minimum of three opportunities to meet certification requirements
   (C) to obtain certification within 1 month of finishing the course
   (D) as much time as they need to meet certification requirements

3. During a survey the nursing assistant should
   (A) try to avoid the surveyors
   (B) stay home, out of the way
   (C) make up care plans to show how much he/she knows
   (D) keep work areas clean and tidy

4. The RAI assists in all of the following except:
   (A) setting payment to the facility
   (B) developing resident care plans
   (C) coordinate staff to better meet resident needs
   (D) determining meal plans

5. Which is not a responsibility of a nursing assistant during a survey?
   (A) Be calm and confident
   (B) Know the residents you care for
   (C) To avoid irritating them, answer questions the surveyors ask you even if you are not sure of your answers
   (D) Use good work habits as you always do

👤 LESSON SYNTHESIS: Putting It All Together

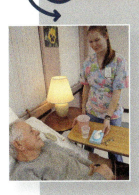

You have just completed this lesson. Now go back and review the Clinical Focus at the beginning of the lesson. Try to see how the Clinical Focus relates to the concepts presented in the lesson. Then answer the following questions.

1. **Why would Mr. McCarver not remain in the acute care facility until he had entirely recovered?**

2. **What services would be provided for Mr. McCarver in the long-term care facility?**

3. **How does the organization of the long-term care facility and the equipment provided for each resident contribute to the comfort, safety, and well-being of the resident?**

4. **How does Medicare relate to the financing of Mr. McCarver's health care? What is the importance of the records that must be kept?**

1 REVIEW

A. Match each term with the proper definition.

a. geriatric care

b. long-term care

c. resident

d. restoration facility

e. terminal

1. _____ rehabilitation

2. _____ last or final

3. _____ care concerned with the medical problems and nursing care of older adults

4. _____ person cared for in long-term care

5. _____ skilled care facility

B. List five community health agencies that provide health care.

6. _____

7. _____

8. _____

9. _____

10. _____

C. Select the one best answer for each of the following.

11. Mr. Jackson has cancer and is not expected to live more than 3 months. He probably would be cared for in

(A) an acute care hospital

(B) a hospice program

(C) a long-term care facility

(D) an outpatient clinic

12. A person being cared for in a long-term care facility is usually called the

(A) patient

(B) resident

(C) client

(D) recipient

13. The care in a skilled care facility is aimed at

(A) acute short-term care

(B) terminal care

(C) restoration

(D) providing a homelike atmosphere

14. Which articles are kept in the "dirty" area of the bedside stand?

(A) denture cup

(B) comb and brush

(C) toothbrush and toothpaste

(D) bedpan, urinal

15. The resident's room is called the

(A) resident's space

(B) resident's bedroom

(C) resident's area

(D) resident's unit

16. The nurses' station is the area where

(A) personal care is given

(B) food is stored

(C) residents' records and charts are kept

(D) residents' clothes are laundered

17. All of the following contain confidential resident records except

(A) resident's chart

(B) Kardex

(C) care plans

(D) policy book

18. OBRA regulations

(A) give nursing assistants recognition through certification and listing in the state registry

(B) require nursing assistants to report to duty on time

(C) require nursing assistants to have some home health experience before working in an acute care facility

(D) allow people with no previous education to work as nursing assistants

19. The expense of long-term care is mostly paid by

(A) private funds

(B) health maintenance organizations

(C) preferred provider organizations

(D) Medicare and Medicaid

20. Surveyors observe to see that standards are being met for everything except

(A) safety

(B) infection control

(C) residents' rights

(D) employee pay scales

21. The Resident Assessment Instrument (RAI) requires facilities to transmit information gathered from all of the following except

(A) Minimum Data Set (MDS3.0)

(B) Care Area Triggers (CAT)

(C) Care Area Assessment protocols (CAA)

(D) Part A, Medicare forms

22. During a survey, how should the nursing assistant answer questions asked by the surveyor?

(A) "I'm new here."

(B) "No one ever told me that."

(C) "I'll find out for you."

(D) "I don't usually work here."

D. Indicate where each of the following areas is found by selecting from the list (items a–d). (More than one answer may apply.)

a. nurses' station

b. dining room

c. resident unit

d. lounge

23. _____ bedside stand

24. _____ medication storage

25. _____ meal service area

26. _____ emesis basin

27. _____ bed

28. _____ group activities area

29. _____ television

30. _____ reports

31. _____ resident's health record

32. _____ Kardex

E. Clinical Experience

Amelia Walters, 85, has lived in the same community all of her life. She has lived alone since her husband died 3 years ago. Her only living relative, a daughter, lives some distance away.

Mrs. Walters had frequent upper respiratory infections and received care from her neighborhood physician.

During wet weather, Mrs. Walters fell and broke her right ankle and both wrists. Mrs. Walters is unable to perform personal care. She requires full-time care. Healing is slow and her generally frail health makes it impossible for her to live independently. Despite care, her condition declines.

Tests ordered by her physician reveal advanced cancer of the colon, a terminal condition. Mrs. Walters insists that she wants to go home and remain there as long as possible. Answer the following questions relating to Mrs. Walters. Select your answers from the list provided.

a. hospice care

b. acute care hospital

c. skilled nursing

d. physician's office

e. home care facility

33. _____ Mrs. Walters received care here for her upper respiratory infections.

34. _____ Care was given here when Mrs. Walters fell, breaking an ankle and both wrists.

35. _____ Mrs. Walters received restorative care here as her ankle and wrists healed.

36. _____ What help may make it possible for Mrs. Walters to go home once more?

37. _____ What kind of care is available to Mrs. Walters during the final stage of her life?

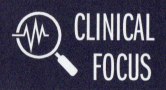

LESSON 2
THE CAREGIVERS

CLINICAL FOCUS

Think about how staff members contribute their special knowledge and expertise to the resident's well-being as you study this lesson.

OBJECTIVES

After studying this lesson, you should be able to:

- Define vocabulary words and terms.
- Name three or more members of the interdisciplinary team.
- Describe the purpose of the interdisciplinary team.
- List the members of the nursing staff.
- State the purpose of the organizational chart.
- Discuss the importance of routine testing of skills and abilities as required by OBRA.

VOCABULARY

activities of daily living (ADL) (ack-TIV-ih-tees of DAY-lee LIV-ing)
adaptive device (ah-DAP-tiv dih-VICE)
administrator (ad-MIN-iss-tray-tor)
ambulation (am-byou-LAY-shun)
assessment (ah-SESS-ment)
assistive device (ah-SIS-tiv dih-VICE)
audiologist (awe-dee-OL-oh-jist)

care plan conference (kair plan KON-fer-ens)
consultant (kon-SUL-tant)
dental hygienist (DEN-tal high-JEE-nist)
dentist (DEN-tist)
diagnosis (die-ag-NOH-sis)
dietitian (die-eh-TISH-un)
environmental services (en-vire-un-MEN-tal SIR-vuhsez)

CASE STUDY

Ms. Esther Patterson is 74 years old and complains every time her shoes are put on her feet and she is assisted to walk. You are asked to help the podiatrist who is visiting her. Consider how this care will help Ms. Patterson become more active.

interdisciplinary health care team (in-ter-DISS-sihplin-air-ee health kair team)
licensed practical nurse (LICE-enst PRACK-tih-kul nurs)
mobility (moh-BILL-ih-tee)
nursing assistant (NUR-sing ah-SIS-tant)
occupational therapist (ock-you-PAY-shun-al THERah-pist)
ophthalmologist (op-thal-MOL-oh-jist)
optometrist (op-TOM-eh-trist)
orthotic device (or-THAW-tick dih-VICE)
physical therapist (FIZ-ih-kul THER-ah-pist)
podiatrist (poh-DYE-ah-trist)

psychiatrist (si-KI-a-trist)
psychologist (si-KOL-a-gist)
registered nurse (REJ-is-terd nurs)
rehabilitation aide (ree-hah-BILL-ah-tay-shun ayd)
social worker (SO-shul WERE-ker)
speech-language pathologist (speech LAN-gwehj pah-THOL-oh-jist)
support services (sup-PORT SIR-vuh-sez)
therapeutic diet (ther-ah-PEW-tick DIE-et)
therapeutic recreational specialist (ther-ah-PEW-tick reck-ree-AY-shun-al SPEH-shul-ist)
total care (TOH-tal kair)

THE INTERDISCIPLINARY TEAM MEMBERS

Many workers help care for the resident. These caregivers represent many professions or "disciplines," and each has a specific function. As a group they are called the **interdisciplinary health care team** (Figure 2-1). Each member of the interdisciplinary health care team helps plan and/or provide for the care of the residents. This process is completed at the resident's **care plan conference**. You will learn more about this in Lesson 6. The team members in the facility who may attend the care plan conference include the:

- Resident
- Resident's family (if resident gives permission)
- Members of the nursing staff
- Members of the rehabilitation staff
- Social worker
- Activities director
- Dietitian or dietary supervisor

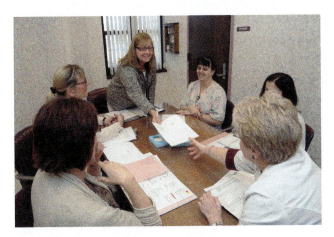

Figure 2-1 The interdisciplinary health care team is responsible for the care of the resident.

By using the interdisciplinary team approach, the residents receive **total care**. This considers the emotional, spiritual, physical, and social needs of each person. The resident and the resident's family are also considered members of the team. If the resident is unable to attend the meeting, the team should make every effort to go to the resident. Most of the direct care is given by the nursing staff. Figure 2-2 defines the jobs of people who are commonly part of the interdisciplinary health care team.

The Nursing Staff

The nursing staff in a long-term care facility includes **registered nurses** (RNs), **licensed practical nurses** (LPNs), and **nursing assistants**. (In some states LPNs are called licensed vocational nurses or LVNs.)

The *Director of Nursing* must be a registered nurse. This person has had, besides nursing education, some additional training in administration. The director of nurses is the head of the nursing staff and is responsible for all nurses, nursing assistants, and residents in the facility. If the facility is very large, there may also be an assistant director of nursing and supervisors, as well as other nurses in charge of education, infection control programs, and quality assurance. These programs ensure that all residents receive appropriate care.

An *Assistant Director of Nursing* works with the director. *Supervisors* are in charge of the entire building during a specific shift. *Charge nurses* are responsible for a nursing unit. There may be one or several nursing units within a facility. *Staff nurses* are in charge of a specific number of residents. They pass medications, perform treatments, and supervise the residents' direct care (Figure 2-3). There may be a *rehabilitation nurse* who coordinates activities between the therapists and the nurses and restorative care. The nursing assistants are responsible for carrying out most of the personal resident care (Figure 2-4).

Each of these disciplines requires a specified course of study (usually a minimum of a college degree and clinical training). Most require either licensing by a state agency or certification from a professional association. Requirements for some disciplines may vary from state to state.

Activities director	Requirements vary. Plans and implements activities for residents to meet the goals on the care plan.
Administrator	Licensed and meets state requirements to provide general administration and supervision of a long-term care facility.
Audiologist	Certified in audiology and qualified to test hearing and prescribe hearing aids.
Chaplain	Provides services to meet the spiritual needs of residents.
Dental hygienist	Licensed by the state and provides dental services under the supervision of a dentist.
Dentist	Licensed by the state to provide services for the prevention and treatment of diseases and disorders of the teeth and oral cavity.
Dietitian	Licensed by the state and responsible for the provision of all nutritional assessments and food services for residents.
Licensed practical nurse (LPN)	Licensed by the state and provides direct resident care under the supervision of a registered nurse. Sometimes called licensed vocational nurse (LVN).
Medical record practitioner	Certified or licensed to review and audit all medical records.
Nursing assistant	Has completed at least 75 hours of a state-approved course and is certified to provide direct resident care under the supervision of a licensed or registered nurse.
Occupational therapist	Licensed to provide rehabilitative services to evaluate and treat persons with physical injury or illness, psychosocial problems, or developmental disabilities. Occupational therapy assistants and aides have completed specified courses of study and work under the supervision of an occupational therapist.
Optometrist	Licensed by the state to examine eyes and prescribe glasses.
Orthotist	Licensed by the state and designs and fits braces and splints for the extremities.
Pharmacist	Licensed by the state and fills prescriptions for medications as ordered by the physician. Resource to nurses and physicians for updates on new medications and for maintaining safe drug therapy for residents.
Physical therapist	Licensed by the state to provide rehabilitative services to evaluate and treat persons with neuromuscular and musculoskeletal problems due to disease, injury, or developmental disability. Physical therapy assistants and aides have completed specified courses of study and work under the supervision of a physical therapist.
Physician	Licensed by the state to diagnose and treat disease and to prescribe medications. The many specialty areas within medicine require additional education.
Podiatrist	Licensed by the state to treat diseases and disorders of the feet.
Prosthetist	Licensed by the state to design and fit artificial limbs for persons who have had amputations.
Psychiatrist (Gero)	A physician who specializes in the study, treatment, and prevention of mental disorders of the elderly.
Psychologist	Licensed mental health professional who is trained in methods of analysis, counseling, and research but may not prescribe medications for clients.

Figure 2-2 Who's who on the interdisciplinary health care team.

(continues)

Registered nurse (RN)	Licensed by the state to make assessments and to plan, implement, and evaluate nursing care. Supervises other nursing staff and may coordinate the interdisciplinary health care team. The many specialty areas within nursing require additional education.
Rehabilitation aide, restorative nursing assistant (RNA)	A certified nursing assistant with additional training to perform procedures under the direction of the licensed physical therapist and licensed occupational therapist.
Resident	The most important member of the interdisciplinary team and has input into the planning and implementation of care. The family may participate with the resident or in place of the resident if the resident is unable to do so.
Respiratory therapist	Licensed by the state to evaluate and treat diseases and problems associated with breathing and the respiratory tract.
Social worker	Licensed by the state to assess and provide services for the nonmedical, psychosocial needs of residents.
Speech-language pathologist or Speech therapist	Licensed by the state to evaluate and provide services for residents with problems in hearing, language, speech production, and swallowing.
Therapeutic recreational specialist	Certified to evaluate and provide recreational services to treat mental and physical disorders.
Unit secretary	Certified nursing assistant with additional training; responsible for clerical duties of nursing staff; may also be a person with no previous health care experience who is trained as a unit secretary for a specific period of time.

In addition to these members of the interdisciplinary health care team, many other employees in the long-term care facility provide services that benefit the quality of life for residents.

- Environmental services staff maintain a clean, comfortable, and homelike environment. These services may include housekeeping, laundry, and building and grounds maintenance.

- The business office handles the personal funds of residents as well as the financial affairs of the facility.

- Assistants in all departments provide services to residents as part of the interdisciplinary team.

- Volunteers may provide direct services to residents and may raise funds to provide equipment for resident care.

Figure 2-2 (Continued)

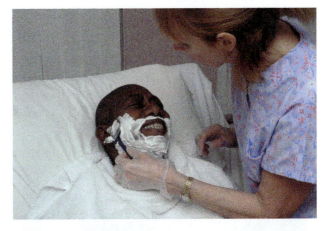

Figure 2-3 Staff nurses pass medications and perform treatments.

Figure 2-4 Nursing assistants provide most of the resident's personal care.

The use of advance practice nurses is becoming more common. An *advanced registered nurse practitioner (ARNP)* or *nurse practitioner (NP)* is licensed as a registered nurse and has completed graduate education with a minimum of a master's degree. In addition, the nurse must pass a national-based certification in their specialty such as geriatrics (GNP), family (FNP), or adult (ANP) and is licensed as an NP through their respective states.

? EXERCISE 2-1

COMPLETION
Complete the following statements by writing in the correct words.

1. The director of nursing must be a _____.
   (social worker) (nurse)
2. The _____ is part of the interdisciplinary team.
   (bookkeeper) (resident)
3. The person who evaluates and treats diseases and problems associated with breathing is called the
   _____.
   (speech therapist) (respiratory therapist)
4. Questions about an assignment should be referred to the _____.
   (physician) (supervising nurse)

The *unit secretary* is responsible for the clerical tasks of the nursing staff. These duties include answering the telephone, writing out daily reports, filing, entering reports into the medical records, making out assignment sheets, and ordering supplies.

Social Services

The social services department provides for many of the nonmedical needs of the residents (Figure 2-5). The department works closely with the nursing staff and in many facilities, are responsible for the admission of new residents. With the new Rules of Participation implemented 2016–2018, social workers must initiate the discharge process for every person admitted, except if it is known the resident will stay at the facility for the rest of their life. With the involvement of managed care, residents become known as "patients" and short-term stays are more and more common. This may involve coordination of community services for the resident, such as making

arrangements for homemaking services or for the services of a home health agency. The social workers may arrange for appointments with dentists, podiatrists, audiologists, or mental health consultants.

The Physician

Each resident has a physician who makes the medical diagnosis and writes medical orders for the resident. In addition to writing new orders, the physician evaluates the health and well-being of the residents at designated intervals. The physician may also participate in care plan conferences.

The Dietitian

A dietitian plans and supervises the preparation of resident meals and therapeutic diets (Figure 2-6). The dietitian performs a nutritional assessment for each resident. Monitoring residents' weights as well as evaluating laboratory tests are duties of the dietitian. Special meals and supplements are provided for residents requiring therapeutic diets (special diets designed to meet a resident's specific needs). Therapeutic diets are ordered by the physician. (Lesson 17 has more details on therapeutic diets.)

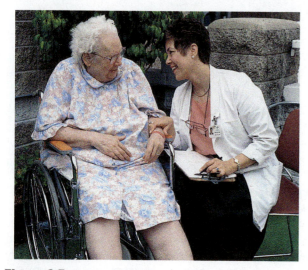

Figure 2-5 The social worker is responsible for ensuring that the resident's discharge plans are complete.

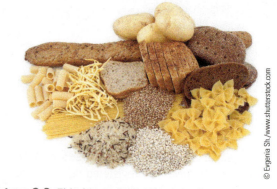

© Evgenia Sh./www.shutterstock.com

Figure 2-6 Elderly people require complex carbohydrates for a healthy diet.

TRUE OR FALSE

Indicate whether the following statements are true (T) or false (F).

1. T F The dietitian performs housekeeping duties.
2. T F The physician defines the diagnosis and writes orders.
3. T F The social worker may arrange for mental health consultations.

Special Therapists

In large facilities, many different types of therapists are in the facility every day. In smaller facilities, the therapists may be **consultants**. In larger facilities, many therapists are part of the staff and do not rotate to other facilities. Consultants come to the facility regularly to evaluate the residents' conditions and recommend treatment.

The **physical therapist** works to improve the **mobility** (ability to move) of the resident (Figure 2-7).

After an initial evaluation, a plan is developed to restore and achieve the next level of physical functioning. This may include teaching the resident how to use an **assistive device**. Canes and walkers are examples of assistive devices. Many times the nursing assistant helps to carry out the program prescribed by the therapist. For example, range of motion exercises are part of daily care. These are ordered by the physician but they are done by the nursing assistant or in the rehabilitation department.

The **occupational therapist** helps residents learn new ways of doing basic self-care (**activities of daily living**, or **ADLs**). For example, the therapist may teach the resident to dress or eat with the use of **adaptive devices**. An adaptive device is a piece of equipment designed to assist a resident to carry out ADL. The occupational therapist may evaluate and fit an **orthotic device** (splint) for a resident's hand. Orthotic devices are appliances used to protect and support a body part. Such a device can hold a paralyzed hand in position or stabilize an ankle, to prevent contractures (permanent deformities) from forming (Figure 2-8).

There may be other members of the rehabilitation team. Physical therapy assistants and occupational therapy assistants must complete 2 years of an approved educational program. They work under

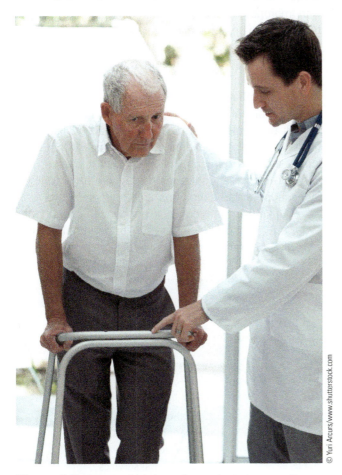

Figure 2-7 The physical therapist works to improve the resident's mobility.

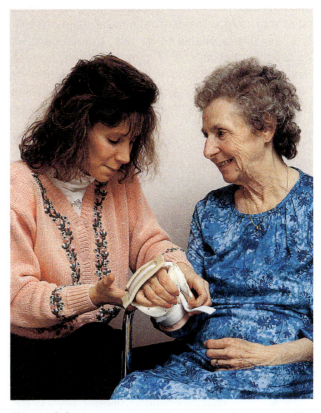

Figure 2-8 The occupational therapist applies an orthotic device to support the resident's weak hand and wrist.

the direct supervision of the therapists. Restorative nursing assistants work under the direction of the RN. Some states allow occupational and physical **rehabilitation aides** to perform some of the less complex, routine procedures. They also work under the direction and supervision of the therapists. The rehabilitation aides are nursing assistants who have taken additional courses to prepare them for this job.

CLINICAL FOCUS

The podiatrist is visiting Ms. Patterson. Think about the role of the podiatrist and what you can do to help Ms. Patterson feel more comfortable during the examination. What can you do to assist the podiatrist?

The activities director or **therapeutic recreational specialist** may direct recreational, educational, spiritual, artistic, or social activities for the resident. Activities aides also work with the resident in doing the activities. Activity Directors must be certified and maintain certification through ongoing education.

The **speech-language pathologist** (speech therapist, or SLT) works with residents who have speech and language problems. The speech-language pathologist may help a resident regain the ability to talk. If a resident is unable to do this, the resident will be taught other means of communication. Speech-language pathologists also work with residents who have trouble swallowing. They do swallowing evaluations and suggest techniques for feeding residents.

Consultants

Some of the services provided by the facility are not needed on a daily basis. Not all residents need all of the services. Consultants are hired to perform these services.

The **audiologist** tests and evaluates hearing. For residents with impaired hearing, the audiologist may prescribe a hearing aid.

Dentists or **dental hygienists** examine and clean teeth. They also evaluate the resident's dental health. Maintaining good nutrition is difficult when teeth are in poor condition. The dentist will recommend dentures or denture repair when needed. Choking is always a concern with improperly fitting dentures. Each facility is required to coordinate dental services for residents, whether that be through a contract where the dentist comes to the facility, or through arrangements at a dental clinic/office where ambulatory residents can go for an evaluation.

The **podiatrist** is another special caregiver who visits periodically. Many older persons have foot and toenail problems that make **ambulation** (walking) difficult. The podiatrist examines and may treat foot problems, such as bunions, hammer toes, calluses, and corns. This increases the resident's comfort and mobility because these conditions are very painful.

An **ophthalmologist** examines the resident's eyes and prescribes glasses. The ophthalmologist may also perform surgery to correct or improve vision

? EXERCISE 2-3

TRUE OR FALSE
Indicate whether the following statements are true (T) or false (F).

1. T F The occupational therapist counsels residents about dental hygiene.
2. T F The physical therapist works to improve the resident's mobility.
3. T F Consultants visit the resident daily.
4. T F A cane is an example of an assistive device.

? EXERCISE 2-4

MATCHING
Match the term on the right with the definition on the left.

Definition	Term
1. _____ special diets designed to meet a specific need	a. assessment
2. _____ basic self-care	b. mobility
3. _____ resident, community, and staff education responsibilities	c. total care
4. _____ messages sent with words	d. therapeutic diets
5. _____ making evaluations	e. activities of daily living (ADL)
6. _____ meeting emotional, spiritual, physical, and social needs	f. educational services
7. _____ ability to get around	g. oral communications

problems. The **optometrist** is licensed by the state to examine eyes and prescribe glasses.

A resident may display signs of anxiety or depression or other mental health problems such as dementia. A **psychiatrist** or geriatric psychiatrist or **psychologist** may be called to aid the staff in identifying appropriate ways to treat the resident. Community mental health counselors are often good resources for residents as well.

BUILDING CULTURAL AWARENESS

The health care facility is staffed with persons from many different ethnic groups. It is important that you examine your ideas about persons who may have different values and traditions from yours. The team effort requires that all persons work together harmoniously.

Support Services

Many other workers provide **support services**. These workers:

- Maintain the building and grounds
- Perform housekeeping duties

- Do the laundry
- Work in the kitchen
- Handle administrative duties
- Manage the financial affairs of the facility

Buildings and grounds, housekeeping, and laundry departments are sometimes called **environmental services**.

ADMINISTRATIVE ORGANIZATION

Each facility has an organizational chart that shows the line of authority or command (Figure 2-9). Each department is represented on the chart. All employees are recognized within these departments. The organizational chart is also used as a guide for communication so all employees know to whom they should report.

The **administrator** of the long-term care facility provides leadership for all departments and employees.

The facility is managed and directed by a board of directors that delegates authority for day-to-day operation to the administrator and department heads.

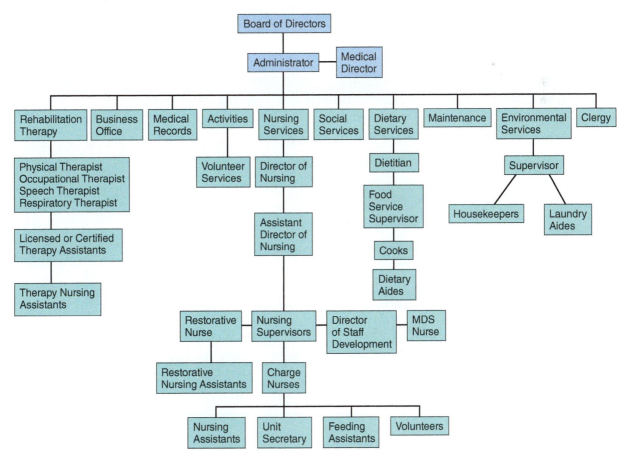

Figure 2-9 Organizational chart.

Your immediate supervisor is the instructor, charge nurse, or staff nurse designated for this role. The supervising nurse will give you your assignment and you will report your observations and the completion of the assigned tasks to this person.

Any questions about your assignment should be directed to your supervising nurse for clarification. *Never attempt to carry out an assignment for which you have not been trained or an assignment you do not fully understand.* Inform the supervisor and ask for help. Never feel embarrassed. It is better to ask for help than to injure a resident.

Educational Services

The term *educational services* includes all forms of educational programs within the health care facility. Resident education, community education, and staff education may all be responsibilities of this department. Employers must provide their staff members with continuing education programs.

All staff members are expected to participate in continuing education programs. This is called *staff development*. Some of the programs will be attended by all members of the interdisciplinary team. Other programs may be presented specifically for nursing assistants. The Omnibus Budget Reconciliation Act (OBRA) requires that all nursing assistants participate in a minimum of 12 hours of continuing education each year. Some states may require more than 12 hours. All states require nursing assistants to work one 8 hour shift every 24 months in order to keep their certification. At these programs, you will learn about:

- New facility policies
- New procedures involving resident care
- Use of new equipment
- Caring for residents with unusual diagnoses or problems
- Issues in health care
- Topics related to residents' rights, safety, and infection control

The more you learn, the better you can care for the residents and the more you will enjoy your work.

⊘N THE JOB

Remember that there are many variations in long-term care facilities. Smaller facilities have fewer staff members and may not employ all the types of workers described in this lesson.

? EXERCISE 2-5

TRUE OR FALSE
Indicate whether the following statements are true (T) or false (F).

1. T F The audiologist examines and cleans the teeth of residents.
2. T F The podiatrist cares for the foot problems of residents.
3. T F The dentist is consulted for vision problems.

COMPLETION
Complete the following statements by writing in the correct words.

1. The staff of _____ maintains a clean and comfortable living facility.
   (business services) (environmental services)
2. The person who provides leadership for all departments and employees is called the _____
   _____.
   (assistant nursing director) (administrator)
3. The person who plans and implements activities for residents to meet the goals on the plan of care is the _____
   _____.
   (chaplain) (activities director)

? EXERCISE 2-6

COMPLETION
Complete the following statements by writing in the correct words.

1. The Omnibus Budget Reconciliation Act (OBRA) requires a minimum of _____ hours of inservice education each year to maintain certification.   (12) (18)

2. Resident, community, and staff education is the responsibility of _____.
(rehabilitation therapy) (educational services)

CLINICAL SITUATION
Select the correct term from the following list to complete each statement.

audiologist   speech therapist
occupational therapist   unit secretary
social services

3. Mrs. Callucci is going home after her 3-month poststroke stay at your facility. Which department will help her with discharge plans? _____

4. The nursing supervisor determines your assignment but you find the list is actually written according to the supervisor's instructions by another person. Who might that be? _____

5. The nurse tells you that Mr. Malik will start work with a team member who will help him learn to use his new adaptive device. What team member might you expect to assist him? _____

6. Mrs. Simpson has shown great progress following her left-sided stroke several months ago, but she is still having difficulty swallowing. She is scheduled for a meeting this morning with a therapist to assist her with this problem. Which therapist can offer this help? _____

7. Mrs. Butler has lost her hearing aid and has great difficulty communicating. In 2 days, her hearing will be retested and she hopes to obtain a new hearing aid. Who will test and evaluate her hearing needs? _____

? EXERCISE 2-7

FACILITY EXPERIENCE
Mrs. Eckland had a stroke that resulted in speech impairment and left-sided paralysis. After a stay in acute care she is admitted to your care facility for restorative care. She is 83 years of age, wears glasses and dentures, and has a hearing aid. During her stay at the long-term care facility, she developed pneumonia. Her physician also identified a heart problem and ordered a special diet. As Mrs. Eckland recovered, she learned to use a cane as an assistive aid. Upon discharge she will need help to recover.

On the figure below, start as Mrs. Eckland is admitted and trace her pathway through her facility experience, noting the team members she met.

(continues)

? EXERCISE 2-7 (Continued)

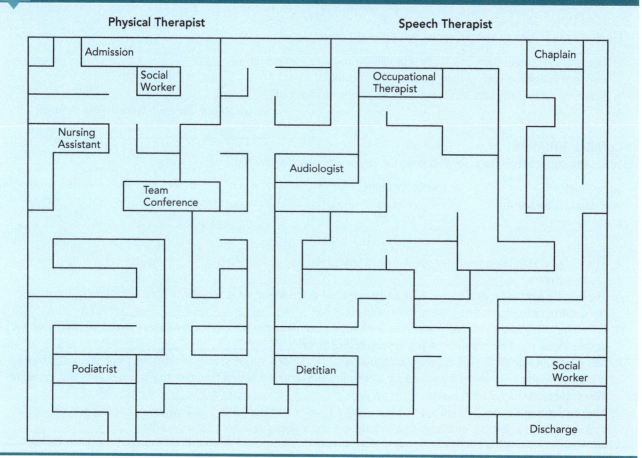

Physical Therapist / Speech Therapist / Admission / Social Worker / Chaplain / Occupational Therapist / Nursing Assistant / Team Conference / Audiologist / Podiatrist / Dietitian / Social Worker / Discharge

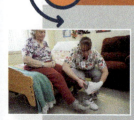

LESSON SYNTHESIS: Putting It All Together

You have just completed this lesson. Now go back and review the Clinical Focus. Try to see how the Clinical Focus relates to the concepts presented in the lesson. Then answer the following questions.

1. What role does each member of the interdisciplinary team play in maintaining and restoring the resident's optimum level of independent functioning?

2. How does the nursing assistant interact with other team members to provide Ms. Patterson with the best care?

3. How do consultants fit into the interdisciplinary team?

4. How are the needs of Ms. Patterson best met when care plans are developed at the care plan conference?

2 REVIEW

A. Select the one best answer for each of the following.

1. The many professions responsible for the care of the resident in the long-term care facility are members of the
   - (A) medical staff
   - (B) interdisciplinary health care team
   - (C) employee council
   - (D) residents' council

2. Employees who attend the resident's care plan conference include all of the following except
   - (A) the resident
   - (B) activities director
   - (C) members of the nursing staff
   - (D) housekeeping staff

3. The person who is responsible for helping residents learn new ways of doing the activities of daily living is the
   - (A) occupational therapist
   - (B) physician
   - (C) pharmacist
   - (D) physical therapist

4. An adaptive device is a
   - (A) piece of equipment designed to assist a resident with activities of daily living
   - (B) cane or walker
   - (C) hearing aid
   - (D) set of dentures

5. A splint is a device that
   - (A) helps the resident walk
   - (B) prevents deformities in an extremity
   - (C) helps the resident breathe
   - (D) restrains the resident

6. The social worker may be responsible for
   - (A) admission and discharge of residents
   - (B) giving medications
   - (C) giving physical therapy
   - (D) supervising nursing assistants

7. Most of the direct care of residents is given by the
   - (A) director of nursing
   - (B) nursing assistants
   - (C) administrator
   - (D) dietitian

8. Which of the following is not a purpose of the organizational chart?
   - (A) To indicate the lines of authority
   - (B) To provide a guide for communication
   - (C) To indicate the chain of command
   - (D) To provide continuing education

9. The housekeeping, laundry, and maintenance departments may be referred to as
   - (A) rehabilitation services
   - (B) food services
   - (C) environmental services
   - (D) nursing services

10. The OBRA requires that all nursing assistants participate in
    - (A) a minimum of 12 hours of inservice education each year
    - (B) annual college courses
    - (C) providing social services
    - (D) food preparation

11. Nursing assistants report to
    - (A) the resident's physician
    - (B) the housekeeping supervisor
    - (C) the administrator
    - (D) a registered nurse or a licensed practical nurse

12. The nursing team *does not* include
    - (A) registered nurses
    - (B) licensed practical or vocational nurses
    - (C) dietitian
    - (D) nursing assistants

B. Match the team members (items a–j) with their responsibilities.

a. physician

b. dietitian

c. physical

d. respiratory therapist

e. administrator

f. audiologist

g. dentist

h. podiatrist therapist

i. ophthalmologist

j. housekeeper

13. _____ cares for residents with mobility problems

14. _____ provides leadership to staff

15. _____ performs housekeeping duties

16. _____ examines and cleans teeth

17. _____ provides eye examinations and prescriptions

18. _____ defines the medical diagnosis and writes orders

19. _____ treats diseases associated with breathing

20. _____ cares for foot problems

21. _____ plans and supervises preparation of meals

22. _____ tests and evaluates residents' hearing

LESSON 3
THE NURSING ASSISTANT IN LONG-TERM CARE

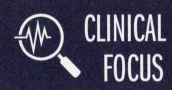

CLINICAL FOCUS

Think about the characteristics that are needed to be a successful nursing assistant as you study this lesson.

OBJECTIVES

After studying this lesson, you should be able to:

- Define vocabulary words and terms.
- Discuss why residents, families, and visitors should expect professional behavior from all members of the health care team.
- List five personal characteristics needed to be a successful nursing assistant in long-term care.
- Describe how a positive mental attitude can impact the physical and mental health of residents.
- Describe why keeping your own personal hygiene is important to residents.
- Describe how to dress properly for work.
- Define the job description.
- List 10 duties that the nursing assistant performs.
- Explain how interpersonal relations influence the effectiveness of resident care.
- Explain why assignments are important to follow.
- List five ways to use time efficiently.
- Identify signs of stress in the resident and nursing staff.
- State ways to deal with violent situations.
- State the responsibilities the nursing assistant has for personal and clinical growth.

CASE STUDY

Ray Rodriquez, who is 20 years old, did not finish high school because he needed to earn money to help at home. Even as a little boy he knew responsibility and the need to be prompt and dependable. He helped his mother care for an elderly grandmother and younger brothers and sisters. He learned to be patient as he helped his grandmother eat. Ray comes from a close and loving family and is putting his skills to positive use.

VOCABULARY

accuracy (ACK-your-ah-see)
assignment (ah-SIGHN-ment)
attitude (AT-ih-tood)
burnout (BURN-out)
compassion fatigue (kum-PASH'un fa-TEEG)
dependability (dee-pen-dah-BILL-ih-tee)
empathy (EM-pah-thee)
harmony (HAR-mun-ee)

integrity (in-TEG-rah-tee)
job description (job dih-SKRIP-shun)
maturity (mah-CHUR-rih-tee)
procedure (proh-SEE-jur)
professionalism (proh-FEH-shun-ul-izm)
sensitivity (sen-sih-TIV-ih-tee)
sympathy (SIM-pa-thee)
violence (VY-oh-lenz)

PROFESSIONALISM

Nursing assistants are expected to function in a professional manner at all times. Professionalism does not come from having a stethoscope around your neck or one or more degrees following your name, although many professional people carry this equipment and have these credentials.

   Professionalism is demonstrated by:

- The security and efficiency with which you carry out your tasks
- Keeping up to date and current with the latest information in your field by reading, taking classes, and attending inservice programs
- The careful way you perform the skills you have been taught
- Paying attention to the safety and comfort of the resident and remembering to protect the resident's dignity
- The gentle way you relate to the resident during care
- Protecting the resident's privacy and offering the resident choices whenever possible
- Keeping all information confidential
- Completing your assignments fully, correctly, and in a timely manner
- Wearing appropriate uniform, including name tag

PERSONAL CHARACTERISTICS

Nursing assistants working in long-term care are very special people. They feel pride in themselves when they fulfill their role with enthusiasm and dedication. They will be successful if they:

- Possess maturity and sensitivity
- Are dependable and accurate
- Can be satisfied with small gains

- Bring a positive attitude to their job
- Carry out an assignment (work to be completed during the shift). Each task is to be performed as it has been taught and in a safe manner
- Maintain integrity by being sincere and honest

Not everyone can be a successful, satisfied long-term care nursing assistant. Nursing assistants care for many people who cannot care for themselves. Some of these residents may be confused; others need a great deal of patience and assistance in carrying out even the most intimate parts of their own personal hygiene.

Sensitivity and Maturity

Because residents have so many needs, the nursing assistant must have the sensitivity to recognize the needs that are expressed and those that are not expressed. The need for dry, clean linen is obvious if the bed is wet. The need for a close human relationship may be less obvious. It is just as important to be aware of and to meet residents' emotional needs as their physical needs (Figure 3-1).

   The sensitive, mature care provider quickly recognizes both the physical and emotional needs of residents and willingly reaches out. Maturity means that you can control your emotions. Angry responses have no place in the facility. You must relate to residents and coworkers with courtesy, kindness, and respect. The mature individual can accept and learn from constructive evaluation and criticism. Maturity and sensitivity are also required to make the observations (assessments) that are part of a nursing assistant's job. Maturity is not a matter of age; it is one of attitude.

   In the acute care hospital, patients who have been very ill or who have had extensive surgery can make rapid, dramatic gains as their health improves. They look forward to returning home. In the past,

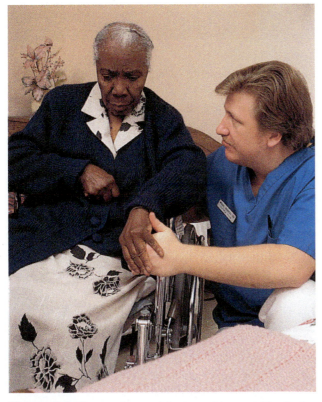

Figure 3-1 The nursing assistant must be sensitive to the resident's needs.

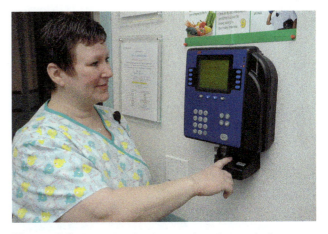

Figure 3-2 Reporting for duty on time demonstrates responsibility.

the resident in a long-term care facility made small strides—for example, relearning to hold a spoon or walking a corridor with the help of a cane. The facility became their home, and often the staff became their only family and friends. A smile or the therapeutic use of touch in the recognition of a resident's successful efforts brightened the day for those being cared for.

Insurance companies and HMOs promote this extension of acute care services in a post acute setting. It is also more economical for private-pay patients who do not have Medicare or private insurance.

Dependability and Accuracy

Dependability and accuracy are also essential qualities of the nursing assistant. You demonstrate these qualities when you:

- Arrive for duty when assigned and on time (Figure 3-2)
- Come prepared to do your job
- Carry out your assignment correctly
- Keep a positive attitude
- Offer assistance to team members as needed

Empathy versus Sympathy

The ability to put yourself in another person's position is called empathy. Being able to see a situation from another person's viewpoint helps you become more sensitive to that person. This understanding is a positive response.

Sympathy, on the other hand, may cause you to cross professional boundaries. When one is sympathetic, the person feels sorrow or pity for the situation or condition of the resident. Sympathy is not considered to be a healthy response for the nursing assistant or the resident.

Just for a moment, pretend you are one of the residents. What qualities do you want in the nursing assistants who care for you? Imagine what it must be like to:

- Have to sit for hours in a chair/wheelchair
- Have thoughts you cannot express in words
- Need to go to the toilet and have to wait for help
- Need help to take a bath
- Not be able to feed yourself
- Have a tube in your bladder to drain urine
- Be separated from family and friends
- Be demeaned by wearing a protective brief for incontinence

As you do this, you will begin to understand the situation of the residents, and your empathy for those in your care will grow.

ATTITUDE

The most important characteristic that you bring to your job is your attitude (Figure 3-3). The other characteristics described here are an outer reflection of your inner feelings, of your attitude about yourself and others.

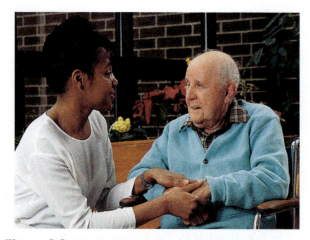

Figure 3-3 Therapeutic relationships with residents in long-term care result when caregiving skills are combined with a positive, caring attitude. Factors affecting the outcome include trust, respect, competent and compassionate care, and promotion of normalcy.

Residents have the right to be cared for in a **calm, unhurried** atmosphere. Your attitude and behavior are critical in providing such an environment.

Attitudes are contagious. To promote a high quality of care and therapeutic relationships with residents, caregiving skills must be combined with a positive, caring attitude. The factors that facilitate these goals include trust, respect, competent and compassionate care, and promotion of normalcy.

Your attitude is reflected in the way you relate to your coworkers as well. Each time you willingly help another worker, you show your shared concern for each other and for the welfare of the residents.

? EXERCISE 3-1

TRUE OR FALSE
Indicate whether the following statements are true (T) or false (F).

1. T F Nursing assistants who work in long-term care facilities are special people.
2. T F Anyone can be a successful long-term care nursing assistant.
3. T F The sensitive nursing assistant recognizes that residents may have unexpressed needs.
4. T F It is permissible for the nursing assistant to lose his or her temper when others are being unfair.
5. T F Residents in long-term care facilities are expected to make rapid and dramatic improvements in their health.
6. T F Attitude is reflected in how people relate to others.
7. T F Nursing assistants are expected to follow the dress code of the facility that employs them.
8. T F The policy book describes how each task should be performed.
9. T F Being friendly and cooperative with members of staff creates a sense of harmony.
10. T F Burnout among those working with the sick and infirmed is common.
11. T F Avoiding violence is preferable to dealing with violence once it erupts.

? EXERCISE 3-2

1. John did not complete his assignment on time and his supervisor told him he must plan more carefully. John said nothing but slammed the door on the way out of the office.
   a. Do you think John responded maturely? _____
   b. How could you tell? _____
   c. Is maturity a matter of age or attitude? _____

2. Even though Carrie's residents could feed themselves slowly, Carrie fed them herself to save time.
   a. Was her method of feeding the best method? _____
   b. Was it more or less satisfying for the residents? _____
   c. How did being fed in this way make the residents feel? _____

3. Eric always comes to work on time, has a pleasant attitude, and finishes his assignment correctly.
   a. What important characteristic does Eric demonstrate by arriving on time? _____
   b. What characteristic does he demonstrate by being sure his assignments are correctly done? _____
   _____

4. Lois is patient with the residents in her care because she says she would find it so hard to need help to go to the bathroom or to have to sit all day. By her actions Lois is demonstrating what important characteristic?
   _____

PERSONAL HYGIENE

The work of a long-term care nursing assistant is physically and emotionally demanding. Because you will be in close contact with the residents, your personal hygiene and grooming must be the very best (Figure 3-4). Good grooming starts with a daily bath or shower and the use of an antiperspirant to control body odor. Careful attention to the cleanliness of teeth and nails is also important; teeth should be cleaned at least twice each day and fingernails kept trimmed and smooth. Wear clear nail polish only. Long nails are unsafe for two reasons: (1) they can injure a resident, and (2) they promote the growth of potentially harmful germs. Hair should be neatly arranged and controlled. Hair should not fall over the face or shoulders. Hair should be pulled up or back neatly. Beards and mustaches should be neatly trimmed. Makeup should be moderate.

Strongly scented aftershave lotions and perfumes can bother many people and cause allergic reactions in others. Do not use them while you are on duty. While gaining in popularity, the wearing of essential oils by the care giver is also discouraged due

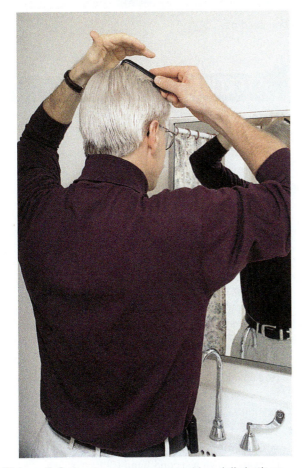

Figure 3-4 Good grooming starts with a daily bath or shower and the use of a deodorant. It also includes teeth that are brushed and clean hair arranged in a neat style.

to potential respiratory issues of residents and other team members.

UNIFORMS

The uniform of nursing assistants in long-term care facilities is often a matter of preference. If your facility has a dress code and specifies how nursing assistants should dress, you must follow that code (Figure 3-5).

The uniform includes shoes and stockings or socks and name tag. Shoes may be white and should be cleaned daily, and white shoelaces should be laundered frequently. Shoes should be closed toed and closed heeled with non-skid soles. Because nursing assistants spend many hours on their feet, good, comfortable, well-fitting shoes are required.

Wear your uniform only while on duty. When you arrive home, remove your uniform, fold it inside out so that the dirtiest part is on the inside, and put it in the laundry. When doing the laundry, use bleach if possible to kill the bacteria that may be present on the uniform.

Wear a fresh, clean uniform each day that you report to work. Make sure that the uniform is presentable, unwrinkled, with no broken zippers, missing buttons, hanging hems, or tears. Ensure that patterned underwear is not visible through the uniform.

Do not smoke while in uniform. Clothing and breath absorb the odor of tobacco, which is offensive to many people. If you do smoke, storing clean uniforms in plastic garment bags at home will help reduce the exposure to smoke.

Accessories

Bracelets, rings, earrings, and necklaces are not to be worn (although most facilities do permit the wearing of a wedding ring and small stud earrings). Other types of body-piercing jewelry should not be worn when in the work setting. Jewelry tends to harbor germs, may scratch or injure a resident, and can easily be lost.

Individual facilities will have policies relating to tattoos. A typical policy may state that tattoos must be completely covered and not visible through the uniform.

A watch with a second hand and an identification badge are part of your official uniform. You will need the watch to do certain procedures. The identification badge lets other staff members know who you are and helps residents remember your name. It should always be worn when you are in uniform so that you are in compliance with state and federal regulations.

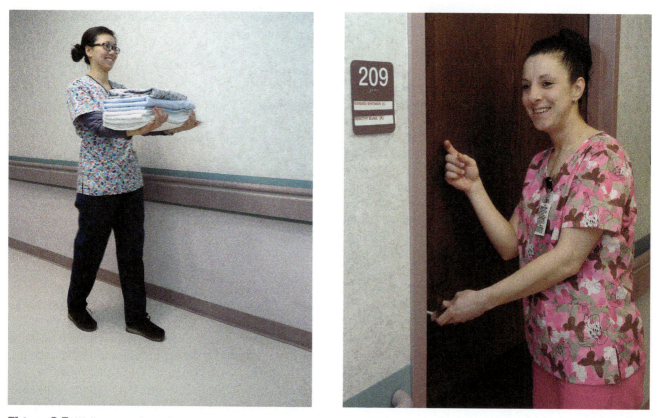

Figure 3-5 Well-groomed nursing assistants wear a fresh, clean uniform each day.

You should keep a pen and a small notepad in your uniform pocket to jot down your observations of the residents and their responses to care.

Pride in Appearance

Always remember that your appearance declares your professionalism and your pride in yourself and your work. Remember that you are a representative of your facility to residents and visitors. You are ready to work if you:

- Demonstrate personal cleanliness
- Use an antiperspirant or deodorant
- Wear an appropriate, clean uniform
- Wear clean shoes and stockings or socks, including clean shoelaces
- Arrange your hair so that it is neat and controlled
- Neatly trim your beard and mustache (if you are a man)
- Trim fingernails smoothly; do not use colored polish or artificial nails
- Do not use strong perfumes or aftershave lotion
- Wear a watch with a second hand
- Carry a pen and notepad in your uniform pocket
- Properly pin identification badge on your uniform
- Do not smoke while in uniform

? EXERCISE 3-3

MULTIPLE CHOICE
Select the one best answer.
1. Professionalism for nursing assistants includes
   (A) earning a degree
   (B) protecting the resident's privacy
   (C) wearing the correct uniform
   (D) attending inservice programs when convenient

2. Which of the following indicates good personal hygiene?
   (A) bathing every 3 days
   (B) using heavy lipstick
   (C) cleaning teeth once a day
   (D) having fingernails trimmed, smooth, and clean

3. Which of the following is usually permitted while in uniform?
   (A) smoking (C) wearing well-manicured artificial nails
   (B) wearing strong perfume (D) wearing a wedding ring

4. Which of the following is not an official part of your uniform?
   (A) watch with a second hand (C) pen/pencil
   (B) necklace (D) name tag

? EXERCISE 3-4

BEST ANSWER

Examine lists A and B, which give characteristics of two nursing assistants. Which long-term care nursing assistant is the best representative of himself or herself and a facility?

List A	List B
Short hair	Long, straggly hair
Smile	Long earrings
Clean uniform	Heavy makeup
Name pin	Cigarette in hand
Pants to top of shoes	Dirty uniform
Clean shoes and laces	No name tag
	Poorly fitting uniform
	Shoes dirty and untied

DUTIES AND RESPONSIBILITIES: THE JOB DESCRIPTION

The duties and responsibilities of nursing assistants in long-term care are stated in the facilities policy book as a job description. During the pre-employment interview, you should review the job description to be sure you can perform the work required before you accept employment. As you learned in Lesson 1, each facility has:

- A policy book that describes what will be done

- A procedure book that describes how each task should be performed

- Job descriptions that state who will do specific tasks

Find each of these books in your unit and become familiar with them. Both books are usually found in the nurses' station.

Basic procedures may be varied in some ways to meet individual needs. You must know any differences in basic procedures preferred by your facility. Differences in procedure may be explained during the orientation period after you are hired. You can also check the procedure book for exact details of how procedures are to be performed.

Be willing to learn new techniques and different ways to perform tasks, taking instruction from your charge nurse or staff development coordinator. If you are asked to perform a procedure that you have not

learned but is within the scope of practice for nursing assistants, ask for a demonstration. You will be supervised until both you and your supervisor are confident in your ability to do the procedure correctly and safely. However, if the adaptation or shortcut is not safe practice or compromises infection control or resident rights, do not do it. Talk with your supervisor to ensure that you are doing things in the right way.

The job description is the basis for specific assignments (Figure 3-6).

⊘N THE JOB

You may find that procedures are carried out in the facility in ways that differ greatly from those you learned in the classroom. You must adapt and learn the procedures according to facility guidelines. Remember, *you* are responsible for performing all procedures correctly.

STAFF RELATIONS (TEAMWORK)

All members of the interdisciplinary health care team are expected to be friendly and to cooperate with each other. This kind of relationship promotes a sense of harmony, which is important to create a calm atmosphere. Older residents are adversely affected by any discord among staff members. While you are in the facility, you must be supportive of and pleasant to everyone in all departments.

If a staff member or resident complains to you about another nursing assistant, tactfully refuse to comment. Never criticize your coworkers to the residents. Suggest that the matter be referred to the charge nurse. Supportive peer review by another nursing assistant can be a positive experience.

Listen to residents and offer to help with legitimate problems according to facility policy. Always remember that the effectiveness of care is affected by interpersonal relationships. Good relationships improve care; poor ones can harm the quality of care.

ASSIGNMENTS

The charge nurse makes out assignments based on the needs of residents and availability of staff and qualifications of the staff members. At times your assignment load will be lighter than usual and at times much heavier. Remember that the staff works as a team. Develop a positive attitude and be ready to help when someone needs it.

? EXERCISE 3-5

Read each statement. Mark Yes (Y) in the space provided if the action will improve staff relationships and No (N) if the action will make staff relationships less pleasant.

1. _____ Ray and Josie are nursing assistants who work together. Ray assists Josie in lifting a heavy resident.
2. _____ Josie tells Ray she is too busy to pick up an extra towel when she gets her own linens.
3. _____ Ray offers to feed one of Josie's residents because his residents do not need help.
4. _____ Josie tells another worker that Ray does not make very good beds.
5. _____ Ray argues with Josie in front of a resident saying his assignment is much harder than hers and it is unfair.
6. _____ Josie offers to help bring residents to the dayroom for daily chair exercises.
7. _____ Josie does only her assignment and ignores other residents' needs even though she notices them.
8. _____ Josie remembers to say "please" and "thank you" when Ray helps her.
9. _____ Ray has a slight lisp to his speech, and Josie teases him about it in front of residents.

Your assignment must be carried out with the resident's personal wishes in mind. Talk with the resident about the care plan so that the resident is involved in making decisions about how and when the plan can best be carried out.

Although you will be responsible for the care of specific residents, do not ignore a resident who needs help but is not part of your assignment. Never allow any resident to be uncomfortable or in danger. For example, a resident who needs assistance to walk becomes impatient waiting in the lounge for her nursing assistant to help her return to her room. She stands up and starts unsteadily down the hall. You see potential danger and without hesitation assist her to her room even though she is not part of your specific assignment (Figure 3-7).

Unfinished Assignments

Be sure to report any difficulty you have in performing a procedure or finishing an assignment. Tell the charge nurse of any tasks that are not completed at the time indicated. This can be very important. For example, you are assigned to have a resident dressed and ready to leave for a physician's appointment before 10:00 a.m.

Some of the tasks performed by nursing assistants include activities that:

1. Protect the rights of residents
   a. Treat resident with respect.
   b. Protect resident's privacy and maintain confidentiality.
   c. Keep call lights within resident's reach and answer promptly.
   d. Give resident choices whenever possible.
   e. Assist in recreational and spiritual activities of resident's choice.

2. Help the unit function smoothly
   a. Report for duty on time and ready to work.
   b. Cooperate with other team members.
   c. Communicate effectively with residents, their families, and other members of the interdisciplinary health care team.
   d. Follow facility policies.
   e. Know and carry out assignments.

3. Protect the safety of residents
   a. Keep units clean and clutter-free.
   b. Know how to operate equipment properly.
   c. Use standard precautions for routine care.
   d. Follow the principles of medical asepsis, including transmission-based isolation precautions when appropriate.
   e. Make beds properly.
   f. Report potential hazards as soon as noted.
   g. Use bed side rails and restraints properly.
   h. Keep call light within reach of resident.

Figure 3-6 Typical nursing assistant tasks. Specific tasks vary depending on state regulations and facility policy.

(continues)

     i. Know and practice the fire safety plan of the facility.
     j. Know and practice the disaster plan of the facility.
     k. Respond promptly to all alarms.
     l. Know and practice emergency procedures for obstructed airway (abdominal thrusts) and cardiopulmonary resuscitation.
     m. Follow oxygen precautions carefully.
     n. Help to implement fall prevention program.

4. Help residents by observing, collecting, and documenting data
     a. Measure and record vital signs (temperature, pulse, respirations, and blood pressure).
     b. Measure weight and height.
     c. Measure intake and output.
     d. Collect specimens.
     e. Document and report observations of resident's condition.

5. Help residents meet personal hygiene needs
     a. Provide skin care.
     b. Give oral hygiene.
     c. Provide denture care.
     d. Provide nail and hair care.
     e. Assist residents to dress and undress.
     f. Shave residents.
     g. Apply support hose.
     h. Assist with makeup.

6. Help residents meet nutritional needs in a pleasant environment
     a. Check food trays (right tray with the right food as prescribed by physician).
     b. Serve food trays.
     c. Assist residents who can help themselves.
     d. Feed dependent residents.
     e. Provide fresh water, nourishments, and supplements.
     f. Provide pleasant conversation.

7. Help residents meet elimination needs
     a. Assist with bedpans, urinals, and commodes.
     b. Empty urine collection bags.
     c. Assure that residents are clean and dry.
     d. Give enemas.
     e. Assist with colostomy care.

8. Help residents with restoration and mobility
     a. Turn and position residents in bed, wheelchair, or geri-chair to prevent complications of immobility.
     b. Assist in transfer activities.
     c. Carry out range of motion exercises.
     d. Use (wedges and pillows) for positioning and restraint alternatives.
     e. Help with ambulation.
     f. Assist with restorative activities.
     g. Encourage independence.

9. Help in carrying out the following special procedures (as defined by the facility):
     a. Admitting, transfer, and discharge
     b. Warm and cold applications
     c. Catheter care
     d. Ostomy care

Figure 3-6 *(Continued)*

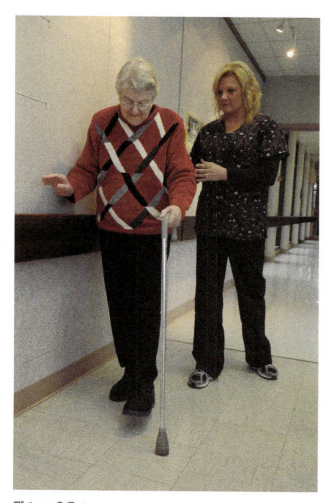

Figure 3-7 A nursing assistant saw that a resident needed help and moved quickly to assist.

You have been very busy with a new admission and will not be able to do this task on time. Tell the charge nurse right away so the resident can receive the necessary care. Always tell the nurse if you believe that you might not be able to complete any part of your assignment. Plan ahead so that someone else may be assigned to take care of it and will have time to do the task. If you should complete your assignment early, check with your coworkers to see if you might assist them. This is called *teamwork*.

SPECIFIC DUTIES

The duties of a nursing assistant can be divided into four groups of activities:

- Assisting in the activities of daily living (ADLs)
- Carrying out special procedures
- Performing support services
- Documenting (keeping records)

⊘N THE JOB

As a nursing assistant, you will be performing intimate procedures for residents. It is important that you accept these tasks and be able to perform them in an objective manner.

Activities of Daily Living

Much of the nursing assistant's duties are centered on helping residents carry out the ADLs that meet their physical, emotional, spiritual, and social needs. The major physical needs of the resident include:

- Cleanliness
- Proper exercise and positioning
- Proper nourishment (Figure 3-8)
- Elimination of wastes

    Remember that each time residents are encouraged to participate in their own care or are able to contribute to making decisions, the residents feel they have some control over their own lives, which minimizes avoidable decline.

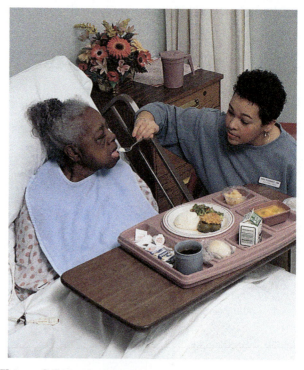

Figure 3-8 Feeding dependent residents is a required nursing assistant task that provides an essential ADL.

Special Procedures

Special procedures are required to care for residents with special needs. Special procedures include:

- Taking vital signs
- Catheter care
- Ostomy care
- Measuring urine
- Giving enemas
- Collecting specimens

Support Services

The third group of tasks does not necessarily involve resident contact. These tasks support needed nursing care and include:

- Supplying drinking water and snacks
- Placing and removing meal trays (Figure 3-9)
- Making beds
- Caring for equipment
- Carrying messages
- Making visitors feel welcome

Each activity makes the nursing care better and more effective. For example, older persons often do not drink enough fluids, and part of your assignment is to encourage them to drink more liquids. Offer them liquids each time you enter the room.

Documentation

The fourth group of nursing assistant tasks involves documentation of observations. These tasks are described in Lesson 6.

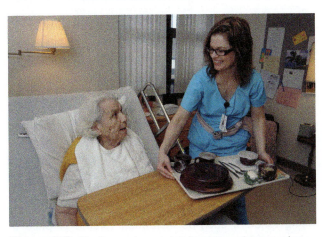

Figure 3-9 Placing and removing food trays is a nursing assistant function.

ORGANIZATION OF TIME

Nursing assistants have many tasks to carry out during their on-duty time. The better organized you are, the more easily you will complete your tasks. You can become more organized by:

- Reporting for duty when assigned and on time
- Listening to report/rounds
- Planning your work
- Working while on duty
- Trying to improve your performance
- Being observant at all times
- Leaving personal problems at home

Report for Duty at the Correct Time

Your job is your first responsibility. People are depending on you. If you are ill, you must call the facility as soon as you know that you will be unable to work, so that someone can cover your responsibilities. Most facilities require at least a 2-hour notice prior to the start of your shift, if you know you're going to be absent. If you have personal responsibilities that might affect your availability, you should discuss these with your employer when you are hired. Be sure that you and your employer agree as to how these responsibilities are to relate to your on-duty time.

Know who you should call if you cannot report for duty. Keep the telephone number and name beside your home telephone and in your wallet.

Listen to the Report/Review Your Assignment

Note any changes in the care plans and any special orders that are to be followed. Make special note of orders that must be carried out at a specific time. Do not assume that because a resident has been at the facility for a long time, orders remain the same.

Plan Your Work and Improve Your Efficiency

Take a few moments to rearrange your plans if something unexpected develops during your shift. Refer to your plan frequently so that you can reorganize if necessary. *Remember that you are employed and paid to work for a whole shift.* Do not waste time chatting with coworkers or talking on the phone. Be on time returning from breaks and lunch and do not leave early without permission. At the end of your shift, review your

? EXERCISE 3-6

MATCHING

Match the long-term care nursing assistant duty on the right with the activity on the left.

Activity

1. _____ making beds
2. _____ answering call lights
3. _____ supplying drinking water
4. _____ caring for residents' dentures
5. _____ irrigating a colostomy
6. _____ shaving residents
7. _____ making oral reports
8. _____ applying an ice bandage
9. _____ bathing residents
10. _____ contributing to evaluation of care
11. _____ cleaning utility room
12. _____ answering telephone
13. _____ giving enema to a resident
14. _____ feeding a resident
15. _____ weighing and measuring residents
16. _____ measuring blood pressures
17. _____ placing and removing meal trays
18. _____ using a mechanical lift to move a resident
19. _____ helping the resident to dress
20. _____ preparing written reports

Duty

a. assisting with ADL

b. carrying out special procedures

c. performing special services (support)

d. documenting

---

assignment. Think of ways you might have used your time and energy more efficiently. Learn to organize activities and tasks in order of importance (prioritize).

WORKPLACE ENVIRONMENT

Part of your responsibility is to maintain a calm, peaceful environment in the facility. However, from time to time, conflict and violence may occur in the facility between residents, residents and staff, residents and family members or other visitors, staff, and staff and visitors.

The International Council of Nurses defines workplace violence as "behavior that humiliates or degrades the dignity of individuals."* One of the fastest growing types of violence in the workplace is bullying. The International Labour Organization, an agency of the United Nations, defines bullying as "offensive behavior through spiteful, cruel, malicious, or humiliating attempts to damage an individual or group of employees."* Bullying can include physical or psychological violence. Psychological bullying is the most common type. According to the American Nurses Association (ANA) 2006 Workplace Abuse and Harassment of Nurses resolution, nurses are advised to report incidents of abuse and should not be afraid of retaliation.

Staff members should be constantly aware of any rising tension, such as increased volume or pitch of voices before actual violence occurs (Figure 3-10).

*Hughes, N. (2010) Environment, health, and safety, *American Nurse Today*, 5(7), 30.

Verbal outbursts

Pacing

Swearing

Increased complaining

Increased body movements

Changes in facial expressions

Figure 3-10 Signs of rising stress.

Avoidance of violence is always preferable to dealing with violence once it erupts (Figure 3-11).

Disagreements Between Staff

Conflicts can arise between staff members because of workload, specific assignments, misunderstandings, or for personal reasons. These conflicts should be handled out of the sound and sight of residents or visitors.

- Seek the help of the supervisor and speak in private.
- Be factual.
- Be open to the other person's point of view, listening carefully.

- Try to solve the problem cooperatively, with each party contributing to the solution.
- Confirm the solution in writing.
- Plan to meet again if the solution is ineffective.
- Put the agreed-upon solution into action.
- Thank the supervisor for meeting with you.

In some facilities there may be a grievance committee to help with severe conflicts.

An Isolated Incident

There may be a single incident in which a resident, feeling frustrated by some event, becomes upset and behaves in an angry way. Try to assess the situation in light of the resident's usual behavior. For example, a resident returns from a tiring therapy session and is feeling despondent about his progress. At this time, his lunch tray is delivered. In a sudden violent response he throws the tray on the floor. You know this is not typical of this resident. Recognize the situation as a temporary emotional response to frustration and stress. Sit with the resident to offer emotional support and provide the resident with an opportunity to express his feelings. Never argue with a resident for any reason. Listen patiently or seek assistance from your supervisor.

The nursing assistant should follow all facility policies and procedures involving safety and security. Other things you can do to prevent potential incidents are:

- Report suspicious individuals or other potential safety hazards to the nurse.
- If you are responsible for a secured area, control access to the area and keep it locked.
- Follow facility policy for locking all entrance doors at a designated time each evening. If your facility has a doorbell, respond to it quickly so oncoming workers are not outside alone in the dark.
- Participate in continuing education programs to learn how to recognize and manage escalating agitation, assaultive behavior, or criminal intent.
- Attend classes on cultural diversity that teach sensitivity on race, gender, religion, sexual orientation, and/or other ethnic issues and differences.
- Report assaults or threats of assaults to the nurse immediately.
- Avoid wearing scarves, necklaces, earrings, and other jewelry that could cause injury if a resident or other individual attacks you.
- Avoid remote, dark areas when you are alone.
- Exercise caution in elevators, stairwells, and unfamiliar areas. Immediately leave the area if you believe a hazard exists.
- If your facility has security personnel, request that they escort you in dark or potentially dangerous areas. If no security personnel are on duty, ask other staff members to accompany you.
- Use the "buddy system" if personal safety may be threatened.
- If a resident or other person is "acting out," or you believe you may be assaulted, do not let the person come between you and the exit.

Figure 3-11 Guidelines for violence prevention.

The Violent Resident

If a resident becomes agitated or violent, signal for help. Some health care facilities have security personnel who can be called for assistance. Move other residents out of the area to safety. Maintain a safe distance between yourself and the disturbed resident. Make sure that you have a safe exit route. Use a calm voice and simple words when speaking to the resident. Do not argue with or contradict the resident but only leave the room after ensuring safety for all involved. You will need to make a report as soon as possible. Refer to Figure 3-11.

Visitors Who Become Violent

Visitors who become violent can be asked to leave the facility. The assistance of security personnel may be necessary, including call the police. Do not take sides in any dispute between residents and their visitors. However, you must be firm and courteous in your insistence that the environment of the facility remain calm. Report all incidents to your supervisor.

SELF-CARE

Caregivers may get so involved in caring for others that they do not pay enough attention to their own well-being. You must take care of your own mental and physical health if you are to have the energy and enthusiasm to work successfully. When people are tired or stressed, they may find it hard to be cooperative, patient, and pleasant. Mistakes are more likely to be made. For your own sake and that of the residents in your care, you need to be at your best.

You will spend much of your time on your feet—walking corridors, pushing wheelchairs, handling equipment, and moving, supporting, and lifting residents—and carrying out detailed procedures. In addition you will be offering emotional support in a variety of situations. All of these activities require physical and emotional energy. To stay fit you will need:

- Sufficient rest
- Good nutrition
- Balanced recreation and exercise

There are some additional actions that you can take to promote your own well-being:

- Have regular physical examinations, including immunizations.
- Limit alcohol intake; do not drink alcohol while on duty or before reporting for duty.
- Avoid the use of illicit drugs.
- Limit or stop smoking.
- Always use proper body mechanics.

- Get help and use mechanical lifts when residents are heavy.
- Practice safe sex.

Career Health

Nursing assistants also need to care for their careers. A nursing assistant who feels insecure in skills and knowledge cannot perform at a high level. You can increase your confidence when you:

- Follow procedures as they are taught
- Do only those activities that are within your job description
- Attend staff development programs
- Seek other opportunities to increase your nursing care knowledge and skills
- Maintain your CNA certification

Following initial certification as a CNA, you are required to participate in continuing education. In order to maintain your registration, the CNA must receive 1.0 or 2.0 hours of in-service education per month, depending upon your particular state requirements. The state may contact the CNA annually to verify the number of in-service education hours that were received. It is imperative that the CNA keep the state registry apprised of any changes in status, such as a change in name or address.

Check with the individual state registry for information relating to exemptions. For example, CNAs on active duty with the Armed Forces may be exempt during a particular calendar year.

Emotional Health

You give so much of yourself to those in your care that you face the risk of burnout.

Burnout is mental and emotional—and sometimes physical—fatigue. People who work with the sick or infirm often experience burnout because of the emotional and physical demands of providing care. You can reduce the stress that leads to burnout by balancing your work with rest and recreation.

Compassion fatigue (CF) is a form of burnout that can affect persons in the health care professions. The affected caregivers expend large amounts of physical and emotional energy day in and day out because they "care too much." They find it difficult to balance objectivity and empathy, and do not take the time to "recharge" themselves. Unlike burnout, the feelings associated with CF do not subside after taking a vacation or a change of activity. Physical or spiritual fatigue and exhaustion take over and the caregiver can experience feelings of apathy, lack of interest, or indifference to what is going on around them. CF can be prevented. Each day caregivers should allocate some time for activities other than those that focus on caregiving. Examples of these activities include spending some quiet time alone (reading or watching TV), participating in some type of enjoyable physical activity, or spending quality time with family or friends discussing nonwork topics. If you as a nursing assistant are feeling overwhelmed, discuss your feelings with your supervisor. It is easier to prevent CF than it is to treat it once it occurs.

You can also learn stress-reducing techniques. Food and cigarettes are used by some people to reduce stress, but these can cause other serious health problems. To reduce stress, try the following:

- Exercise at least three to five times a week, doing something you enjoy.
- Sit for a few moments with your feet up.
- Shut your eyes and take deep breaths.
- With your eyes shut, picture a special place you like, and be there in your mind.
- Take a warm relaxing bath.
- Listen to quiet music.
- Carry out a specific relaxation exercise.
- Make yourself a cup of herbal tea and sip it slowly.
- Find a hobby that you really enjoy.
- Take a few minutes to talk with a friend (Figure 3-12).
- Meditate on your higher power or value belief system.

SEXUAL HARASSMENT

People cannot perform at their best when they are subjected to insensitive remarks or inappropriate behavior by coworkers or supervisors. The anxiety these situations produce is increased by the fear of losing a job if action is taken against the person responsible.

Sexual harassment may be expressed by actions, words, or implied threats. These behaviors create an

EXERCISE 3-7

MULTIPLE CHOICE
Select the one best answer.

1. The duties and responsibilities of the nursing assistant are stated in the
   (A) work order
   (B) daily assignment
   (C) job description
   (D) physician's orders
2. A good way to reduce stress is to
   (A) work an extra shif
   (B) find a hobby you really enjoy
   (C) discuss the residents with a neighbor
   (D) smoke a cigarette
3. If you cannot report to duty on time, you should
   (A) call a friend to cover for you
   (B) go in late, a few minutes will not matter
   (C) call your supervisor
   (D) do not go to work at all if not on time
4. Which of the following is *not* a good way to handle violence?
   (A) listen to the other person's point of view
   (B) avoid taking sides in any dispute between residents and their visitors
   (C) call security personnel if a resident becomes agitated
   (D) exaggerate the facts to make sure you get your point across

environment that is hostile and nonproductive. Examples of sexual harassment can include:

- The administrator makes sexual advances when you deliver reports to the office.
- A coworker rubs your neck as you document your completed tasks in the nurses' station.
- A coworker repeatedly tells off-color jokes in your presence even though you have asked him or her not to do so.
- A coworker makes remarks related to the size of your breasts, buttocks, or genitalia.
- Sexually explicit cartoons are posted on the staff bulletin board.
- A coworker reads and shows pornographic magazines during lunch.
- A charge nurse tells you that your assignments will be reduced if you agree to a date.

It is important to understand that you have the right to work in an environment that is free of sexual harassment. However, handling these situations requires

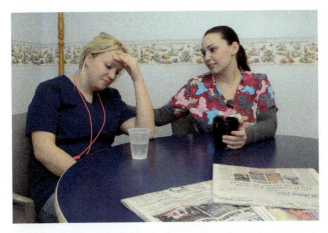

Figure 3-12 A quiet moment relaxing with a friend is a good way to reduce stress.

sensitivity and tact. First, be sure that the situation is truly sexual harassment. Then:

- Tell the offender that you are displeased with the action. Be blunt and ask them to "Stop."
- Document the incident so the details stay fresh in your mind.
- Report the situation to your supervisor.
- If the offender is your supervisor, follow the chain of command upward.

CONTINUE TO GROW

Your training program prepares you to perform as a beginning level nursing assistant. You have a responsibility to continue your education and personal growth (Figure 3-13). If you are willing to do so, you may learn much from team leaders, charge nurses, and other nursing assistants.

The procedure and policy books kept at the nursing station are ready references when you have questions about a new procedure or how to handle a new

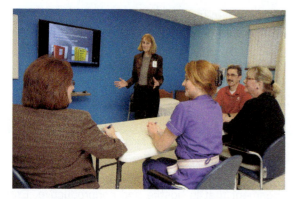

Figure 3-13 Once employed, take advantage of staff development programs to advance your education.

situation. Become familiar with each of these sources and with the medical dictionary on your unit. Use the dictionary/Google to look up and learn the correct spelling of medical words. Learn at least two new words each week and practice using them. Always ask for help when in doubt. Always be ready to learn.

Many facilities have professional magazines for staff use. Take advantage of this opportunity to increase your knowledge.

Care planning conferences can be an excellent way to expand your knowledge. Listen carefully. Remember, learning is a lifelong challenge.

Some long-term care facilities may provide career ladder incentives that will help nursing assistants upgrade their training and seek career advancements. Many states have career ladder initiatives that allow the nursing assistant to receive additional training and become authorized to perform advanced skills. Certified medication aides (CMAs) and qualified medication aides (QMAs) receive additional preparation and take a competency evaluation in order to become certified to administer medications in a variety of long-term care settings. Depending on state requirements, continuing education in medication administration and annual recertification may be required to maintain certification and to function as a CMA or QMA. The continuing education for medication administration is in addition to the basic continuing education requirements to maintain nursing assistant certification. Another opportunity for practice that requires additional skill training for the nursing assistant is referred to as a senior certified nursing assistant, or team lead. After meeting the minimum experience requirements, the CNA must attain the required number of hours of advanced instruction and pass a competency test in order to function as a role model and resource person for entry level CNAs.

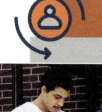

LESSON SYNTHESIS: Putting It All Together

You have just completed this lesson. Now go back and review the Clinical Focus. Try to see how the Clinical Focus relates to the concepts presented in the lesson. Then answer the following questions.

1. How do Ray's attitude and maturity affect the level of care the residents receive?

2. How does the pride Ray has in himself show in his own appearance and work?

3. What important contributions do nursing assistants make to the well-being of residents through the tasks and duties they perform?

4. What responsibility does a nursing assistant have to maintain personal mental and physical health?

3 REVIEW

A. Match each term (items a–e) with the proper definition.

a. accuracy
b. attitude
c. burnout
d. empathy
e. harmony

1. _____ friendly, cooperative atmosphere

2. _____ ability to put yourself in another person's position

3. _____ total emotional and mental fatigue

4. _____ outer reflection of inner feelings

5. _____ performing correctly

B. Select the one best answer for each of the following.

6. Recognizing needs that are expressed and those that are not expressed shows that the nursing assistant is

(A) dependable
(B) mature
(C) sensitive
(D) accurate

7. Maturity is related to

(A) age
(B) attitude
(C) accuracy
(D) energy

8. The nursing assistant should bathe

(A) daily
(B) once a week
(C) twice each week
(D) every other day

9. Which of the following is a proper part of your uniform?

(A) earrings
(B) bracelets
(C) identification badge
(D) necklace

10. The nursing assistant is ready for work when

(A) fingernails are polished bright red
(B) strong aftershave lotion is applied
(C) wearing a watch with a second hand
(D) wearing bracelets

11. The activities and responsibilities of nursing assistants are

(A) stated in the procedure manual
(B) called a job description
(C) located in the nurses' manual
(D) the same all over the country

12. Nursing assistant assignments are based on

(A) the needs of the assistant
(B) the needs of the residents
(C) the wishes of visitors
(D) the wishes of social workers

13. The nursing assistant's uniform is

(A) worn on shopping trips
(B) worn for 3 days without washing it
(C) folded so the dirtiest side is on the outside when it is put into the laundry
(D) worn only on duty

14. Sean, the nursing assistant, notices that a resident who is not assigned to him is walking unsteadily down the hall. He should

(A) ignore the situation
(B) assist the resident as needed
(C) notify the supervisor
(D) inform the assigned nursing assistant of the situation

15. Sabrina, the nursing assistant, has not had the time to carry out the exercises that had been ordered for Mr. Martinez. It is now time to go off duty. She should

    (A) tell another assistant to do the exercises

    (B) go off duty because it is not really important that the exercises be done

    (C) tell the supervisor right away

    (D) plan to do double the amount of exercises the next day

16. Mrs. Angdon is very upset. Her voice is rising and she is swearing (something she never does under ordinary circumstances). She is also making threats. Roseanne, the nursing assistant, should

    (A) speak loudly

    (B) hold Mrs. Angdon in her chair

    (C) make sure there is a clear exit for herself

    (D) ask her roommate to help

17. Peter and Doug are angry with one another because Doug feels Peter's assignment is lighter than his. This situation is best handled by

    (A) discussing it with a resident

    (B) discussing it in the hall

    (C) discussing it in the dining room

    (D) discussing it with the supervisor in private

18. In a professional relationship with the resident, Emily should display _____ toward Anna Chung, who has fallen and fractures her hip.

    (A) sympathy

    (B) empathy

    (C) sensitivity

    (D) tact

C. For each of the following duties, indicate if it is a duty of the nursing assistant by answering yes (Y) or no (N).

19. Y N giving bed baths

20. Y N measuring temperatures

21. Y N serving trays

22. Y N starting intravenous fluids

23. Y N making beds

24. Y N applying sterile dressings

25. Y N calling physicians for orders

26. Y N weighing residents

27. Y N carrying messages

D. Clinical Experiences

Read each case history and answer the questions.

28. Mary was assigned to make the bed of a resident who was able to get out of bed. The supervisor was not satisfied with the way the bed was made and told Mary she would have to remake the bed. Mary was very angry. After the supervisor left, she complained to the resident.

    a. Did Mary show maturity in her reaction?

    b. How should Mary have reacted?

29. Mrs. Randolph is a very slow eater. She had a stroke and lost the use of her left side. She is naturally left-handed. Star, the nursing assistant, can feed Mrs. Randolph faster than she can feed herself, but Star lets Mrs. Randolph feed herself.

    a. Do you think Star has a special reason for letting Mrs. Randolph feed herself?

    b. What do you think her purpose is?

30. John did not complete his assignment on time and his supervisor told him he must plan more carefully. John said nothing but slammed the door on the way out of the office.

    a. Do you think John responded in a mature way?

    b. How can you tell?

    c. Is maturity a matter of age or attitude?

31. Even though they can feed themselves slowly, Carrie feeds her residents to save time.

    a. Is her method of feeding best?

    b. Is it more or less satisfying to the resident to be fed?

    c. What benefit is there in allowing residents to feed themselves?

32. Eric always comes to work on time, has a pleasant attitude, and finishes his assignment correctly.

    a. What important characteristic does Eric show by arriving on time?

    b. What characteristic does he show by being sure his assignments are done correctly?

33. Lois is very patient with the residents in her care because she says she would find it so hard to need help to go to the bathroom or to have to sit all day.

    a. By her actions Lois is showing what important characteristic?

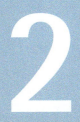

2

Communication Skills

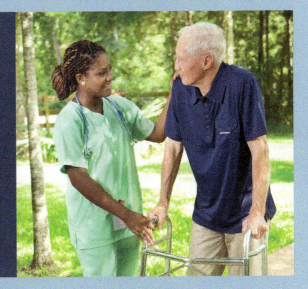

COMMUNICATION AND INTERPERSONAL SKILLS

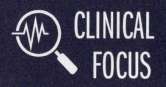

CLINICAL FOCUS

Think about how effective messages are sent and received and how people communicate with one another as you study this lesson.

OBJECTIVES

After studying this lesson, you should be able to:

- Define and spell vocabulary words and terms.

- Identify barriers to effective communications with residents.

- State two ways in which people communicate.

- Describe situations when nursing assistants must communicate with other staff members.

- List general guidelines for communicating with residents.

- Describe ways in which a nursing assistant can improve communications with residents who have impaired hearing, impaired vision, aphasia, disorientation, or decreased level of consciousness.

VOCABULARY

aphasia (ah-FAY-zee-ah)
articulation (are-tick-you-LAY-shun)
body language (BAH-dee LAN-gwihj)
Braille (brayl)
care plan (kair plan)
communication (kom-myou-nih-KAY-shun)
disorientation (dis-oh-ree-en-TAY-shun)
medical chart (MED-ih-kul chart)

memo (MEM-oh)
nonverbal communication (NON-ver-bal kom-myou-nih-KAY-shun)
shift report (shift ree-PORT)
symbol (SIM-bull)
verbal communication (VER-bal kom-myou-nih-KAY-shun)

CASE STUDY

Doris Greene, age 83, broke her hip and had no one to care for her at home. She has been a resident in long-term care for 4 years. She has no immediate family and her only sister lives 3,000 miles away. The staff and residents have become her family and friends.

THE COMMUNICATION PROCESS

Communication involves the exchange of information (Figure 4-1). For successful communication, you must have a:

- Sender
- Message
- Receiver
- Feedback

As a nursing assistant, you can assist in this process by using effective methods of communication with residents and coworkers. Some of the residents you care for will have barriers to effective communication. These may be caused by difficulties in hearing, seeing, or understanding what is being communicated. You can improve the quality of life for residents by communicating appropriately with each one (Figure 4-2). This may be enhanced by visiting with family and friends. When residents speak a different language, you may need an interpreter to communicate effectively.

The two ways to communicate are:

- Verbally—using spoken or written language
- Nonverbally—using body language, gestures, and symbols

Verbal Communication

Verbal communication uses words, both spoken and written. Written communication also depends on the use of symbols. Words are symbols of language. Visual signs, such the Standard Precautions or Biohazard logos, are also symbols. These symbols tell health care workers to wash their hands before and after procedures or to take extra precautions when handling soiled items. You will be using words to explain to residents what you plan to do when carrying out a procedure and how they can help. The oral report to the nurse after your assignment is completed also involves the use of words. When using written forms of communication, it is important to use the correct word with the correct spelling. Choose words carefully so that your message is clear.

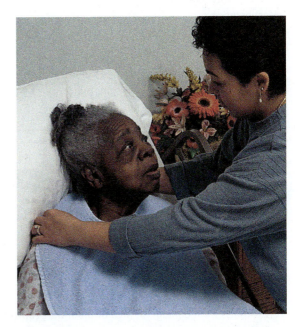

> ## ⊘N THE JOB
>
> As a health care worker, you may be communicating with persons who are not able to talk or hear, with persons who speak a different language, or with persons who are disoriented. Communication is the foundation for successful health care.

Oral communication includes more than the words you speak. How you say the words also sends a message to the listener. When communicating verbally with others, be aware of:

- The tone of your voice
- Loudness (volume) of your voice
- Articulation
- Words or phrases with double meanings or cultural meanings
- Swearing or the use of slang

The tone of voice you use and its volume can convey a message of happiness, anger, sadness, or caring. Keep the volume of your voice at a moderate level. A harsh, loud voice is disturbing to others.

Articulation is the clarity with which you pronounce words. If you do not articulate (speak clearly), others will not be able to understand you.

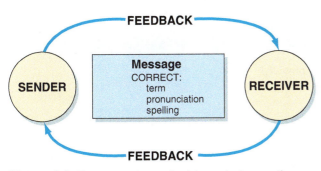

Figure 4-1 The message can be interpreted correctly only if the words are chosen carefully and pronounced and spelled correctly.

Figure 4-2 The nursing assistant is listening to the resident.

You will be caring for residents from many cultures and ethnic groups. Remember that certain words in your culture may have an entirely different meaning to someone else. Occasionally a resident may use swear or curse words in conversation. It is important that the nursing assistant remain calm and refrain from responding in a like manner. Swearing by staff members is never permissible in a health care facility. Slang is another form of communication that is not appropriate to be used in conversation with residents or coworkers.

Nonverbal Communication

Your nonverbal communication or body language can sometimes say more than words. Be aware of the message that is being sent through your:

- Body posture/position
- Body movements
- Facial expressions
- Activity level
- Overall appearance
- Proximity
- Silence

Your body movements send messages that can give the receiver either a negative or positive reaction about you. Your appearance gives others

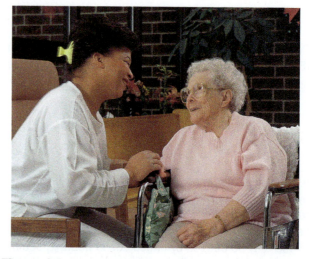

Figure 4-3 Nonverbal communication involves the use of facial expressions, body language, gestures, eye contact, and touch to convey messages or ideas.

their first impression about you. Since this impression is usually lasting, it is important that it be positive. As you work in the facility, be aware that your body language is sending messages to those around you (Figure 4-3). Remember that residents may be looking at you when you are not aware of their attention.

? EXERCISE 4-1

Define the following by selecting the correct term from the list provided.

communication
articulation
body language
symbol

1. communicating through body movements _____
2. object used to represent something else _____
3. exchanging information _____
4. ability to speak clearly _____

? EXERCISE 4-2

Define the following by selecting the correct term from the list provided.

aphasia
disorientation
stroke

1. Unaware of time and place _____
2. Results from damage to area of brain that controls speech _____
3. Common cause of aphasia _____

? EXERCISE 4-3

COMPLETION

Select the correct term(s) from the following list to complete each statement.

activity level	caring	overall appearance
anger	sadness	tone
articulate	double	slang
body movements	facial expressions	
body position	happiness	
body posture	loudness	

1. When communicating verbally, remember to:
   a. Control the _____ of your voice.
   b. Control the voice _____.
   c. Be aware of the way you _____.
   d. Avoid _____ meanings or cultural meanings.
   e. Not use informal language or _____.
2. Loudness and tone of your voice can convey a message of:
   a. _____
   b. _____
   c. _____
   d. _____
3. Six ways a message can be sent through body language include:
   a. _____
   b. _____
   c. _____
   d. _____
   e. _____
   f. _____

COMMUNICATING WITH STAFF MEMBERS

In Lesson 2 you learned that the organizational chart is a guide for communication. The organizational chart tells you the lines of authority. All facilities have an organizational chart that illustrates how each department relates to other departments. Some larger departments, such as nursing, have their own chart that indicates the line of authority within the nursing department (Figure 4-4). You will need to develop methods of communication with other staff members in nursing and with members of other departments.

ORAL COMMUNICATIONS

Oral reports are used frequently to communicate information about residents. When you first come on duty, you may listen to a **shift report**. The nurse who worked the previous shift will report to staff coming on duty. This report will include:

- Changes in residents' conditions
- Information about new residents
- Names of residents who were discharged or passed away
- Any incidents that occurred to residents
- New orders
- Special events for the residents that will occur during your shift

Listen carefully to the report because it will help you plan your assignment (Figure 4-5A & B). Your assignment includes:

- The residents you will care for during your shift
- The procedures you will need to do for these residents

Your supervising nurse will then give you additional information about your assignment based on

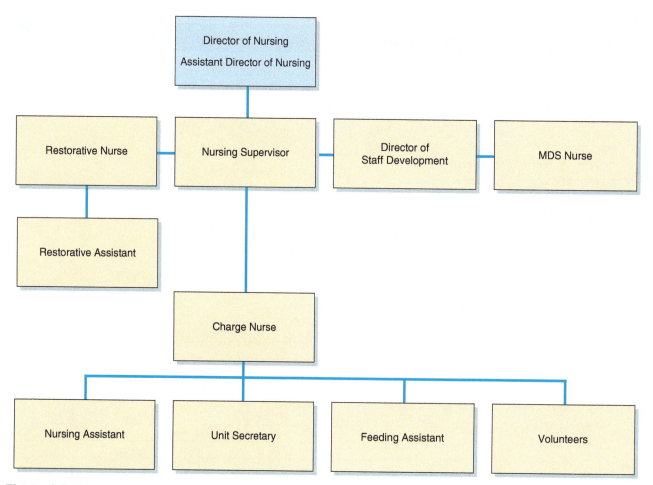

Figure 4-4 Nursing organizational chart.

CNA ASSIGNMENT SHEET 10/12/XX														
Room	Resident Name	Bath	Position Schedule	Range of Motion	Vital Signs	Weight	Toileting	B & B	ADL Program	Ambulate	Transfer or Gait Belt	Restraint or Alternative	Safety	I & O
300A	Mary King	S	X	PROM			X					Wedge in chair	X	
300B	Susan Kowalski	WP	X	PROM			X						X	
301A	June Lee		X	PROM		X			X					
301B	Elena Hernandez	BB	X	PROM	X							Side rails	X	X
302	John Murray			AROM					X	X	X			
303A	Albert Strong	S		AROM	X					X				X
303B	Norman Jones		X	PROM			X					Lap buddy	X	
304	Hazel Urich	TB		AROM		X		X		X	X			

Figure 4-5A The nurse gives daily assignments based on the problems, goals, and needs listed in the care plan for each resident. Use the assignment to set priorities for your shift. If you believe you will be unable to complete your assignment, inform the nurse promptly.

the shift report. This information may include orders to complete procedures for specific residents:

- Take temperature, pulse, and respirations on designated residents
- Obtain weights on designated residents

- Allow a resident to remain in bed because of a change in condition
- Make observations on a resident who has had a change of condition

Nursing Assistants' Daily Assignments

DATE: _10/12/XX_

UNIT: _3rd Floor_

Everyone must participate in passing food trays and feeding residents so that hot food is served

Cindy Res. group 1 300A- 304	John Res. group 2 305A- 309B	Mary Res. group 3 310- 314B	Susan Res. group 4 315A- 320A	James Res. group 5 320B- 325	Norma Res. group 6 326A- 330B
Break time: 8:30	Break time: 8:45	Break time: 9:00	Break time: 8:30	Break time: 8:45	Break time: 9:00
Meal time: 10:45	Meal time: 11:15	Meal time: 12:30	Meal time: 10:45	Meal time: 11:15	Meal time: 12:30

SPECIAL ASSIGNMENTS
Fresh Water Pass
(AM & PMs)

John AM

Norma PM

Mealtime Assignments

James - hall trays

Norma - feeders

Others to main
dining room

Water Pitcher Collection (PM)

Tub Room/Shower Room
Cindy

Utility Rooms/Soiled Linen
Mary

Deliver Nourishments
Susan

Utensil Collection (PMs)

Fill Humidifiers

CHARGE NURSE NOTES:

Bible Study - 10:00

Current Events - 11:00

Bingo - 2:00

All beds made by

10 AM please

RESIDENT APPOINTMENTS:

304 - Beauty shop 9:30

317B - Daughter picking up 11:00
    for lunch

323A - Dentist - 2:00

TREATMENTS:

WEIGHTS:	INTAKE/OUTPUT:
301A -	301B -
321B -	303A -
329 -	312 -
VITAL SIGNS:	317B -
301B -	324B -
316A -	326B
321A -	329A -

See Routine Equipment Cleaning Assignment Form on clipboard

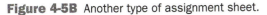

Figure 4-5B Another type of assignment sheet.

Many skilled nursing facilities are eliminating the shift report and, instead, a task list is printed for each resident. If your facility does not use shift reports or a task list you must go to the team leader for assignments. At this time, you may ask about any unusual occurrences or admissions that took place while you were away from the facility.

During your shift you will give oral reports to the nurse about procedures you have completed and observations you have made. Often, this is when you would enter documentation in the computer. At the end of the shift you will summarize your assignment to the nurse so that the information can be included in the shift report for the employees coming on duty when you leave. When leaving the nursing unit for any reason during your shift, always report to the nurse.

At the end of the shift, or during the shift, if possible, be sure that you have also fully documented the care you provided to residents. Sign each entry. Remember that if the care is not documented, it is considered not done.

Telephone Etiquette

Many telephone calls come into a long-term care facility. Families call to ask about the condition of a loved one. Physicians call to leave new medical orders. The laboratory may call to give results of diagnostic tests. Remember that nursing assistants are not allowed to take physician's orders or results of diagnostic tests or to give information to families. You must call the nurse to do this. If you answer the telephone:

- Smile as you answer the telephone; it will give your voice a pleasant, professional sound to the person listening.
- Identify the nursing unit: "third floor, north," for example.
- Identify yourself and your position: "Mary Smith, nursing assistant, how may I help you?"
- Ask the caller's name and ask the caller to wait while you locate the person called.
- If the person is unavailable, take a message (Figure 4-6) and write down the following information:
  - Date and time of call
  - Caller's name and telephone number
  - Message left by caller
  - Whether the person is to return the call or whether the caller will telephone again later
  - Your signature

Some facilities have more complex telephone systems. You will be taught how to transfer calls or to voice page. Most facilities do not allow employees to make or receive personal telephone calls while they are on duty.

Recent advances in the use of technology have made cell phones and pagers prevalent in our society. Your facility will have a clear policy about the use of your personal devices during work hours. The majority of agencies prohibit cell phone use; the phone must be turned off when you enter the facility. Personal calls may only be made when you are taking a rest or lunch break. Failure to follow the cell phone policy may result in disciplinary action.

The use of cell phones among residents is also becoming popular. You should never use a resident's cell phone for your personal use or borrow their charger for your personal use.

WRITTEN COMMUNICATIONS

Many situations rely on written communications. The ability to accurately write or read the communication is essential to the care of the resident.

Memos

A memo (Figure 4-7) is a brief communication that informs or reminds employees of:

- Changes in policies or procedures
- Upcoming meetings or staff development classes

Figure 4-6 Telephone messages must be accurate and clear.

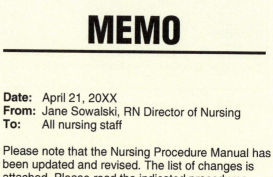

Figure 4-7 Memos are brief but contain important information.

- Admission of new residents
- Promotions of staff members

Be sure you know where memos are posted so that you will be aware of the facility activities. Some facilities may use electronic messaging.

Manuals

All facilities have several manuals that provide information about policies and procedures (Figure 4-8). These may include:

- Employee personnel handbook—describes all the personnel policies and benefits
- Disaster manual—gives directions for actions to take for fire or other disasters
- Procedure manual—gives directions for all procedures performed for residents
- Quality assurance manual—describes all quality control policies and procedures
- Nursing policy manual—describes rules and regulations pertaining to care of residents

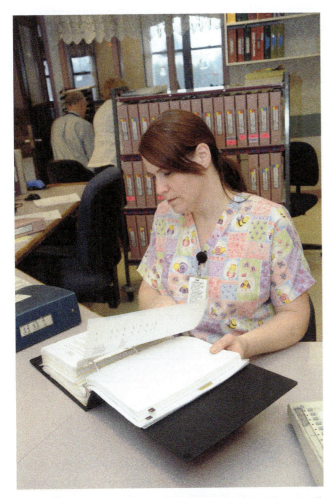

Figure 4-8 The procedure manual gives information on all nursing procedures performed in the facility.

- Dietary manual—explains therapeutic diets
- Infection control manual—identifies practices to prevent the spread of infection

You are not expected to memorize all the information contained in the manuals, but you should know where they are kept on the nursing unit and be able to look up information when it is needed. Some facilities may provide the information on a computer network.

The Resident Care Plan

Each resident has a Minimum Data Set (MDS) care plan that has been developed by the interdisciplinary health care team (Figure 4-9). The care plan:

- Lists the resident's medical diagnoses
- Identifies the resident's problems
- Gives directions for resolving the resident's problems
- Lists the expected outcomes for resolving the problems
- Is updated regularly

Your assignment is based on the resident's care plan. You will learn more about the care plan in Lesson 6.

The Resident's Medical Chart

Each resident has a **medical chart** or record (Figure 4-10). The medical chart contains:

- The physician's medical orders for that resident—medications, treatments, diagnostic tests
- The medical history of the resident—summary of all past illnesses and surgeries
- Results of physical examinations
- Results of all diagnostic tests—blood tests and x-rays
- Progress notes from the physician and from all disciplines involved in the resident's care—brief, periodic descriptions of the resident's condition and response to treatment
- Assessments from all disciplines—identifies the resident's problems
- Nursing notes—information that describes the resident's condition, nursing care given, and the resident's response to the care
- Consultant notes

The information entered into the chart is called *documentation*. The chart is a legal document. It may be used to:

- Determine payments by insurance companies
- Determine settlement of lawsuits

MARYSVILLE CARE CENTER	CARE PLAN	02/06/20XX
		FORM # 280L

PROBLEM	SHORT TERM GOAL	APPROACH

(1) Potential for impaired skin integrity
  a) Related to altered circulation in legs
 	
  b) Related to flexion contracture of neck
 	
ONSET 02/06/20XX TARGET 05/07/20XX RESOLVE / /
	(1) Will remain ulcer free (legs) through 05/07/20XX
	
	BEGIN 02/06/20XX TARGET 05/07/20XX RESOLVE / /
	
	(2) Skin intact lower neck through 05/07/20XX
	
	BEGIN 02/06/20XX TARGET 05/07/20XX RESOLVE / /
		(1) R.N. check legs q a.m.
		  DISC: NSG
		
		(2) Elevate legs when up in w/c.
		  DISC: NA
		
		(3) Wash and dry area b.i.d.
		  DISC: NA
		
		(4) Apply 4 x 4 to separate skin surfaces.
		  DISC: NSG NA
		
		(5) Use Mycalog cream for increased redness prn.
		  DISC: NSG

(2) Alteration in comfort
  a) Related to impaired circulation
  b) Related to joint pain
 	
ONSET 02/06/20XX TARGET 05/07/20XX RESOLVE / /
	(1) 2 nocs/week without leg cramps by 05/07/20XX
	
	BEGIN TARGET 05/07/20XX RESOLVE / /
	
	(2) States relief of pain with heat packs through 05/07/20XX
	
	BEGIN 02/06/20XX RESOLVE / /
		(1) Administer Procardia as ordered and assess effectiveness
		  DISC: NSG
		
		(1) Heat packs to neck, shoulder, knees 5x/wk.
		  DISC: RA

PHYSICIAN / ALT. PHYSICIAN	PHONE NO.	ALLERGIES / NOTES					
WASHINGTON, JAMES M.D. KEELEY, JANICE M.D.	(555) 555-8888	PENICILLIN, ASPIRIN					
RESIDENT	STATION / ROOM / BED	ADMISSION NUMBER / DATE	SEX	DATE OF BIRTH	CARE PLAN DATE	PAGE #
JAMES, FIONA	NORTH-222-B	33652 10/18/20XX	F		02/06/20XX	1

Figure 4-9 The care plan gives information for the resident's care.

This means that all entries must be made in blue or black ink and signed. The entries are considered permanent and should never be scratched through or changed using white-out. At the end of the shift, or as often as possible, during the shift, the nursing assistant is responsible for fully documenting the care provided for the resident. You are to sign each entry. *Remember that if the care is not charted, it is considered not done.*

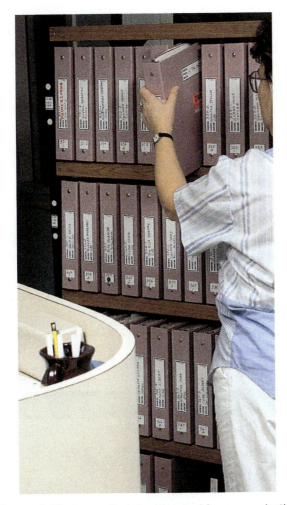

Figure 4-10 The medical chart is a tool for communication.

Electronic Communication

Various health care agencies have been using computers for billing for years. Pharmacies and clinical laboratories associated with various health care agencies have been relaying medication orders and laboratory findings. Increasingly, computers are being used to store data based on the care given by clinicians: doctors, nurses, nursing assistants, various therapists, and other professionals in both acute care and long-term care facilities.

Some facilities use the computer for documentation of care given, administration and charting of medications, and developing and storing nursing care plans. All data collection and storage must adhere to the guidelines developed under HIPAA. The use of the computer for documentation improves legibility of records, can enhance MDS compliance with timely recording, improves communication within the health care team, and can allow more time to care for the residents by decreasing the time associated with completing the "paper work." More discussion of this topic takes place in Lesson 6.

More discussion of this topic takes place in Lesson 6.

> **? EXERCISE 4-4**
>
> **YES OR NO**
> Indicate whether the following oral messages fit the action described by circling yes (Y) or no (N).
> 1. Y N Dorothy rubs her head with her hand and tells you she does not have a headache.
> 2. Y N Ellen sits with her arms and legs crossed, has turned her wheelchair toward the window, and tells you she is happy to meet her new roommate.
> 3. Y N Aimee makes a face when you feed her and says she hates chocolate pudding.
> 4. Y N Mary appears on duty with dirty shoes and untidy hair and says she is proud to be a nursing assistant.
> 5. Y N Emma keeps moving about the room and says she feels calm about her transfer to another facility.
> 6. Y N Nichole says she is interested in her residents. She often looks out the window and seldom makes eye contact when residents speak.
> 7. Y N Carrie and Terry claim to care about residents and often talk "over" them as they work together giving care.
> 8. Y N Tim describes himself as a caring nursing assistant but often interrupts residents when they are talking.
> 9. Y N Fernando says he is sensitive to residents' feelings and stands about 2 feet away when conversing with them.
> 10. Y N Greg is careful to show caring by never discussing personal activities with other staff members in the presence of residents.

COMMUNICATING WITH RESIDENTS

The ability to communicate with a resident is a skill that will develop with experience. It is not always the words you choose that are important, but the way in which they are said. Your tone of voice, facial expression, and even the way you touch a resident all communicate a sense of honest caring, or lack of caring, to the resident. Looking directly at the resident as you speak and addressing the person respectfully by name are also indications of caring. (See "Guidelines for . . . Communicating with Residents.")

Listening actively is a special skill requiring more than just being physically present. When you listen actively, all of your attention is focused on the speaker. You maintain eye contact and do not interrupt while the other person is speaking. You ask questions that encourage the speaker to continue and respond to specific questions being asked. To communicate effectively:

- Face the resident.
- Speak slowly.
- Be at eye level.
- Maintain appropriate eye contact.
- Listen carefully.
- Be patient and take your time.
- Use touch appropriately.
- Be aware of your body language.
- Do not sit or stand too close to the resident.
- Avoid finishing their sentences for them.

🌐 BUILDING CULTURAL AWARENESS

You should be aware that not all cultures view direct eye contact as meaning interest, attention, and courtesy. Some Asian and Native American cultures view sustained, direct eye contact as rude. People from these cultures normally would not look at a speaker directly for any length of time, nor would they stare at a person they were addressing. To do so is considered a sign of disrespect in their cultures. Do not make assumptions about the behavior of the residents in your care. If they are not of your culture, find out as much as you can about their culture. Refer to the resident assessment and care plan for information that is resident-specific. This may be done if people from specific cultures are residents in the facility.

? EXERCISE 4-5

COMPLETION

Select the correct term(s) from the following list to complete each statement regarding touch.

not
identify   startled
best   sexual
patronizing   substitutes

1. Residents can interpret a pat on the head as being _____.
2. Some residents consider touching as only a prelude to _____ intercourse.
3. Residents who have been abused in the past may _____ want to be touched.
4. Disoriented or blind residents may be _____ if you touch them unexpectedly.

⚠ GUIDELINES FOR... COMMUNICATING WITH RESIDENTS

Remember these guidelines when you are communicating with residents.

SENDING A MESSAGE

First, be aware of the message you are sending to the resident:

1. Use nonthreatening words or gestures.
   - Be calm. Avoid rapid, jerky movements.
   - Speak clearly and courteously.
   - Use a pleasant, low-pitch tone of voice.
   - Use the name of the resident's choice. Some residents may wish to be called by Mr., Mrs., or Miss with the last name. Others will ask you to use their first names. Avoid using names like "dear" or "honey."

2. Use appropriate body language.
   - This includes your general appearance. Think about the first impression that you make. Do your uniform and grooming show pride in yourself and your work?
   - Your posture and movements will tell the residents whether or not you are enthusiastic about your work.

3. Show interest and concern when the client is talking.
   - Use eye contact that is natural.

(continues)

⚠ GUIDELINES FOR... COMMUNICATING WITH RESIDENTS (Continued)

- Try to communicate at *eye level*. Many clients use wheelchairs, so you may need to squat down or sit to do this.
- Remain at a comfortable distance from the resident. For most people, this is about 2 to 4 feet away. If a resident is disoriented, this may be too close (Figure 4-11).

4. Be considerate when you are working with clients.
   - Do not talk as if the resident is not present. Include the resident in the conversation.
   - Do not discuss personal activities with other staff members in the presence of the clients.
   - Converse with the resident on topics they can relate to.
   - Do not interrupt when the resident is speaking.
   - Ask for clarification if you do not understand the resident.

5. Give the resident only factual information, not your personal feelings, opinions, or beliefs. Your responsibility as a nursing assistant is to listen in a nonjudgmental manner. Remember:
   - Do not give orders or advice to clients.
   - Do not use threats or warnings to get clients to do what you want them to do.

- Do not criticize or make fun of clients' beliefs or ideas.

6. Information concerning the resident's condition, medications, and treatments should be given only by the nurse. This information is regulated by the HIPAA laws; see Lesson 1.

RECEIVING A MESSAGE

Be sensitive to the message you are receiving from the resident.

1. Be alert to the resident's needs to communicate with you. Allow time for the resident to talk and respond.

2. Observe the resident's body language. This is especially important if a resident is unable to communicate verbally.
   - Does the resident's posture indicate the presence of pain?
   - Do the resident's gestures and movements indicate that the resident may be anxious or frightened (Figure 4-12)?

3. Consider whether the resident can see and hear you. A resident may have difficulty paying attention if there are many distractions in the environment. This includes other people, televisions, and radios.

4. Report problems to the nurse if you are concerned about the resident's statements. Do not argue or try to talk a resident out of a belief.

5. Ask for clarification if you are unsure of what the resident is saying.

6. Reflect the feelings and thoughts of the resident by rewording the resident's statements into questions.

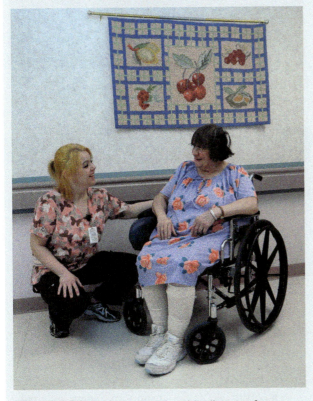

Figure 4-11 Remain a comfortable distance from the resident.

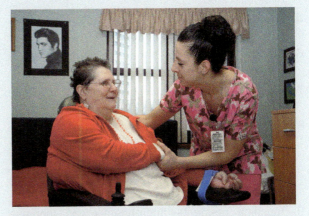

Figure 4-12 This resident's body language indicates fear and anxiety.

COMMUNICATING THROUGH THE USE OF TOUCH

All human beings have a need to touch and be touched by others. Infants go through a "bonding" process when they are held close to another human being. This human contact is essential to the growth and development of infants and children. The need for touching is never outgrown. However, as people age, there are fewer opportunities for touching. Many older people no longer have a spouse. As one gets older, the circle of friends and relatives becomes smaller.

Appropriate Touch

Nursing assistants can learn to use touch appropriately with residents. First, you must know the residents. The way people touch each other may mean different things to different people. This is because everyone comes from a different background. Cultural meanings may be attached to touching. Be aware of these factors:

1. You will touch residents frequently while you are giving care. Be gentle and patient.
2. Touching others is not just physical contact. We touch others with our eye contact, facial expressions, and body language.
3. Some residents may have been physically abused in the past. They may associate all forms of physical contact with abuse. It may be difficult for them to accept nonthreatening forms of touch. Always explain procedures and actions before placing hands on patients.
4. Some individuals view touching only as a preliminary to sexual intercourse. You will need to avoid touching these individuals in a way that can be misinterpreted.
5. Touching can be patronizing. An example of this is patting a client on the head.
6. Holding a resident's hand can demonstrate a sense of caring (Figure 4-13).
7. For some residents, a hug may be suitable (Figure 4-14).
8. Disoriented residents may be startled if you touch them unexpectedly. They may react aggressively. Be sure they are aware of your approach and never approach someone from behind.
9. Touching residents appropriately can increase their self-esteem. It gives the message that you accept and care about them.

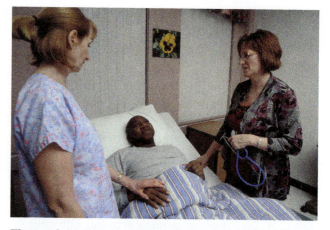

Figure 4-13 Holding a resident's hand can show a sense of caring.

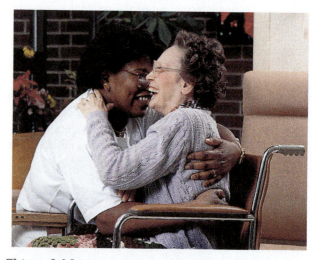

Figure 4-14 Some residents may appreciate a hug.

? EXERCISE 4-6

COMPLETION

Select the correct term(s) from the following list to complete each statement regarding hard of hearing residents.

slowly	cover
see	shout
best	facial

1. Make sure residents can _____ you clearly.
2. Stand on the residents' _____ hearing side.
3. Do not _____ your mouth when speaking.
4. Speak _____, distinctly, and naturally.
5. Use _____ expressions, gestures, and body language to help express your meanings.

COMMUNICATING WITH RESIDENTS WHO HAVE SPECIAL NEEDS

Some residents may have difficulty communicating with you. This may be caused by:

- Hearing impairment
- Vision impairment
- Aphasia
- Disorientation
- Unconscious state
- Altered level of consciousness

CLINICAL FOCUS

Think about Doris Greene and how you might use the sense of touch to communicate with her.

Be aware that the resident who is unconscious may not be able to respond to you but may still be able to hear. Studies have shown that hearing is the last sense to leave us—that is why we always act like residents can hear us and are aware of our intentions. Always make the resident aware of your presence. Knock on the door and greet the resident by name before touching him or her. While you are present in the room, inform the resident of what you are doing and always tell him or her when you are leaving and when you will return.

Always check the care plan before attempting to communicate with a resident who has special communication needs. Specific approaches may be established for all staff members to use with the client. Lack of consistency in the use of these approaches is confusing and frustrating to the resident.

Communicating with Residents Who Have Hearing Impairment

Many older adults lose some of their hearing. Some of them may wear hearing aids. Even those who do may still have problems understanding others when they speak.

1. Get the resident's attention first.
   - Make sure the resident sees you.
   - Touch the resident lightly to indicate you wish to speak.
2. If the resident uses a hearing aid, be sure the client is wearing it and that the hearing aid is on.
3. If the resident has a "good" ear, stand or sit on that side when you are talking.
4. Do not chew gum, eat, or cover your mouth while you are talking.

5. The light should be behind the resident, so your face can be clearly seen.
6. Face the resident; many persons with hearing impairments can read lips or interpret your facial expressions.
7. Reduce outside distractions. Turn off the television and move the resident to a quieter place.
8. Speak quietly and calmly.
9. Keep your voice pitch low.
10. Speak slowly, distinctly, and naturally.
11. Start conversation with a key word or phrase to identify the topic for the resident.
12. Form words carefully, use familiar words, and keep sentences short.
13. Pronounce words clearly. If a hearing-impaired resident has difficulty with letters and numbers, say: "M as in Mary," "T as in twins," "B as in boy." Say each number separately: "five six" instead of fifty-six. Remember that *m, n; 2, 3, 56, 66*; and *b, c, d, e,* and *v* sound alike.
14. Rephrase words as needed.
15. Avoid shouting, exaggerating words, or speaking very slowly. It is harder for the resident to understand you.
16. Keep a notepad handy and write your words if the resident does not understand. Sometimes a small, dry erase board is very helpful in communicating with those with hearing impairments.
17. Use facial expressions, gestures, and body language to help express your meanings.
18. Some residents with hearing impairment use sign language.
    - Signing depends upon hand and finger movements and facial expressions.
    - This is a skill that requires learning and practice.
    - There are different forms of sign language, just as there are different spoken languages; American Sign Language is the most common form used in the United States.
    - There are some basic signs that may be helpful (Figure 4-15).
19. Residents who have been hearing impaired for several years may have speech that is difficult to understand.
20. Some persons with hearing impairment are embarrassed to tell you when they do not understand you. Watch the resident's facial expressions. You may be able to tell whether your message was understood.
21. People who cannot hear may appear confused when they are not.
22. Never walk away leaving a hearing-impaired resident puzzling over what you said and possibly thinking that you do not care.

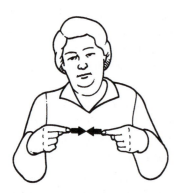

A. HURT, PAIN, ACHE, SORE

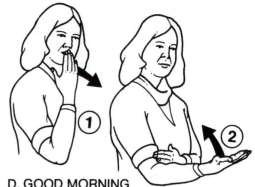

(REPEAT MOVEMENT)

B. NO

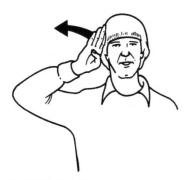

C. HELLO, HI!

D. GOOD MORNING

Figure 4-15 Signing. (A) Palms facing chest, index fingers extended toward, but not touching, one another. Thrust them toward one another several times: *hurt, pain, ache, sore*. (B) Extend index and middle fingers, bringing them down to meet the thumb in two quick movements: *no*. (C) Start with the index finger of the right hand at the right temple, palm forward and fingers pointing up. Bring the hand outward to the right: *hello, hi*. (D) Start with the fingertips of the right open hand toward face. Touch lips and bring hand down, bending elbow. Touch inner elbow with left open hand as the right hand is brought upward: *good morning*.

Communicating with Visually Impaired Residents

As people age, vision changes usually occur. These can generally be corrected with glasses. However, some older people have eye diseases that may seriously impair their vision. Even though they are not completely blind, they may be unable to see clearly.

Having a visual impairment does not necessarily mean the resident will have problems with communication. However, some actions you can take will make the resident feel more at ease.

? EXERCISE 4-7

COMPLETION

Select the correct term(s) from the following list to complete each statement regarding the visually impaired resident.

audio	identify	objects	see	specific
radio	cover	lightly	patronizing	short
substitutes	TV			

1. Describe the environment and _____ around the resident to establish a frame of reference.
2. Touch the resident _____ on the hand to avoid startling the resident.
3. Be _____ when giving directions.
4. When entering a room _____ yourself and your purpose.
5. Make sure residents are aware of the availability of _____ book format.
6. Encourage residents to listen to _____ and _____ to keep up with current events.

1. When approaching a resident who has a visual impairment, address the person by name and then touch him or her lightly on the hand or arm to avoid startling.

2. After you speak to the resident, identify yourself and explain why you are there. "Hello, Mr. Smith. My name is Mary Jones and I would like to check your blood pressure."

3. Be specific when giving directions: "I am putting your mail on the right side of your bedside stand."

4. When giving directions for locating an area in the building, tell the resident how many doors to pass and when the resident should turn right or left.

5. When you leave the resident, make sure you announce your departure, "I am leaving your room now. May I get you anything else?"

6. Offer to read mail to residents who have visual impairments (Figure 4-16).

7. Help the resident use a telephone by counting the numbers on the dial or number pad or otherwise guiding the resident verbally to make calls.

8. Tactfully inform a person who has visual impairment if clothing is soiled, unmatched, or in need of repair.

9. Encourage the resident to listen to the radio or television to keep up with news and current events.

10. Make sure the resident is aware of the Talking Book format available through the National Library Service. This service is offered free of charge and is now accessible in digital format. Digital Talking Books are available through Braille and Audio Download (BARD); thousands of books are available. Inform the social worker or the activities director of the resident's interest. Some residents may own a digital reader; the technology is available through a number of vendors. In some areas of the United States, books for download may be available through the public library at no charge; they also are available for purchase from many distributors.

11. Describe the environment and objects around the resident. This helps avoid disorientation. Never change the location of items on the bedside stand or furniture without discussing it with the resident.

12. Describe the food served to the resident. Use an example of a clock. "Your meat is at 12:00, the peas are at 3:00, and the potato is at 9:00."

Using Braille

Some residents with impaired vision may know how to read Braille. This is a system in which each letter of the alphabet and numbers 0 through 9 are translated into a unique pattern of raised dots. Rather than reading the printed letters with their eyes, those who know Braille "read" with their fingers as they touch the raised dots and spell out words. Many books and other printed materials are produced in Braille. In addition, most elevator controls are marked in Braille. Braille telephones are also available. Room numbers in facilities may also be marked in Braille and residents with visual impairments may have their names marked in Braille outside their rooms.

Communicating with Residents Who Have Aphasia

Aphasia is a condition that results from damage to the area of the brain that controls speech. This can happen after a stroke or a severe brain injury. Some

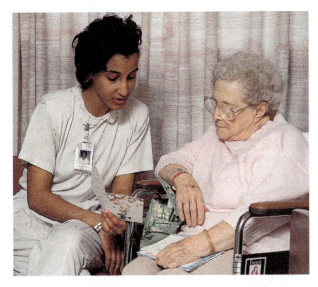

Figure 4-16 Offer to read mail to residents who have visual impairments.

? EXERCISE 4-8

COMPLETION

Select the correct term(s) from the following list to complete each statement regarding aphasic residents.

abstract	focused	shout
patronizing	short	TV
eye	nonverbal	praise

1. Use questions that require _____ answers.

2. Use _____ cues to reinforce spoken communication.

3. Make _____ contact before speaking.

4. Repeat what the resident has said to help the resident keep _____.

5. Do not _____ to try to make the resident understand.

chronic diseases can also cause aphasia, and this impairment can take many forms. Some residents with aphasia:

- Have trouble expressing themselves
- Express themselves better than they can understand others
- May have lost control of the muscles needed for speech
- May not be able to understand what is said
- May have intact muscle control, but lack the memory of how to say the word
- May understand what is said but not have the ability to communicate accurately
- Be confused; other residents with aphasia are not confused but may not be able to speak clearly and correctly

Be patient with anyone who has a communication impairment.

Aphasia can be frustrating to the resident and the caregivers. To communicate more effectively with residents who have aphasia, follow these suggestions:

1. Face the resident and make eye contact before speaking (Figure 4-17).
2. Say the resident's name and include a social greeting ("Good morning, Mrs. Jones.") before asking questions or giving instructions.
3. Speak slowly and clearly. Use short, complete sentences.
4. Pause between sentences to allow the resident time to understand and interpret what you said.
5. Check the resident's comprehension before you proceed. Ask a question based on information you just gave the resident.

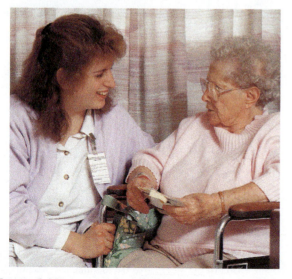

Figure 4-17 Sit at the resident's eye level and maintain eye contact during the conversation.

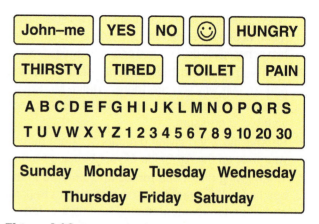

Figure 4-18 Communication boards are tools the resident can use to communicate wants and needs.

6. Use nonverbal cues to reinforce spoken communication. Gestures, facial expressions, or pictures are helpful.
7. Ask questions that require only short responses or answers that can be made nonverbally.
8. Repeat what the resident just said to help the resident keep focused on the conversation.
9. Find out if the speech therapist has devised methods of nonverbal communication, such as communication boards, ipads or picture books. See Figure 4-18.
10. Do not avoid talking to persons with aphasia. Do not shout to try to make them understand.
11. If you sense frustration, let the resident know that you are aware of the frustration. Suggest that you talk about something else for a while and then try again.

Communicating with Residents Who Are Disoriented

Some residents in long-term care facilities are disoriented. **Disorientation** means the resident is not aware of time and place. This may be permanent, as a result of a mental impairment such as Alzheimer's disease. Sometimes disorientation is temporary. This is common in new clients until they get used to their new surroundings. Residents who have an acute illness such as an infection may also be temporarily disoriented. You can improve communication with disoriented residents when you:

1. Begin a conversation by identifying yourself and calling the resident by name. Do not ask the resident if he remembers you or knows who you are. This puts the resident "on the spot" and may embarrass him.
2. Talk to the resident at eye level and maintain eye contact.
3. Maintain a pleasant facial expression while you are talking and listening.

? EXERCISE 4-9

COMPLETION

Select the correct term(s) from the following list to complete each statement regarding the disoriented resident.

abstract	focused	radio
best	lengthy	one
short	substitutes	praise

1. Ask the resident to do only _____ task at a time.
2. Use word _____ if they have meaning for the resident.
3. Be specific in speech and avoid being _____.
4. Avoid _____ explanations.
5. Use nonverbal _____ freely and respectfully.

4. Place a hand on the resident's arm or hand unless this causes agitation.
5. Make sure the resident can hear you.
6. Use a lower tone of voice.
7. Provide a calm and quiet environment.
8. Use short, common words and short, simple sentences.

9. Give the resident time to respond.
10. Ask only one simple question at a time. If you must repeat it, say it exactly the same way.
11. Ask the resident to do only one task at a time.
12. Residents with dementia will eventually be unable to understand any verbal communication. Use pictures; point, touch, or hand things to the resident. Demonstrate the action when you want the resident to complete a task. For example, put the washcloth in your hand and make face-washing movements. Then instruct the resident to do the same. If this does not work, use a hand-over-hand technique.
13. Understand the word substitutes used by the resident. If these are consistent, find out what they mean. Use them yourself to see if the resident understands you better.
14. Avoid abstract, common expressions that may be misunderstood. For example, "You can hop into bed now," may mean just that to the resident. The resident may really try to hop into bed.
15. Repeat the resident's last words to help stay on track during conversation.
16. Do not try to force the resident to understand. Avoid lengthy explanations and excessive verbal communication. This tends to agitate people who are disoriented.
17. Use nonverbal praise freely and always respect the resident's feelings.

? EXERCISE 4-10

Complete the nursing organizational chart using the names presented.

Feeding Assistants	Nursing Supervisor
Charge Nurses	MDS Nurse
Nursing Assistants	Director of Nursing

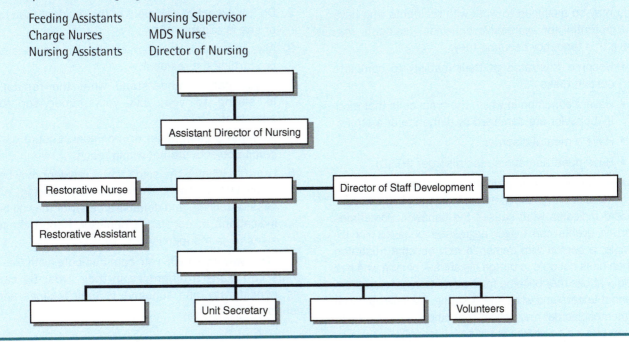

Communicating with the Residents Who Are Unconscious

Persons with an altered level of consciousness may not be able to respond. Since hearing is the last sense to be lost, they undoubtedly can hear you even though they may not be able to respond. These residents also are sensitive to pain and touch. When approaching an unconscious resident:

1. Knock on the door to make them aware of your presence.
2. Greet the resident by name before touching him or her.

3. Tell the resident in a normal tone of voice what you will be doing, giving a bath or making the bed, and so on. Talk them through the activity as you proceed.
4. Inform family and friends to talk to the resident even if he or she does not respond.
5. Inform them when you are finished and are leaving the room.
6. Tell the resident when you or the next CNA will return.
7. Place the call light in the palm of their hand regardless of response level of resident.

? EXERCISE 4-11

MULTIPLE CHOICE
Select the one best answer.
1. To find information about care to be given to an individual resident, you should consult the
   (A) resident's medical chart
   (B) procedure manual
   (C) nursing care plan
   (D) nursing policy manual
2. For the most up-to-date information about the resident's condition, check the
   (A) resident's medical chart
   (B) nursing policy manual
   (C) procedure manual
   (D) resident's care plan
3. The resident's chart
   (A) is not a permanent document
   (B) is used to determine law suits
   (C) is properly written in pencil
   (D) may be used only while the resident is part of the facility

COMMUNICATING WITH THE POTENTIALLY VIOLENT RESIDENT

You may be assigned to work with residents who have the potential for aggressive behavior. Residents may have this tendency because they:

- Become frustrated at their inability to complete certain tasks
- Have a condition in which the brain cells that modify behavior are damaged by dementia or a stroke
- Have a mental disorder
- Have posttraumatic stress disorder (PTSD)
- Are affected by a form of chemical abuse

Check with your supervisor to find out if the medical record indicates what causes the behavior. Sometimes certain events can trigger aggressive behavior. For example, a person with dementia may become frustrated when he is not able to button his shirt. A person who has had a stroke may become frustrated when her caregivers cannot understand what she is saying. An individual with a mental disorder may believe that others are planning to harm him, so he strikes out in self-defense.

To avoid aggressive behavior:

1. Prevent situations that you know may trigger this behavior.
2. Do not expect or ask more of the resident than he or she is capable of.
3. Always use a calm approach and avoid surprising or startling the resident.
4. If you cannot understand what the resident is saying to you, ask your supervisor for assistance.
5. Maintain a calm, quiet environment. Ensure dangerous objects are not within reach.
6. Learn to identify the signs that a resident may become violent. For example, constant pacing, excessive talking, and defensive behavior may all be indications of escalating behavior. Report these signs to your supervisor.

The way in which you communicate with residents can make a difference in their lives. Be caring, considerate, and sensitive to their feelings and needs.

LESSON SYNTHESIS: Putting It All Together

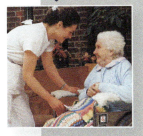

You have just completed this lesson. Now go back and review the Clinical Focus. Try to see how the Clinical Focus relates to the concepts presented in the lesson. Then answer the following questions.

1. How can Doris Greene meet her physical, emotional, and social needs if communications with the staff are ineffective?

2. How can the nursing assistant improve the flow of communication or make it more difficult?

3. What special situations may make communications especially difficult with this resident?

4. What can the nursing assistant do to improve communications in the situations listed for question 3?

5. Why is it especially important for communications to be open with Doris Greene?

? EXERCISE 4-12

Which staff behaviors would be appropriate for the staff as they interact with Doris Greene? Indicate **A** if appropriate and **I** if inappropriate.

1. _____ "You had better eat your breakfast or we will have to put a tube in your stomach."
2. _____ "Perhaps I could get something you would enjoy more for breakfast."
3. _____ "Let me help you move up in bed."
4. _____ "Get out of this room now and walk. You need some exercise!"
5. _____ "I don't think you should give your granddaughter such an expensive gift."
6. _____ "It's foolish to believe in life after death."

4 REVIEW

A. Select the one best answer for each of the following.

1. Successful communication requires all but which of the following?

   (A) sender
   (B) message
   (C) receiver
   (D) telephone

2. Verbal communication includes

   (A) talking and listening
   (B) facial expressions
   (C) writing reports
   (D) using a fax machine

3. Verbal communication is influenced by all but which of the following?

   (A) tone of voice
   (B) choice of words used
   (C) handwriting
   (D) articulation

4. Examples of nonverbal communication include

(A) gestures and body language

(B) answering the telephone

(C) listening to shift report

(D) conversing with residents

5. A nursing assistant may give or take which information over the telephone?

(A) report of a resident's condition

(B) physician's orders

(C) results of laboratory tests

(D) name of person leaving the message

6. The shift report is given by the

(A) administrator

(B) physician

(C) nurse who worked the previous shift

(D) director of nursing

7. The purpose of the shift report is to

(A) give information about all the residents on the nursing unit

(B) discuss the social activities of the staff

(C) tell the nursing assistants when they are scheduled for days off

(D) rest before starting work

8. You must report to the nurse when you

(A) take a break or go to lunch

(B) have completed each assigned task

(C) wash your hands

(D) have any contact with a resident

9. One purpose of a memo is to inform staff of

(A) meetings or educational programs

(B) clients' conditions

(C) physicians' new orders for specific clients

(D) weather conditions

10. Examples of manuals that are found on nursing units include

(A) salary manual

(B) disaster manual

(C) employee evaluation manual

(D) physician's procedure manual

11. The resident's care plan provides information for

(A) the nursing assistant assignments

(B) employee benefits

(C) procedure for fire drills

(D) dietary procedures

12. The resident's medical record or chart is

(A) used only by the physician

(B) used by all members of the interdisciplinary health care team

(C) a temporary record

(D) a report of the nursing assistant's competencies

13. Which of the following is an example of verbal communication?

(A) The resident is crying.

(B) The resident is sleeping.

(C) The resident states, "I am having chest pain."

(D) The resident is shaking a fist at you.

14. If a resident is disoriented, it means the resident is

(A) mentally ill

(B) unaware of the environment and the time

(C) unable to communicate with you

(D) unable to hear

15. Aphasia means the resident

(A) has an infection of the respiratory tract

(B) is hearing-impaired

(C) is disoriented

(D) is unable to speak or to understand the spoken language of others

16. When working with residents who have hearing impairments, you should

(A) speak in a calm, quiet manner

(B) talk louder

(C) avoid speaking if possible

(D) speak very slowly

17. When working with residents with aphasia, it is best to

(A) use only hand gestures to communicate

(B) speak louder

(C) avoid communication if at all possible

(D) face the resident and make eye contact before speaking

18. Residents who are visually impaired should

    (A) stay in their rooms to avoid getting lost in the facility

    (B) have identification on their clothing so everyone realizes they are visually impaired

    (C) learn to use sign language

    (D) be given directions for locating various areas in the building

19. When working with clients who are disoriented, you should

    (A) ask the resident if she remembers you or knows who you are

    (B) try to make the resident understand you

    (C) avoid distractions of noise and activity when communicating with them

    (D) get as close as possible to the resident when talking or giving care

20. Touching the resident can be a successful method of communication if you

    (A) are gentle and caring

    (B) use stern gestures and facial expressions

    (C) restrain a resident's hand

    (D) avoid eye contact

21. Persons who cannot express themselves verbally or understand verbal communications have _____.

22. Loss of recognition of time, place, location, or person is called _____.

23. The exchange of information given by the nurse going off duty to those coming on duty is called the _____.

24. The _____ is a legal document.

25. A brief, written message that provides information is a _____.

26. _____ is an example of nonverbal communication.

27. The record that contains a description of the resident's problems, the goals for resolving the problems, and the approaches used is the _____.

28. Sign language is an example of _____.

29. Talking orally is _____.

30. _____ may be used by persons who are visually impaired.

A. Fill in the blanks by selecting the correct word or phrase from the list provided.

aphasia	medical chart
body language	memo
Braille	nonverbal communication
care plan	shift report
disorientation	verbal communication

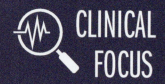

LESSON 5
THE LANGUAGE OF HEALTH CARE

CLINICAL FOCUS

Think about how your knowledge of the language of health care and the human body can improve your understanding of the conditions of the residents in your care as you study this lesson.

OBJECTIVES

After studying this lesson, you should be able to:

• Define vocabulary words and terms.

• List the meanings of common suffixes and prefixes.

• Use combining forms to develop new words.

• Write terms and abbreviations commonly used in health care communications and documentation.

• Describe the location of body parts and organs, using the proper anatomic terms.

• Explain the organization of the body into cells, tissues, organs, and systems.

• List body systems and their functions.

VOCABULARY

abbreviation (ah-BREE-vee-ay-shun)
abdominal (ab-DOM-ih-nal)
anatomic position (an-ah-TOM-ick poh-ZISH-un)
anatomy (ah-NAT-oh-mee)
anterior (an-TEER-ee-or)
cardiac muscle (KAR-dee-ack MUS-ell)
cavity (KAV-ih-tee)
cell (sell)

connective tissue (kuh-NECK-tiv TISH-you)
connective tissue cell (kuh-NECK-tiv TISH-you sell)
cutaneous membrane (kyou-TAY-nee-us MEM-brain)
distal (DIS-tal)
dorsal (DOR-sal)
epithelial cell (ep-ih-THEE-lee-al sell)
epithelial tissue (ep-ih-THEE-lee-al TISH-you)
gerontology (jer-on-TOL-oh-jee)

CASE STUDY

Georgina England, 74 years old, has just been admitted to your facility because she can no longer care for herself. Her Hx reveals long-term arthritis, cardialgia, and recurrent cystitis. Her current admission Dx is ASHD, arthritis, and UTI. Part of her care plan includes: ass't c̄ ADL, Amb & Ass't c̄ cath care, I & O, VS q4h.

inferior (in-FEER-ee-or)
kidney (KID-nee)
lateral (LAT-er-al)
medial (MEE-dee-al)
medical terminology (MED-ih-kul ter-mih-NOL-oh-jee)
membrane (MEM-brain)
meninges (meh-NIN-jeez)
mucous membrane (MYOU-kus MEM-brain)
mucus (MYOU-kus)
muscle cell (MUS-ell sell)
muscle tissue (MUS-ell TISH-you)
nerve cell (nurv sell)
nervous tissue (NUR-vus TISH-you)
organ (OR-gan)
pancreas (PAN-kree-as)
pathology (pah-THOL-oh-jee)
pericardium (pair-ih-KAR-dee-um)
peritoneum (pair-ih-toh-NEE-um)

physiology (fiz-ee-OL-oh-jee)
pleura (PLOOR-ah)
posterior (pos-TEER-ee-or)
prefix (PREE-fix)
proximal (PROX-ih-mal)
quadrant (KWAHD-rant)
serous membrane (SEE-rus MEM-brain)
skeletal muscle (SKEL-eh-tal MUS-ell)
smooth muscle (smooth MUS-ell)
suffix (SUF-fix)
superior (soo-PEE-ree-or)
synovial membrane (sih-NOH-vee-al MEM-brain)
system (SIS-tum)
tissue (TISH-you)
umbilicus (um-BILL-ih-kus)
ventral (VEN-tral)
word combinations (werd kom-bi-NAY-shuns)
word root (werd root)

THE LANGUAGE OF HEALTH CARE

The study of medical terminology can aid you in understanding the names of specific diseases or conditions that residents may experience. You have learned that people communicate information to one another in different ways. It is important that the sender and receiver understand the same message.

Two ways to help keep the message clear in written and oral communications are:

- Choosing the correct word or term to express the message
- Spelling or pronouncing the word properly

Health care has its own language and sometimes one or two letters can change the entire meaning. For example:

- *Ilium* is part of the pelvic bone.
- *Ileum* is part of the intestinal tract.
- *Perineum* is an area of the body between the vagina and anus.
- *Peritoneum* is a membrane that lines one of the body cavities.

You can see how important it is to use the correct scientific terms and to spell them accurately.

WORD PARTS

The language of health care is formed by building on common word parts (Figure 5-1).

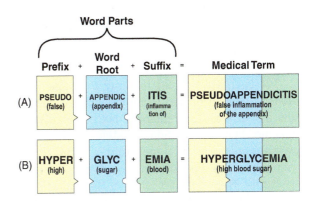

Figure 5-1 Prefixes, suffixes, and word roots can be used to form and interpret the meaning of a word. Word roots sometimes incorporate the use of a term for a body part, as in example A, or use another term, as in example B.

These parts include:

Word root. The word root (or root word) provides the basic meaning or foundation of the word. Word roots can be defined as main words or parts to which prefixes and suffixes can be added. Sometimes, *but not always*, the word root describes a part of the body that is involved. Note the formation of new words in Figure 5-1. A list of common word roots is given in Table 5-1.

⊘N THE JOB

Poor communications can result in injury to a resident and liability for you.

Root	Meaning	Root	Meaning	Root	Meaning
abdomin(o)	abdomen	gloss(o)	tongue	pharyng(o)	throat
aden(o)	gland	glyc(o)	sugar	phleb(o)	vein
angi(o)	vessel	gynec(o)	female	pneum(o)	lung, air
arteri(o)	artery	hem(o)	blood	proct(o)	rectum
arth(o)	joint	hemat(o)	blood	psych(o)	mind
bronch(i)(o)	bronchus	hepat(o)	liver	pulm(o)	lung
cardi(o)	heart	hydr(o)	water	py(o)	pus
cephal(o)	head	hyster(o)	uterus	rect(o)	rectum
cerebr(o)	brain	lapar(o)	abdomen, flank, loin	rhin(o)	nose
chol(e)	bile	laryng(o)	larynx	splen(o)	spleen
col(o)	colon	lith(o)	stone	stern(o)	sternum
crani(o)	skull	mamm(o)	breast	thorac(o)	chest
cyst(o)	bladder, cyst	mast(o)	breast	thromb(o)	clot
cyt(o)	cell	men(o)	menstruation	tox(o)	poison
dent(i)(o)	tooth	my(o)	muscle	trache(o)	trachea
dermat(o)	skin	myel(o)	bone marrow, spinal cord	ur(o)	urine
encephal(o)	brain	nephr(o)	kidney	urethr(o)	urethra
enter(o)	small intestine	neur(o)	nerve	urin(o)	urine
erythr(o)	red	ocul(o)	eye	uter(i)(o)	uterus
fibr(o)	fiber	ophthalm(o)	eye	ven(o)	vein
gastr(o)	stomach	oste(o)	bone		
geront(o)	elderly	ped(i)(o)	child		

Table 5-1 Word Roots

Prefix. The word part found at the beginning of a word to change or add to its meaning. It does not stand alone. Prefixes frequently, *but not always*, indicate time, number, location, or status. The prefix is always accompanied by a root word, a suffix, or both. Common prefixes are listed in Table 5-2.

Suffix. The word part found at the end of a word to change or add to its meaning. It does not stand alone. Suffixes usually, *but not always*, indicate condition, procedure, disorder, or disease. The suffix is combined with a root word, a prefix, or both. Commonly used suffixes are listed in Table 5-3.

Word combinations. Table 5-4 shows common examples of how the different elements are joined to form words. For example, the word form *cyte* means cell. It is a common word root because the human body is made up of many different kinds of cells. *Cyt* is seen in different positions in many words.

Look at the following examples carefully:

- *Cytology*—(prefix) study of the cell
- *Erythrocyte*—(suffix) red blood cell
- *Granulocytoma*—(root word) a tumor made up of cells called granulocytes

Prefix	Meaning	Prefix	Meaning	Prefix	Meaning
a-, an-	without, not	hemi-	half	peri-	around
ab-	away from	hyper-	high, above, excessive	poly-	many
ad-	toward	hypo-	low, below normal	post-	after
ante-	before	inter-	between	pre-	before
anti-	against	intra-	inside, within	pseud-	false
bi-	double, two	leuk-	white	retro-	backward
bio-	life	micro-	small	semi-	half
brady-	slow	neo-	new	septic-	infection
circum-	around	non-	not	sub-	under, below
dys-	difficult, abnormal	pan-	all	tachy-	fast
epi-	on, over	per-	by, through		

Table 5-2 Prefixes

Suffix	Meaning	Suffix	Meaning	Suffix	Meaning
-algia	pain	-megaly	enlargement	-pnea	breathing
-alysis	analyze	-meter	instrument that measures	-ptosis	sagging, falling
-ectomy	surgical removal	-ostomy	surgical opening	-rrhagia	excessive flow
-emia	blood	-otomy	surgical opening	-rrhea	discharge
-gram	record	-pathy	disease	-scope	instrument that examines
-itis	inflammation of	-penia	deficiency	-stasis	constant
-logy	study of	-phasia	speaking	-therapy	treatment
-lysis	destruction of	-plegia	paralysis	-uria	condition of urine

Table 5-3 Suffixes

? EXERCISE 5-1

PREFIXES
Underline the prefix in each of the following words. Define the prefix and define the word.

	Define Prefix	Define Word
Example:		
Leukocyte	white	white blood cell
1. bradycardia	_____	_____
2. pericardium	_____	_____
3. antiembolism	_____	_____
4. epigastric	_____	_____
5. hypotension	_____	_____
6. polycystic	_____	_____
7. postoperative	_____	_____
8. noninvasive	_____	_____
9. neoplasm	_____	_____
10. hypertension	_____	_____

? EXERCISE 5-2

SUFFIXES
Underline the suffix in each of the following words. Define the suffix and define the word.

	Define Suffix	Define Word
Example:		
Nephroptosis	falling/sagging	downward displacement of a kidney
1. Proctoscopy	_____	_____
2. Apnea	_____	_____
3. Hematuria	_____	_____
4. Hemiplegia	_____	_____
5. Oximeter	_____	_____
6. Tracheotomy	_____	_____
7. Bronchitis	_____	_____
8. Mastectomy	_____	_____
9. Hematology	_____	_____
10. Thrombocytopenia	_____	_____

Medical Term	Prefix	Root	Suffix	Meaning
antiseptic	anti-	septic		against infection
arthritis		arthr	-itis	inflammation of joints
cardiology		cardi	-ology	study of the heart
colostomy		col	-ostomy	surgical opening into the colon
dyspnea	dys-		-pnea	difficult breathing
hemiplegia	hemi-		-plegia	paralysis in one half of the body
hypoglycemia	hypo-	glyc	-emia	low blood sugar
glycosuria		glyc	-uria	sugar in urine
leukemia	leuk-		-emia	condition of white blood cells
urinalysis	urin-		-alysis	analysis of the urine

Table 5-4 Combining Word Parts to Form Medical Terms

EXPANDING YOUR VOCABULARY

During your career you will continue to add to your understanding and ability to use scientific terms. Here are some ways to help yourself.

- Use the facility medical dictionary to check new words.
- Look up new words; note spelling, meaning, and pronunciation.
- Get a medical dictionary and keep it available at home.
- Keep a notebook of new words, writing down:
  - Definitions
  - Spelling
  - Pronunciation
- Practice writing new words until you spell them correctly without checking your notebook or the dictionary.
- Try to use each new term correctly three times in the next month. If you succeed, you can claim it as your own. You might do this in your conversation, in your documentation, or by explaining the word to a coworker.

- Be willing to accept your teacher's or supervisor's suggestions as to proper pronunciation and usage. Remember, this is a learning process and everyone needs a guide.

ABBREVIATIONS

An **abbreviation** is the shortened form of a word. Abbreviations are often used to save space and time in charting. Some abbreviations are a combination of letters that form a word such as *IDDM* to mean *insulin-dependent diabetes mellitus*. Many medical terms are derived from Latin. The abbreviation p.o. meaning *per os* is frequently used (*per* comes from Latin meaning *through*, *os* is also a Latin derivative meaning *mouth* or *opening*). So when we use the term p.o. or *per os*, we mean *to give something by mouth*.

Specific abbreviations may have different meanings in different parts of the country and in different facilities. For example, *drg* in one facility may mean

? EXERCISE 5-3

COMBINATIONS
Define the following suffixes. Using the prefix *nephro*, add the suffixes to see how many new words can be formed. Check the words against the text glossary or a dictionary.

Suffix	Definitions
1. — otomy	_____
2. — itis	_____
3. — ectomy	_____
4. — scopy	_____
5. — ology	_____

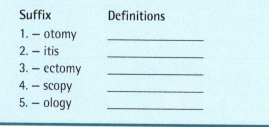

? EXERCISE 5-4

ABBREVIATIONS
I. Body Parts
Write the name of the body part indicated by the abbreviation.

Abbreviation	Body Part
1. B & B	_____
2. GI	_____
3. GU	_____
4. abd	_____
5. ax	_____
6. vag	_____
7. Lt	_____
8. RA	_____

(continues)

? EXERCISE 5-4 (Continued)

II. Orders and Charting

Write the appropriate words for the abbreviations listed.

Abbreviation	Orders/Charting
9. ac	_____
10. BID	_____
11. hs	_____
12. pc	_____
13. q2h	_____
14. am	_____
15. ad lib	_____
16. amb	_____
17. BM	_____
18. ht	_____
19. D/C	_____
20. I&O	_____
21. HOB	_____
22. liq	_____
23. NPO	_____
24. NKA	_____

III. Medical Diagnosis

Write the medical diagnosis in the spaces provided for each abbreviation listed.

Abbreviation	Medical Diagnosis
a. MS	_____
b. CVA	_____
c. TB	_____
d. MI	_____
e. MRSA	_____
f. VRE	_____
g. RA	_____
h. URI	_____
i. UTI	_____
J. DM	_____

drainage, yet in another facility it is used to mean *dressing*. Table 5-5 lists commonly used abbreviations. However, check the policy and/or procedure manuals where you work to determine which abbreviations are approved for use in that facility.

UNDERSTANDING THE BODY

The reasons for the type of care given to residents are based on an understanding of how the body is made, how it functions normally, and the changes caused by age and disease.

These reasons, or principles, are derived from four sciences:

- **Anatomy**: the study of the structure of living organisms
- **Physiology**: the study of the function of living organisms
- **Gerontology**: the study of aging
- **Pathology**: the study of disease

ANATOMIC TERMS

Special terms are used to describe the location and relationship of body parts and organs. Knowing these terms will help you to study and learn more easily. You will also be able to communicate more accurately as you report and record your observations.

The Anatomic Position

Health care providers must use the same frame of reference when describing the resident's body, position, and actions to be taken. For example, everyone who works with the resident must understand and describe precisely where the back of the resident's left wrist is and which is the resident's right hand.

It is helpful to view the resident as if he or she were standing in the **anatomic position**. This means the resident:

- Is standing
- Is facing the observer
- Has hands at the sides
- Has palms forward (Figure 5-2)

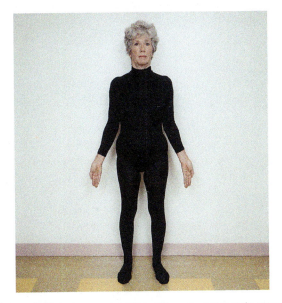

Figure 5-2 In the anatomic position, the person is standing, facing forward, with palms forward.

Abbreviation	Meaning	Abbreviation	Meaning
ā	before	C1, C2, C3, etc.	first cervical vertebrae, second cervical vertebrae, third cervical vertebrae, etc.
AAROM	active assistive (assisted) range of motion		
abd	abdomen	CA	cancer
ABT, ABX	antibiotic therapy	CAD	coronary artery disease
ā c̄	before meals	cal, kcal	calorie
ACT	active, actively, activities	cath	catheter
AD	Activity Director	CBB	complete bed bath
ADA	American Dietetic Association, American Diabetic Association	CBC	complete blood count
		CC	chief complaint
add.	adduction	CHF	congestive heart failure
ad lib	as desired	ck, ✓	check
ADLs	activities of daily living	ck or ✓ freq	check frequently
adm	admission	cl liq	clear liquid
AEB	as evidenced by	CMA	certified medication aide
AFO	ankle/foot orthosis	can	certified nursing assistant or certified nurse administrator
AIDS	acquired immune deficiency syndrome		
		c/o	complains of
aka	above-the-knee amputation, also known as	COLD, COPD	chronic obstructive lung (pulmonary) disease
alt	alternate, alternating	CP	care plan, clinical pathway, critical pathway
am	morning		
AMA	against medical advice	CPM	continuous passive motion machine
amb	ambulate	CPR	cardiopulmonary resuscitation
amt	amount	C & S	culture and sensitivity
ant	anterior	CVA	cerebrovascular accident, stroke
A&P	anatomy and physiology	CXR	chest x-ray
AROM	active range of motion	DDS	Doctor of Dental Surgery (dentist)
ASAP	as soon as possible	dep	dependent
assist	assistance	dept.	department
as tol	as tolerated	diab	diabetes, diabetic
ax	axillary (under the arm)	DJD	degenerative joint disease
B, (B),Ⓑ	bilateral, both	DNR	do not resuscitate
B&B	bowel and bladder	DO	Doctor of Osteopathy
BB	bed bath	DOA	dead on arrival
bid	twice a day	DOB	date of birth
bilat	bilateral	DPM	Doctor of Podiatric Medicine
BKA	below-the-knee amputation	DR, D/R	dining room
BLE	both lower extremities	Dr.	doctor
BM	bowel movement	DSD	dry sterile dressing
BP, B/P	blood pressure	DSM	Dietary Services Manager
BPM	beats per minute	DT	dietetic technician
BR	bed rest, bathroom	DVT	deep vein thrombosis (blood clot)
BRP	bathroom privileges	Dx	diagnosis
BS	blood sugar	E	enema
BSC	bedside commode	ECG, EKG	electrocardiogram
BSE	breast self-examination	EENT	eye, ear, nose, and throat
BUE	both upper extremities	ENT	ear, nose, and throat
C	Celsius, centigrade	ER, ED	emergency room, emergency department
c̄	with		
cm	centimeter	ESRD	end stage renal disease

Table 5-5 Common Abbreviations

(continues)

Abbreviation	Meaning	Abbreviation	Meaning
et	and	isol	isolation
ETOH	ethanol (often used to refer to alcoholic beverages)	IV	intravenous
		K, K⁺	potassium
eval	evaluation	L	liter, left
ex.	exercise	L1, L2, etc.	first lumbar vertebra, second lumbar vertebra, etc.
exam	examination		
ext.	extension, extremity, external	lab	laboratory
F	Fahrenheit	lat	lateral
FB	foreign body	lb	pound
FBS	fasting blood sugar	LBP	low back pain
FE	Fleet's enema	LE	lower extremity
FF	force fluids	lg, lge	large
flex	flexion	liq	liquid
freq	frequently	LL	left leg
FS	frozen section, finger stick	LLE	left lower extremity
FSBS	finger stick blood sugar	LLQ	left lower quadrant
FU, F/U	follow up	LOC	loss of consciousness, level of consciousness, level of care
FUO	fever of unknown origin		
FWB	full weight bearing		
Fx	fracture	LPN	licensed practical nurse
G	good	lt	left
g/c, GC	geriatric chair	LTC	long-term care
GERD	gastroesophageal reflux disease	LTCF	long-term care facility
GI	gastrointestinal	LTG	long-term goal
G/T, GT	gastrostomy tube	LUQ	left upper quadrant
gtt	drop	LVN	licensed vocational nurse
GU	genitourinary	m	meter
Gyn	gynecology	MA	medication aide
H	hydrogen	max	maximum
HAV, HBV, HCV, etc.	hepatitis A virus, hepatitis B virus, hepatitis C virus, etc.	MD	muscular dystrophy, medical doctor
		MDR	main dining room
hemi	half, hemiplegia	MDS	Minimum Data Set
Hg	mercury	mech soft	mechanical soft
HIV	human immunodeficiency virus	med rec	medical records
H₂O	water	meds	medications
H₂O₂	hydrogen peroxide	MI	myocardial infarction (heart attack)
HOB	head of bed	min	minimum, minimal, minute
HOH	hard of hearing	mL or ml	milliliter
H & P	history and physical	mm	millimeter
hr	hour	mmHg	millimeters of mercury
ht	height	mod	moderate
Hx	history	MRSA	methicillin-resistant *Staphylococcus aureus*
Ⓘ, ind.	independent, independently		
ID	initial dose	MS	multiple sclerosis
IDCP	interdisciplinary care plan	mult.	multiple
IDDM	insulin-dependent diabetes mellitus	NA, N/A	not applicable, nursing assistant (meaning determined by context)
IDT	interdisciplinary team		
IM	intramuscular	Na⁺	sodium
I & O	intake and output	NACEP	Nurse Aide Competency Evaluation Program
int.	internal		
IPPB	intermittent positive pressure breathing	NAR	no adverse reaction
		NAS	no added salt

Table 5-5 (Continued)

Abbreviation	Meaning	Abbreviation	Meaning
NATCEP	Nurse Aide Training and Competency Evaluation Program	qt	Quart
N/C, no c/o	no complaints	quad	quadrant, quadriplegic
neg, -, Θ	negative	R	rectal, respiration, right
NG	nasogastric	RA	rheumatoid arthritis, right arm
NGT	nasogastric tube	RAI	Resident Assessment Instrument
NIDDM	non–insulin-dependent diabetes mellitus	RCP	Respiratory Care Practitioner
		RD	Registered Dietitian
NKA	no known allergies	re:	Regarding
NN	nurse's notes	reg	regular, regulation
NPO	nothing by mouth	rehab	rehabilitation
N/S, NSS	normal saline, normal saline solution	res, Res	resident
		resp, R	respirations
N & V	nausea and vomiting	RL	right leg
NVD	nausea, vomiting, and diarrhea	RLE	right lower extremity
NWB	nonweight-bearing	RLQ	right lower quadrant
O_2	oxygen	rm	room
OA	osteoarthritis	RN	registered nurse
obj	objective	RNA	restorative nursing assistant
OBS	organic brain syndrome	R/O	rule out
obs	observations	ROM	range of motion
occ	occasional	rot.	rotation
OOB	out of bed	rt, R	right
ORIF	open reduction, internal fixation	RT	respiratory therapy
os, o	mouth	r/t	related to
OT	occupational therapy	RUE	right upper extremity
Oz	ounce	RUQ	right upper quadrant
$\overline{P}$	after	Rx	prescription, therapy, treatment
P	pulse, poor	$\overline{S}$	without
B, PBB	partial bath, partial bed bath	SBA	standby assistance
$\overline{PC}$	after meals	semi	Half
PCT	Patient Care Technician	sm	small
PE	physical examination	SNF	skilled nursing facility
peds, pedi	pediatrics	SNU	skilled nursing unit
per	by, through	SOB	shortness of breath
pm	afternoon or evening	spec	specimen
PN	progress notes, practical nurse	SS	social service
po	by mouth	S/S, S & S	signs and symptoms
pos, +, ⊕	positive	SSE	soapsuds enema
PPE	personal protective equipment	S/T	skin tear
PPS	post polio syndrome, prospective payment system	ST	speech therapy
		stat	immediately
preop	preoperative	Std prec	standard precautions
prep	prepare	STG	short-term goal
prn	as needed	STNA	state tested nursing assistant
prog	prognosis, progress	sup	suppository
PROM	passive range of motion	SW	social worker
pt or Pt	Patient	Sx	symptoms
PT	physical therapy	T, temp	temperature
PUD	peptic ulcer disease	T1, T2, etc.	first thoracic vertebra, second thoracic vertebra, etc.
PVD	peripheral vascular disease	TB	tuberculosis
PWB	partial weight bearing	TF	tube feeding

Table 5-5 (Continued)

Abbreviation	Meaning	Abbreviation	Meaning
TIAN	toilet in advance of need	w/c	wheelchair
TID, tid	three times a day	WFL	within functional limits
TKO	to keep open	WNL	within normal limits
TLC	tender loving care	wt	weight
TPN	total parenteral nutrition	x, X	times
TPR	temperature, pulse, respiration	XR, X/R	x-ray
trach	tracheostomy	yr	year
TT	therapeutic touch	↑	up, increase
TTWB	toe-touch weight bearing	↓	down, decrease
Tx	traction, treatment	1°	first, primary, first degree
UA, U/A	urinalysis	2°	second, secondary, secondary to, second degree
UE	upper extremity		
URI	upper respiratory infection	3°	third, tertiary, third degree
UTI	urinary tract infection	i, ii, iii, iv, etc.	one, two, three, four, etc.
vag	vaginal	=	equals, equal to
vc, VC	verbal cues	±, +/−	plus or minus
VRE	vancomycin-resistant Enterococcus	Δ (triangle)	change, change to
		°	degrees
VS	vital signs	0	zero, or numeric 0
WA, W/A	while awake	*	important
WB	weight bearing	♀	female
WBAT	weight bearing as tolerated	♂	male

Table 5-5 (Continued)

The following abbreviations were removed by the Joint Commission (formerly, the Joint Commission on Accreditation of Healthcare Organizations [JCAHO]) in 2004 because they can be misinterpreted and lead to critical errors. It has been suggested that facilities keep a list of the approved and unapproved abbreviations at the nurse's station: cc, cubic centimeter; D/C, DC; discontinue, discharge; hs, bedtime (hour of sleep); q, each, every; qd, every day; qh, every hour; q2h, q3h, q4h, etc., every 2 hours, every 3 hours, every 4 hours, etc.; qhs, every night at bedtime; qm, qam, every morning; qod, every other day; @, at; >, greater than, <, less than.

Source: The Joint Commission. "Do Not Use List" retrieved from http://www.jointcommission.org/assets/1/18/official_do_not_use_list_6_111.pdf and Institute for Safe Medicine Practices. "List of Error Prone Abbreviations, Symbols, and Dose Designations" retrieved from http://www.ismp.org/tools/errorproneabbreviations.pdf.

This means that the heels will always be toward the back, even if the resident is resting on the abdomen or lying on the side. The breasts will always be described as facing front even if she is sitting in a wheelchair or walking away from you. Notice also that the resident's left hand will be on the same side as your right hand. It is the same as looking at a mirror image.

Descriptive Terms

Imaginary lines drawn through the body (Figure 5-3) can provide us with other reference terms.

- A line drawn down the center of the body from head to foot divides the body into equal right and left sides. This line is called the midline or midsagittal line. Note that the body has the same parts on either side. For example, there is an arm, a leg, an eye, and half of a nose on each side of the line.
- Parts close to this line are medial to the line.
- Parts farther away from the line are lateral to the line.
- For example, in the anatomic position, the thumbs are more lateral to the line and the little fingers are more medial to the line.

Another line drawn parallel to the floor divides the body into upper and lower parts. This line can be drawn at any level on the body as long as it is parallel to the floor. This is the transverse line.

- Parts located above this line are superior to the line.
- Parts located below this line are inferior to the line.
- For example, if the line is drawn between the knees and ankles, the knees are superior to the ankles and the ankles are inferior to the knees.

A third line can be drawn to divide the body into front and back.

- Parts in front of this line are anterior or ventral to the line.
- Parts in back of this line are posterior or dorsal to the line.

Points of Attachment

The arms and legs are called the extremities of the body. The arms are attached to the body at the shoulders. The legs are attached to the body at the hips. Two terms are used to describe the relationship between

? EXERCISE 5-6

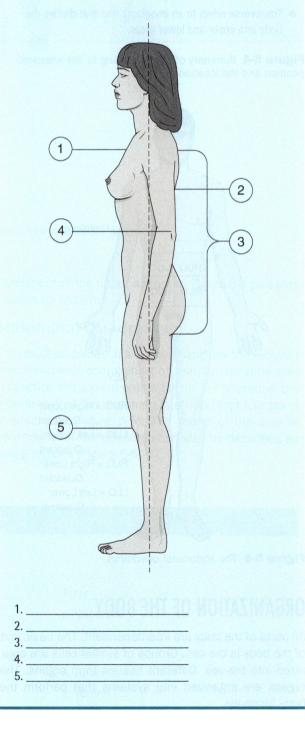

1. _____
2. _____
3. _____
4. _____
5. _____
6. _____

TISSUES

Groups of similar cells are organized into tissues. The basic tissue types are:

- Epithelial tissue
- Connective tissue
- Nervous tissue
- Muscle tissue

? EXERCISE 5-7

Refer to the figure below. Write the terms for the body parts or areas shown. Select the proper term from the list provided.

    anterior
    lower extremities
    posterior
    torso
    upper extremities

1. _____
2. _____
3. _____
4. _____
5. _____

? EXERCISE 5-8

Refer to the accompanying figure. Select the correct word for each body region from the list provided.

- epigastric
- hypogastric
- left lower quadrant
- right lower quadrant
- umbilical
- left upper quadrant
- right upper quadrant

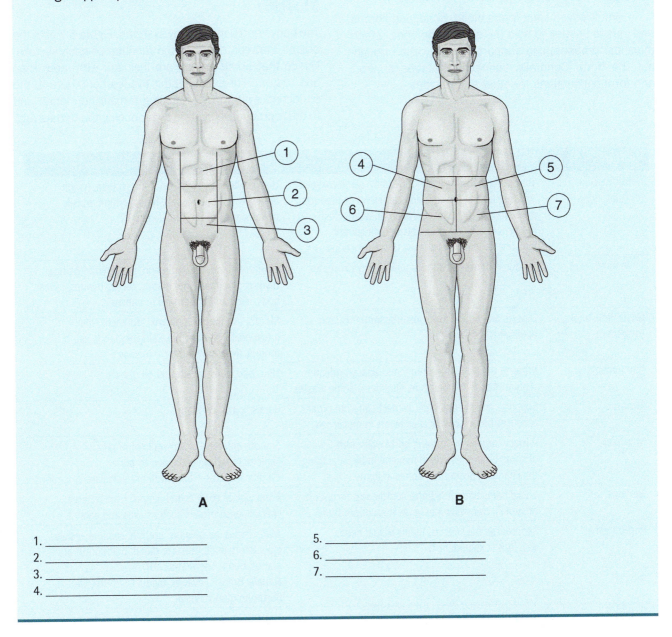

A   B

1. _____   5. _____
2. _____   6. _____
3. _____   7. _____
4. _____

Epithelial tissue is made up of a specialized group of cells that form the skin, as well as line the body cavities and the various tubes that lead outside the body. These cells have the ability to absorb, secrete (produce) fluids, excrete (eliminate) waste products, and protect.

Nervous tissue forms the brain and spinal cord and the nerves throughout the body. This tissue is also found in the special sense organs such as the eyes, ears, and taste buds. The activities of the rest of the body are directed and coordinated through the nervous tissues.

Three kinds of **muscle tissue** are found in the body:

- **Skeletal** muscle is attached to bones for movement.
- **Cardiac muscle** forms the heart wall.
- **Smooth muscle** (visceral) forms the walls of body organs such as the stomach and intestines.

Connective tissue forms blood, bone, and fibrous and elastic tissues to hold the skin on the body, attach muscles to bones, and support delicate cells throughout the body. Generally, connective tissues support and form connections for other tissue types.

ORGANS

Each **organ** is made up of more than one kind of tissue and performs special functions that contribute to the function of the body systems. Some organs, like the **kidneys**, are found in pairs. Some single organs contribute to more than one system. For example, the **pancreas** contributes secretions to both the endocrine and digestive systems.

SYSTEMS

The body has 10 major body systems. Figure 5-7 lists the organs that contribute to the function of each **system**. Notice that some organs are included with more than one system. For example, the ovaries contribute to the endocrine system by producing female hormones and to the reproductive system by producing the female egg.

System	Function	Organs
Cardiovascular (circulatory)	Transports materials around the body; carries oxygen and nutrients to the cells and carries waste products away; part of the immune system that provides protective cells and chemicals to fight current infections and protect against future infections	Heart, arteries, capillaries, veins, spleen, lymph nodes, lymphatic vessels, blood, lymph, tonsils, thymus, specialized blood cells
Endocrine	Produces hormones that regulate body processes	Pituitary gland, thyroid gland, parathyroid glands, thymus gland, adrenal glands, testes, ovaries, pineal body, islets of Langerhans in pancreas
Gastrointestinal (digestive)	Digests, transports food, absorbs nutrients, and eliminates solid wastes	Mouth, esophagus, pharynx, stomach, small intestine, large intestine, salivary glands, teeth, tongue, liver, gallbladder, pancreas
Integumentary	Protects the body from injury and against infection, regulates body temperature, eliminates some wastes	Skin, hair, nails, sweat and oil glands
Skeletal	Supports and shapes body, protects internal organs, produces blood cells, acts as levers in movement	Bones, joints, cartilage
Muscular	Protects organs by forming body walls, forms walls of some organs, assists in movement by leveraging the changing position of bones at joints	*Smooth* muscles—form walls of organs *Skeletal* muscles—attached to bones *Cardiac* muscles—form wall of heart Fascia, tendons
Nervous	Coordinates body functions, coordinates reception of stimuli, transmits messages throughout body	Brain, spinal cord, spinal nerves, cranial nerves, special sense organs such as eyes and ears
Reproductive	Reproduces the species, fulfills sexual needs, develops sexual identity	*Male:* Testes, epididymis, urethra, seminal vesicles, ejaculatory duct, prostate gland, bulbourethral glands, penis, spermatic cord *Female*: Breasts, ovaries, oviducts, uterus, vagina, Bartholin glands, vulva
Respiratory	Brings in oxygen and eliminates carbon dioxide	Sinuses, nose, pharynx, larynx, trachea, bronchi, lungs
Urinary	Manages fluids and electrolytes of body, eliminates liquid wastes	Kidneys, ureters, urinary bladder, urethra

Figure 5-7 Systems of the body.

? EXERCISE 5-9

Match the system on the right with the function on the left.

Function System

1. _____ coordinates body activities through nervous stimuli
2. _____ controls reproduction and sexual activity
3. _____ carries materials around the body
4. _____ digests, transports, and absorbs nutrients
5. _____ brings gases into and out of the body
6. _____ protects body and helps control body temperature
7. _____ protects vital organs and moves the body
8. _____ produces hormones
9. _____ eliminates liquid wastes from the body

a. Reproductive
b. Respiratory
c. Endocrine
d. Urinary
e. Gastrointestinal
f. Musculoskeletal
g. Nervous
h. Circulatory
i. Integumentary

MEMBRANES

Membranes are sheets of epithelial tissues supported by connective tissues. Membranes:

- Cover the body
- Line body cavities
- Produce some body fluids

Important membranes include:

- **Mucous membranes**
  - Produce a fluid called **mucus**
  - Line body cavities that open to the outside

Because the respiratory, digestive, and genitourinary systems all open to the outside, they are lined with mucous membranes. The eyelids are also lined with a mucous membrane; a mucous membrane covers the eyeballs.

- **Synovial membranes**
  - Produce synovial fluid
  - Line joint cavities

The synovial fluid is a clear fluid resembling the white of an egg. It reduces the friction between the bones of active joints and the tendons.

- **Serous membranes**
  - Produce serous fluid
  - Cover the organs and line the closed cavities of the body

Serous fluid reduces friction as the organs work and move. Important serous membranes are the:

- **Pericardium**—surrounds the heart
- **Pleura**—surrounds the lungs and lines the thoracic cavity
- **Meninges**—cover the brain and spinal cord and line the dorsal cavity
- **Peritoneum**—covers the digestive organs and lines the abdominal cavity
- **Cutaneous membrane** (skin)
  - Protects the body
  - Covers the entire body
  - Helps control body temperature
  - Eliminates wastes through sweat glands
  - Produces vitamin D when exposed to sunlight

Special epithelial cells in this membrane, called *glands*, secrete perspiration and oils.

? EXERCISE 5-10

COMPLETION

Select the correct term(s) from the following list to complete each statement. Some words may be used more than once.

absorb	excrete	meninges	outside	secrete
body	heart	movement	ovaries	serous
brain	kidneys	mucous	pericardium wall	spinal cord
closed	lungs	open	peritoneum wastes	testes
connect	membranes	organs	pleura	

(continues)

? EXERCISE 5-10 (Continued)

1. The organs that eliminate liquid waste from the body are the _____.
2. The organs that exchange gases (oxygen and carbon dioxide) for the body are the _____.
3. The organ that pumps blood around the body is the _____.
4. The organs that produce the female hormones are the _____.
5. The organs that produce the male hormones are the _____.
6. Epithelial tissue is specialized in the ability to _____, _____ fluids, and _____ waste products.
7. Connective tissues serve to _____ and support body parts.
8. Muscle tissue is attached to bones for _____, forms the _____ of the heart and the wall of body _____.
9. Nervous tissue forms the _____ and _____ and the nerves throughout the body.
10. Sheets of epithelial tissue supported by connective tissue form _____.
11. A membrane that produces the fluid called mucus is called a _____ membrane.
12. The type of membrane described in the previous question (11) lines body cavities that _____ to the _____ of the body.
13. Serous membranes produce _____ fluid.
14. Serous membranes cover _____ and line _____ body cavities.
15. Cutaneous membrane covers the entire _____, eliminates _____, and produces vitamin _____.
16. The membrane that covers the lungs is called the _____.
17. The membrane covering the brain and spinal cord is called the _____.
18. The membrane lining the abdominal cavity is called the _____.
19. The membrane covering the heart is called the _____.

CAVITIES

The body seems like a solid structure, but cavities (spaces) within it contain the organs. Figure 5-8 lists the two main cavities, the dorsal cavity and the ventral cavity. Each of these cavities is lined by and divided into other cavities by serous membranes. These other cavities are also listed in Figure 5-8, as are the organs contained in each. Figure 5-9 is a simple drawing of the location of these cavities.

	Cavity	Organs	
Dorsal cavity	Cranial	Brain, pineal body, pituitary gland	
	Spinal	Nerves, spinal cord	
	Thoracic	Lungs, heart, great blood vessels, thymus gland	
	Abdominal Peritoneal	Stomach, small intestine, most of large intestine, liver, gallbladder, pancreas, spleen	
Ventral cavity	Pelvic	*Male* Seminal vesicles, prostate gland, ejaculatory ducts, urinary bladder, urethra, rectum	*Female* Uterus, oviducts, ovaries, urinary bladder, urethra, rectum
	Retroperitoneal space	Kidneys, adrenal glands, ureters	

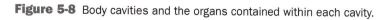

Figure 5-8 Body cavities and the organs contained within each cavity.

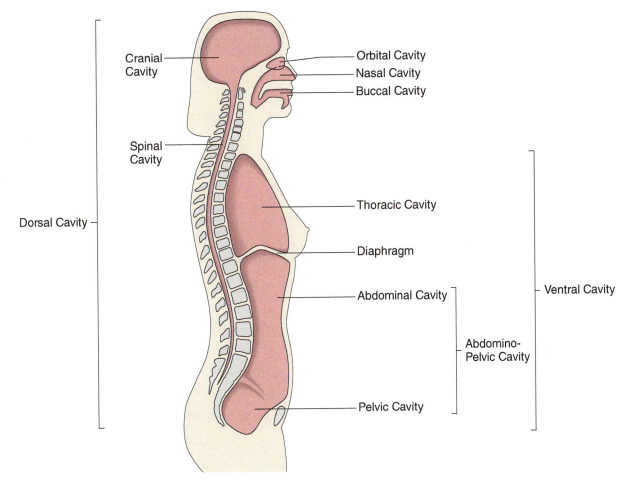

Figure 5-9 Lateral view of body cavities.

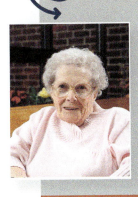

LESSON SYNTHESIS: Putting It All Together

You have just completed this lesson. Now go back and review the Clinical Focus. Try to see how the Clinical Focus relates to the concepts presented in the lesson. Then answer the following questions.

1. What health problems has Mrs. England had before her present problem?
2. What health problems have made admission to the long-term facility necessary?
3. Which activities would you be performing as part of Mrs. England's care?
4. What value to you, as a nursing assistant, is knowing the language of health care?

5 REVIEW

A. Complete the definition by crossing out the incorrect term in each sentence.

1. The word part found at the end of a word to change or add to its meaning is the (prefix) (suffix).

2. A word that means the study of aging is (gerontology) (pathology).

3. The term that means the front of the body is (ventral) (dorsal).

4. The term meaning closest to the point of attachment is (distal) (proximal).

5. Cells that are specialized to produce body fluids like mucus are called (nerve cells) (epithelial cells).

B. Based on the prefixes in each of the words, match the correct meaning (items a–e) with the word.

a. excessive urine
b. high blood pressure
c. painful urination
d. rapid pulse
e. slow pulse

6. _____   bradycardia

7. _____   hypertension

8. _____   dysuria

9. _____   tachycardia

10. _____   polyuria

C. Based on the suffixes in each of the words, match the correct meaning (item a–e) with the word.

a. excision of a breast
b. record produced by electrocardiography
c. inflammation of the bronchi
d. study of blood
e. insufficient quantity or quality of blood

11. _____   electrocardiogram

12. _____   mastectomy

13. _____   hematology

14. _____   bronchitis

15. _____   anemia

D. Match the tissue with its function.

Tissue

a. connective
b. epithelial
c. muscle
d. nervous

Function

16. _____   coordinates body activities

17. _____   attached to bones for movement

18. _____   forms the walls of the stomach and intestines

19. _____   connects and supports body parts

20. _____   specialized in its ability to excrete waste products

21. _____   found in the eyes, ears, and taste buds

22. _____   specialized in its ability to absorb

23. _____   forms the heart wall

24. _____   forms blood and bone

25. _____   forms nerves

E. Match the organ to the system of which it is a part.

System

a. cardiovascular
b. respiratory
c. endocrine
d. digestive

e. reproductive

f. urinary

Organ

26. _____   kidney

27. _____   uterus

28. _____   small intestines

29. _____   heart

30. _____   lungs

31. _____   urinary bladder

32. _____   mouth

33. _____   thyroid gland

34. _____   veins

35. _____   gallbladder

F. Using your knowledge of combining forms, prefixes, and suffixes, write a medical word that means each of the following. Then check to see if you can find it in the glossary at the back of the book.

36. without infection _____

37. instrument for inspecting the ear _____

38. study of the cells _____

39. tumor containing fibrous tissue _____

40. after surgery _____

G. Name the areas indicated in the diagram. Select from the list provided.

left lower quadrant   right lower quadrant
left upper quadrant   right upper quadrant

41. _____

42. _____

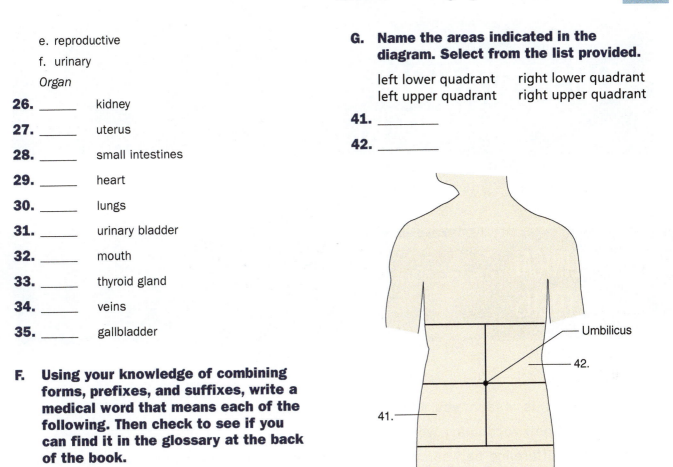

OBSERVATION, DOCUMENTATION, AND REPORTING

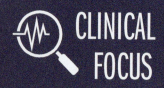

CLINICAL FOCUS

Think about using your vision, hearing, sense of smell, and sense of touch to learn about the residents as you study this lesson.

OBJECTIVES

After studying this lesson, you should be able to:

• Define and spell vocabulary words and terms.

• Explain the difference between an objective observation and a subjective observation.

• Explain the difference between signs and symptoms.

• Describe one observation to make for each body system.

• List the information to include when reporting off duty.

• List the guidelines for documentation.

• Name the four components of the interdisciplinary health care team process.

• Describe the responsibilities of the nursing assistant for each component of the interdisciplinary health care team process.

VOCABULARY

approach (ah-PROHCH)
document (DOCK-you-ment)
evaluation (ee-val-you-AY-shun)
goal (gohl)
implementation (im-plih-men-TAY-shun)
intervention (in-ter-VEN-shun)
Minimum Data Set (MDS 3.0) (MIN-ih-mum DAY-tah set)
nurse's notes (NUR-sez nohts)

nursing diagnosis (NURS-ing die-ag-NOH-sis)
objective observation (ob-JECK-tiv ob-sir-VAY-shun)
observation (ob-sir-VAY-shun)
PAINAD Scale (pan-ad)
resident care plan (REZ-ih-dent kair plan)
sign (sighn)
subjective observation (sub-JECK-tiv ob-sir-VAY-shun)
symptom (SIMP-tum)

CASE STUDY

Mrs. Sara Bass was admitted to the facility from the local hospital after having surgery for a fractured hip. She is going to therapy every day in the hope that she will be able to return to her home. The hospital reported that she was disoriented after surgery.

OBSERVATION

One of the most important skills you will develop is the ability to make accurate observations. An observation is something you note about the resident by using your senses: seeing, hearing, smelling, or touching. Some observations must be reported immediately. Other observations may be reported later to the nurse. Always carry a pen and note pad with you to record your observations if they are not immediately communicated to the nurse. If you rely on your memory, you may forget some vital information when you give your report. You will use your senses to observe in the following manner:

- You use your eyes to see observations:
  - Blood in the urine
  - Bruises, redness, or breaks in the skin
  - The resident crying
  - A change in the way the resident walks
- Your ears to hear observations:
  - Wheezing when the resident breathes
  - Pulse or blood pressure with a stethoscope
  - Comments from the resident such as "I am very tired today"
- Your nose to smell observations:
  - Body odor
  - Stool or urine when the resident is incontinent
- Your hands and fingers to use your sense of touch:
  - A lump under the resident's skin
  - Radial pulse
  - Warmth or coolness of the resident's skin

Signs and Symptoms

The things you notice are called signs and symptoms. A sign is objective evidence of disease. These are facts that can be seen or measured by the observer (Figure 6-1). Examples of signs are:

- Rashes, bruises, pressure ulcers
- Elevated temperature
- Vomiting
- Rapid heartbeat

When you observe a sign, you are making an objective observation.

Symptoms are subjective evidence of disease. These are facts that need to be relayed from the resident to the observer; that is, the resident tells you either verbally or through body language (Figure 6-2). Examples of symptoms are:

- The resident tells you he has nausea.
- Anxiety—may be noted by the resident's behavior such as pacing or the resident may tell you she is nervous.

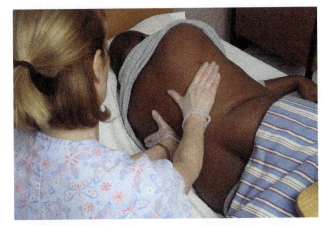

Figure 6-1 The nursing assistant observes for bruises, breaks in the skin, rashes, or other skin conditions while giving a backrub.

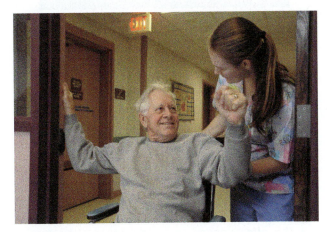

Figure 6-2 The resident's body language and facial expression are examples of subjective observations.

- Pain may be noted by the resident's position or facial grimace, or he may tell you he has pain.

🌐 BUILDING CULTURAL AWARENESS

Remember that persons of different cultures may express their symptoms in different ways. It is very important that you closely observe body language and facial expressions. Report exactly what you observe and do not assume anything.

When a resident reports a symptom to you, you are making a subjective observation.

Observations provide evidence of:

- A change in the resident's physical condition. Example: A resident with diabetes may be having an insulin reaction.

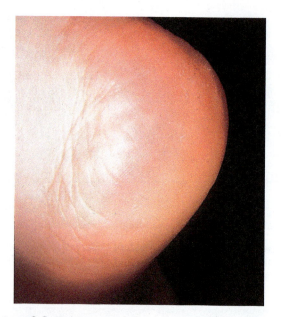

Figure 6-3 The first sign of a pressure ulcer should be reported immediately.

- A new condition that is developing. Example: A pressure ulcer may be noted (Figure 6-3).
- A change in the resident's mental condition. Example: A resident who has shown no signs of disorientation is now wandering about, saying he does not know where he is.
- A change in the resident's emotional condition. Example: A resident is crying and says she "does not want to continue living."
- The effectiveness of a medication or treatment. Example: A resident may be taking an antibiotic for a urinary tract infection. If the signs and symptoms of the infection are not going away, then the medication may not be effective and the physician will need to change the order.
- A change in the resident's ability to function. Example: The resident may not be able to walk as far or may not be able to complete an activity of daily living independently.

Remember that observations:

- Must be accurate and timely
- Are reported to the nurse immediately (Table 6-1)
- Are documented in the resident's record by either you or the nurse

Making Initial Observations

To make accurate observations, you must first know what is expected or normal for an individual. For this reason, baseline information is collected when the resident is admitted to the facility. If you help admit a resident, make observations while you are completing your assignment. It is especially important to note any signs of injury or skin breakdown. Think of the body systems as an organized way of making observations. This information will provide you with a basis for making future comparisons. For example, one resident may have a blood pressure of 110/68 on admission. If you take the resident's blood pressure later and it is 140/88, you should report this to the nurse, because this is not the usual blood pressure for this person.

? EXERCISE 6-1

Identify the following observations as objective or subjective by marking each statement with an O for Objective (observed by you) or S for Subjective (reported to you by the resident either verbally or through body language).

1. _____ The resident has a temperature of 100°F.
2. _____ The resident did not finish his or her food. The resident said he is not hungry.
3. _____ The resident pulls back when you try to move his or her arm.
4. _____ The resident's face is flushed.
5. _____ The resident says she has back pain.
6. _____ The resident is pacing.
7. _____ The resident has his legs drawn up, maybe he has cramps.
8. _____ The resident has a dry, frequent cough.
9. _____ There is bleeding from the left nostril.
10. _____ The resident chews the food but has difficulty swallowing.

? EXERCISE 6-2

DIFFERENTIATION

Differentiate between signs and symptoms by writing each observation under the proper label in the space provided.

	Sign	Symptom	Observation
1.	_____	_____	nausea
2.	_____	_____	vomiting
3.	_____	_____	pain
4.	_____	_____	restlessness
5.	_____	_____	dizziness
6.	_____	_____	cold, clammy skin
7.	_____	_____	incontinence
8.	_____	_____	elevated blood pressure
9.	_____	_____	anxiety
10.	_____	_____	cough

Chest pain	Nausea or vomiting	Excessive thirst
Shortness of breath	Diarrhea	Lethargy
Difficulty breathing	Cough	Unusual drainage from a wound or body cavity
Weakness or dizziness	Cyanosis or change in color	Changes in vital signs
Headache	Pain	Change in mental status

System or Problem	Observation to Report
Signs/symptoms of infection	Elevated temperature Sweating Chills Skin hot or cold to touch Skin flushed, red, gray, or blue Inflammation of skin as evidenced by redness, edema, heat, or pain Drainage from wounds or body cavities Any unusual body discharge, such as mucus or pus
Evidence of pain	Chest pain Pain that radiates Pain upon movement Pain during urination Pain when having a bowel movement **Pain is not normal; all complaints of pain should be reported to the RN**
Cardiovascular (circulatory) system	Abnormal pulse below 60 or above 100 Blood pressure below 100/60 or above 140/90 (Figure 6-4) Unable to palpate pulse or hear blood pressure Chest pain Chest pain that radiates to neck, jaw, or arm Shortness of breath Headache, dizziness, weakness, vomiting Cold, blue, or gray appearance Cold, blue, painful feet or hands Shortness of breath, dyspnea, or abnormal respirations Blue color of lips, nail beds, or mucous membranes

Table 6-1 General Signs and Symptoms of Illness that Should Be Reported to the RN

(continues)

System or Problem	Observation to Report
Respiratory system	Respiratory rate below 12 or above 20 Irregular respirations Noisy, labored respirations Dyspnea Shortness of breath Gasping for breath Wheezing Coughing Retractions Blue color of lips, nail beds, or mucous membranes
Integumentary system	Rash Redness in the skin that does not go away within 30 minutes after pressure is relieved Pressure sores, blisters Irritation Bruises Skin discoloration Swelling
Integumentary system (continued)	Lumps Abnormal sweating Excessive heat or coolness to touch Open areas/skin breakdown Drainage Foul odor Complaints such as numbness, burning, tingling, itching Signs of infection Unusual skin color, such as blue or gray color of the skin, lips, nail beds, roof of mouth, or mucous membranes Abrasions, skin tears Skin growths Poor skin turgor/tenting of skin Sunken, dark appearance around eyes
Gastrointestinal (digestive) system	Sores or ulcers inside the mouth Difficulty chewing or swallowing food Unusual or abnormal appearance of bowel movement Blood, mucus, or other unusual substances in stool Unusual color of bowel movement Hard stool, difficulty passing stool Complaints of pain, constipation, diarrhea, bleeding Frequent belching Changes in appetite Excessive thirst Fruity smell to breath Complaints of indigestion or excessive gas Nausea, vomiting Choking Abdominal pain Abdominal distention Coffee-grounds appearance of emesis or stool

Table 6-1 (Continued)

System or Problem	Observation to Report
Genitourinary system	Urinary output too low Oral intake too low Fluid intake and output not balanced Abnormal appearance of urine: dark, concentrated, red, cloudy (Figure 6-5) Unusual material in urine: blood, pus, particles Complaints of difficulty urinating or inability to urinate Complaints of pain, burning, urgency, frequency, pain in lower back Urinating frequently in small amounts Sudden-onset incontinence Edema of the face, hands, or feet; the sacral area in a bedfast resident Sudden weight loss or gain Respiratory distress Change in mental status
Nervous system	Tremors on one side or of both hands Change in level of consciousness, orientation, awareness, or alertness Increasing mental confusion
Nervous system (continued)	Progressive lethargy Loss of sensation Numbness, tingling Change in pupil size; unequal pupils Abnormal or involuntary motor function Loss of ability to move a body part Poor coordination
Musculoskeletal system	Pain Obvious deformity Edema Immobility Inability to move arms and legs Inability to move one or more joints (Figure 6-6) Limited/abnormal range of motion Jerking or shaky movements Weakness Sensory changes Changes in ability to sit, stand, move, or walk Pain upon movement
Mental status	Change in level of consciousness, awareness, or alertness Changes in mood or behavior Change in ability to express self or communicate Mental confusion Excessive drowsiness Sleepiness for no apparent reason Sudden onset of mental confusion Threats of harm to self or others

Table 6-1 (Continued)

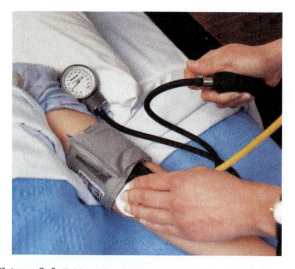

Figure 6-4 Taking blood pressure provides important information about the circulatory system.

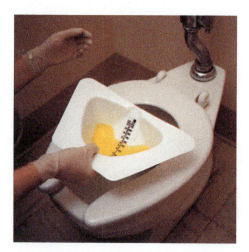

Figure 6-5 Before discarding urine, check the amount, color, clarity, and the presence of blood and sediment.

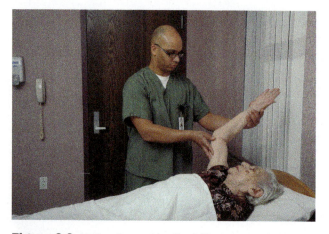

Figure 6-6 Noting the resident's ability to move the joints is an observation of the musculoskeletal system.

Body System Observations

Try to establish a routine way of making observations. Keep in mind the age and known illness of the resident. It may be helpful to think of each body system and note the following observations to report.

Observations of Pain and Behavior

You also need to note facts related to the resident's pain and behavior.

- Pain: location, type (sharp, burning, dull, aching), constant or intermittent (stopping and starting) or related to specific activities
- Behavior: actions, conduct, functioning

A resident's complaints of pain should never be ignored. Pain is a subjective symptom but it is important that health care workers consistently evaluate the resident's response to pain and to the treatment of that pain. Be objective when you report observations of pain and behavior. Never try to judge whether a resident really has pain or how severe it is. Some persons are expressive about pain and others try not to show their discomfort. Never compare residents. One person may seem to have more pain than another person with the same diagnosis. It is not appropriate to think that they should both respond in the same way. A person's culture or ethnic background may influence the way he or she responds to pain. Some persons may be stoic (not demonstrating pain with facial expressions or complaints because it is considered a sign of weakness); however, persons from other cultures may cry, moan, and scream. Others may believe that pain is a punishment from a higher power.

Constantly be alert to changes in the resident. Recall that pain is not *normal*; the cause must always be investigated. Is the resident grimacing, crying, moaning, or screaming? Does he or she rub or splint a body part, refusing to move it? Also note any physical changes: blood pressure may be elevated and the pulse and respirations may be increased; the skin may be moist and pale.

The nurse may use a pain scale to help assess and manage the resident's pain. The scale is a tool for communication. Figure 6-7 shows examples of several types of pain scales used in health care. Because a variety of scales are used to measure the intensity of pain, your facility may use one that is the same or different from the ones shown. Note that some scales use numbers, words, or pictures to help the resident describe the intensity of the pain. The nurse is responsible for assessing the level of the resident's pain; however, the resident may tell you that he or she is experiencing pain at "level 9" an hour after receiving medication for the pain. It is your responsibility to

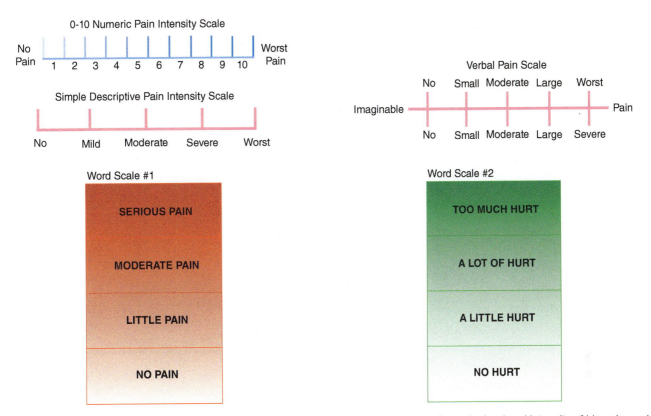

Figure 6-7 The resident will select the pain scale that best helps him or her communicate the level and intensity of his or her pain.

immediately report this finding to the nurse, because a serious problem may be occurring with the resident that must be reassessed.

When you report to your supervisor about the resident's behavior, do not use "labels" based on your judgment of the resident. Describe only what you see and hear. Refer to Figure 6-8 for examples of how certain behaviors should be reported.

You will make additional observations that are related to the resident's medical diagnoses. For example, if a resident has a kidney condition, you will look for edema (swelling) of the face, hands, and ankles.

You will also monitor the person's fluid intake and output. You will learn more about observations related to medical diagnoses as you study these conditions.

In some situations you may be expected to report "normal" observations. This information tells the nurse and physician whether the resident's condition is improving. For example, if a resident has a respiratory tract infection and the signs and symptoms have decreased, it is important to report that "no coughing or respiratory distress is noted."

It is a challenge to assess for the location and severity of pain in a resident who may be cognitively

Resident's Actions	What You Will Report
agitating other residents	0300 Out of bed, talking to roommates, attempting to get them out of bed.
confused	0210 States over and over that he "wants to go to Maywood to see his mother."
disoriented	0100 States "I want to go to church today because it is Sunday."
combative	2130 Hit nursing assistant 2x on upper arm with fist when nursing assistant attempted to change incontinent pad.
uncooperative	1300 Refused to get up from chair when nursing assistant tried to take to bathroom.
verbally abusive	1420 Called resident in next bed a "stupid, ignorant idiot."
physically abusive	1000 Scratched nursing assistant on face when bed was being changed.

Figure 6-8 When reporting observations of residents' behavior, you will report only what you see and hear (second column). The words in the first column are judgments, opinions, or assumptions.

? EXERCISE 6-3

MATCHING 1

Match the observation on the left with the system or problem on the right to which it best relates (some answers will be used more than once).

Observation

1. _____ pain upon movement
2. _____ disoriented
3. _____ rash
4. _____ elevated blood pressure
5. _____ jaundiced skin
6. _____ unable to walk without assistance
7. _____ elevated temperature
8. _____ difficulty breathing
9. _____ coughing frequently
10. _____ unable to respond with words

System or Problem

a. circulatory
b. integumentary
c. musculoskeletal
d. infection
e. nervous
f. respiratory

? EXERCISE 6-4

MATCHING 2

Match the observation on the left with the system or problem on the right to which it best relates (some answers will be used more than once).

Observation

1. _____ cloudy urine
2. _____ bruises
3. _____ difficulty passing stool
4. _____ wheezing
5. _____ belching frequently
6. _____ chest pain
7. _____ pressure sores
8. _____ progressive lethargy
9. _____ inability to urinate
10. _____ loss of sensation
11. _____ sudden mood change

System or Problem

a. gastrointestinal
b. mental status
c. respiratory
d. nervous
e. genitourinary
f. cardiovascular
g. integumentary

impaired (Alzheimer's or other dementias). The nurse may use a scale that has been specifically developed to rate pain in a person with advanced dementia. This scale is referred to as the PAINAD Scale. The scale is depicted in Table 6-2.

REPORTING

When you make observations, you must report your findings to the nurse. Be specific when you describe your observations. If you are relaying a subjective

Items*	0	1	2	Score
Breathing independent of vocalization	Normal	Occasional labored breathing Short periods of hyperventilation	Noisy labored breathing Long periods of hyperventilation Cheyne-Stokes respirations	
Negative vocalization	None	Occasional moan or groan Low-level speech with a negative or disapproving quality	Repeated troubled calling out Loud moaning or groaning Crying	
Facial expression	Smiling or inexpressive	Sad Frightened Frown	Facial grimacing	
Body language	Relaxed	Tense Distressed pacing Fidgeting	Rigid posture Fists clenched Knees pulled up Pulling or pushing away Striking out	
Consolability	No need to console	Distracted or reassured by voice or touch	Unable to console, distract, or reassure	
*Five-item observational tool.			TOTAL**	
** Total scores range from 0 to 10. The higher score indicates more severe pain. (0 = "no pain" to 10 = "severe pain.")				

Table 6-2 Pain Assessment in Advanced Dementia (PAINAD) Scale

Reprinted from Journal of the American Medical Directors Association, 4, 1, Warden, V., Hurley, A.C., and Volicer, L., Development and Psychometric Evaluation of the Pain Assessment in Advanced Dementia (PAINAD) Scale, pp 9–15, copyright 2003, with permission from Elsevier.

observation (something the resident has told you), repeat it exactly the way the resident told it to you. Here are examples:

- "Mr. Jones in 249 says it hurts every time he urinates."
- "Mrs. Bernetti says her heart is racing and feels like it's skipping beats."
- "Mrs. Goldberg was wandering around in the hall and said she did not know where she was."

When you report off duty at the end of your shift, report to the nurse:

- The condition of each of the residents you cared for
- The care you gave each resident
- Observations you made while giving care
- Any tasks not completed

⊘ ON THE JOB

The resident's treatment is frequently based on the signs and symptoms that are reported to the physician by the nurse. It is extremely important that you report your findings promptly and accurately.

DOCUMENTATION

In most facilities you will be expected to document your observations on the resident's medical chart, or electronically through a desktop or wall-mounted computer, often referred to as a kiosk. A chart or electronic document is a legal record. The resident's care, response to treatment, and progress are documented (charted) in the resident's chart. To **document** means to write out your findings. Nursing assistants may document on flow sheets in the chart or on the **nurse's notes** (sometimes called nurse's progress notes, Figure 6-9). The charting must:

- Address the problems listed in the resident's care plan
- Describe the interventions listed in the care plan and note whether the interventions are effective
- Indicate the progress the resident is making toward meeting the goals on the care plan
- Describe the extent of assistance required with activities of daily living or document level of independence

Recording Observations— Charting Guidelines

The medical record or resident's chart is a legal document that can be subpoenaed and used in court.

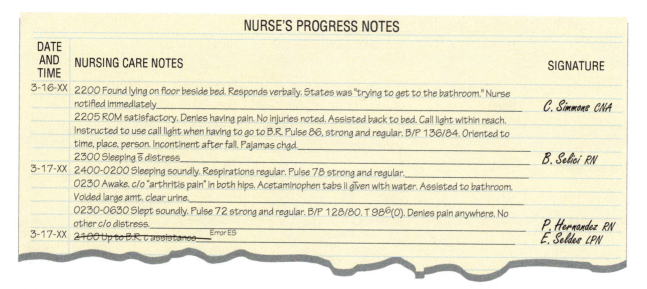

Figure 6-9 Documentation on the nurse's notes in the resident's chart.

This data is usually kept in a special notebook or binder in the nurse's station, or stored electronically on a desktop computer. Policies vary as to who is responsible for recording information in the chart. However, documentation of care given is important and should be taken seriously. There is a common rule in health care regarding documentation: "If it is not charted, it was not done." All entries to the chart should be objective, clear, concise, and easy to read. Many facilities use a combination of narrative notes (see Figure 6-9) and flow-sheet charting (Figure 6-10). Know and follow your facility's policy.

Notes on the narrative pages of the chart are recorded in chronological order, by date and time of entry. Many facilities allow the use of only blue or black ink. Notes are *never* made in pencil; no erasures are permitted. If an error is made, draw a single line through the entry and label it "Error" followed by your initials (see Figure 6-9). Leave no blank spaces or lines between entries. Sign your first initial, last name, and job title to all entries. Flow sheets that are used to record the resident's care apply to a whole month. Be careful to record the appropriate data in the column under the specific date the care was given and sign your initials where indicated. A signature page accompanies the monthly flow sheet where you sign your name and your initials. If any questions arise relating to the care of a resident, it is possible to determine who gave care on that specific day.

Most health care facilities use international (24-hour) time (Figure 6-11) to avoid confusion between am and pm. With international or military time, the 24 hours of each day are identified by the numbers 0100 (1:00 AM) through 2400 (12:00 AM, midnight).

? EXERCISE 6-5

24-HOUR CLOCK
Write the international time equivalent for each of the following times.

1. 6:30 AM _____
2. 8 AM _____
3. 11 AM _____
4. 12 noon _____
5. 4:30 PM _____
6. 5 PM _____
7. 7:20 PM _____
8. 9 PM _____
9. 11:16 PM _____
10. 12 midnight _____

The last two digits indicate the minutes of each hour from 01 to 59. Thus 0101 is 1 minute after 1:00 AM; 12:10 is 10 minutes after 12 PM (noon); 1658 is 4:58 PM, and so on.

Computerized Medical Records

The use of computers is becoming more prevalent in long-term care facilities. They are useful as efficient and cost-effective tools that can help simplify some activities. Large amounts of data can be stored, processed, and retrieved.

Nursing departments are using the computer to complete the information for the **Minimum Data Set**

NURSE ASSISTANT CARE RECORD—A.M. SHIFT

(Reference tags: F309, F310, F312, F315–F318, F327; Cross reference tags: F221, F222, F241, F241, F246–F247)

INSTRUCTIONS: Identify the appropriate code for each item listed under the correct date column. Unless otherwise indicated refer to the following response key: Y = Yes; N = No; I = Independent; A = Assist; D = Dependent; — = Not Applicable. Initial each day's documentation and identify your initials by signing (one time) on the reverse where indicated. Additional notes and comments should also be documented on the reverse.

			1	2	3	4	5	6	7	8	9	10	11	12	13	14	15	16	17	18	19	20	21	22	23	24	25	26	27	28	29	30	31
Month		Year																															
FEEDING	Breakfast	% Eaten																															
	Lunch	% Eaten																															
	Self/Assisted/Fed	S-A-F																															
	Ate in-Bed/Room/Dining Room/Chair	B-R-D-C																															
	Nourishment-Taken/Refused	T-R																															
BODY CARE	Bath-Bed/Shower/Tub/Partial/Whrpl/Shampoo	B-S-T-P-W-SH																															
	Nail Care-Fingers/Toes	F-T																															
	Skin-Clear/Other (Report "O" to Nurse)	C-O																															
	Positioned qh	¼-½-1-2 / I-A-D																															
	Pads-Air/Water/Foam/Synthetic	A-W-F-S																															
	Continent-Bedpan/Urinal/BRP/Commode	P-U-B-C																															
BLADDER	Incontinent	# Times																															
	Catheter	C-N																															
	Intake	cc's																															
	Output	cc's																															
BOWEL	Continent-Bedpan/BRP/Commode	P-B-C																															
	Incontinent	# Times																															
	Enema-Tap Water/Soap/Fleets	T-S-F																															
	Loose Stool	# Times																															
BEHAVIOR	Cooperative-Accepts Assist	C-N																															
	Resistant-Refuses Assist	R-N																															
	Alert-Oriented to Reality	Y-N																															
	Confused/Noisy/Agitated (if ✓'d note reason on reverse)	Y-N																															
	Behavior Monitored (specify)	# Times																															
RESTORATIVE CARE	Feeding Program	Y-N																															
	Oral Hygiene	I-A-D																															
	Hair Care	I-A-D																															
	Shave	I-A-D																															
	Dressing/Undressing with ROM	I-A-D																															
	Range of Motion-Passive/Active	P-A																															
	Transfers	I-A-D																															
	Bowel & Bladder Program	Y-N																															
	Up in Chair	I-A-D																															
SAFETY DEVICES	Restraints-Bed/Wheelchair	B-W																															
	Ambulation-Walker/Cane/Assist/Self	W-C-A-S																															
	Scheduled Activities-Attended/Refused	A-R																															
	Side Rails Up/Down/Release	U-D-R																															
	Geri Chair/Vest/Wrist/Waist/Pelvic	G-V-W-WA-P																															
	Safety Device/Restraint-Released qh	2-1-½																															
OTHER	Checked q 30 minutes	✓																															
	Positioned qh	½-1																															
	CHARGE NURSE NOTIFIED (record reason on back)	Y-N																															
	OUT OF FACILITY	Y-N																															
AIDE INITIALS																																	

NAME—Last   First   Middle   Attending Physician   Chart No.

NURSE ASSISTANT CARE RECORD
A.M. SHIFT

Figure 6-10 Most long-term care facilities use flow-sheet charting to record daily care.

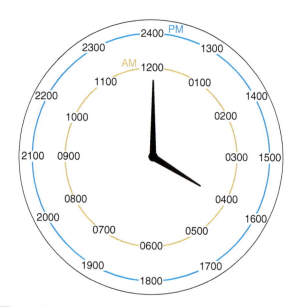

Figure 6-11 The 24-hour clock.

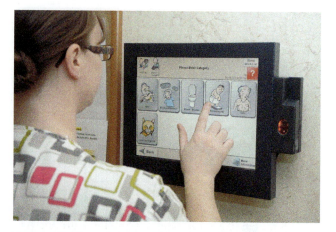

Figure 6-12 Wall-mounted touch screen.

for Medicare. Special programs for documentation of routine care for the resident have been created; these programs are different from the word processing programs that you may use. Some facilities generate daily work assignments. If your facility uses the computer to record data about the resident's care, you will be instructed in the use of this technology. One of the benefits of using computer technology is that it will allow you to spend more time with the resident while completing your documentation activities with more accuracy.

Figure 6-12 depicts one type of computerized system for documenting resident care. The wall-mounted touch screens are situated at selected locations throughout the facility. This placement allows the CNA to document care at point of service throughout the shift. The CNA selects the picture on the wall screen to match the care provided such as Activities of Daily Living (ADLs): dressing, walking, continence and nutritional information, and so on. Intake and output, weight changes, and behavioral patterns also can be documented.

In addition, the nurses and licensed staff can retrieve the information about an individual resident or a group of residents, at any time. The data can be used for a variety of purposes: MDS 3.0 data, developing care plans, preparing for change of shift report, as well as use by the billing departments to accurately charge for services, data collection by the management team to develop timely and appropriate in-service education programs.

? EXERCISE 6-6

TRUE OR FALSE

Indicate whether the following statements are true (T) or false (F).

1. T F The resident's record is a legal document.

2. T F Blank spaces are not to be left between entries when charting in a resident's medical record.

3. T F Sign your first initial, last name, and job title to all entries.

4. T F In some facilities, some parts of the documentation may be assigned to the nursing assistant.

5. T F Written documentation describes resident responses to the care plan goals.

6. T F Documentation can be written in pencil.

7. T F Errors in the resident's record are corrected by erasing them.

8. T F Each entry in the record must be timed, dated, and signed.

9. T F If it isn't charted, it wasn't done.

10. T F Residents' charts may be used in court in legal situations.

THE INTERDISCIPLINARY HEALTH CARE TEAM PROCESS

The interdisciplinary health care team provides the right care for the residents. The members of the team are responsible for completing activities that will result in a care plan for each resident. To do this, the team members must have a foundation of knowledge on which to base their recommendations. The team members and other staff are accountable for implementing the care. Nursing assistants help in each step of this process.

In addition to the Interdisciplinary Team Process, nurses communicate with each other by way of a similar process termed the *nursing process*. The nursing process involves similar steps: assessment, nursing diagnosis, planning, implementation, and evaluation. This process develops an orderly method for communicating and administering nursing care to residents. The term **nursing diagnosis** is used to identify specific, unique problems and the probable cause for each resident based on the assessment data. The information obtained through the MDS 3.0 can help the nurse in this process. Here are some examples of nursing diagnoses:

- Impaired physical mobility related to pain and stiffness due to osteoarthritis
- Diarrhea related to tube feedings
- Imbalanced nutrition related to inability to ingest food

Step 1: Assessment

Assessment means to make an evaluation of the resident's mental, physical, and emotional status. The CNA reports observations to the nurse, who then assesses the resident. This evaluation is completed by gathering information about the resident's past and present problems. The information is called *data*. Each discipline completes an assessment when the resident is admitted and annually. This assessment is called the Minimum Data Set (MDS 3.0) and is required by law. A less complex assessment is repeated every 3 months. If the resident's condition changes, the assessment is again completed. In addition to the MDS 3.0, the resident may be evaluated for specific risk factors. Examples include:

- Pressure ulcer risk assessment. If data indicate the resident is at risk of developing pressure ulcers, a preventive program is initiated.
- Safety assessment. If the resident is at risk of falling or wandering, a program to prevent incidents is initiated.

- Mental status examination. This is done to determine the resident's orientation to time and place and mental capabilities.

Data for the MDS 3.0 and the other assessments are collected by the nurse and other members of the team from many sources:

- Interviewing the resident, the family, and nursing staff on all shifts
- Reading the results of the physician's history and physical examination and progress notes
- Reading the results of all diagnostic tests
- Performing a physical assessment (Figure 6-13)
- Performing a functional assessment

Nursing Assistant Responsibility: Assessment

The nursing assistant's responsibility for Step 1: Assessment is to:

- Make accurate and thorough observations.
- Report and document observations factually.

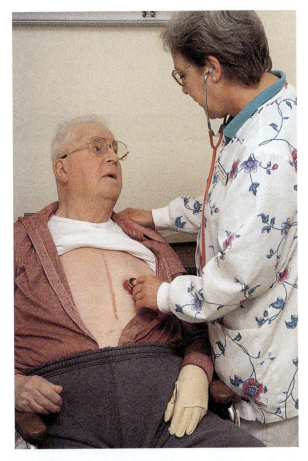

Figure 6-13 The registered nurse collects information by doing a physical assessment of the resident.

Step 2: Planning

The new Rules of Participation, enacted 2016–2019 require a care plan be written within 48 hours of admission. The observations the CNA makes in these first 2 days are critical to the development of this care plan. After the assessments are completed and the nursing diagnoses have been developed, the long-term care plan is written. The **resident care plan** is the "blueprint" for giving care. Members of the interdisciplinary team attend the care plan conference. The resident is invited to attend. Family members are also invited to participate if the resident agrees. At the care plan conference the team:

- Establishes goals for the resident. A **goal** is an outcome; it states what the team (including the resident) plans for the resident to accomplish or be able to do. The goals are developed by determining the resident's potential. For example, if one of the nursing diagnoses is impaired mobility, the team would set goals to maintain or improve mobility. In some situations goals may come from more than one discipline. A mobility problem may involve goals from both the physical therapist and the nursing staff. The goals must be realistic and measurable. A nursing goal for impaired mobility might be: that the resident will walk 100 feet with a walker and one assistant two times a day by a certain date. Goals may be restorative (improvement), preventive (prevent complications such as pressure ulcers or infection), or maintenance (the resident's current state will not change).

- Determines the approaches or interventions to use to help the resident meet the goals. The **approach** or **intervention** states exactly which members of the team are responsible for the approach—what they will do, how they will do it, and when. The approach for the impaired mobility goal might be: to place a transfer belt on the resident, assist to standing position, place walker in front of resident, and instruct resident to use three-point gait to walk, to be done by nurse or nursing assistant after breakfast and before supper.

Nursing Assistant Responsibility: Planning

The nursing assistant responsibility for Step 2: Planning is to:

- Give suggestions to the nurse if you think a specific approach may be successful. Example: Mrs. Donetti becomes agitated when you try to give her a shower. You tell the nurse you think Mrs. Donetti might prefer a tub bath instead.

- Attend care plan conference if you have the opportunity to do so.

? EXERCISE 6-7

BRIEF ANSWERS
Briefly answer the following.

1. The four steps of the interdisciplinary health care team process are:
   a. _____
   b. _____
   c. _____
   d. _____

2. The assessment completed by each discipline on admission and annually is called the _____
   _____.

3. At what other times is the MDS 3.0 revised? _____

4. What is the nursing diagnosis? _____

5. What is the name given to the "blueprint" for care giving? _____

6. During the care conference, "goals" are established. These are _____.

7. Approaches that explain the goal and how it can be reached are called _____.

8. Putting the care plan into practice is known as _____.

9. Determining how well the goals are being met is called _____.

10. Regarding MDS completion, a less complex assessment must be completed every _____.

Step 3: Implementation

Implementation is putting the care plan into practice. Members of the interdisciplinary team carry out the approaches listed on the care plan.

Nursing Assistant Responsibility: Implementation

The nursing assistant responsibility for Step 3: Implementation is to:

- Read the residents' care plans.
- Carry out the approaches assigned to nursing assistants consistently and correctly.

Step 4: Evaluation

The purpose of **evaluation** is to determine whether or not the resident is meeting the goals as set forth in the care plan. If the goals are not met, the problems are not resolved. The resident's condition may be deteriorating; there may be complications or decreasing functional abilities. The team needs to determine why the resident is unable to meet the goals. Then different goals will be written or different approaches will be used.

Nursing Assistant Responsibility: Evaluation

The nursing assistant responsibility for Step 4: Evaluation is to:

- Report to the nurse when you are unable to carry out an approach as stated in the care plan.
- Relay to the nurse any ideas you have about why there is a problem.
- Report to the nurse the resident's progress toward meeting the care plan goals.

? EXERCISE 6-8

CLINICAL SITUATION

1. Mrs. Cohen, one of your residents, is suffering from renal failure (a kidney condition). What two special observations should you make relating to her?

   a. _____

   b. _____

3. Mr. Burgdorf is making a rapid recovery from an upper respiratory infection. He is breathing easily and is no longer coughing. How might you document this information? _____

4. Mrs. Vanderhooten is being admitted to your facility. As the interdisciplinary team makes its assessment and carries out the care process, indicate how the nursing assistant could be of assistance.

STEP NURSING ASSISTANT ACTION

   a. Assessment _____

   _____

   b. Planning _____

   _____

   c. Implementation _____

   _____

   d. Evaluation _____

   _____

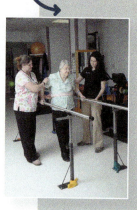

LESSON SYNTHESIS: Putting It All Together

You have just completed this lesson. Now go back and review the Clinical Focus. Try to see how the Clinical Focus relates to the concepts presented in the lesson. Then answer the following questions.

1. Which systems would be most important in making observations for Mrs. Bass?
2. Which members of the interdisciplinary health care team would attend Mrs. Bass's care plan conference?
3. Which senses would you use to determine whether Mrs. Bass was disoriented?
4. What information could you gain by observing her facial expressions and body language?

6 REVIEW

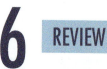

A. Select the one best answer for each of the following.

1. Which of the following examples is a subjective observation?

   (A) Mrs. Pochoski tells you she feels sick to her stomach.

   (B) You take Mr. Johnson's temperature and it is 99.6°F.

   (C) Miss Dominick has a reddened area around her tailbone.

   (D) Mr. Flores has a blood pressure of 126/84.

2. Which of the following examples is an objective observation?

   (A) You feel a lump when you are giving Mrs. Smith her bath.

   (B) Mrs. Smith tells you she has a lump in her breast.

   (C) Mr. Johnson tells you he thinks he has a fever.

   (D) Miss Dominick says she has pain in her tailbone.

3. When you make observations, one of the following is not recommended practice:

   (A) must be accurate and timely

   (B) reported to the nurse immediately

   (C) documented in the resident's record by you or the nurse

   (D) errors can be erased

4. Initial observations or baseline information is collected when the resident

   (A) is discharged from the facility

   (B) is admitted to the facility

   (C) has a care plan conference

   (D) has a change in condition

5. When observing the integumentary system, you would note the

   (A) resident's ability to move his arms and legs

   (B) resident's blood pressure

   (C) color of the resident's skin

   (D) resident's ability to respond

6. When you observe the resident's breathing, you are observing the resident's

   (A) circulatory system

   (B) digestive system

   (C) respiratory system

   (D) reproductive system

B. Answer each statement true (T) or false (F).

7. T F Charting is done in pencil in case you make a mistake and need to erase.

8. T F Each statement in the chart begins with the word *resident*.

9. T F The resident and the resident's family (if the resident agrees) are invited to attend the care plan conference.

10. T F The nursing diagnosis is the physician's statement of the resident's problem.

11. T F Goals must be realistic and measurable.

12. T F Residents are quick to report pain when it begins.

13. T F A low urine output should be reported.

14. T F Sudden onset of mental confusion need not be reported, because the resident may just be tired.

15. T F A report of level 8 pain indicates a moderate amount of pain being experienced.

C. Fill in the blanks by selecting the correct word or phrase from the list.

approach	intervention
assessment	nurse's notes
baseline	objective
goal	planning
implementation	subjective

16. A sign is a/an _____ observation.

17. A symptom is a/an _____ observation.

18. Making initial observations provides _____ information.

19. The MDS 3.0 is used to make a/an _____ of the resident.

20. The second step of the interdisciplinary health care team process is _____.

21. Carrying out the instructions on the resident's care plan is called _____.

22. Nursing assistants may be expected to document on the _____ in the resident's medical record.

23. A statement of what the interdisciplinary team plans for the resident to be able to accomplish is called a _____.

24. The actions taken by members of the interdisciplinary team to help the resident is called a/an _____ or a/an _____.

25. Change the following times to international time (24-hour clock system).

    a. 6:35 AM

    b. 9:10 AM

    c. 11:25 AM

    d. 1:15 PM

    e. 3:24 PM

    f. 6:42 PM

    g. 9:25 PM

    h. 11:59 PM

3

Protecting Residents' Rights and Safety

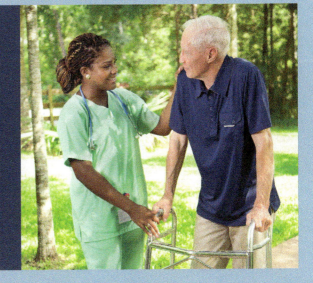

LESSON 7
RESIDENTS' RIGHTS

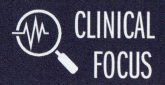

CLINICAL FOCUS

Think about the basic rights guaranteed to each resident as you study this lesson.

OBJECTIVES

After studying this lesson, you should be able to:

- Define and spell vocabulary words and terms.
- Describe the purpose of the Residents' Rights document.
- State the differences between physical abuse, sexual abuse, mental abuse, and verbal abuse.
- Describe the term *involuntary seclusion*.
- Give two examples of neglect.
- List four situations when the nursing assistant should provide privacy for the resident.
- Explain the nursing assistant's responsibilities for meeting (accommodating) the resident's needs.
- List five situations in which the resident can make choices.
- Describe four ways the nursing assistant can help residents meet their psychosocial needs.

VOCABULARY

abandonment (a-BAN-don-ment)
advance directives (ad-VANS dih-RECK-tivs)
advocate (AD-voh-kit)
artificial nutrition (are-tih-FISH-al new-TRIH-shun)
assault (ah-SALT)
battery (BAT-er-ee)

cardiac arrest (KAR-dee-ack ah-REST)
cardiopulmonary resuscitation (CPR)
  (kar-dee-oh-PUL-moh-nair-ee ree-sus-ih-
  TAY-shun)
chemical restraint (KEM-ih-kal ree-STRAYNT)
corporal punishment (KOR-poh-ral PUN-ish-ment)

CASE STUDY

Stanley Davidson has no close relatives and has chosen you to be a confidant. He has shared many personal facts that he would not want anyone else to know.

defamation of character (def-eh-MAY-shun of KAIR-ack-ter)
ethics (ETH-icks)
false imprisonment (falls im-PRIHS-on-ment)
financial abuse (fy-NAN-shul ah-BYOUSE)
grievance (GREE-vans)
hospice (HAHS-piss)
hot-line number (hot-line NUM-ber)
incontinent (in-KON-tin-ent)
informed consent (in-FORMD kon-SENT)
invasion of privacy (in-VAY-shun of PRY-vah-see)
involuntary seclusion (in-VOL-un-ter-ee sih-KLUE-zhun)
legal guardian (LEE-gul GAR-dee-un)
libel (LIE-bul)
living will (LIV-ing will)
mental abuse (MEN-tal ah-BYOUSE)
neglect (neh-GLECKT)

no-code (DNR) (do not resuscitate) (NO-kohd) (do not ri-sus-i-TATE)
ombudsman (OM-buds-man)
physical abuse (FIZ-ah-kul ah-BYOUSE)
physical restraint (FIZ-ah-kul ree-STRAYNT)
power of attorney for health care (POW-er of ah-TUR-nee for helth kair)
prosthesis (pros-THEE-siss)
reprisal (ree-PRY-zul)
Self-Determination Act (self dee-ter-mih-NAY-shun akt)
sexual abuse (SEX-you-al ah-BYOUSE)
sexuality (sex-you-AL-ih-tee)
slander (SLAN-der)
terminal condition (TER-mih-nal kon-DIH-shun)
theft (theft)
verbal abuse (VER-bal ah-BYOUSE)

PURPOSE OF THE RESIDENTS' RIGHTS DOCUMENT

The Older Americans Act (OAA) that was signed into law in 1965 included the Residents' Bill of Rights for long-term care settings and the Patient's Bill of Rights for acute care settings. This legislation was designed to protect senior citizens from maltreatment in nursing homes as well as all persons in acute health care settings. The bill also included the provision for Medicare for elders under the Social Security Administration. In 1978, the OAA strengthened the law by requiring that each state establish the Long-Term Care Ombudsman program that would oversee that the rights of residents were not violated (more discussion will be found later in this chapter). The Omnibus Budgeting Reconciliation Act (OBRA) of 1987 further strengthened the legislation by mandating that nursing facility residents must have direct and immediate access to ombudsmen whenever protection or advocacy services are needed. The resident and family or court-appointed representative of the resident (legal guardian) must be given a copy of the Resident's Rights document at the time of admission to the facility (Figure 7-1). With the new Rules of Participation enacted in 2016 to 2018, all agency numbers, including state and federal, must be posted and explained to all new admissions.

All citizens in the United States have certain rights (e.g., the right to vote) that are guaranteed by law. Health care consumers have rights to ensure that they will receive quality care. Any questions they

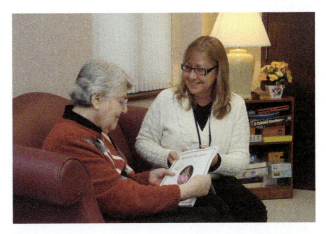

Figure 7-1 The resident must receive a full explanation of the Residents' Rights document before admission to the facility.

have should be discussed with the staff member who is coordinating the admission. Copies of these rights also are posted in prominent places throughout the facility.

🌐 BUILDING CULTURAL AWARENESS

There may be major cultural differences among the residents you care for. These differences may be reflected in their beliefs about health and illness and health care practices. These beliefs must always be respected regardless of your own personal feelings.

The resident rights are written in simple language that all residents can understand. In communities with a large population of non–English speaking residents, the rights are translated into the prevalent language of the area. All persons working in the facility should be familiar with the document. The nursing assistant is in a unique position to assist all residents in exercising their rights. Residents who are physically or mentally unable to exercise their rights must be protected to ensure their rights are not violated. A summary of the resident rights is listed in Table 7-1.

- Residents have the right to exercise all their rights as citizens of the state and citizens of the United States, as well as any other rights given them by law.
- The facility must explain the rights to residents both verbally and in writing in a language that the residents understand.
- Residents cannot be discriminated against because of age, sex, race, ethnic origin, religion, or disability.

Privacy, Dignity, and Respect
- Residents have a right to privacy.
- Residents will be treated with consideration, dignity, and respect.
- The resident's likes, dislikes, and special needs and preferences must be considered in the services provided by the facility. This is called reasonable accommodation.
- Personal and clinical records must be kept confidential. Residents have the right to refuse to allow others to see these records. Permission to release records is given in writing.
- Residents have the right to communicate both verbally and in writing with anyone of their choosing. This includes family members, other visitors, the ombudsman, attorneys, and representatives of governmental agencies.
- Residents have the right to send and receive personal mail unopened. Residents may request that staff assist them to open and read their mail when it arrives.

Safety and Security
- Residents have the right to a safe environment.
- Residents have the right to care that is free from *misappropriation of property* (theft).

Medical Care and Treatment
- Residents have the right to choose their own physicians. They have the right to be informed of matters affecting their care and to make decisions regarding their care.
- Medical problems must be explained to residents in a language they understand.
- Residents may refuse treatment. If they do refuse treatment, they have the right to be informed of the consequences of their refusal.
- Residents have a right to voice problems and complaints about their care without fear of reprisal, or retaliation. The facility is required to respond to these complaints.
- Residents have the right to make choices to withhold life-sustaining treatment in the event of terminal illness.
- Residents may designate someone else to make treatment decisions for them in the event they become unable to make these decisions themselves.

Freedom from Restraint, Abuse, Neglect, and Misappropriation of Property
- Residents have the right to be free from abuse, neglect, and misappropriation of property. The facility is responsible for caring for the resident's health, well-being, and personal possessions.
- Drugs cannot be given for discipline or convenience of the nursing home staff. Any mood-altering drugs given are only for the treatment of a medical condition.
- Residents cannot be punished, scolded, abused, neglected, or secluded. Their privileges cannot be taken away and they cannot be physically, mentally, or sexually abused.
- Residents cannot be restrained by physical means except for their own safety, the safety of others, during certain medical procedures, or in an emergency.

Financial Matters
- Residents have the right to manage their own financial affairs or may choose another person to manage their money.
- Facilities must account for and properly manage resident money deposited with them.

Table 7-1 Residents' Rights

(continues)

Freedom of Association
- Residents have the right to have visitors at any reasonable hour.
- Residents do not have to talk to or see anyone they do not want to visit.
- Residents may make and receive private phone calls.
- Married couples have the right to share a room.
- Residents have the right to organize and participate in resident and family councils.
- Residents may meet with others outside the facility.
- Residents may leave the facility for visits or shopping trips, with physician approval.
- Family members may meet with families of other residents in the nursing home.
- Residents have the right to plan and execute their daily activities.
- Residents have the right to vote in elections.

Work
- Residents may choose to work in the facility as part of their activity plan. They have the right to be paid the prevailing rate for the same type of work in the community. Residents may also perform certain duties without pay, if they choose to do so.

Personal Possessions
- Residents may wear their own clothing.
- Residents may bring in furnishings and personal belongings from their own homes.

Grievance
- If residents have problems or complaints, they have the right to speak to those in charge. The complaints may be about care or failure to receive expected services. Residents have the right to a response.
- Residents have the right to contact the ombudsman for the facility and the state survey and certification agency. The ombudsman is a resident advocate. He or she can provide information on how to find a facility and how to get quality care. An ombudsman can help solve problems and will assist the resident to file a grievance, or complaint, if requested.
- The facility may not retaliate against residents who have complained.

Admission, Transfer, and Discharge
- The facility must advise residents about eligibility for Medicaid. If Medicaid or Medicare pays for any items or services, the resident cannot be charged additional money for these services.

Admission, Transfer, and Discharge
- In the event of the resident's death, the facility must give an accounting of money in the resident's personal account to the person responsible for the estate.
- Residents may not be asked to give up their rights to benefits under Medicaid or Medicare.
- The facility is required to have the same policies and practices regarding services, transfer, or discharge for all individuals, regardless of the source of payment.
- The facility may be required to hold the resident's bed for a specified period if the resident is hospitalized or goes on a therapeutic pass.
- The facility cannot make the resident leave or move to another room unless:
  - The health and safety of the resident or others are affected.
  - The facility cannot meet the resident's needs.
  - The resident's condition has improved so that services are no longer required.
  - The resident has not paid the bill and the facility has given the resident reasonable notice of discharge.
- Residents must be given a 30-day written notice before they can be transferred unless there are medical reasons, or the life, safety, and health of the resident or others is endangered. Residents may waive the right to the 30-day waiting period if they choose.

Table 7-1 (Continued)

RESIDENTS' RIGHTS

The Right to Free Choice

The resident has the right to make choices regarding medical treatment, including:

- The right to choose an attending physician. If the attending physician refuses to obey certain federal regulations regarding the resident's care, the facility may replace the physician after notifying the resident and utilize the medical director contracted with the facility.

- The right to full advance information about changes in care or treatment that affect the resident. This includes the right to refuse treatment. Treatment refers to procedures ordered by the physician. The resident must be consistent and persistent in refusing treatment. State laws must be followed. For example, if a resident cannot take in food and fluids, the resident may refuse to have a feeding tube inserted (artificial nutrition). In this case, the specific laws of that state would be obeyed. Whenever a resident refuses treatment, the nurse or physician must explain the possible consequences of the refusal.

- The right to be part of the assessment and care-planning process. This means the resident must be told of the evaluations made by the members of the care team. The resident and the family (if the resident agrees) are invited to the care plan conference so they may help with the planning process (Figure 7-2).

- The resident may self-administer medications if the assessment demonstrates that this is possible and the resident wishes to do so. The nurse is responsible for overseeing this process.

- The interdisciplinary team must make the determination if self-administration of medication is a reasonable choice for the resident. If the resident refuses to take a medication, an explanation of the possible consequences must be provided. The survey team refers to this as a risk/benefit analysis. The nurse must periodically offer the medication again. If the resident continues to refuse, the nurse must contact the physician to attempt to find an alternative solution. If it is determined that residents can self-administer, approved medications must be kept locked in a container at bedside, with the access key signed out only to the resident.

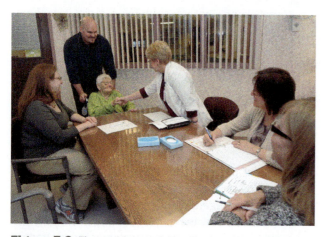

Figure 7-2 The resident and family are invited to participate in the care planning conference.

- The right to consent to participate in experimental research. Research that personally affects the resident cannot be done without the resident's consent. In order for a facility to conduct experimental research, there must be a current, written contract between the research company and the facility.

The Right to Freedom from Abuse and Restraints

The term *abuse* refers to mistreatment of a person. Residents may be abused by staff members, family members, other residents, or visitors. The different forms of abuse are physical abuse, sexual abuse, verbal abuse, mental abuse, and financial abuse. Improperly used or applied restraints are another form of abuse.

One of your most important concerns as a nursing assistant is to help the resident maintain dignity. That means that each person must be treated as having worth, no matter what the individual's physical or mental abilities might be. Prevention of abuse is one way to preserve dignity.

Physical abuse is:

- Hitting, slapping, pinching, or kicking
- Any physical contact that intentionally causes pain or discomfort
- Corporal punishment—inflicting pain on residents to force them to follow orders

Sexual abuse is:

- Using physical means or verbal threats to force a resident to perform any sexual act, including fondling, kissing, or sexual intercourse.
- Tormenting or teasing a resident with sexual gestures or words

Verbal abuse is:

- Talking to the resident in a sarcastic or rough manner
- Using crude slang or swearing
- Using gestures that are considered demeaning or obscene

Mental abuse is:

- Making verbal threats to hurt or punish a resident (e.g., telling a resident you will put him in a restraint if he does not obey you, or telling a resident he will not receive his meal if he doesn't cooperate)
- Humiliating a resident (e.g., embarrassing a resident who is incontinent)
- Separating a resident from other residents against the resident's will (involuntary seclusion), unless

this action is part of a therapeutic plan and is documented. Involuntary seclusion may be used if a resident's actions endanger or offend other residents, such as cursing or being physically aggressive.

Financial abuse is:

- Misuse of a resident's money or property by family, friends, or staff

Physical and psychosocial neglect may be considered forms of abuse. **Neglect** is the failure to provide safe care. Some examples are:

- Not meeting the resident's physical need for food, fluids, rest, activity, oxygen, cleanliness, shelter, and elimination. This is physical neglect.
- Actions by staff that make the resident agitated or depressed. This is psychosocial neglect.

No resident deserves to be abused or live in fear. Preventing all forms of abuse is everyone's responsibility. If staff members, family members, volunteers, or visitors appear to be abusive or on the verge of becoming so, report this immediately to your supervisor. If you witness abuse and do not report it, you are also guilty. Health care workers are legally mandated to report abuse to residents. Every facility is required to post the name and number of the abuse prevention coordinator, who general is the Administrator of the facility. Failure to report abuse is considered a misdemeanor and may incur a financial penalty as well. Family members are also under a great deal of stress and may need counseling. Promptly report any bruises or wounds that you observe or any statements of the resident that may possibly be a result of abuse.

Caring for residents requires patience and tolerance. If you feel yourself becoming tense or short-tempered, take action to calm yourself. Take a short break and some deep breaths. If you notice coworkers who appear "uptight," help them to regain their composure. Staff members need to care for each other as well as the residents. Working together with a true team spirit can help prevent abuse.

There are two forms of restraints:

- Chemical restraints
- Physical restraints

Chemical Restraints

At times, medications to alter behavior are needed. These situations must be carefully evaluated by the interdisciplinary team, resident, and family. **Chemical restraints** are medications that affect the resident's behavior so that mental powers such as thinking are changed. Residents receiving such medications are monitored for unusual reactions. The ordering and dispensing of medications are not the responsibility of the

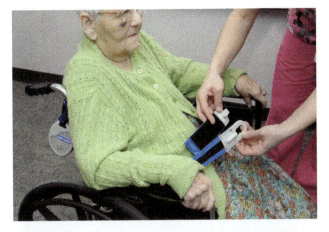

Figure 7-3 A physical restraint is a device that inhibits the resident's movements.

nursing assistant. The nursing assistant should report a resident's unusual behavior or a change in behavior.

Physical Restraints

A **physical restraint** (Figure 7-3) is any device that:

- A resident cannot easily remove
- Restricts a resident's movement
- Does not allow resident normal access to his or her own body

Physical restraints are discussed in Lesson 8.

The Right to Privacy

The right to privacy includes:

- Privacy during medical treatment and nursing care
- Receiving and sending unopened mail
- Privacy during telephone calls
- Privacy when visitors are present

Here are some suggestions for ensuring the resident's right to privacy:

- Always knock before entering a resident's room, whether the door is closed or open (Figure 7-4). Introduce yourself and wait for a response before entering.
- Close the door, the window curtain, and pull the privacy curtains when you are working with residents in their rooms (Figure 7-5).
- Keep residents covered as much as possible when you perform procedures.
- No other people should be present when you are helping the resident to go to the bathroom, to dress, or to complete personal care procedures. The exceptions are times when more than one staff person is required to complete a procedure (e.g., to position a dependent person).

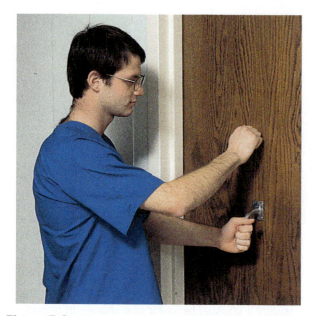

Figure 7-4 Always knock and wait for permission before you enter a resident's room.

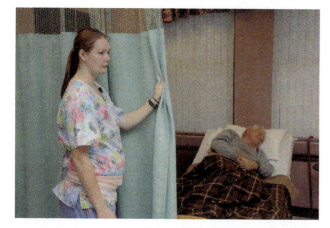

Figure 7-5 Pull the privacy curtain when you are working with a resident in her room.

- Close the doors to tub rooms, showers, and bathrooms when these areas are in use.
- The HIPAA regulations discussed in Lesson 1 further protect residents' privacy.

The Right to Confidentiality of Personal and Clinical Records

This means that information about the resident is available only to those who need the information to provide care. This includes information on the resident's chart and care plan. It also includes any information about the resident's personal life and relationship with the family. The caregivers who receive this information must keep the information confidential.

To protect this right:

- Avoid talking about residents or families during breaks or when you are off duty. When you have to discuss a resident with a coworker, do so in private. Family members, other residents, and visitors should not be able to overhear your conversation. Also remember that not all family members have access to information. It is necessary to know who is authorized to be given updates and who is not.
- Shift reports and other conferences should be held in areas of privacy.
- If a resident or family member wishes to see the medical records, relay the request to the nurse.
- Avoid talking about residents to other residents in the facility.

The Right to Accommodation of Needs

This includes the right to make choices about life that are important to the resident. This includes activities, schedules, and health care that are consistent with the resident's interests and care plan.

This right means the resident may make choices about:

- Nutrition and eating
- Times for getting up and going to bed
- Clothing, use of makeup, hair style
- Bath or shower and when to take it
- Use of free time
- Visitors

Accommodation of Needs

The resident has the right to expect the assistance of the staff in meeting both physical needs and psychosocial needs.

Physical Needs

As a nursing assistant, you help residents meet their physical needs when you:

- Assist residents to maintain personal hygiene and cleanliness.
  - Give baths or showers.
  - Clean and trim fingernails and toenails.
  - Shave daily.
  - Give shampoos and allow residents to wear the hair style of their choice.
  - Give regular and thorough oral hygiene.
  - Allow residents to choose their own clothing (Figure 7-6).

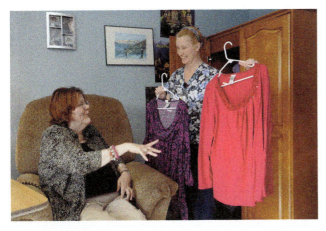

Figure 7-6 Allow residents to choose their own clothing.

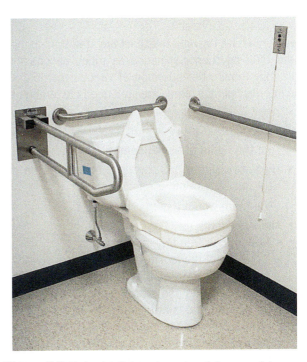

Figure 7-7 Raised toilet seats and grab bars assist residents to be more independent.

- Provide clothing that is:
  - Clean.
  - In good repair and fits properly.
  - Appropriate for the season and the weather.
  - Appropriate for the resident's age and gender.
- Assist residents with toileting needs as necessary.
  - Take residents to the bathroom as needed or at regularly scheduled times. The bathroom is designed to meet the physical needs of the residents, with grab bars and elevated toilet seats (Figure 7-7).
- Attend to **incontinent** residents (those unable to control bladder or bowel) immediately.
- Assist residents to remain adequately nourished.
  - Consider the residents' food choices as much as possible.
  - Give residents the assistance necessary to eat independently.
  - Feed residents who cannot feed themselves in a dignified manner.
  - Never force residents to eat.
  - Provide access to fresh drinking water often throughout the day (Figure 7-8).
  - Give dependent residents drinks of fresh water regularly.
- Assist residents with the use of devices to meet their needs.
  - Make sure they have their eyeglasses and that the glasses are clean and in good repair.
  - Assist residents with insertion of hearing aids and report improperly functioning hearing aids to the proper person.
  - Assist with the use of canes and walkers.
  - Help residents with a **prosthesis** (artificial body part) or other positioning devices or adaptive equipment.

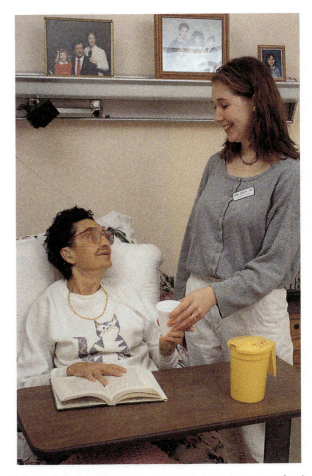

Figure 7-8 Residents should always have access to fresh drinking water.

Psychosocial Needs

Residents have the right to expect the staff to help them meet their psychosocial needs as much as possible. This may require the attention of various members of the interdisciplinary team. The staff needs to remember:

- The medical condition of a resident when providing these rights
- That the rights of all residents are equal
- That no resident has the right to infringe on the right or safety of other residents

  The team works together to:
- Allow residents to:
  - Spend their free time as they wish
  - Move about the facility (if their medical condition permits) as long as they respect the privacy of other residents and staff members
  - Participate, if desired, in structured activities offered by the facility (Figure 7-9)
  - Visit other residents in the facility
- Allow married couples who both reside in the facility to share a room, if they both so desire and if it is medically appropriate (Figure 7-10).

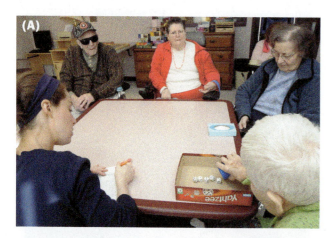

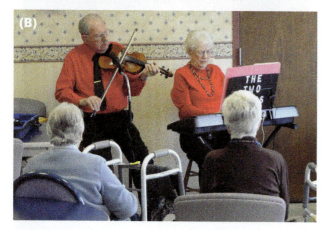

Figure 7-9 Facilities must offer an activity program to all residents.

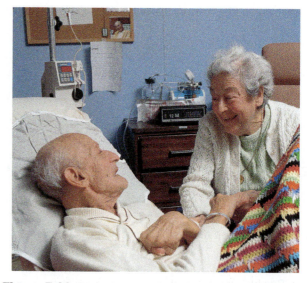

Figure 7-10 A married couple in a long-term care facility has the legal right to share a room if both members of the couple are residents in the facility.

- Respect the **sexuality** and sexual needs of the resident. Sexuality is one aspect of human psychosocial needs. Whether married to each other or not, residents have the right to express their needs and to experience satisfaction as long as this is mutually agreeable. Residents must be mentally and physically able to agree to the relationship.

CLINICAL FOCUS

Family members frequently assist residents and do things for them to increase the resident's enjoyment. Because Mr. Davidson has no close relatives, what are some issues that the staff may need to think about?

Environmental Needs

The resident has the right to expect that the environment will be adapted to meet the needs of individuals with disabilities. This means:

- The residents must be able to safely move about and function within the facility. This requires:
  - Handrails attached to corridor walls (Figure 7-11)
  - Elevators for resident use
  - Ramps that allow wheelchair access into and out of the facility
  - Permanent grab bars in bathrooms and elevated toilet seats
  - Signal lights in the residents' rooms and in the bathrooms and showers
  - Safety measures for residents who wander

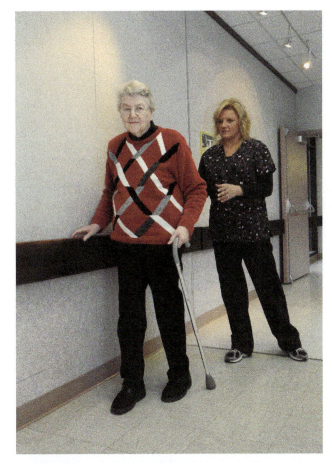

Figure 7-11 Handrails attached to the wall allow residents more independence.

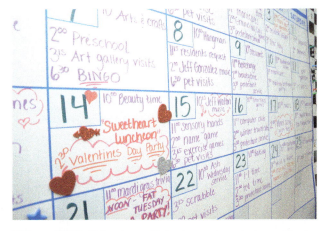

Figure 7-12 Calendars with large numbers help residents remain oriented.

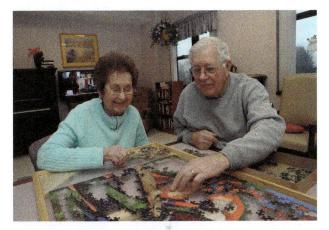

Figure 7-13 Facilities should have comfortable visiting areas.

- Clocks and calendars with large numerals located throughout the building to help residents remain oriented (Figure 7-12)
- The facility environment is expected to be home-like and to allow social interaction, including:
  - Furniture arrangements in public areas that allow for visiting (Figure 7-13)
  - The use of color, plants, and artwork to create a cheerful environment

Advance Directives

Residents also have the right to make **advance directives**. In 1990, the federal government passed a law called the **Self-Determination Act**. This law states that all competent adults have the right to:

- Accept or refuse any medical treatment, including life-sustaining treatments
- Be adequately informed about:
  - Their medical condition
  - Treatment alternatives

? EXERCISE 7-1

IDENTIFICATION 1

Determine which needs are being met as residents make choices about each activity by indicating A for psychosocial needs or B for physical needs.

1. _____ walking in the hallways
2. _____ getting up at 8:30 AM
3. _____ eating spinach instead of broccoli
4. _____ playing cards
5. _____ taking a shower rather than a tub bath
6. _____ listening to the radio
7. _____ wearing a green sweater
8. _____ watching news programs
9. _____ participating in facility activities
10. _____ shutting off the lights to sleep at 10 PM
11. _____ speaking with a priest
12. _____ reading mystery novels
13. _____ visiting with friends
14. _____ shaving daily
15. _____ sharing a room with a spouse

EXERCISE 7-2

IDENTIFICATION
Identify five environmental adaptations in the figure below that help residents meet disability needs.

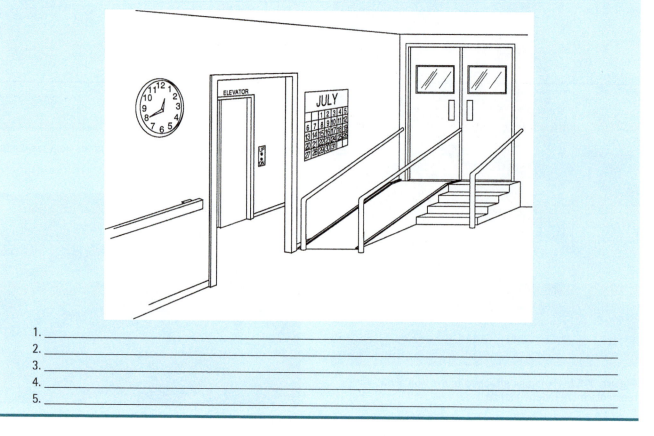

1. _____
2. _____
3. _____
4. _____
5. _____

- Likely risks of each treatment alternative
- Benefits of each alternative
- Possible consequences of each alternative

The law applies to competent adults entering hospitals, nursing homes, home health care, or **hospice** (an agency that provides care for terminally ill persons). The law requires that residents:

- Be informed of what kinds of advance directives are available to ensure that their wishes are carried out when they are no longer able to make or communicate their decisions
- Be informed that it is the right of every competent adult to choose whether he or she wants to execute an advance directive

There are two types of advance directives:

- **living will** (Figure 7-14)
- **power of attorney for health care** (Figure 7-15)

A living will:

- Allows individuals to describe their wishes about discontinuing procedures that delay death if they

have a **terminal condition**. This means that death is expected soon and the person's condition is incurable and irreversible.

- Is legal in most states
- Must be witnessed by two people who will not benefit from the resident's death. (In most facilities, the nursing assistant should not be a witness for the signing of legal forms.)

A durable power of attorney for health care:

- Permits a person (called the *principal*) to delegate to another person (called the *agent*) the power to make any health care decision that the principal is unable to make

Even though these advance directives have been completed, the resident must still make decisions regarding other support measures.

In addition to advance directives, a program called Physician Orders for Life Sustaining Treatment (POLST) has been developed (Figure 7-16). The POLST creates a standardized medical order form that is printed on brightly colored paper. These orders identify

INSTRUCTIONS	FLORIDA LIVING WILL – PAGE 1 OF 2
PRINT THE DATE	Declaration made this ______ day of ______________, ________, (day) (month) (year)
PRINT YOUR NAME	I, ______________________________________, willfully and voluntarily make known my desire that my dying not be artificially prolonged under the circumstances set forth below, and I do hereby declare that :
PLEASE INITIAL EACH THAT APPLIES	If at any time I am incapacitated and ______ I have a terminal condition, or ______ I have an end-stage condition, or ______ I am in a persistent vegetative state and if my attending or treating physician and another consulting physician have determined that there is no reasonable medical probability of my recovery from such condition, I direct that life-prolonging procedures be withheld or withdrawn when the application of such procedures would serve only to prolong artificially the process of dying, and that I be permitted to die naturally with only the administration of medication or the performance of any medical procedure deemed necessary to provide me with comfort care or to alleviate pain. It is my intention that this declaration be honored by my family and physician as the final expression of my legal right to refuse medical or surgical treatment and to accept the consequences for such refusal. In the event that I have been determined to be unable to provide express and informed consent regarding the withholding, withdrawal, or continuation of life-prolonging procedures, I wish to designate, as my surrogate to carry out the provision of this declaration:
PRINT THE NAME, HOME ADDRESS AND TELEPHONE NUMBER OF YOUR SURROGATE	Name: ______________ Address: ______________ ______________ Zip Code: ______ Phone: ______________
© 2005 National Hospice and Palliative Care Organization 2006 Revised	

(A)

	FLORIDA LIVING WILL - PAGE 2 OF 2
	I wish to designate the following person as my alternate surrogate, to carry out the provisions of this declaration should my surrogate be unwilling or unable to act on my behalf:
PRINT NAME, HOME ADDRESS AND TELEPHONE NUMBER OF YOUR ALTERNATE SURROGATE	Name: ______________ Address: ______________ ______________ Zip Code: ______ Phone: ______________
ADD PERSONAL INSTRUCTIONS (IF ANY)	Additional instructions (optional):
SIGN THE DOCUMENT	I understand the full import of this declaration, and I am emotionally and mentally competent to make this declaration. Signed: ______________
WITNESSING PROCEDURE	Witness 1: Signed: ______________ Address: ______________
TWO WITNESSES MUST SIGN AND PRINT THEIR ADDRESSES	Witness 2: Signed: ______________ Address: ______________
© 2005 National Hospice and Palliative Care Organization 2006 Revised	*Courtesy of Caring Connections* *1700 Diagonal Road, Suite 625, Alexandria, VA 22314* *www.caringinfo. , 800/658-8898*

(B)

Figure 7-14 A living will is a legal document that allows an individual to state what measures should or should not be taken to prolong life.

specifically the types of life-sustaining treatments that are to be performed or not to be performed on the severely ill resident who chooses to use this format. This medical order form is part of the resident's chart and follows him or her into any type of care setting such as the emergency room, long-term care, or hospice. This program has proven to be an effective communication tool among health professionals. As of mid-2010, 32 states have implemented or are developing the POLST program. It is important that the POLST document is reviewed by resident, family, and physician to ensure the choices for life-sustaining treatments have not changed.

Cardiopulmonary Resuscitation (CPR)

- The resident must inform the physician whether **cardiopulmonary resuscitation** is to be administered if **cardiac arrest** occurs. In most states, the law requires that all persons be resuscitated unless they have previously made their wishes known.
- The physician must write the order on the resident's chart if a resident or the person with a power of attorney for health care determines that CPR should not be administered. This is called **no-code or DNR (do not resuscitate)** order.

When there is a DNR order, resuscitation is not performed when the resident stops breathing. The resident is allowed to die with peace and dignity. All personnel should be aware when a DNR order is written. It is often difficult to carry out a DNR order when you have come to know and love the resident. Try to remember that life needs to be meaningful and that quality of life is limited for a person on life support systems.

If a resident has chosen to be resuscitated in the event that cardiac arrest occurs, then every effort is made to keep the resident alive. A "code" is called and CPR is initiated. An ambulance is called to transport the resident to the hospital for additional life support measures.

Hospitalization

- Some technical procedures cannot be performed in the long-term care facility.

Part I. Durable Power of Attorney for Health Care

• If you do NOT wish to name an agent to make health care decisions for you, write your initials in the box [Initials]

This form has been prepared to comply with the "Durable Power of Attorney for Health Care Act" of Missouri.

1. Selection of agent. I appoint:
Name:_____
Address:_____

> It is suggested that only one Agent be named. However, if more than one Agent is named, anyone may act individually unless you specify otherwise.

Telephone:_____
as my Agent.

2. Alternate Agents. Only an Agent named by me may act under this Durable Power of Attorney. If my Agent resigns or is not able or available to make health care decisions for me, or if an Agent named by me is divorced from me or is my spouse and legally separated from me, I appoint the person(s) named below (in the order named if more than one):

First Alternate Agent

Name:_____
Address:_____
_____
Telephone:_____

Second Alternate Agent

Name:_____
Address:_____
_____
Telephone:_____

> This is a Durable Power of Attorney, and the authority of my Agent shall not terminate if I become disabled or incapacitated.

Part I. Durable Power of Attorney for Health Care (Continued)

3. Effective date and durability. This Durable Power of Attorney is effective when two physicians decide and certify that I am incapacitated and unable to make and communicate a health care decision.

• If you want ONE physician, instead of TWO, to decide whether you are incapacitated, write your initials in the box to the right. [Initials]

4. Agent's powers. I grant to my Agent full authority to:

A. Give consent to, prohibit, or withdraw any type of health care, medical care, treatment, or procedure, even if my death may result;

• If you wish to AUTHORIZE your Agent to direct a health care provider to withhold or withdraw artificially supplied nutrition and hydration (including tube feeding of food and water), write your initials in the box to the right. [Initials]

• If you DO NOT WISH TO AUTHORIZE your Agent to direct a health care provider to withhold or withdraw artificially supplied nutrition and hydration (including tube feeding of food and water), write your initials in the box to the right. [Initials]

B. Make all necessary arrangements for health care services on my behalf, and to hire and fire medical personnel responsible for my care;

C. Move me into or out of any health care facility (even if against medical advice) to obtain compliance with the decisions of my Agent; and

D. Take any other action necessary to do what I authorize here, including (but not limited to) granting any waiver or release from liability required by any health care provider, and taking any legal action at the expense of my estate to enforce this Durable Power of Attorney.

5. Agent's Financial Liability and Compensation. My Agent acting under this Durable Power of Attorney will incur no personal financial liability. My Agent shall not be entitled to compensation for services performed under this Durable Power of Attorney, but my Agent shall be entitled to reimbursement for all reasonable expenses incurred as a result of carrying out any provision hereof.

Part II. Health Care Directive

• If you DO NOT WISH to make a health care directive, write your initials in the box to the right, and go to Part III. [Initials]

I make this HEALTH CARE DIRECTIVE ("Directive") to exercise my right to determine the course of my health care and to provide clear and convincing proof of my wishes and instructions about my treatment.

If I am persistently unconscious or there is no reasonable expectation of my recovery from a seriously incapacitating or terminal illness or condition, I direct that all of the life-prolonging procedures which I have initialed below be withheld or withdrawn.

I want the following life-prolonging procedures to be withheld or withdrawn:

> • artificially supplied nutrition and hydration (including tube feeding of food and water) . . . . [Initials]

• surgery or other invasive procedures. . . . . [Initials]
• heart-lung resuscitation (CPR) . . . . [Initials]
• antibiotic. . . . . [Initials]
• dialysis. . . . . [Initials]
• mechanical ventilator (respirator). . . . . [Initials]
• chemotherapy. . . . . [Initials]
• radiation therapy. . . . . [Initials]

• all other "life-prolonging" medical or surgical procedures that are merely intended to keep me alive without reasonable hope of improving my condition or curing my illness or injury. . . . . [Initials]

However, if my physician believes that any life-prolonging procedure may lead to significant recovery, I direct my physician to try the treatment for a reasonable period of time. If it does not improve my condition, I direct the treatment be withdrawn even if it shortens my life. I also direct that I be given medical treatment to relieve pain or to provide comfort, even if such treatment might shorten my life, suppress my appetite or my breathing, or be habit forming.

IF I HAVE NOT DESIGNATED AN AGENT IN THE DURABLE POWER OF ATTORNEY, THIS DOCUMENT IS MEANT TO BE IN FULL FORCE AND EFFECT AS MY HEALTH CARE DIRECTIVE.

Part III. General Provisions Included in the Directive and Durable Power of Attorney

YOU MUST SIGN THIS DOCUMENT IN THE PRESENCE OF TWO WITNESSES. IN WITNESS WHEREOF, I have executed this document this_____day of _____, year____.

_____
Signature

Print name _____
Address _____

The person who signed this document is of sound mind and voluntarily signed this document in our presence. Each of the undersigned witnesses is at least eighteen years of age.

Signature_____   Signature_____
Print name _____   Print name _____
Address _____   Address _____

> ONLY REQUIRED FOR PART I — DURABLE POWER OF ATTORNEY

STATE OF MISSOURI   )
) as
_____OF _____   )

On this _____day of _____, year_____, before me personally appeared to me known to be the person described in and who executed the foregoing instrument and acknowledged that he/she executed the same as his/her free act and deed.

IN WITNESS WHEREOF, I have hereunto set my hand and affixed my official seal in the County of _____, State of Missouri, the day and year first above written.

_____
Notary Public

My Commision Expires:

Figure 7-15 A durable power of attorney or designation of health care surrogate is a legal document that allows an individual to appoint another person to make health care decisions if the individual is unable to make his or her own decisions.

HIPAA PERMITS DISCLOSURE OF POLST TO OTHER HEALTH CARE PROVIDERS AS NECESSARY

Physician Orders for Life-Sustaining Treatment (POLST)

First follow these orders, then contact physician. This is a Physician Order Sheet based on the person's current medical condition and wishes. Any section not completed implies full treatment for that section. A copy of the signed POLST form is legal and valid. POLST complements an Advance Directive and is not intended to replace that document. Everyone shall be treated with dignity and respect.

EMSA #111 B
(Effective 4/1/2011)

Patient Last Name:	Date Form Prepared:
Patient First Name:	Patient Date of Birth:
Patient Middle Name:	Medical Record #: *(optional)*

A

Check One

CARDIOPULMONARY RESUSCITATION (CPR): *If person has no pulse and is not breathing.*
When NOT in cardiopulmonary arrest, follow orders in Sections B and C.

☐ **Attempt Resuscitation/CPR** (Selecting CPR in Section A **requires** selecting Full Treatment in Section B)

☐ **Do Not Attempt Resuscitation/DNR** (**A**llow **N**atural **D**eath)

B

Check One

MEDICAL INTERVENTIONS: *If person has pulse and/or is breathing.*

☐ **Comfort Measures Only** Relieve pain and suffering through the use of medication by any route, positioning, wound care and other measures. Use oxygen, suction and manual treatment of airway obstruction as needed for comfort. *Transfer to hospital __only__ if comfort needs cannot be met in current location.*

☐ **Limited Additional Interventions** In addition to care described in Comfort Measures Only, use medical treatment, antibiotics, and IV fluids as indicated. Do not intubate. May use non-invasive positive airway pressure. Generally avoid intensive care.
    ☐ *Transfer to hospital __only__ if comfort needs cannot be met in current location.*

☐ **Full Treatment** In addition to care described in Comfort Measures Only and Limited Additional Interventions, use intubation, advanced airway interventions, mechanical ventilation, and defibrillation/cardioversion as indicated. *Transfer to hospital if indicated. Includes intensive care.*

Additional Orders: _____

_____

C

Check One

ARTIFICIALLY ADMINISTERED NUTRITION: *Offer food by mouth if feasible and desired.*

☐ No artificial means of nutrition, including feeding tubes.   Additional Orders:_____
☐ Trial period of artificial nutrition, including feeding tubes.   _____
☐ Long-term artificial nutrition, including feeding tubes.   _____

D

INFORMATION AND SIGNATURES:

Discussed with: ☐ Patient (Patient Has Capacity)   ☐ Legally Recognized Decisionmaker

☐ Advance Directive dated _____ available and reviewed →   Health Care Agent if named in Advance Directive:
☐ Advance Directive not available   Name: _____
☐ No Advance Directive   Phone: _____

Signature of Physician
My signature below indicates to the best of my knowledge that these orders are consistent with the person's medical condition and preferences.

| Print Physician Name: | Physician Phone Number: | Physician License Number: |
| Physician Signature: *(required)* | | Date: |

Signature of Patient or Legally Recognized Decisionmaker
By signing this form, the legally recognized decisionmaker acknowledges that this request regarding resuscitative measures is consistent with the known desires of, and with the best interest of, the individual who is the subject of the form.

Print Name:	Relationship: *(write self if patient)*
Signature: *(required)*	Date:
Address:	Daytime Phone Number:	Evening Phone Number:

SEND FORM WITH PERSON WHENEVER TRANSFERRED OR DISCHARGED

Materials used with permission from the Coalition for Compassionate Care of California, www.coalitionccc.org.

Figure 7-16 POLST form: Standardized medical record form.

(continues)

HIPAA PERMITS DISCLOSURE OF POLST TO OTHER HEALTH CARE PROVIDERS AS NECESSARY

Patient Information			
Name (last, first, middle):		Date of Birth:	Gender: **M F**

Health Care Provider Assisting with Form Preparation		
Name:	Title:	Phone Number:

Additional Contact		
Name:	Relationship to Patient:	Phone Number:

Directions for Health Care Provider

Completing POLST

- Completing a POLST form is voluntary. California law requires that a POLST form be followed by health care providers, and provides immunity to those who comply in good faith. In the hospital setting, a patient will be assessed by a physician who will issue appropriate orders.
- POLST does not replace the Advance Directive. When available, review the Advance Directive and POLST form to ensure consistency, and update forms appropriately to resolve any conflicts.
- POLST must be completed by a health care provider based on patient preferences and medical indications.
- A legally recognized decisionmaker may include a court-appointed conservator or guardian, agent designated in an Advance Directive, orally designated surrogate, spouse, registered domestic partner, parent of a minor, closest available relative, or person whom the patient's physician believes best knows what is in the patient's best interest and will make decisions in accordance with the patient's expressed wishes and values to the extent known.
- POLST must be signed by a physician and the patient or decisionmaker to be valid. Verbal orders are acceptable with follow-up signature by physician in accordance with facility/community policy.
- Certain medical conditions or treatments may prohibit a person from residing in a residential care facility for the elderly.
- If a translated form is used with patient or decisionmaker, attach it to the signed English POLST form.
- Use of original form is strongly encouraged. Photocopies and FAXes of signed POLST forms are legal and valid. A copy should be retained in patient's medical record, on Ultra Pink paper when possible.

Using POLST

- Any incomplete section of POLST implies full treatment for that section.

Section A:

- If found pulseless and not breathing, no defibrillator (including automated external defibrillators) or chest compressions should be used on a person who has chosen "Do Not Attempt Resuscitation."

Section B:

- When comfort cannot be achieved in the current setting, the person, including someone with "Comfort Measures Only," should be transferred to a setting able to provide comfort (e.g., treatment of a hip fracture).
- Non-invasive positive airway pressure includes continuous positive airway pressure (CPAP), bi-level positive airway pressure (BiPAP), and bag valve mask (BVM) assisted respirations.
- IV antibiotics and hydration generally are not "Comfort Measures."
- Treatment of dehydration prolongs life. If person desires IV fluids, indicate "Limited Interventions" or "Full Treatment."
- Depending on local EMS protocol, "Additional Orders" written in Section B may not be implemented by EMS personnel.

Reviewing POLST

It is recommended that POLST be reviewed periodically. Review is recommended when:

- The person is transferred from one care setting or care level to another, or
- There is a substantial change in the person's health status, or
- The person's treatment preferences change.

Modifying and Voiding POLST

- A patient with capacity can, at any time, request alternative treatment.
- A patient with capacity can, at any time, revoke a POLST by any means that indicates intent to revoke. It is recommended that revocation be documented by drawing a line through Sections A through D, writing "VOID" in large letters, and signing and dating this line.
- A legally recognized decisionmaker may request to modify the orders, in collaboration with the physician, based on the known desires of the individual or, if unknown, the individual's best interests.

This form is approved by the California Emergency Medical Services Authority in cooperation with the statewide POLST Task Force. For more information or a copy of the form, visit **www.caPOLST.org**.

SEND FORM WITH PERSON WHENEVER TRANSFERRED OR DISCHARGED

© 2011 Coalition for Compassionate Care of California (CCCC)

Figure 7-16 (Continued)

- When residents become acutely ill, hospitalization may be necessary if lifesaving measures are to be taken.
- Residents may choose not to go to the hospital, but to remain in the facility for supportive care only.

Feeding Restrictions

- Residents who are terminally ill frequently do not wish to eat or drink.
- The physician may suggest inserting a feeding tube into the stomach.
- In most states this procedure will not be done if the resident has made his wishes clear in the advance directives.

In an advance directive, the resident may state that this procedure is not to be performed. Most states will honor this statement and not insert a feeding tube.

Medication and Treatment Restrictions

The resident has the right to refuse:

- Life-sustaining medications such as chemotherapy or antibiotics
- Blood transfusions
- Surgery
- Being placed on a ventilator
- Any medical treatment

Residents always have the right to change their minds. For example, if the advance directives state that a feeding tube is not to be inserted, the resident may change this directive if the time comes.

The Right to Voice Grievances

This means the resident may voice **grievances** (complaints) to the facility without fear of retaliation (**reprisal**) or discrimination. The facility must take prompt action to resolve the grievances (Figure 7-17).

The resident may have a grievance about:

- The way in which care is given
- Treatment or care that is not given

As a nursing assistant, you can help avoid problems by following these guidelines.

- Relay concerns of the resident to the nurse in charge.
  - Carry out all instructions you may be given for solving the problem.
  - Never withhold care or attention from a resident because of grievances or complaints voiced by the resident.

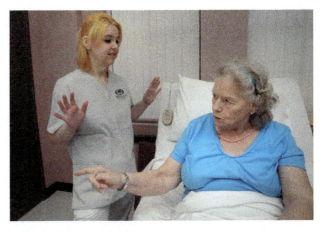

Figure 7-17 Residents have the right to voice grievances.

- Avoid discussing grievances with other staff members unless there is a valid need for such discussion. You may, for example, discuss a grievance at a care plan conference as a way of trying to solve the problem.

The Right to Organize and Participate in Family and Resident Groups

This means:

- The facility must provide space for meetings.
- A staff member from the facility will attend if invited.
- The staff will address written recommendations from the meetings that concern decisions affecting the resident's care and life in the facility.

Most long-term care facilities have resident councils. These councils meet regularly and all residents are invited to participate in the meetings. The councils give the residents a way to communicate with each other and with staff in a constructive and organized manner.

To assist in providing these residents' rights, you can:

- Cooperate in assisting residents to attend council meetings.
  - Help residents to get dressed to attend the meeting.
  - Arrange residents' care so it does not interfere with their attendance at the meetings.
  - Toilet residents if necessary before they go to the meeting.
  - Help transport residents to and from the meeting if necessary.
- Cooperate in carrying out recommendations of the council that are implemented by the facility administration.

The Right to Participate in Social, Religious, and Community Activities

Social Activities

Someone from the activities staff meets with each resident shortly after admission to the facility. Residents are given an opportunity to express their choices for activities. Monthly calendars are posted in resident rooms and throughout the facility so residents and family members are aware of events for each day. Activities must include:

- Empowerment activities
  - Activities that increase self-respect by providing opportunities for self-expression such as doing artwork or creative crafts
  - Activities that require personal responsibility and choices. Voting is an example of this type of activity. Residents have the right to vote in all local, state, and federal elections. Residents are given the opportunity to vote by absentee ballot or they are taken to the polls.
  - Some facilities may provide for resident access to computers for email or other computer-related activities.
- Maintenance activities
  - Maintenance activities promote physical, mental, social, and emotional health.
  - Maintenance activities include physical exercise, current events discussion groups, picnics, and musical or dramatic presentations.
- Supportive activities
  - Supportive activities provide stimulation to residents with severe mental or physical disabilities who cannot participate in other types of programs.

As a nursing assistant, follow these guidelines for supporting the residents' participation in activities.

- Cooperate with the activities staff schedule of events. Schedule resident care so it does not interfere with the residents' attendance.
- Be aware of the activities that are scheduled. Give residents information if they ask about the nature and time of the activities being offered.

   Residents also have the right to refuse to participate in any of these activities. They can develop their own individual activities, for example, reading or doing needlework or crossword puzzles.

Religious Activities

Worship and religious activities are an important aspect of living in a long-term care facility. Freedom of worship must be allowed for each resident.

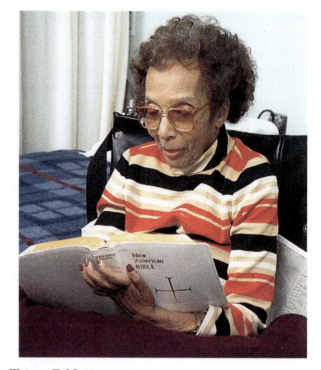

Figure 7-18 The resident has the right to keep religious items in the room.

- Respect the residents' religious beliefs and practices.
- Assist residents to attend church services and other religious activities within the facility.
- Treat religious articles such as Bibles, crucifixes, and rosaries with respect (Figure 7-18).
- Provide privacy for residents' visits with the clergy (such as priest, pastor, or rabbi).
- Allow residents privacy for prayer and meditation.
- Remember that the resident also has the right to not have religious beliefs or practices.

Community Activities

Involvement with the community can be important for the residents' interest and enthusiasm. Many long-term care facilities have large vans or buses with wheelchair access that enable residents to attend community events. These activities might include entertainment, educational, religious, or recreational programs. Groups from the community visit the long-term care facility to provide these events for residents who cannot leave the facility.

The Right to Examine Survey Results and Correction Plans

Surveys of all facilities are completed on a regular basis by regulatory agencies. Federal regulations mandate that the results from the survey must be displayed in a prominent place at all times. The surveyors write up their findings from the survey and if any problems are found, the facility must write a plan of correction that states how the problems will be solved. The resident (or family, if the resident wishes) may inspect these records during normal business hours or by special appointment.

The Right to Manage Personal Funds

This means:

- The resident may request the facility to manage the funds. The resident must give written authorization.
- If the account exceeds $50, it must earn interest, which is given to the resident.

The Right to Information About Eligibility for Medicare/Medicaid Benefits

This means:

- The resident has the right to receive these benefits if the resident is eligible for the benefits, and the facility participates in the programs.

The Right to File Complaints About Abuse, Neglect, or Misappropriation of Property

This means:

- If the resident believes there has been abuse, neglect, or property stolen, the resident can file a complaint with the state agency that inspects the facility.

The Right to Information About Advocacy Groups

An ombudsman seeks to improve the quality of life of residents of long-term care facilities (skilled care, nursing homes, assisted living, and personal care homes). The Ombudsman program is governed by the federal OAA and by state law where the resident resides.

This means that an ombudsman:

- Investigates and works to resolve problems that can affect residents in long-term care settings
- Visits long-term care facilities to talk with residents
- Identifies problems and advocates for change

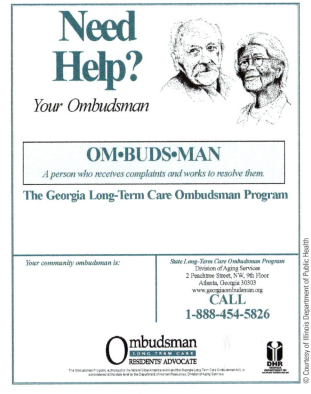

Figure 7-19 Each resident must have access to the hot-line number.

- Investigates and works to resolve problems and/or complaints
- Participates in resident and family council meetings, upon invitation by the Council
- Provides in-service education for staff in long-term care facilities about Resident Rights and other issues
- Promotes involvement in long-term care by residents, families, and community
- Helps to coordinate activities of other agencies concerned with long-term care needs.

The telephone numbers of advocacy groups must be available to residents. Each facility must post a **hot-line number** that can be used to register complaints about a facility or a caregiver (Figure 7-19).

The Right to Unlimited Access for Immediate Family or Relatives

This also includes:

- The long-term care ombudsman
- Government agency representatives
- The attending physician

The resident may also withdraw consent to visit with any of these people.

The Right to Share a Room with Spouse

If spouses are residents in the facility, they may share a room. This may not be possible if there are medical reasons to keep one of the couple in a special unit.

The Right to Perform or Not Perform Work for the Facility

The resident may perform work at the facility if it is medically appropriate for the resident to do so. In addition:

- The resident must formally agree to any work arrangement.
- If the work is for pay, the resident earns the prevailing rate for the services.

The Right to Remain in the Facility

The resident can remain in the facility unless one or more of the following items applies:

- The resident no longer needs the care.
- The resident's welfare requires transfer.
- The facility no longer meets the resident's needs.
- The health or safety of others in the facility is endangered.
- The resident fails to pay for services.
- The facility ceases to operate.
- In these cases, 30 days' notice must be given except when health is improved, there is an emergency, or there is danger to the health or safety of individuals in the facility.

The Right to Use Personal Possessions

Personal possessions means:

- Personal clothing and jewelry (Figure 7-20)
- Personal furnishings when these can be used in accordance with health and safety regulations

The residents' right to retain and use personal possessions ensures that the residents' environment is homelike. Using personal possessions gives residents some control over their lives. The facility is responsible for taking reasonable measures to safeguard residents' belongings. Each resident's record contains a personal possession list. It must be noted on this list any time an item is brought into the facility or any time an item is removed from the facility. Nursing assistant responsibilities include the following:

- Encourage residents to display pictures and family photos in their rooms.

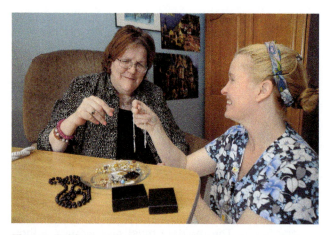

Figure 7-20 Residents can wear their own jewelry and clothing.

- Assist residents to arrange their personal items if they need help.
- Report any lost items immediately and take measures to find the items.
- Do not rearrange furniture in a resident's room without the person's permission, unless there is a valid health or safety reason.
- Do not go through dresser drawers, closets, lockers, or purses without the resident's permission.
- Be careful what you throw out when tidying the room.

The Right to Notification of Change in Condition

This means the facility will notify the resident's attending physician, legal representative, and family member of:

- An accident involving the resident
- A significant change in the resident's condition
- A need to alter treatment significantly
- A decision for transfer or discharge

The members of the interdisciplinary team work together to provide the residents with the rights expressed in this document.

Legal Aspects of Health Care

The Residents' Rights document has a legal foundation. Contained within the document are several rights which, if violated, could result in legal action against the facility or care provider. This action may be a fine or imprisonment for the offender. Each employee is responsible for personal actions. The OBRA legislation requires that a facility report any case of abuse and

? EXERCISE 7-3

COMPLETION 1

Select the correct term(s) from the following list to complete each statement.

asked	exploitation	regularly
cleaned	fed	resident
closed	free	style
covered	labeled	time
death	personal	throw out
equal	personal possessions	

1. When working with a resident, curtains should be _____ for privacy.
2. Residents should be kept _____ as much as possible when giving care.
3. Do not open or read a resident's mail unless _____ to do so by the _____.
4. If a resident is in a terminal condition, then _____ is likely.
5. Psychosocial needs can be met by encouraging residents to make choices of how they use free _____.
6. Residents have the right to wear their hair in a(an) _____ of their own choosing.
7. Incontinent residents must be _____ after each incontinent episode.
8. Residents who cannot feed themselves must be _____ by the staff.
9. Dependent residents must be given fresh water _____ throughout the day.
10. The rights of all residents are _____.
11. Residents are _____ to move about the residence as long as they respect the privacy of others.
12. Residents have the right to bring some _____ items from home.
13. When personal items are brought into the facility, they should be listed on the _____ list.
14. Be careful when tidying a room so as not to _____ personal possessions of value to resident.
15. All personal possessions of a resident should be _____.

? EXERCISE 7-4

COMPLETION 2

Select the correct term(s) from the following list to complete each statement. Some terms may be used more than once.

carry out	exercise	Power of Attorney for Health Care
choose	free	resident
communicating	hotline	right
complaint	living will	self-respect
councils	not	staff
durable	personal	supportive

1. A grievance is a(an) _____ that a resident may have with respect to treatment or care.
2. A(An) _____ allows individuals to state their wishes about discontinuing death-delaying procedures if they have a terminal illness.
3. Resident groups are often called resident _____.
4. Resident councils give staff and residents a method of _____ with one another.
5. The facility is required to name a(an) _____ person to provide assistance and response to the resident council.
6. The nursing assistant cooperates with the resident council by helping to _____ recommendations implemented by administration.
7. Family and visitors also have the _____ to meet with other family members in the facility.
8. Empowerment activities increase _____ and require _____ responsibility and choices.

(continues)

? EXERCISE 7-4 (Continued)

9. Residents who cannot generally benefit from either maintenance or empowerment activities are provided with _____ activities for stimulation.
10. A direct line to a state-appointed agency to report complaints is called the _____.
11. A document that gives legal permission to another person to make medical decisions when a person is unable to make these decisions is called a(an) _____.
12. Any _____ may use the hotline.
13. Advocacy services are _____ of charge.
14. Residents have the _____ to refuse to participate in activities.
15. Residents have the right to _____ the activities in which they wish to participate.
16. Provisions must be made for residents to _____ their right to vote.
17. Residents have a right to _____ have a religious practice or belief.
18. Taking advantage of someone for your own benefit is called _____.

the names of the persons involved. Each state has a designated agency that investigates such reports.

Assault and Battery

Assault and battery are examples of actions that violate the residents' rights and are criminal offenses. Any type of abuse of a resident may be a form of assault or battery. Assault is a threat or an attempt to harm another person. An assault of a resident may lead to a felony. Threatening to restrain a resident if he does not stay in bed is an example of assault. Battery is touching another person without that person's consent. Grabbing a resident to give him a bath when he does not want one is battery. To protect the caregivers, legal permission is required from the resident, family, or legal guardian for certain procedures. This permission must be obtained with the informed consent of the resident. This means the resident fully understands the procedure. This formal consent is not required for routine personal care and procedures. However, you must explain what you are going to do to the resident before you do it. If the resident objects, discuss the situation with the nurse.

False Imprisonment

The unauthorized use of restraints can be considered false imprisonment (detaining an individual without a reason and against that individual's will). Consult the care plan before using restraint devices.

Invasion of Privacy

Violating a resident's right to privacy and confidentiality of personal and medical records is an example of invasion of privacy.

Defamation of Character

If a person spreads false information about a resident, then that person may be guilty of defamation of character. If the false information is verbal or spoken, it is called slander. If it is written, it is called libel.

Neglect

Neglect may also be considered a criminal offense. Neglect is discussed earlier in this lesson.

Theft

The resident has the right to use personal possessions. To take anyone's personal possessions is theft.

You will avoid problems as a health care provider if you:

- Always do the very best job possible.
- Treat the resident with respect.
- Remember the rights of the resident.
- Do only those tasks that you are legally qualified to perform.

Abandonment

Abandonment means leaving or walking off the premises without permission and failing to provide continuity of care. The nursing assistant must notify the nurse if he or she must leave the facility for any reason. If the nursing assistant leaves and an equally qualified person has not been designated as a replacement, the nursing assistant can be accused of abandonment. Loss of CNA certification may be the outcome of this type of action.

? EXERCISE 7-5

BEST ANSWER

Answer the following statements about nursing assistants' actions with A for Appropriate or I for Inappropriate. If the action is inappropriate, write the appropriate action in the space provided.

1. _____ Ms. Blair tells the nursing assistant that Mr. Richards pinches her every time she wheels her chair by him. The nursing assistant ignores the report because she likes Mr. Richards. _____
_____

2. _____ Mr. Jones, a resident, tells Nancy (the nursing assistant) that another nursing assistant roughly turns him so that it hurts. Nancy reports the complaint to the charge nurse. _____
_____

3. _____ Joe, a nursing assistant, notices that every time another nursing assistant begins to give a particular resident care, the resident pulls away and does not want to be touched by the nursing assistant. Joe does nothing because he was not assigned to care for this resident. _____
_____

4. _____ A resident complains to the charge nurse because Mike (a nursing assistant) was rude. Another nursing assistant found this resident wet and soiled even though Mike was supposed to change the resident. The nursing assistant knows that the resident has been neglected but says nothing because Mike is a friend. _____
_____

5. _____ A nursing assistant notices bruises that look like finger marks on a resident's arms. The nursing assistant reports their presence to the charge nurse. _____
_____

Good Samaritan Laws

Health care workers and private citizens who render *emergency aid* to an injured person are protected from civil liability by the Good Samaritan Laws in each state if they are not reimbursed for their services. In most states, a person is not obligated to give first aid unless it is part of their job description. However, any person may be considered negligent if they do not at least call for help.

ETHICS AND THE HEALTH CARE PROVIDER

The term **ethics** refers to principles of conduct or behavior. Every profession has a code of ethics for its members. These codes are especially important in health care. Persons receiving care are dependent on caregivers to meet many of their physical, mental, and emotional needs. Whether you are following the ethics of your profession is determined by the behavior you exhibit while you are working. For example:

- Report for work when scheduled, unless you have a truly justifiable reason for being absent. Your absence may mean that residents will not be given the care they deserve. If you cannot report for work, call in well in advance so a substitute can be found or assignments can be rearranged.

- Report to work on time. When you are late, it can upset the resident's schedule for the rest of the day.

- Health care providers do not accept tips in the form of money or gifts. If these are offered, thank the resident and explain that you are not allowed to accept them.

- Do not take supplies or items that belong to the facility, to residents, or to other staff members.

- Accept your assignments willingly and help others as needed.

- Always be honest. If you make a mistake, report it to your supervisor immediately. If you do not know how to perform a task, ask for help so that you do not harm anyone.

⊘N THE JOB

You may be assigned to work with employees who do not follow the rules of ethical behavior. For instance, if you work with someone who is dishonest or who does not follow skill procedures. How do you report this type of misconduct? You may want to discuss these issues with your supervisor.

- Avoid horseplay, joking around, and loud laughter when you are working. Humor is necessary but should be appropriate. Never make fun of a resident.
- Do not discuss your personal problems at work. If you have problems that may affect your work, discuss them with your supervisor.
- Avoid gossiping and griping. A negative attitude from one person can affect the morale of everyone else.
- Use only language that the resident understands.
- Your physical appearance reflects your attitude. Follow the dress code of your employer and follow the rules of personal hygiene and grooming.

? EXERCISE 7-6

TRUE OR FALSE

Indicate whether the following statements are true (T) or false (F).

1. T F A resident's room should be considered his or her private space.
2. T F If a door is open, it is not necessary to knock or announce your presence before entering.
3. T F It is permissible to read residents' mail that is not sealed.
4. T F It is appropriate to allow a visitor to remain when assisting the resident with the commode.
5. T F The tub room door should be left open during bathing in case you need help.
6. T F It is alright to listen to a resident's telephone conversation in case the resident says something about you and you need to defend yourself.
7. T F Two or more assistants may be present during personal care when the resident is difficult to turn and position.
8. T F When visited by clergy, the resident should be provided with privacy.
9. T F It is alright to leave a resident's door open when giving an enema as long as no visitors are present.
10. T F It is alright to leave a resident's door open when emptying the urinary drainage bag at the end of the shift.
11. T F It is alright to make comments in front of a resident in a language he or she does not understand when the comment has nothing to do with the resident.

? EXERCISE 7-7

IDENTIFICATION 3

Determine the appropriateness of a nursing assistant's behavior by indicating C for Correct or I for Incorrect.

1. _____ listening to visitors' conversations
2. _____ discussing a resident's physical status with a relative
3. _____ making shift reports so that residents cannot hear
4. _____ reading a resident's record to satisfy your curiosity
5. _____ sharing the medical records with the resident's minister
6. _____ telling a resident that his or her roommate has a terminal condition
7. _____ telling another nursing assistant that a resident eats best when fed from the right side
8. _____ sharing information with another staff member that the resident is incontinent
9. _____ telling another resident that a roommate has dirty toenails
10. _____ mentioning that a resident has beautiful white hair to his or her roommate
11. _____ accepting a tip from a resident's family

LESSON SYNTHESIS: Putting It All Together

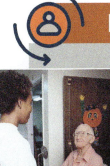

You have just completed this lesson. Now go back and review the Clinical Focus. Try to see how the Clinical Focus relates to the concepts presented in the lesson. Then answer the following questions.

1. Why is it necessary to know and actively protect Mr. Davidson's rights?
2. How do the rights of Mr. Davidson differ from those that every citizen enjoys?
3. What nursing assistant actions would interfere with the rights of a resident?
4. When a resident is unable to make decisions, how may his or her rights be protected?
5. How could you protect Mr. Davidson's right of privacy?

7 REVIEW

A. Select the one best answer for each of the following.

1. The purpose of the Residents' Rights document is to
   (A) separate the resident from the community
   (B) provide a moderately comfortable environment
   (C) help the resident maintain the highest level of well-being possible
   (D) restrict some resident choices

2. The right to free choice means the resident
   (A) will be assigned a room by the facility
   (B) must use one of the facility physicians
   (C) can choose which nursing assistants will provide his or her care
   (D) will be able to read the evaluation report but not participate in care planning

3. An example of mental abuse is
   (A) not taking the resident to the bathroom when she needs to go
   (B) swearing at the resident
   (C) slapping the resident when she refuses to eat
   (D) fondling the resident's breasts

4. Corporal punishment means
   (A) isolating the resident without providing care
   (B) using chemical restraints
   (C) using painful treatment for correction of behavior
   (D) using physical restraints

5. Involuntary seclusion is
   (A) helping the resident to his room and closing the door when the resident wants to lie down
   (B) isolating the resident when it is not part of a therapeutic plan
   (C) placing a resident with a communicable disease in isolation
   (D) giving the resident medication to put him to sleep

6. A chemical restraint
   (A) is a medication that influences behavior
   (B) is any device that enhances the resident's mobility
   (C) has no effect on the resident's behavior
   (D) is administered by the nursing assistant

7. The resident has the right to privacy when

(A) walking down the hall

(B) receiving nursing care or medical treatment

(C) talking to the housekeeper

(D) being served a meal tray

8. The right to confidentiality means

(A) the resident cannot see her chart or medical record

(B) that only the physician can read the chart

(C) information about the resident is available only to those who need it to provide care

(D) that nursing assistants cannot read the chart

9. Accommodation of needs means that the staff must

(A) provide the resident with fresh fruit at every meal

(B) escort the resident to the church of his or her choice

(C) give every resident a private room with bath

(D) assist the resident to maintain personal hygiene and cleanliness

10. Residents are not allowed to

(A) move about the facility

(B) visit other residents

(C) enter another resident's room without permission of that resident

(D) have visitors in their rooms

11. If a husband and wife are both admitted to the facility, they are

(A) not allowed to have sexual activity

(B) allowed to share the same room if their medical conditions permit

(C) expected to help take care of each other

(D) not allowed to have the same physician

12. Providing an environment to meet the needs of the residents means that

(A) the resident can choose the color of his room and drapes

(B) there are permanent grab bars in the bathrooms

(C) there must be wall-to-wall carpeting throughout the facility

(D) the residents' personal furnishings are not allowed

13. A living will provides instructions for

(A) who will inherit the resident's money

(B) how the resident will pay her bill

(C) carrying out the resident's wishes if she has a terminal illness

(D) the resident's funeral in the event of her death

14. A person who has durable power of attorney for health care

(A) must be a lawyer

(B) makes decisions for the resident even if he is able to do so himself

(C) can make health care decisions if the resident is unable to do so

(D) can decide how the resident's money is spent

15. A grievance is a

(A) complaint

(B) sad feeling

(C) lawsuit

(D) casual remark

16. An ombudsman

(A) is the person who has durable power of attorney for health care

(B) visits facilities to make sure residents are receiving adequate care

(C) is the administrator

(D) has an office in the facility

17. The hot-line number is used

(A) by a resident or family member to call a state agency to register a complaint about the facility

(B) to call the fire department in the event of fire

(C) to order meals to be sent in to the resident

(D) by staff members to register complaints about their supervisors

18. Assault is the legal term for

(A) touching another person without consent

(B) a threat or an attempt to harm another person

(C) placing a restraint on a resident

(D) invasion of privacy

19. The term *slander* means

    (A) spreading false information about a resident verbally

    (B) writing false information about a resident

    (C) mental abuse

    (D) false imprisonment

20. Which situation would be considered unethical?

    (A) accepting a tip from a resident

    (B) accepting a homemade cookie from the resident's daughter

    (C) calling in sick when you have an elevated temperature and the flu

    (D) asking another nursing assistant to help you get a heavy resident out of bed

B. Match the resident right (items a–e) with the nursing assistant actions that protect that right.

    a. freedom from abuse

    b. providing privacy

    c. ensuring confidentiality

    d. accommodating individual needs

    e. participation in religious activities

21. _____ encouraging the resident to feed himself

22. _____ frequently visiting a disoriented resident

23. _____ informing the nurse that the resident wishes a visit from a clergy-person

24. _____ knocking before entering a room

25. _____ refusing to discuss one resident's condition with another

26. _____ assisting the resident to the telephone

27. _____ gently handling the resident when turning him

28. _____ leaving all written notes regarding residents in the facility

29. _____ drawing the curtains during a bed bath

30. _____ encouraging residents to choose their own clothing

C. Fill in the blanks by selecting the correct word or phrase from the list.

chemical restraints

empowerment

maintenance

physical restraint

supportive care

31. Medications that affect the resident's behavior and alter thinking are called _____.

32. A device that restricts a resident's movement and does not allow normal access to the body is called a _____.

33. An activity that promotes self-respect by providing opportunities for self-expression is a/an _____ activity.

34. _____ activities promote physical, mental, social, and emotional health.

35. Providing comfort measures to a person who is dying is called giving _____.

LESSON 8
SAFETY

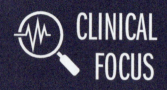

CLINICAL FOCUS

Think about the role the nursing assistant can play in ensuring a safe environment for each resident as you study this lesson.

OBJECTIVES

After studying this lesson, you should be able to:

- Define vocabulary words and terms.
- List the ergonomic factors that may lead to work-related musculoskeletal disorders.
- List the ergonomics techniques you can use to prevent incidents on the job.
- Demonstrate the correct use of body mechanics.
- Describe the types of information contained in Safety Data Sheets (SDSs). Formerly MSDSs or Material Safety Data Sheets, revised in 2012.
- Describe safe equipment use.
- Describe three safety rules for when oxygen is in use.
- Identify residents who are at risk of having incidents.
- Describe four precautions to take when the side rails of the bed are down.
- List three alternatives to the use of physical restraints.
- Describe the guidelines for the use of restraints.
- Differentiate between enablers and restraints.
- Demonstrate the correct application of restraints.
- Describe three measures for preventing resident incidents: accidental poisoning, thermal injuries, skin injuries, falls, and choking.
- List four measures to follow for safe wheelchair use.
- Describe three procedures to follow in the event of fire, tornado, hurricane, or bomb threat.

CASE STUDY

Debra Polluck is a nursing assistant at the Great Neck Nursing Center. Each month, Debra and members of the staff carry out a fire drill. This practice means that they will all be prepared to act promptly in case of a real emergency.

VOCABULARY

aspiration (ass-pih-RAY-shun)
body mechanics (BAH-dee mih-KAN-icks)
chemical restraints (KEM-i-kul ri-STRAINTS)
ergonomics (er-goh-NOM-icks)
incident (IN-sih-dent)
laceration (lass-er-AY-shun)

Material Safety Data Sheet (MSDS) (mah-TEER-ee-alSAYF-tee DAY-tah sheet)
Occupational Safety and Health Administration (OSHA) (ock-you-PAY-shun-alSAYF-tee and helth ad-min-iss-TRAY-shun)
physical restraints (fiz-i-kul ri-STRAINTS)
restraints (ri-STRAINTS)

SAFETY IN HEALTH CARE FACILITIES

A major concern in health care facilities is the prevention of injuries to residents, employees, volunteers, and visitors. An incident (accident) is any unexpected situation that can cause a resident, employee, or any other person harm. Prevention of incidents depends on:

- Employees knowing their jobs and all policies and procedures related to safety
- Maintaining a safe environment
- Knowing the residents and using safety measures to decrease their risk of injury

When an incident occurs, it must be reported immediately to your supervisor who will offer guidance and follow the policy of your facility.

EMPLOYEE SAFETY

Health care workers are required to perform many physical tasks. You must learn how to use your body correctly while you are completing your assignments. This is called using good body mechanics. This means you are using your muscles correctly when you lift or move residents or heavy objects. If you always apply the rules of body mechanics, you will avoid injury to yourself and to the residents.

Ergonomics

The word ergonomics means adapting the environment and using techniques and equipment to prevent injury to the body. The Occupational Safety and Health Administration (OSHA) is a part of the federal government under the Department of Labor. This agency is responsible for overseeing the health and safety of all employees in the country. For health care employees, work-related disorders of the musculoskeletal system are a major concern. These types of injuries can result in permanent disability, preventing the individual from performing job duties and personal responsibilities. Ergonomic programs are designed to prevent injuries

by educating employees about potential hazards of the job, risk factors that may result in injury, techniques to use to prevent injuries, and reporting procedures.

If certain risk factors are present, it is likely that an ergonomic (work-related) problem will occur. These risk factors include:

- Performance of the same motion or motion pattern every few seconds for more than 2 to 4 hours at a time
- Being in a fixed or awkward posture for more than 2 to 4 hours
- Using forceful hand movements for more than 2 to 4 hours at a time
- Doing heavy lifting, unassisted, for more than 1 to 2 hours

The Bureau of Labor Statistics reported that the highest incidence of musculoskeletal disorders (MSD) and injuries are reported among nursing aides, orderlies, and attendants. Because the extent of MSD among U.S. workers is high, the American Nurses Association (ANA) has been instrumental in calling attention to the issue. Even though OSHA requires employers to maintain records of serious workplace illnesses and injuries, the statistics do not reflect the seriousness of the issue. Musculoskeletal disorders are largely the result of repetitive movement over time and are likely to go unreported.

The United States has been slow to adopt a "no lift" policy. The ANA developed the "Handle with Care" program in 2003. This program recommends changes to the nursing curriculum related to lifting procedures, as well as encouraging legislation to discourage the practice. Thus far, 11 states have enacted "Safe Patient Handling." The initiative is referred to as Safe Patient Handling and Movement (SPHM) because the legislation applies to both acute care as well as long-term care settings. As of July 2010, enacted legislation is in place in 11 states and legislation will be introduced in 10 additional states.

The emphasis of the SPHM is to develop programs within a facility that create "no lift" policies and

⚠ GUIDELINES FOR... USING ERGONOMIC TECHNIQUES TO REDUCE THE RISK OF HAVING AN INCIDENT

1. Use correct body mechanics at all times, at work and when you are off duty.

2. Raise the beds to a comfortable working height (remember to lower the beds when you finish your task).

3. Use a mechanical lift (Figure 8-1) when you need to transfer very heavy or dependent residents into or out of bed.

4. Get another person to help when you need to transfer a resident who is not full weight bearing. Use a transfer belt when ordered.

5. Use a cart to move heavy items (Figure 8-2).

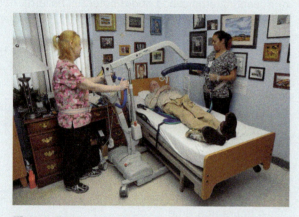

Figure 8-1 Use a mechanical lift to protect your back.

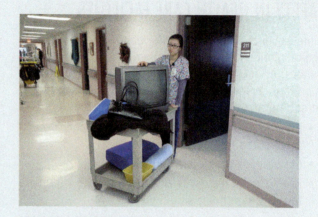

Figure 8-2 Use a cart to move heavy items.

to secure appropriate handling equipment and lifts, trains staff in the proper use of the equipment, and creates a comprehensive injury tracking system of MSD injuries. Implementation of this type of policy can benefit the patient and resident as well by preventing injuries such as skin tears and falls.

Body Mechanics

The use of proper body mechanics at all times can prevent fatigue and body injury. Good body mechanics means to:

- Maintain good standing posture.
  - Stand with your feet flat on the floor.
  - Separate your feet about 12 inches (shoulder width apart).
  - Bend your knees slightly.
  - Keep your back straight.
  - Tighten your abdominal muscles.
- Use the weight of your body to help to push or pull an object.
- Use the strongest muscles to do the job.
  - It is easier to bring the resident or object toward you than to lift the resident or object away from you.

- Use stronger muscles (leg muscles) rather than weaker muscles (back muscles) when lifting, pushing, or pulling.
- Avoid twisting your body and overreaching as you work.
- Avoid bending for long periods of time.
- Use the method that has been ordered to move a resident. For example, if the care plan states that two people are needed to transfer a resident from bed to chair, always get another person to help you.
- Follow the eight commandments of lifting to greatly decrease the risk of injuring yourself:
  - Plan your lift and test the load (Figure 8-3A).
  - Ask for help (Figure 8-3B).
  - Get a firm footing (Figure 8-3C).
  - Bend your knees (Figure 8-3D).
  - Tighten your stomach muscles (Figure 8-3E).
  - Lift with your legs (Figure 8-3F).
  - Keep the load close (Figure 8-3G).
  - Keep your back upright (Figure 8-3H).
- Ask your physician or a physical therapist for specific exercises for the back that can help prevent injuries.

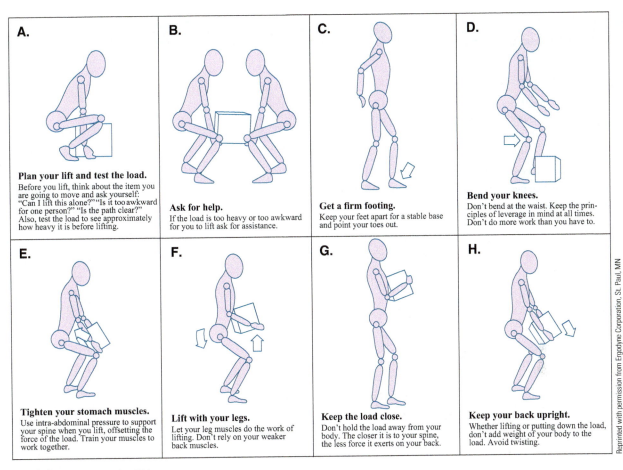

Figure 8-3 Eight rules for lifting.

- Warm up before working to help prevent strains. Perform the exercises shown in Figure 8-4 before each work shift. Remember that you can avoid many problems if you also:
  - Exercise every day. Get outside if possible and take several deep breaths.
  - Eat a nourishing, well-balanced diet.
  - Get adequate sleep.
- Avoid alcohol, tobacco, and drug use and too much caffeine.
- Wear comfortable shoes with good support and nonskid soles.
- Remember that most back injuries can be prevented if you follow the rules for good body mechanics and if you complete all lifting procedures correctly.

? EXERCISE 8-1

TRUE OR FALSE
Indicate whether the following statements are true (T) or false (F).

1. T F *Ergonomics* refers to the resident's ability to pay for health care.
2. T F *Mechanics* refers to using the body like a machine.
3. T F *OSHA* is responsible for overseeing the health and safety of employees.
4. T F When lifting, keep your back straight.
5. T F Bending from the waist rather than the hips or knees provides better control.
6. T F Leg muscles are weaker than back muscles.
7. T F Bending for long periods can be fatiguing.
8. T F Good standing posture includes feet being about shoulder width apart.

(continues)

MULTIPLE CHOICE

Select the one best answer.

9. To decrease the risk of injury when required to lift, you should
   (A) keep your knees straight
   (B) lift with your arms
   (C) flex your back
   (D) tighten your stomach muscles

10. Strains may be avoided if you do some extra activities such as
    (A) diet to keep thin
    (B) exercise every day
    (C) stay up late at night
    (D) wear shoes with heels

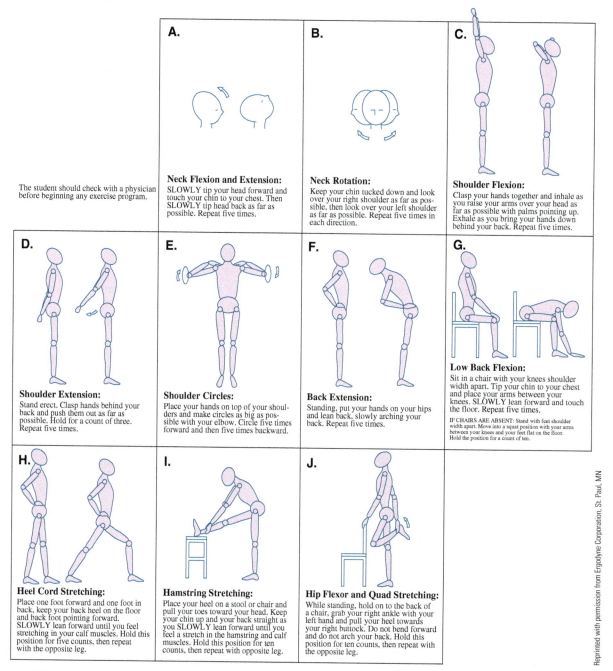

The student should check with a physician before beginning any exercise program.

A. Neck Flexion and Extension:
SLOWLY tip your head forward and touch your chin to your chest. Then SLOWLY tip head back as far as possible. Repeat five times.

B. Neck Rotation:
Keep your chin tucked down and look over your right shoulder as far as possible, then look over your left shoulder as far as possible. Repeat five times in each direction.

C. Shoulder Flexion:
Clasp your hands together and inhale as you raise your arms over your head as far as possible with palms pointing up. Exhale as you bring your hands down behind your back. Repeat five times.

D. Shoulder Extension:
Stand erect. Clasp hands behind your back and push them out as far as possible. Hold for a count of three. Repeat five times.

E. Shoulder Circles:
Place your hands on top of your shoulders and make circles as big as possible with your elbow. Circle five times forward and then five times backward.

F. Back Extension:
Standing, put your hands on your hips and lean back, slowly arching your back. Repeat five times.

G. Low Back Flexion:
Sit in a chair with your knees shoulder width apart. Tip your chin to your chest and place your arms between your knees. SLOWLY lean forward and touch the floor. Repeat five times.

IF CHAIRS ARE ABSENT: Stand with feet shoulder width apart. Move into a squat position with your arms between your knees and your feet flat on the floor. Hold the position for a count of ten.

H. Heel Cord Stretching:
Place one foot forward and one foot in back, keep your back heel on the floor and back foot pointing forward. SLOWLY lean forward until you feel stretching in your calf muscles. Hold this position for five counts, then repeat with the opposite leg.

I. Hamstring Stretching:
Place your heel on a stool or chair and pull your toes toward your head. Keep your chin up and your back straight as you SLOWLY lean forward until you feel a stretch in the hamstring and calf muscles. Hold this position for ten counts, then repeat with opposite leg.

J. Hip Flexor and Quad Stretching:
While standing, hold on to the back of a chair, grab your right ankle with your left hand and pull your heel towards your right buttock. Do not bend forward and do not arch your back. Hold this position for ten counts, then repeat with the opposite leg.

Figure 8-4 Warm-up exercises.

HAZARDS IN THE WORK ENVIRONMENT

Chemical Hazards

All health care facilities have hazards that may injure employees. Many of these items are chemicals that you may have in your own home (e.g., chlorine bleach). A nursing unit may contain cleaning supplies, disinfectants, and other hazardous products. Injuries can be prevented if you know what the hazards are and how to protect yourself and others. OSHA requires that all manufacturers of these items supply Safety Data Sheets (SDS) with all hazardous products they sell. The SDS provide hazard information that explains:

- What precautions to take in the presence of a hazard (e.g., wearing personal protective equipment)
- Instructions for safe use of the potentially dangerous substance
- How to clean up and dispose of the hazardous product
- First aid measures to use if exposure occurs

⊘N THE JOB

It is possible that you will be assigned to work with someone who does not always follow the precautions for preventing work-related injuries. For example, the person may want to take shortcuts in an effort to save time. Remember that, in the end, what little time is saved may result in painful injuries.

OSHA has established other rules for a safe environment. Employers are required to inform employees of:

- The location of the SDS
- The hazards in the work environment and where they are in the building
- The location of information related to the hazards
- How to read and understand chemical labels and hazard signs
- What type of personal protective equipment should be worn if working with these hazards and where the personal protective equipment is stored
- How to manage spills and where cleaning equipment is stored

All hazardous products must be kept in the original container with the original label intact and legible. Long-term care facilities must keep all chemicals in locked cabinets.

Equipment Safety

Learn to use equipment correctly. Report equipment that is broken or in need of repair. Your facility may have a system of tagging equipment that needs repair. The tag will have the words "DO NOT OPERATE." *Never* attempt to use equipment that has been tagged. Your facility designates who is responsible for removing the tag. The equipment is returned to service only after it has been repaired and tested.

- Beds
  - The wheels of the bed should always be locked, unless you need to move the bed.
  - Raise the bed to a comfortable working height when giving resident care.
  - Put the bed in the lowest horizontal position when you are finished giving care.
  - Make sure latch handles on manually operated beds do not stick out.
  - Do not attach restraints, supports, drainage bags, or tubing to side rails.
  - Ensure that all therapeutic, support, and protective devices are attached securely and properly to the bed. These devices include bed cradles, side rail pads, wandering alerts, special mattresses, overhead trapezes, and pads.
- Signal cords (call lights)
  - Check call lights to make sure they are in working order.
  - Residents must always have access to caregivers. If a resident is physically or mentally unable to use a signal cord, the resident must be monitored frequently. The call light must still be within reach.
  - Answer call lights promptly.
- If a resident suffers from arthritis or has difficulty using a traditional call light, soft-touch systems are available that require very little effort to activate. Alarm systems also are available in the form of jewelry, pendants, or watches. If used, chair or bed monitoring systems are cordless and designed to be placed beneath the mattress or chair cushion. These alarm systems are not visible and hence there is less chance of tampering with the system. (See Figure 8-16A–D later in the chapter.)
- Other equipment
  - Use equipment only if you know how to use it correctly.
  - Report needed repairs promptly, such as:
    Lost screws
    Frayed straps or cords
    Loose wheels
    Broken control knobs

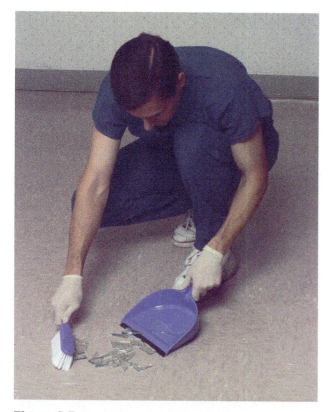

Figure 8-5 Small pieces of glass may be swept into a dustpan using a small brush.

Latches that do not hook
Side rails that do not fasten correctly
Rips or tears in fabric of wheelchair

- Avoid injury from "sharps." These are needles, blades, disposable razors, or instruments that can puncture your skin.
  - Dispose of needles and blades in puncture-resistant, leakproof containers that are labeled or color coded. (This is described further in Lesson 11.)
  - Never handle broken bits of glass with your bare hands. Before cleaning up broken glass, put on disposable gloves or utility gloves. Use a brush and dustpan to sweep up the broken glass. Discard the glass according to facility policy (Figure 8-5).

Oxygen Safety

All health care facilities have oxygen in the building. Oxygen is provided through a system installed in the walls of the facility with outlets in the residents' rooms (Figure 8-6A) or by portable oxygen tanks (Figure 8-6B). Oxygen concentrators are used in many long-term care facilities. These devices use room air to deliver oxygen to residents (Figure 8-7).

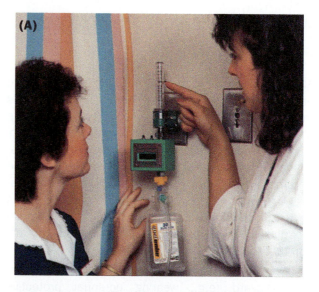

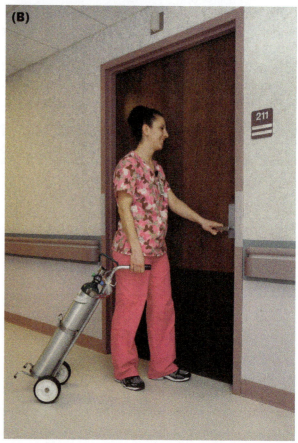

Figure 8-6 (A) Oxygen is piped into the resident's room and attached to a flow meter. (B) Small portable tanks of oxygen are kept on hand.

Oxygen is flammable in the presence of a spark or open flame. For safety when a resident is using oxygen, remember:

- Do not allow smoking.
- Do not use woolen blankets because they can discharge status electricity.

? EXERCISE 8-2

TRUE OR FALSE

Indicate whether the following statements are true (T) or false (F).

1. T F Signal lights must be kept in working order.

2. T F All chemicals and cleaning solutions should be kept in locked cupboards.

COMPLETION

Select the correct term(s) from the following list to complete each statement. Not all terms are used.

raised	hands
comfortable	tightened
locked	flat on floor
wiped	

3. Bed should be _____ to a _____ working height.

4. Before giving care, always be sure the bed is _____.

5. Never handle broken glass with your bare _____.

6. Spills should be _____ up immediately.

? EXERCISE 8-3

MULTIPLE CHOICE

Select the one best answer.

1. MSDS stands for
    (A) medical standard direction sheets
    (B) material safety data sheets
    (C) material standard detection supervision
    (D) medical safety defect supports

2. The MSDS provides communications that explain
    (A) location of the MSDS
    (B) information related to medical diagnosis
    (C) where hazards are in the building
    (D) instructions for safe use of the potentially dangerous substance

3. Hazardous products
    (A) must be kept in the original container with the label intact
    (B) need not be kept in locked closets
    (C) may have a new handwritten label attached when necessary
    (D) may be transferred to smaller unlabeled containers

4. Equipment that is "tagged" should
    (A) always be used first
    (B) not be operated
    (C) be used if no other equipment is available
    (D) none of these

5. When caring for the resident receiving oxygen, remember to
    (A) permit smoking in the room
    (B) turn down oxygen flow rate when using electrical equipment
    (C) not adjust the liter flow rate
    (D) use only woolen blankets

6. The best way to clean up a broken drinking glass is to
    (A) pick up the large pieces with your fingers
    (B) use several thicknesses of damp paper towels in your gloved hand to pick up pieces
    (C) use a broom to sweep pieces into a dustpan
    (D) use a newspaper

- Do not allow an open flame such as matches, lighters, or candles.
- Disconnect oxygen before using electrical equipment.
- Do not adjust the liter flow.
- Be sure the oxygen source (if a tank) is secure.

- Post oxygen safety signs.
- Do not use electric razors in the presence of oxygen.
- Do not use petroleum jelly for dry lips or skin where oxygen is in use.

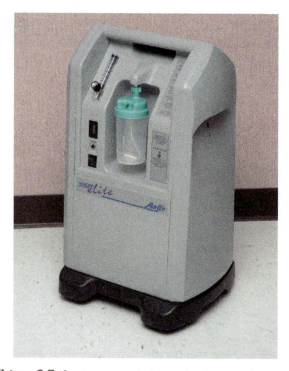

Figure 8-7 Oxygen concentrators extract oxygen from room air for delivery to a resident.

RESIDENT SAFETY

You can contribute to resident safety by performing procedures as taught and correctly following orders. Review the care plans for the residents in your care as soon as you receive your assignments after the shift report. This will allow you to see any changes in the orders for the residents. For example, on your previous shift, a resident was up and about with minimal supervision; now the resident is anxious and disoriented because of a slight stroke during the night.

All staff members in long-term care facilities are responsible for monitoring residents as they move about the building.

Risk Factors for Incidents

Residents in long-term care facilities are at risk for incidents. There are several reasons why residents may have incidents:

- The changes in vision and hearing that most older people experience cause a loss of "warning systems." They are unaware of dangerous situations.
- Problems with mobility result from arthritic changes. These changes cause the joints to be less flexible.
- Dehydration may weaken the resident and lead to confusion that can affect perception.
- Residents may tire more easily. This increases the risk of an incident.

- Inner ear changes can cause a loss of balance and coordination.
- Frequency of urination often leads to fear of incontinence. This can result in unsafe toileting habits.
- Disorientation can cause residents to have poor judgment and an inability to recognize unsafe conditions.
- Some elderly persons experience dizziness when they stand up too quickly. This can cause them to fall.
- Certain medications can affect mental status, balance, and coordination.
- Residents may use assistive mobility devices (canes, walkers) unsafely.
- Residents who suffer from a form of dementia, such as Alzheimer's disease, may be more prone to incidents.

Restraints

Restraints (safety or protective devices) were used to prevent injury to the resident. However, it is rare to see a restraint of any type used in a long-term care facility any longer. This is because the risks of harm far outweigh any benefit. At times, a restraint may be applied to a specific body part to prevent removal of tubes or wound coverings, or to maintain anatomical alignment to prevent deformity. Restraints are classified as physical or chemical.

Physical restraints are defined as any technique or device (physical or mechanical) attached or adjacent to the resident's body that cannot be easily removed by the client. Physical restraints restrict freedom of movement and normal access to one's own body. Federal regulations prevent the use of physical restraints without a specific physician's order with a limited time frame. **Chemical restraints** are any medications (drugs) that are used in order to prevent harm to the resident or to others. These drugs control the resident's mood or behavior, are not required to treat the resident's medical condition. Licensed nurses and advanced care practitioners are authorized to administer medications. This section focuses on the use of physical restraints, as well as enablers and restraint alternatives and the responsibilities of the nursing assistant.

In the past, restraints were routinely used as preventive measures to avoid falls. As mentioned, research has shown that restraints pose greater risks than benefits. The negative consequences of restraint use may lead to serious injury and even death. There is no study that has shown the use of restraints to be beneficial. Restraints should *only* be used for physical safety of the resident and *only* with a physician's order. *Never* use restraints to relieve staff workload, as a form of discipline, or as an alternative to treating an underlying medical problem. With the passage of the OBRA regulations, definitions as to the use of physical and chemical restraints in long-term care facilities have been clearly outlined. The Residents' Rights state that "residents have the right to be free from physical and chemical restraints." Many devices qualify as restraints if the resident does not have the physical or mental ability to easily remove the restraint. Examples of restraints include:

- Wrist/arm
- Vests
- Jackets
- Hand mitts (Figure 8-8)
- Geriatric and cardiac chairs (Figure 8-9)
- Wheelchair safety belts, boards, and tables (Figure 8-10)
- Bed rails (if they meet the definition of a restraint)

Restraints are medical devices. They should never be used as a form of punishment or for the convenience of the nursing staff. Restraint application must be considered very seriously and avoided

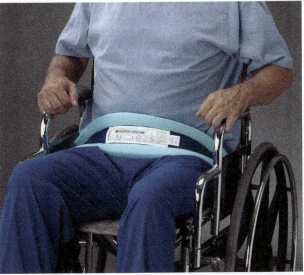

Figure 8-10 Wheelchair safety belts, bars, and tables are considered restraints if the resident does not have the physical or mental ability to remove them.

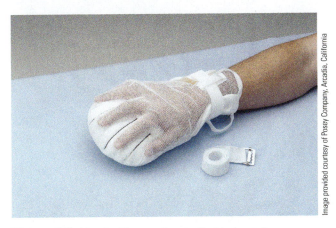

Figure 8-8 Hand mitts may be applied to keep the resident from injuring himself or pulling on tubes.

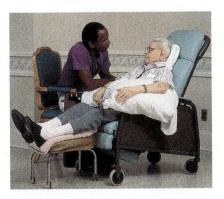

Figure 8-9 Geriatric chairs are restraints in some circumstances.

whenever possible. Potential complications associated with the use of restraints are listed in Table 8-1.

If restraints are indicated, *the least restrictive restraint required to keep the resident safe should be selected.* The restraint should be used as infrequently as possible. Using restraints requires careful assessment, planning, and monitoring. Studies have proved that it takes more time to care for residents in restraints than to care for residents who are not restrained. The physician must agree to the use of the restraints and write an order before they can be used. The care plan will provide information about the type of restraint to use, the time the restraint is to be applied, and other special information and instructions. Refer to the guidelines for using restraints. Restraints are rarely used in long term care facilities and must be ordered and approved by a physician.

Before using restraints, the staff must assess the resident's capabilities and the reasons for use of the restraint. If the cause of the problem can be identified and corrected, the need for a restraint may be eliminated. For example, if restraints are being considered to prevent falls, the resident's individual risk factors associated with falls are assessed. Some risk factors can be eliminated or modified; this reduces the risk of falls and restraints may not be necessary. An elderly male resident who is unsteady on his feet may get up to use the bathroom at night, but does not call for help. His risk of falls may be modified by making sure his urinal is within reach and emptied regularly.

Potential Physical Problems	Potential Psychosocial Problems
Decreased independence	Worsening of behavior problems
Increased dependence on staff	
Pressure ulcers	Withdrawal, loss of social contact
Weakness	
Decreased range of motion	Depression
Muscle wasting	Forgetfulness
Contractures (frozen, deformed joints)	Fear
Loss of ability to ambulate	Anger
Edema of ankles, lower legs, feet, fingers	Shame
	Agitation
Decreased appetite, weight loss	Mental confusion
Dehydration	Combativeness
Distended abdomen	Restlessness
Urge to void frequently, dribbling	Sense of abandonment
Incontinence	
Urinary tract infection	Loss of self-esteem
Constipation	Crying
Fecal impaction	Screaming, yelling, calling out
Lethargy	
Shortness of breath	Loss of dignity
Pneumonia	Boredom
Bruising, redness, cuts	Feelings of hopelessness
Falls	
Impaired circulation	Feelings of helplessness
Blood clots	
Choking	Irritability
Death	Ritualistic behavior

Table 8-1 Complications of Restraints

Enablers

Devices that empower residents and assist them in functioning at their highest possible level are referred to as enablers (Figures 8-11, 8-12, and 8-13). The use of an enabler may help improve the resident's self-esteem by allowing the person to perform activities for himself that would normally require assistance by staff members. Postural supports that are used to maintain body position and alignment are considered to be enablers unless they fit the description of a restraint.

Enablers frequently function as restraint alternatives. The wheelchair lap tray is a restraint alternative that is also used as an enabler. The tray is simple to use: it is attached to the back of the wheelchair with Velcro straps. Residents can lean on the tray, and its surface can hold personal items or reading and writing supplies. The tray may enable the resident to feed herself by moving the food closer so she can reach it. The tray also reminds the resident not to stand up. If the tray allows the resident to perform a task, it is an enabler. If it is used strictly to keep the resident in

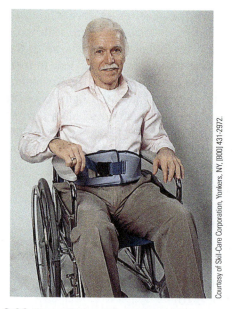

Figure 8-11 The self-release belt serves as a reminder to call for help before rising. It is not a restraint if the resident has the physical and mental ability to release the Velcro fastener.

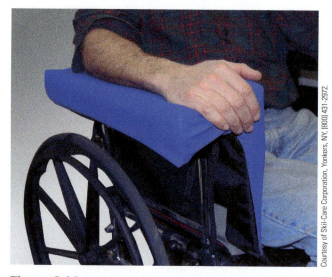

Figure 8-12 Some residents lean to the side, necessitating restraint to keep them upright in the chair. The lateral armrest supports and keeps the resident upright, making restraint unnecessary.

the chair, and he does not have the physical or mental ability to remove the tray, it is considered a restraint. If the tray can be removed by the resident, it is a restraint alternative (Figure 8-14).

Side Rails as Restraints

By definition, side rails are restraints. However, when the top two side rails are in the up position, many residents use the rails to position and turn themselves in bed. In that instance, the side rails act as an enabler or a positioning device.

Courtesy of Skil-Care Corporation, Yonkers, NY, (800) 431-2972.

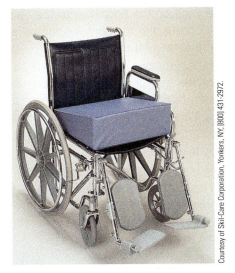

Figure 8-13 Some residents slide forward to the edge of the chair and must be restrained to keep their hips back. The wedge cushion prevents sliding. A piece of gripper can be placed on top of the wedge for additional security.

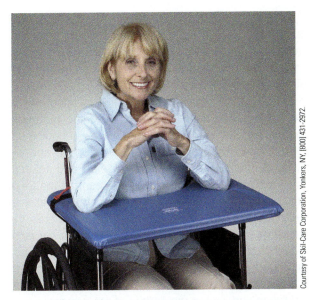

Figure 8-14 The lap tray is an enabler if it improves function, permitting the resident to eat independently. This tray has a soft, a nonslip surface that holds the dishes in place. The tray is a restraint if it is used to keep the resident in the chair and she cannot remove it by herself.

? EXERCISE 8-4

BRIEF ANSWERS
Provide brief answers to complete each statement.

1. Physical restraints are any device that:
   a. _____
   b. _____
   c. _____

2. Types of physical restraints include:
   a. _____
   b. _____
   c. _____
   d. _____
   e. _____
   f. _____

3. The nursing staff must understand what the restraint order covers in regard to:
   a. _____
   b. _____
   c. _____
   d. _____

4. Devices that empower residents and assist them to function at their highest possible level are referred to as enablers. List at least four types of devices that may be enablers.
   a. _____
   b. _____
   c. _____
   d. _____

As mentioned earlier, studies have shown that serious injuries can occur if residents attempt to climb over side rails and fall. This is a common cause of fractures in confused, elderly residents. Leaving the side rails down may be a safer alternative.

If a quarter side rail is used, it is important to check the space between the rail and the mattress. Hospital-type beds are permanent pieces of equipment that are used for years. Mattresses wear out and are replaced. There have been cases of injury and death in which residents became trapped between the mattress and the side rails because the replacement mattress was not the same size as the original. *Make sure the gap between the mattress and the side rail is not large enough to cause injury.* Figure 8-15 shows areas of potential entrapment. Padded foam barriers may be used to reduce the space between the mattress, side rails, and bed frame and lessen the danger of entrapment.

Facilities and commercial manufacturers have developed many excellent alternatives to the use of side rails. Each resident's care plan will provide instruction regarding the use of restraints, side rails, or alternative devices. *The nurse will give you clear instructions before asking you to apply a device of any type to the resident.* Make the environment as safe and user-friendly as possible. Other possible alternatives to the use of side rails include:

- Using a bed that can be raised and lowered close to the floor
- Keeping the bed in the lowest possible position with the wheels locked

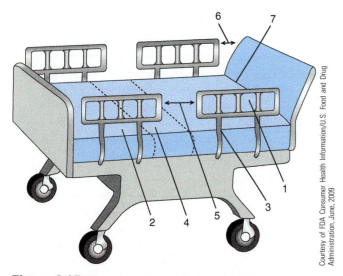

Figure 8-15 Entrapment between the mattress and the side rail occurs in one of the following 7 bed system zones: (1) through the bars of an individual side rail (zone 1); (2) through the space between split side rails (zone 5); (3) between the side rail and mattress (zones 2, 3, and 4); or (4) between the headboard or footboard, side rail, and mattress (zones 6 and 7).

Courtesy of FDA Consumer Health Information/U.S. Food and Drug Administration, June, 2009

- Placing mats on the floor next to the bed so that if a fall occurs, the resident will fall on a padded surface instead of the hard floor
- Anticipating reasons the resident will use to get up from the bed, including the need to use the bathroom, hunger, thirst, restlessness, and pain; meeting these needs promptly and providing calm interventions when you are in the room
- Using side rail bolster cushions
- Using pressure-sensitive alarms that emit a sound when a resident attempts to get up (Figure 8-16A–D). These must be used selectively as the noise can startle and anger some residents, causing them to strike out or become combative.

Alternatives to the Use of Restraints

Alternatives to restraints should be tried before restraints are even considered. Restraints are used only as a last resort when the resident may harm himself or others. Nursing assistants can perform a number of actions to help reduce the need for restraints.

- Care for residents' personal needs promptly.
- Take residents to the bathroom regularly.
- Provide adequate food and fluids to prevent hunger and thirst.
- Report signs and symptoms of pain or illness promptly.
- Follow all instructions for positioning and for assisting residents with exercise.
- Be sure the residents have their eyeglasses and hearing aids if they need them.
- Answer call signals promptly.
- Check residents often to see if they need anything.
- Provide appropriate exercise and activities (Figure 8-17).
- Know which residents are at risk for falling. Monitor these residents regularly during your shift.
- Observe residents who walk and transfer independently. Sometimes falls occur because residents use incorrect or unsafe methods. Report these situations and learn how to teach residents the correct way. Therapy is often called upon to evaluate gait issues.
- Report immediately any physical or mental change that could increase the risk of an incident, such as:
  - Disorientation (resident does not know time, place, or self)
  - Complaints of dizziness
  - Problems with balance and coordination
- Maintain a safe, quiet, calm, environment.

⚠ GUIDELINES FOR... USING RESTRAINTS

- Each facility has policies and procedures for the use and application of restraints. Know and follow your facility policies.
- Restraints are never used for staff convenience. They are used in rare cases for the safety of the resident and others.
- Restraints are applied only with a physician's order and for a specific medical reason.
- The resident and family should clearly understand the purpose of the restraint. Emphasize safety; restraints are not used for punishment.
- The need for restraints is assessed by members of the interdisciplinary team, and alternatives are considered.
- The least restrictive type of restraint is used to keep the resident safe.
- The restraint is applied for the least time possible.
- Restraints are applied only according to manufacturers' directions.
- The proper size restraint must be used for the resident's weight and body size.
- Check the care plan for instructions on using restraints. The care plan will specify the type of restraint to use, the length of time it is to be applied, the reason for the restraint, when to release the restraint, and any special information.
- Check the restraint before using it. If it is worn, torn, cut, or frayed, discard it and obtain another restraint that is in good repair.
- Restraints used on the torso area of the body are always applied over clothing. They should not be applied directly against the skin. Extremity restraints are applied either over or under clothing on the arms and legs, but are padded to prevent restriction of circulation.
- The restraint straps should be smooth. Avoid twisting.
- When applying a restraint to a female resident, make sure the breasts are not under the strap to the restraint.
- After a restraint is applied, check the fit by slipping two or three fingers under the strap to be sure it is not too loose or too tight.
- The skin under the restraint is closely monitored to observe for signs of redness, irritation, or breakdown from the restraint.
- Check the skin above and below the restraint for signs of impaired circulation, such as blue or abnormal color and swelling.
- If the resident is restrained in the chair, the feet must be supported to prevent pain and circulatory problems.
- Restraints are tied in slipknots or bows so the health care provider can release them quickly in an emergency.
- The resident should be positioned using good body mechanics and good posture while in a restraint. Props and supports may also be necessary to keep the resident in good alignment.
- When the resident is restrained in a chair, the hips should be kept back. The purpose of the restraint is to keep the hips down. Restraint straps applied to the waist area instead of the hips may be incorrectly applied. Check the manufacturer's recommendations. The restraint should be at a 45° angle to keep the hips back.
- Most restraints are tied under the chair to the frame. Avoid tying them around the back of the chair, unless the manufacturer's directions clearly give this direction.
- When the resident is restrained in a wheelchair, the brakes should be locked when the chair is parked. The large part of the small front wheels of the chair should face forward. This changes the center of gravity of the chair, making the chair more stable and preventing tipping. The resident's feet should be supported.
- Facility policies vary on visual checks of residents in restraints, but a general rule is that the resident should be visually checked every 15 minutes while restrained.
- The resident should have the call signal, water, and other needed items within reach while restrained. Provide an alternative type of call signal, such as a manual bell, if the resident cannot use the regular call signal.
- The restraint is released every 2 hours for 10 full minutes. During this time the resident is repositioned, exercised, ambulated, and taken to the bathroom.
- Report any changes in behavior or side effects from the restraint.
- Restraint use must be recorded on the medical record. A flow sheet is commonly used for this purpose.

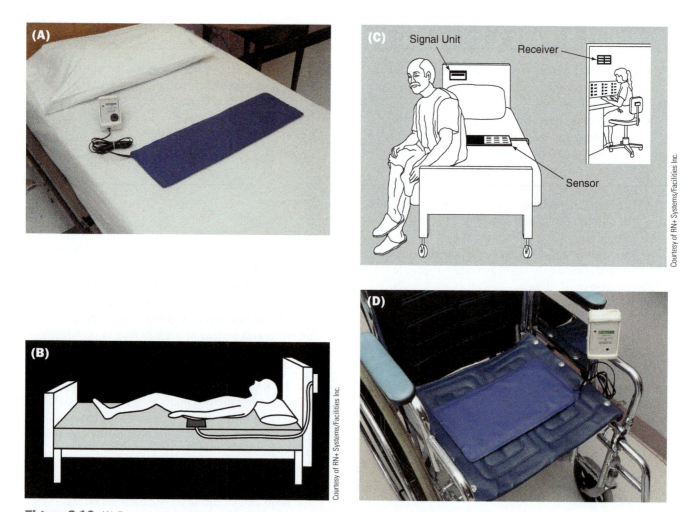

Figure 8-16 (A) Pressure-sensitive pads emit an alarm when a resident attempts to get up. (B) The pressure-sensitive pad is placed under the sheet. (C) The pressure-sensitive pad is placed under the sheet. The signal unit is placed in the room. When the resident relieves pressure from the pad, a distinctive alarm sounds at the desk. The alarm sound is optional in the resident's room. (D) This pressure-sensitive pad is placed on the seat of a wheelchair. When resident attempts to rise, the alarm will sound.

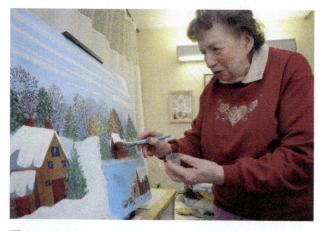

Figure 8-17 Providing appropriate activities can reduce the need for restraints.

- Provide comfortable chairs. Use supportive devices as necessary.
- Use security devices that are designed to prevent falls and eliminate the need for restraints. These devices are described earlier in this section.
- Use magnetic sensor bracelets (Figure 8-18) for residents who are able to walk around unaided but may encounter harm by wandering from the facility or into dangerous areas. The bracelet is usually applied to the dominant wrist, and it sets off an alarm if the resident crosses the magnetic detector. If a resident can self-disable a body alarm system, it is futile to attempt to use this type of system. Reassess the resident at frequent intervals for falls and monitor for wandering.

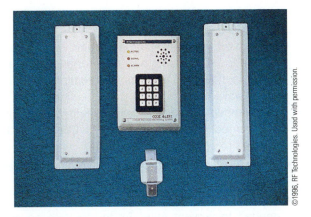

©1996, RF Technologies. Used with permission.

Figure 8-18 The magnetic sensor bracelet is used to allow cognitively impaired residents to wander within the unit. The door alarm will sound if the resident tries to exit.

The inappropriate use of restraints or safety devices can lead to physical and psychosocial complications. The nursing assistant plays an important role in knowing the residents' needs and making recommendations for restraint alternatives.

Preventing Accidental Poisoning

Residents who are disoriented may eat poisonous substances. Persons with dementia may eat or drink items that other residents have in their rooms, such as shaving lotion, cologne, nail polish, denture cleaning tablets, and plants. Residents may store food in their rooms until it spoils. Because of poor vision and reduced ability to taste and smell, they are unaware of spoilage. To prevent accidental poisonings:

- Keep all chemicals and cleaning solutions in locked cupboards (OSHA requirement).
- Use only nonpoisonous plants in the facility.
- The facility may provide residents with refrigerator space for perishable food items. Label containers with the residents' names, room numbers, and

---

? EXERCISE 8-5

COMPLETION

Select the correct term(s) from the following list. Complete the statements in the spaces provided to indicate ways to protect residents from abuse and provide proper care when residents are restrained.

ambulated	order
breakdown	quickly
call signal	redness
exercised	repositioned
feet	slipknot
impaired circulation	toileted
least restrictive	2
irritation	15 to 30
manufacturer's	water

1. When residents are restrained, the _____ type of restraint is used to keep the resident safe.

2. The physician must write a(an) _____ for the restraint.

3. The restraint must always be applied following the _____ directions.

4. All restraints must be able to be released _____ in an emergency.

5. Most restraints should be tied in a _____.

6. If the resident is restrained in a chair, the _____ must be supported.

7. Restrained residents must be checked every _____ minutes.

8. The restrained resident must be released every _____ hours.

9. The restraint is released every 2 hours for 10 minutes, during this time the resident is: _____, _____, _____, and _____.

10. Check skin above and below the restraint for signs of _____.

11. The skin under the restraint should be observed for _____, _____, and _____.

12. Give the resident _____. Always place the _____ within the resident's reach.

date. Remind residents that food is being kept for them in the refrigerator.

Preventing Thermal Injuries

Thermal injuries (those caused by heat or cold) occur less frequently than other injuries but are still a source of concern.

- Follow procedures accurately when administering warm or cold treatments.
- Water temperature is usually regulated but check it before placing a resident in the tub or shower. Turn the hot water on last and turn it off first.
- Check food temperatures before feeding residents. Using a microwave oven to reheat food can be dangerous because of the uneven temperatures. If residents have tremors (shaking of the hands), use a special cup or fill the cup only half-full with a hot liquid to prevent accidental spills.
- Store smoking materials in a safe place and supervise residents while they smoke.

Preventing Skin Injuries

Residents may receive lacerations (cuts or breaks in the skin) or skin punctures. To prevent these injuries:

- Store knives, scissors, razors, and tools in locked cupboards.
- Store needles and syringes in locked cupboards. Syringes and needles should be disposed of immediately after use in the proper sharps container.
- Clean up broken glass immediately, using the methods described earlier.

Preventing Falls

It is estimated that each year 50% to 60% of all residents in long-term care facilities fall. To reduce the number of falls, the environment can be altered to meet the needs of elderly persons. In Section 4, you will learn more about the changes of aging and how to adapt the environment to these changes.

- Do not obstruct open areas with supplies and equipment. Place equipment on one side only of the hallway so residents do not have to navigate through an obstacle course.
- Wipe up spills immediately.
- Encourage residents to use rails along corridor walls when walking.
- Monitor residents for signs of weakness, fatigue, dizziness, and loss of balance. Observe their

actions to detect unsafe habits. Give instructions when necessary:

- Residents who self-propel their wheelchairs need instructions on how to enter and leave elevators, how to use ramps, and reminders to use the brakes.
- Dependent residents may benefit by learning some techniques of self-transfer. Check with the nurse to see if this is possible.

- Provide adequate lighting in all resident areas. Avoid glare.
- Rearrange furniture in the resident's room as needed to prevent falls. Try to simulate an environment as close to their home environment as possible.
- Eliminate noise and other environmental distractions. Noise can increase confusion and create anxiety even in alert individuals.
- Do not leave residents alone in the tub or shower. All tubs and showers should have chairs so residents can remain seated throughout the procedure. Lifts for tubs minimize the risk of injuries in getting in and out of the tub. Avoid using oils that make the tub bottom slippery.
- Check residents' clothing for fit. Loose shoes and laces, long robes, and slacks that drag on the floor increase the risk of falling. Residents should always wear properly fitted, nonskid shoes when walking and during standing transfers. Some residents may prefer to wear "gripper" socks at night.
- Side rails are a frequent cause of falls. This is discussed earlier in this section.
- Care for residents' personal needs promptly. This may prevent residents from attempting unsafe transfers or ambulation.
- Always use the correct techniques for transferring residents. Use a gait belt (transfer belt) when it is ordered. Use lift sheets when moving residents in bed to prevent skin tears from friction.
- Use of body alarms for residents who wander may be effective.
- Be certain the resident wears his or her glasses and hearing aids if indicated. The facility is required to make sure the resident has been evaluated by an audiologist and an eye doctor to assure that they have optimum eye and hearing functions.

Preventing Choking

Aspiration is the accidental entry of food or a foreign object into the trachea (windpipe). This causes the resident to choke. Because swallowing becomes

EXERCISE 8-6

TRUE OR FALSE
Indicate whether the following statements are true (T) or false (F).

1. T F *Lacerations* refer to a nursing assistant's physical abuse to a resident.
2. T F Because temperatures are regulated in facilities, there is no need to check water before placing a resident in a tub.
3. T F Residents are adults, so they do not need supervision when smoking.
4. T F Reheating food in the microwave oven can be unsafe because of uneven heating.

COMPLETION
Select the correct term(s) from the following list to complete each statement. Not all terms are used.

falls	locked	brakes
method	gloves	ramps
handrails		

5. Residents should be encouraged to use _____ along corridor walls when walking.
6. Residents who self-propel wheelchairs need instruction on how to use _____ and reminders to use the _____.
7. Noise can contribute to confusion that can contribute to _____.
8. Use the _____ that has been ordered to move a resident.

---

less efficient as people age, choking occurs more often in the elderly. Residents with dementia have an increased risk of choking. To prevent incidents of choking or aspiration:

- Be aware of residents who have problems with swallowing. Follow all instructions for giving feeding assistance to these residents.
  - Cut food into small pieces.
  - Feed slowly.
  - Offer fluids carefully between solid foods.
  - If the resident has had a stroke, place the food in the unaffected side of the mouth.
  - Use drinking straws judiciously; the resident may be predisposed to aspiration.
  - Make sure dentures fit well.
  - Remind residents to swallow.
  - Incorporate findings from swallowing studies for individual residents: know high-risk foods and thicken liquids as instructed.
- Place residents upright in good position before meals. Have them remain in this position for at least 30 minutes after eating.
- At the end of the meal, give oral care to residents who are known to keep food in their mouths. Food may remain in the mouth for several minutes after a meal and be accidentally aspirated if the resident coughs.

- Monitor disoriented residents for placing nonedible items in their mouths. Remove such items from the environment.
- Know how to administer the procedure for obstructed airway (see Lesson 9).

WHEELCHAIR SAFETY

Many residents can propel their own wheelchairs. This increases their independence and allows them to move from one part of the facility to another. Whether a resident can propel a wheelchair or a care provider does it, safety measures must be followed.

- Place the casters (smaller front wheels) in forward position for balance and stability.
  - To do this, go forward and then back up so the casters swing to the forward position.
  - Remind the resident to keep the wheelchair locked when it is not moving and when the resident wishes to get up or sit down.
  - The footrests must be removed when the resident is getting in or out of the wheelchair. Footrests are usually removed if the resident can propel the wheelchair independently by foot.
- It is not safe for the resident in a wheelchair to attempt to pick up an object from the floor. If the

resident has a reaching aid or "grabber," then small items can be picked up. The wheelchair should be moved next to the object to be picked up and the small front wheels turned forward and the large wheels locked. The resident should not attempt to pick up an item using a reaching aid by leaning over and reaching between the knees. If the resident does not have a reaching aid, the resident should be instructed to ask for assistance in picking up an object from the floor.

- A wheelchair should never be used as a seat in a motor vehicle unless the vehicle is equipped for wheelchairs.
- If a resident does not use the foot pedals on the wheelchair because they self-propel themselves using their feet, make sure the resident is aware to hold their feet up if they are being pushed by another person. Failure to lift the legs may result in serious foot, ankle, or leg injury. If the feet are caught by some obstruction on the floor it is also possible for the resident to be thrown from the wheelchair.
- Use care when pushing a resident through a doorway to ensure that toes and feet do not hit the door frame. In order to prevent arm and hand injury, keep the resident's hands in their lap and elbows inside the armrests when pushing the resident through a doorway.
- A wheelchair should be pulled backwards through outside doorways, on to elevators and down ramps.
- Most long-term care facilities have been designed for wheelchair use. However, if it is necessary to manipulate curbs, ramps, or enter elevators with a wheelchair, be sure to back the wheelchair down the curb or ramp and back the wheelchair into and out of the elevator.

FIRE SAFETY

Three things are needed to start a fire: heat, fuel, and oxygen (Figure 8-19). Every staff member must know and practice the fire and evacuation procedures for the facility.

- You must know:
  - The facility fire procedure
  - Evacuation routes
  - Locations of extinguishers, fire alarms (call boxes), fire doors, and fire escapes
  - How to use fire extinguishers
- Participate in facility fire drills.
- Be alert to fire hazards and report:
  - Frayed electrical wires
  - Overloaded circuits

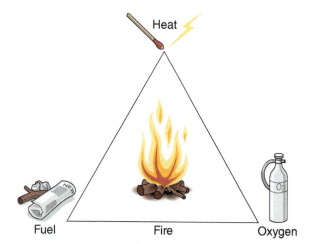

Figure 8-19 The fire triangle represents the elements needed for combustion (burning).

  - Improperly grounded plugs
  - Accumulated clutter
  - Inadequate steps to prevent fire during oxygen therapy
  - Uncontrolled smoking
  - Matches and cigarette lighters
  - Unsafe smoking habits of staff, residents, or visitors
  - Oily rags and paint rags
- Remember the *RACE* steps if fire occurs (Figure 8-20):
  - *Remove* all residents, staff, and other people in the immediate vicinity of the fire.
  - *Activate* the alarm and notify other staff members that a fire exists.
  - *Contain* the fire and smoke by closing all doors in the area.
  - *Extinguish* the fire, if it is very small, or allow fire department to extinguish fire.
- Be sure that you know evacuation procedures:
  - Read evacuation plan.
  - Know the whereabouts of residents in your care.
  - Know the method of transport for residents in your care.
  - Know emergency exit routes.

R	Remove resident
A	Activate alarm
C	Contain fire
E	Extinguish (put out) fire

Figure 8-20 The RACE system: Remember the sequence of critical actions in case of a fire.

Safety in the long-term care facility is the responsibility of all staff members. Teamwork prevents injuries to employees and residents.

Fire Extinguishers

There are many different types of fire extinguishers. Each is used for a different type of fire:

- Type A extinguishers are filled with water and are used to put out paper and wood fires.
- Type B extinguishers are used for grease and oil fires.
- Type C extinguishers are used for electrical fires.
- Extinguishers marked ABC may be used on all three types of fires.

It is important that you learn:

- The location of the extinguishers
- The type of fire for which they are used
- How to use them properly. Always carefully follow the manufacturer's instructions for the use of a fire extinguisher.

SAFETY ISSUES FOR DISASTERS/THREATS

Many emergency situations require rapid and effective responses from the staff. Tornados, hurricanes, earthquakes, floods, and bomb threats are examples of disasters that are possibilities in various parts of the country. Each facility should have its own procedures for dealing with these emergencies. You should become familiar with the procedures as quickly as possible.

Should evacuation from the facility or even within the facility be required, remember that altering the routine and environment for the resident is likely to be traumatic. Many residents may have difficulty communicating or moving; there is the potential for injury and/or psychological distress. Try to remain calm as you carry out your duties. In most facilities, the staff will immediately be assigned to 12-hour shifts. All staff remains at the facility until replacement staff provides relief. Sometimes this may entail of staying at work for 24 hours or longer. Periods of respite are provided to the staff during this time.

Natural Disasters

Tornados

Tornados can occur anywhere if the atmospheric conditions are right. Become familiar with the policies for caring for residents during a natural disaster situation. An alert, either a tornado watch or tornado warning, is issued by the National Weather Service. A *tornado watch* means that the weather conditions are such that a tornado may develop. When a tornado has actually been spotted in an area, a *tornado warning* is issued. During a tornado watch, someone is designated to monitor all weather updates, but the residents are not evacuated. Once a tornado warning is reported, residents are moved to the safest areas in the facility, usually internal hallways away from windows. Because tornados strike with little or no warning, it is important to quickly carry out the evacuation procedures.

Each facility will conduct periodic drills of the procedures to follow in the event of an emergency like a tornado, so that you may become familiar with your responsibilities. Always protect the resident from debris (flying glass). Move the residents away from windows to the designated area. You may be instructed to cover the resident with blankets to further protect them from injury. Residents may be transported in their beds or wheelchairs depending upon their mobility status. Always close all windows and doors, including the fire doors. Power failures are common during severe storms, so it is important that you know the location of flashlights to use during the emergency.

Hurricanes

Unlike tornados, hurricanes can be predicted, so there is adequate time to prepare for evacuation before the hurricane strikes. All facilities in coastal areas prone to hurricanes have an agreement with another facility that is located further inland to temporarily house the residents who may be displaced because of the storm. If the facility management gives the order to evacuate, the residents, medications, and charts are all moved to the safer location. Follow evacuation procedures as outlined by the management.

If residents are not evacuated, they are moved to interior hallways or rooms to protect them from flying debris, as during a tornado watch. Close all resident room doors as well as fire doors, but avoid blocking emergency exits.

Earthquakes

The earth shakes or trembles during an earthquake. Building destruction and fires are sometimes caused by severe earthquakes. Because earthquakes occur suddenly and without warning, broken glass and various objects in the environment can fly around. If you should experience an earthquake, remain calm. Protect yourself by standing in a doorway (within the door frame) or take cover under a heavy object.

Following the earthquake, check the residents for potential injury. Do not move an injured resident unless you are instructed to do so by the nurse and the resident is in danger. Mop any spills from the floor to prevent falls by employees and residents. Use flashlights for light and battery-operated radios for updates of the emergency information. Avoid using electrical appliances, candles, smoking cigarettes, or open flames of any kind because of the danger of ruptured gas lines. Be prepared for aftershocks following the initial earthquake; these may occur in the hours or days following the initial tremors. Follow the disaster plan for your agency following such an occurrence.

Floods

The potential for flooding may lead to the necessity of evacuating the facility. Residents may be relocated to other, safer areas within the facility or to other facilities in the area. During a flooding event there is likely to be disruption if basic utilities such as, gas, electricity, telephone, and water. Facilities that are known to be located in a "flood plain" area should have bottled water available for use until a supply of safe drinking water is available. Water for external use will also be in short supply. Disposable linens may need to be used until there is sufficient water to provide for adequate laundry activities.

Power Outages Caused by Natural Disasters

Disruption in power is common with many types of storms and other natural disasters. The CNA must be prepared to assist during this type of emergency. Many new facilities will be equipped with generators, which help to make the situation somewhat easier to deal with. Back-up generator systems usually only provide power for critical areas, resident rooms, appliances such as refrigerators, and exit lights. Facilities are required by the state to have a 96-hour supply of food and beverages that do not require refrigeration or heat preparation.

In the event the outage occurs in *cold weather*, a staging process occurs:

- Barrier protection (blankets, etc.) is placed at the base of all exterior doors
- Doors to resident rooms are closed; extra blankets are added to the bed and clothing may be layered to conserve body heat
- Draw blinds and drapes, unless the area is "sun" exposed
- Extra surveillance may be needed because all door alarms will be inactivated. Particular attention must be given to residents who have a tendency to wander.
- Automatic door locks will be inactivated, therefore entry of unauthorized persons may be possible.

In the event of *warm weather*:

- Offer water and fluids frequently to prevent dehydration
- Open windows to encourage cross ventilation
- Draw shades on the "sun" exposed windows
- Monitor for heat-related illnesses
- Provide cool baths, showers or wet towels as needed.

Other Potentially Serious Events

Bomb Threats

A long-term care facility may be the target for a bomb threat. Any warning of such a threat should be taken seriously. Fire and law enforcement officials will be notified. Follow all procedures that are advised by the management; this usually involves evacuation of the facility. Remain calm and reassure the residents. Following a search of the facility, law enforcement authorities will indicate when it is safe to reoccupy the facility.

Concealed Weapons/Active Shooter

All states have laws regarding the carrying of concealed weapons. Become familiar with the laws for your state. In many states, law enforcement personnel are the only persons authorized to carry weapons into a health care facility; all other persons are required to place any weapons in the trunk of their car before entering the facility. If you should notice any individual carrying a handgun or any other weapon, immediately notify the nurse.

Bioterrorism

Since the events following September 11, 2001, the United States has been aware of the need for vigilance and protection against agents that may be used to terrorize its citizens. The Centers for Disease Control and Prevention (CDC) defines *bioterrorism* as the deliberate release of biological agents such as viruses, bacteria, or other germs that could be used to cause illnesses and death in people, animals, or plants. Biological agents can be spread through the air, in food or water supplies. These agent are extremely difficult to detect, it may take several hours, days, or even years to identify the agent(s).

An anthrax outbreak occurred in the latter part of 2001. Following a study of the outbreak, in an attempt to link the cases, it was determined that the cases were not passed from infected to susceptible persons. The anthrax spores had been mixed with powder and sent in letters through the mail by potential terrorists. This transfer of spores occurred when opening an envelope or even through seepage of the spores through small holes in unopened envelopes. A number of persons became ill and several people died as a result of exposure to the powder. Because the cases occurred in more than one state and the materials were sent through the United States Postal Service, the Federal Bureau of Investigation (FBI) and the CDC investigated the cases.

Anthrax spores can enter the body through the skin or by inhaling the material into the lungs. It also can be spread by handling contaminated animal products or by ingesting undercooked meats from infected animals. Cutaneous anthrax is the least serious type but gastrointestinal anthrax can lead to fatalities.

Smallpox is another disease that can become a biological terror agent. Mass immunizations will be offered if this disease becomes a threat because the disease can be easily transmitted from person to person. Other agents that may be responsible for causing outbreaks of disease include tularemia, plague, botulism, brucellosis, and hemorrhagic fevers. Health care facilities regularly update procedures for disaster preparedness and have plans to deal with these types of emergency situations. You will receive inservice education programs to keep you prepared should you need to deal with any type of disaster situation.

LESSON SYNTHESIS: Putting It All Together

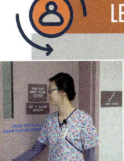

You have just completed this lesson. Now go back and review the Clinical Focus. Try to see how the Clinical Focus relates to the concepts presented in the lesson. Then answer the following questions.

1. Why are residents in long-term care particularly at risk for injury due to accidents such as falls?
2. Why are fire drills carried out routinely in long-term care facilities?
3. Explain how the principles of safety applied to resident care also apply to the protection of the nursing assistant.
4. What actions can the nursing assistant take to avoid the need for restraints?

8 REVIEW

A. Select the one best answer for each of the following.

1. The word that means adapting the environment to prevent body injury is
   (A) body mechanics
   (B) incident
   (C) ergonomics
   (D) RACE

2. One principle of body mechanics is to
   (A) bend from the waist when lifting
   (B) keep your feet close together when lifting
   (C) use the muscles of your arms and legs for lifting
   (D) keep the load as far from your body as possible

3. Material Safety Data Sheets (MSDS)

(A) explain whether you need personal protective equipment when using the product

(B) require that all spills be cleaned up by housekeeping staff

(C) describe a system of tagging all chemical agents

(D) require that hazardous materials be kept in unlocked cabinets

4. Which of the following residents is not at risk for having an incident?

(A) Mrs. Smith who has frequency of urination because of a bladder infection

(B) Mr. James who has terminal cancer and is on bed rest

(C) Mr. Edwards who is ambulatory and has stable diabetes

(D) Mrs. Porter who has a fractured leg and is in bed in traction

5. Which of the following contributes to unsafe conditions in the facility?

(A) equipment sitting in the halls

(B) chemicals in locked cupboards

(C) allowing residents to smoke only with supervision

(D) teaching residents how to use assistive devices such as canes and walkers

6. When oxygen is in use, you should

(A) use woolen blankets on the resident's bed

(B) allow smoking in the room

(C) adjust the liter flow

(D) be sure the oxygen source is secure

7. Which of the following could cause a resident to fall?

(A) taking residents to the bathroom promptly

(B) answering call lights promptly

(C) pulling the side rails up on every resident's bed

(D) monitoring residents' ambulation abilities

8. Resident falls can be prevented by

(A) keeping the side rails up at all times

(B) using restraints when the resident is up

(C) encouraging the resident to stay in bed

(D) caring for physical needs promptly

9. Physical restraints may be used for residents who

(A) wander about the building

(B) are disoriented

(C) refuse to eat or take medication

(D) may harm other residents

10. Fire safety in the facility means that

(A) only the administrative staff needs to know the evacuation plan

(B) knowing how to operate the fire extinguishers is optional

(C) every staff member must take part in fire drills

(D) the fire alarm is activated by a supervisor only

11. A severe weather alert has been issued for possible tornados in your area. What should you do?

(A) Call and make sure your family is safe.

(B) Activate the fire alarm.

(C) Participate in the facility disaster plan.

(D) Take cover in the linen closet.

12. A widespread power outage has occurred in your town. The outdoor temperatures are hovering around 30°F. Which of the following activities is *not* important for the CNA to perform?

(A) Close doors to resident rooms

(B) Layer resident clothing to retain body heat

(C) Be alert to wandering residents since door alarms are inactivated

(D) Close blinds and drapes on sun-exposed windows

B. Fill in the blanks by selecting the correct word or phrase from the list.

ABC	laceration
aspiration	mechanical lift
body mechanics	Safety
call light	Data Sheets
earthquake	(SDS)
ergonomics	OSHA
hips and knees	physical restraint
incident	RACE

13. Using your body correctly while you are working is called _____.

14. Basic rules for lifting include bending from the _____ and not from the waist.

15. An unexpected situation that can cause harm to an employee, a resident, or a visitor is called a/an _____.

16. Adapting the environment and using techniques and equipment to prevent body injury is called _____.

17. You should use a _____ when you need to transfer very heavy or dependent residents.

18. All residents must have access to a _____ because it may be the only way they have to summon help.

19. All manufacturers must supply _____ with the hazardous products they sell.

20. The section of the federal government that oversees employee safety is called _____.

21. A cut or break in the skin is called a/an _____.

22. Any device that restricts a resident's movement is called a/an _____.

23. _____ is the accidental entry of food or a foreign object into the trachea (windpipe).

24. The acronym used to remember the sequence of critical actions in case of fire is _____.

25. The type of extinguisher that can be used on all types of fires is the _____ extinguisher.

26. An example of a disaster involving a long-term care facility would be a/an _____.

LESSON 9
EMERGENCIES

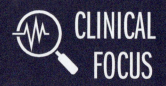

CLINICAL FOCUS

Think about ways you can help prevent incidents to residents as you study this lesson.

OBJECTIVES

After studying this lesson, you should be able to:

• Define words and terms.

• List general measures to take in the event of an emergency.

• Describe the actions to take for the emergencies discussed in the lesson: cardiac arrest, obstructed airway, hemorrhage, falls, seizures, shock, stroke, burns, orthopedic injuries, accidental poisoning, and fainting.

• Demonstrate the following:

Procedure 9-1   Assisting the Conscious Person with Obstructed Airway—Abdominal Thrusts
Procedure 9-2   Obstructed Airway, Unconscious Person
Procedure 9-3   One-Rescuer CPR, Adult
Procedure 9-4   Positioning the Resident in the Recovery Position
Procedure 9-5   Hemorrhage
Procedure 9-6   Care of Falling Resident

VOCABULARY

aspiration (ass-pih-RAY-shun)
aura (AWE-rah)
automatic external defibrillator (awe-tuh-MAT-ik eks-TURN-uhl dee-FIB-rill-ay-tur)
cardiac arrest (KAR-dee ack ah-REST)

cardiopulmonary resuscitation (CPR) (kar-dee-oh-PUL-moh-nair-ee ree-sus-ih-TAY-shun)
defibrillation (dee-fih-bryl-AY-shun)
dislocation (dis-loh-KAY-shun)
do not resuscitate (DNR) (do not ree-SUS-ih-tayt)

CASE STUDY

Selina Lattini lives at the Community Nursing and Rehabilitation Center. She recently suffered a stroke but is able to walk with a cane. Since the stroke she receives medication for seizures but still occasionally has a seizure. She is disoriented at times and is not always able to remember recent events.

emergency (ee-MER-jen-see)
Emergency Medical Services (EMS) (ee-MER-jen-see
  MED-ih-kul SIR-vih-sez)
fracture (FRACK-shur)
Heimlich maneuver (HIGHM-lick mah-NEW-ver)
hemorrhage (HEM-or-ij)

recovery position (rih-KUV-er-ee puh-zih-shun)
respiratory arrest (RES-pih-rah-tor-ee ah-REST)
seizure (SEE-zhur)
sprain (sprayn)
strain (strayn)
syncope (SIN-koh-pee)

GENERAL MEASURES TO FOLLOW FOR EMERGENCIES

An **emergency** is any unexpected situation that requires immediate action. In a true emergency, prompt action is needed to prevent further complications and injuries and to save the victim's life. It is important that you know the signs and symptoms of an emergency and that you are able to initiate immediate actions.

The instructions here are for emergencies in the long-term care facility. In some emergency situations the resident may be transferred by ambulance to a hospital. In other cases, the nurses will handle the emergency and the resident will remain in the facility. The following guidelines are basic actions to follow in any emergency.

CARDIAC ARREST

A person may stop breathing but still have a heartbeat. This is called **respiratory arrest**. If the situation is not reversed, the heart will stop beating. **Cardiac arrest** is the term used when the heart has stopped beating. When the heart and lungs are not functioning, blood and oxygen are not circulated to the brain and the rest of the body. The person is clinically dead. Permanent damage to the brain and other

organs occurs within 4 to 6 minutes. Indications of cardiac arrest are:

- Loss of consciousness
- Abnormal breathing
- No breathing
- No pulse

Cardiac Chain of Survival

There are four steps to the cardiac chain of survival, which is designed to assist a victim of cardiac arrest. These steps include:

1. Early recognition of the emergency and use of 911 or the local emergency number
2. Cardiopulmonary resuscitation with an emphasis on chest compressions
3. Rapid defibrillation with an automated external defibrillator (AED) by a qualified person
4. Advanced life support by trained professional health personnel

The *first step* in the chain is to identify the resident in cardiac arrest and activate the emergency number (911 or local). The *second step* is cardiopulmonary resuscitation (CPR), a procedure designed to rescue a resident in cardiac arrest. The *third step* in the chain of survival is the use of the AED. If this device is available in the facility, someone must bring it to the room and prepare it for use while step two is being performed. This device has been proved to increase survival. It is operated by someone specially trained in this function.

The instrument is designed to automatically administer an electrical shock to the resident's heart after proper placement of the conduction patches. The machine analyzes the resident's heart rhythm and determines if a shock is needed. The machine will announce "stand clear" if a shock will be delivered. Make sure your body and uniform are not in contact with the resident or equipment attached to the resident's body when the shock is delivered. If the shock is successful, the resident's heart beat is reestablished, although ventilation assistance may be required.

Many communities have recognized the value of placing AEDs in areas where many people gather, such

? EXERCISE 9-1

TRUE OR FALSE
Indicate whether the following statements are true (T) or false (F).

1. T F An emergency is an unexpected situation that requires immediate action.
2. T F Whenever an emergency occurs, the resident will be immediately transferred to an acute care hospital.
3. T F It is important to stay calm whenever an emergency occurs.

as airports, schools, and sports facilities. This is an important and growing trend.

ON THE JOB

Emergencies require prompt action. Do not be tempted to overstep your knowledge base or authority.

The *fourth step* is intervention by trained health care personnel, who provide advanced respiratory support, medications, and other services during transport to the hospital.

CPR

Cardiopulmonary resuscitation or **CPR** (Figure 9-1) is a procedure used to maintain blood circulation throughout the body until the EMS can respond to the emergency. New CPR guidelines were initiated in 2017. The previous **A-B-C** (**A**irway, **B**reathing, **C**hest compressions) has been changed to **CVR** (Compression–Ventilation ratio). More emphasis is now placed on chest compressions to keep the heart pumping the blood throughout the body prior to opening the airway and initiating breathing. New guidelines state that after 20 chest compressions at a rate of 100 to 120 per minute, give two rescue breaths. Some oxygen remains in the bloodstream following the last breath that was inhaled.

You must never perform CPR unless you have completed an approved course, taught by an approved instructor from the American Red Cross or the American Heart Association. You must also know whether CPR is to be initiated. Many residents in long-term care facilities are very old and have been ill for a long time. They are ready for death. These residents may have indicated that they do not wish to be resuscitated. The physician must write the order "**do not resuscitate (DNR)**" or "no codes" (Figure 9-2). Other residents may indicate that they wish full life support measures in the event of cardiac arrest. For these individuals, the EMS system is activated and CPR is started immediately. CNAs should always know if the resident they are caring for has DNR orders.

ON THE JOB

Be aware that not all attempts at resuscitation are successful, especially if the resident is advanced in years. A resident may die even though vigorous efforts are made to maintain life.

⚠ GUIDELINES FOR... RESPONDING TO AN EMERGENCY

- Always remember the priorities of any emergency:
  - Chest compressions
  - Airway
  - Breathing
- Stay calm. Nothing is accomplished and more problems can result if the people at the scene of an incident become flustered and agitated. If you are calm, you will be a calming influence on the resident.
- Know what to do to summon immediate help; you need to get the nurse to the scene as soon as possible. Stay with the resident and call out for help.
- Stay with the resident until the person in charge gives you permission to leave.
- Know your limitations. Be aware of what procedures nursing assistants are qualified to perform in an emergency. Never attempt a procedure unless you have received the appropriate training.
- Do not move the resident involved unless the resident is clearly in danger by staying where he or she is.
- Know the procedures to follow for emergencies. Most health care facilities have code names for various emergencies. Know what these are and how to announce a code.
- Know the procedures for activating the **Emergency Medical Services (EMS)** system. In most parts of the country this is done by dialing 911. You will need to give the address and be able to describe what has happened (e.g., a resident was burned or has had cardiac arrest).
- Keep the person warm. Cover with blankets.
- Do not give the person any fluids or food.
- If the person starts to vomit, turn his or her head to one side to avoid aspiration.
- If the person is conscious, assure him or her that help has been called and is on the way.
- Protect the person's privacy. Keep other residents and visitors away from the scene.
- Remember that many emergencies involve bleeding. There is potential for contact with blood, body fluids (except sweat), and secretions from non-intact skin or mucous membranes. Apply principles of standard precautions and use personal protective equipment.

? EXERCISE 9-2

TRUE OR FALSE

Indicate whether the following statements are true (T) or false (F).

1. T F When an incident occurs do not leave the resident alone.

2. T F In most parts of the country the emergency medical services (EMS) can be activated by dialing 888.

3. T F It is all right to move the resident if the resident is not clearly in danger.

4. T F A calm person has a soothing influence on those around them.

MULTIPLE CHOICE

Select the one best answer.

5. When activating the EMS system you will need to
   (A) describe what happened   (C) give fluids
   (B) keep the resident cool   (D) take the victim's temperature

6. A person who has stopped breathing but still has a heartbeat
   (A) requires full cardiopulmonary resuscitation (CPR)
   (B) is in respiratory arrest
   (C) is in cardiac arrest
   (D) is clinically dead

7. Permanent damage to the brain during a cardiac arrest can occur within
   (A) 1 to 2 minutes   (C) 4 to 6 minutes
   (B) 3 minutes   (D) 7 minutes

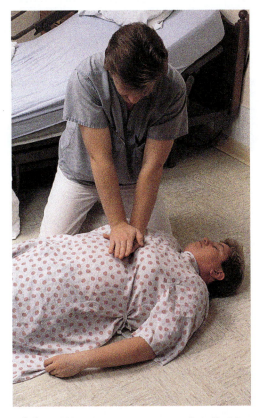

Figure 9-1 CPR is an emergency procedure that is performed only by persons who have completed an approved course.

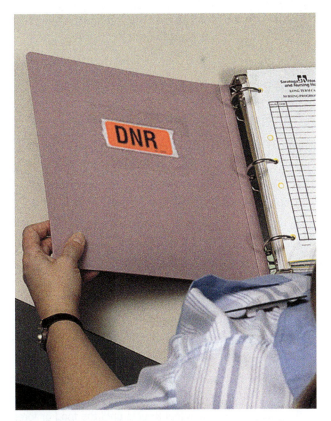

Figure 9-2 DNR on a resident's chart means that the resident does not wish to be resuscitated in the event of cardiac arrest.

CLINICAL SITUATION
Read the following situations and answer the questions.

1. Rebecca Newhart is 97 years of age and has diabetes, emphysema, and congestive heart failure. She has had both legs amputated because of gangrene and is emphatic that no resuscitation be used when her "time" comes. A DNR order has been written.

   a. What do the letters DNR stand for? _____
   b. Will the EMS system be activated if she ceases to breathe? _____
   c. How does this make you feel? _____

FOREIGN BODY AIRWAY OBSTRUCTION (CHOKING)

NOTE: If time permits, gloves should be worn for emergency procedures. Other personal protective equipment may also be needed.

Aspiration means the accidental entry of food or a foreign object into the trachea (windpipe). This causes the resident to choke. Choking occurs more readily in older persons because the swallowing mechanism is less efficient. Aspiration can occur during vomiting. When a resident begins to vomit, it is important to:

- Stay with the resident until the vomiting has ceased and you are sure the resident is out of danger.

- If the resident is in bed, turn the head to one side to allow the vomitus to drain out of the mouth instead of going into the trachea. Wipe the mouth as necessary.

- If the resident is in a chair, help the resident flex the neck to allow the vomitus to drain out of the mouth. Wipe the mouth as necessary.

When choking occurs, immediate action is necessary. There are two procedures you must know. The Heimlich maneuver (or abdominal thrusts) is used for persons who are choking but are still conscious. The other procedure is cardiopulmonary resuscitation. You should be instructed and approved for performing these procedures.

PROCEDURE 9-1
Assisting the Conscious Person with Obstructed Airway—Abdominal Thrusts

1. Ask the resident if he or she can speak or cough.

2. Call for help.

3. Do not attempt to interfere if the resident is coughing or is able to speak.

4. If the resident cannot speak, is not coughing, or shows the universal distress sign (both hands clutching throat) (Figure 9-3), take immediate action. Tell the resident you are going to help and call for the nurse.

5. Stand behind the resident. Wrap your arms around the resident's waist. Avoid placing pressure on the resident's ribs with your forearms.

6. Clench your fist. Tuck the tip of your thumb inside your fist (Figure 9-4).

7. Place your fist, thumb side in, against the resident's abdomen between the navel and the tip of the sternum (Figure 9-5).

8. Grasp your fist with your other hand and press your fist into the resident's abdomen with quick inward and upward thrusts (Figure 9-6).

9. Repeat the abdominal thrusts until the food or foreign object is expelled.

   If the object remains in the airway, the resident will eventually lose consciousness. If this happens, you must proceed with the procedure for Obstructed Airway, Unconscious Person.

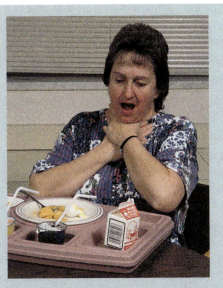

Figure 9-3 Immediate action is required if the resident cannot cough or speak, or if she shows the universal distress sign.

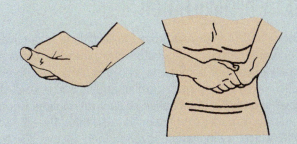

Figure 9-4 Clench your fist, keeping your thumb straight.

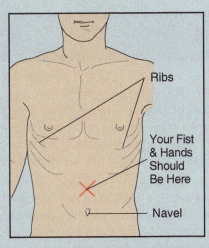

Ribs

Your Fist & Hands Should Be Here

Navel

Figure 9-5 Place your fist, thumb side in, against the resident's abdomen between the navel and the tip of the sternum.

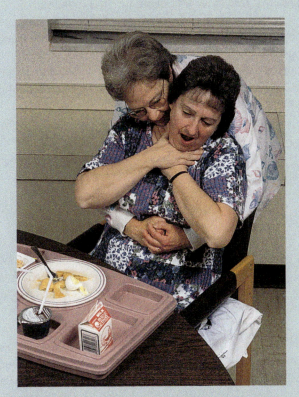

Figure 9-6 Grasp your fist with your other hand and press your fist into the resident's abdomen with quick inward and upward thrusts.

THE RECOVERY POSITION

If the resident is unresponsive but is breathing and has a pulse, he or she should be positioned in the recovery position to prevent complications. The recovery position is a modified lateral position (see Figure 9-7). Avoid pressure on the lower arm. The resident's position must be stable and must avoid pressure on the chest. The airway must remain open. Continue to monitor the resident according to facility policy to ensure that the pulse and respirations remain adequate.

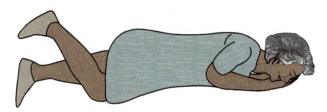

Figure 9-7 Recovery position.

EARLY DEFIBRILLATION

Early **defibrillation** has proved to be critical to survival in cardiac arrest. Defibrillators are placed in various locations in the community and are used by trained rescuers in the event of cardiac arrest. Some studies have shown that the chance of survival doubles when early access to defibrillation is available. The speed with which defibrillation is performed is the key to success. Early defibrillation (within 5 minutes) is a high-priority goal in the community. In health care facilities, the goal is to defibrillate within 3 minutes.

Automatic external defibrillators (AEDs) are computerized devices that are simple to learn and operate. The AED is used only when a resident is unresponsive, not breathing, and pulseless. When the device is attached to the victim's chest, the unit determines if an electrical shock is necessary to reestablish or regulate the heartbeat. Several different models are available, and the operating instructions are slightly different for each. The four basic steps to using an AED are:

1. Turn the power on to the unit.
2. Apply the electrode pads to the resident's chest.
3. All rescuers stand back to allow the machine to analyze the heart rhythm.
4. All rescuers continue to stand back; the operator of the unit presses the shock button and/or follows the unit's instructions, which are usually audible through a voice-synthesized message.

If your facility purchases an AED, employees will be trained in its use. Although the AED is simple to operate, only those who are properly trained may use it. CPR and use of the AED are included in basic life support classes for health care professionals.

PROCEDURE 9-2
Obstructed Airway, Unconscious Person

1. If the resident loses consciousness, place him or her on the back with face up and arms at sides.

2. Open the mouth with tongue-jaw lift method and sweep deeply into the mouth to remove the foreign body, if possible (Figure 9-8). To perform a tongue-jaw lift, grasp the tongue and lower jaw between your thumb and fingers and lift the jaw. To sweep, insert the index finger of your other hand deep into the resident's throat at the base of the tongue. With a hooking motion, attempt to remove the obstruction. Take care not to push the obstruction farther into the throat.

3. If the foreign body cannot be removed, open the resident's airway with the head-tilt/chin-lift method. First, extend the neck (Figure 9-9). Then, place your upper hand on the resident's forehead. Apply pressure to tilt the head back. Place the fingertips of your other hand under the bony part of the resident's lower jaw near the chin. Lift the chin while keeping the mouth partially open. Apply the barrier device to the face, covering both the nose and mouth. Seal the device tightly by placing the thumb and index finger of your top hand on the top of the mask. Place the thumb of your other hand on the lower part of the mask. Place the remaining fingers of your hand on the jaw to keep it in position. Sealing the mask is an important step that prevents air from leaking around the sides.

4. Attempt to ventilate through the mask. If the resident's chest does not rise, reposition the head and attempt to ventilate a second time.

5. Straddle the resident's thighs. Place the heel of one hand against the resident's abdomen midway between navel and xiphoid process (bottom of sternum) as in Figure 9-10.

6. Place your second hand on top of first hand (Figure 9-11). Press into the abdomen with quick, upward thrusts. Perform five thrusts.

7. If the foreign body is still not expelled, repeat steps 2 through 6 until the foreign body is expelled or until help arrives.

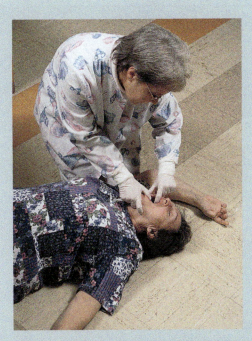

Figure 9-8 Open the resident's mouth with tongue-jaw lift method and sweep deeply into the mouth with your finger to remove the foreign body, if possible.

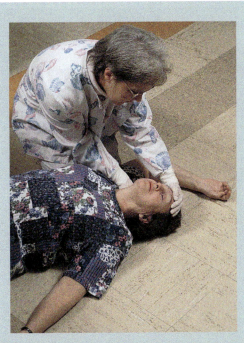

Figure 9-9 If the foreign body cannot be removed, open the resident's airway with head-tilt/chin-lift method. Extend the neck first.

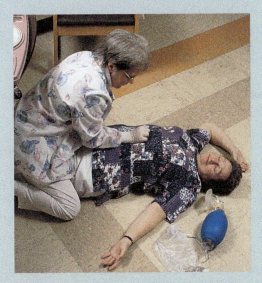

Figure 9-10 Straddle the resident's thighs. Place heel of one hand against the resident's abdomen midway between the navel and the xiphoid process.

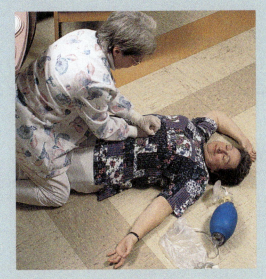

Figure 9-11 Place second hand on top of first hand.

NOTE: If the foreign body is not expelled and breathing does not resume, the resident will probably go into cardiac arrest.

The obstruction must be removed for further emergency procedures to be effective. If the obstruction is removed, immediately evaluate the resident for breathing and pulse. Your facility will have an established procedure for this type of emergency. Follow your facility policy and practices. If permitted, it may be necessary for you to begin the steps of the CPR procedure. To be effective, the resident's upper torso must be on a firm surface during CPR. *This information is presented for your information and understanding. Do not perform this procedure unless you have been properly trained to do so.*

? EXERCISE 9-4

TRUE OR FALSE

Indicate whether the following statements are true (T) or false (F).

1. T F The instrument designed to automatically administer an electrical shock to the resident's heart is a pacemaker.

2. T F A resident sitting in a wheelchair begins to vomit. Help him by extending his neck or tilting his head back.

3. T F After choking on some food, the resident continues to cough. You should initiate the Heimlich maneuver.

4. T F The purpose of an automated external defibrillator is to reestablish the resident's heartbeat.

MULTIPLE CHOICE

Select the one best answer.

5. Aspiration is more apt to occur in older persons because
   (A) they cannot tolerate spicy food
   (B) swallowing is less efficient
   (C) tastebuds are less effective
   (D) sense of smell is diminished

6. When a resident chokes, immediate action is necessary. You should
   (A) use the Heimlich maneuver or abdominal thrusts if he or she is conscious.
   (B) use cardiopulmonary resuscitation only.
   (C) call a nurse for help.
   (D) stay with him or her until vomiting has ceased.

7. Defibrillation
   (A) should be used only on residents who are breathing and have a pulse
   (B) should occur within 7 minutes
   (C) has proved to double chances of survival
   (D) should occur only in health care facilities

HEMORRHAGE

Hemorrhage is the rapid loss of a large amount of blood from the body. Death will occur if the hemorrhage is not stopped. Hemorrhage may be internal or external. Internal hemorrhage is suspected when the resident's:

- Pulse becomes weak, rapid, and irregular
- Blood pressure is falling
- Skin is dusky gray, cold, and clammy

Call the nurse immediately if these signs are present. Internal hemorrhage requires immediate action by the physician.

External hemorrhage is more obvious and is noted by the obvious loss of blood. Bleeding may be from an artery or from a vein. Blood coming from an artery will spurt and be bright red. A large amount of blood can be lost in a very short time from an artery. Blood coming from a vein will ooze out and have a bluish tinge.

Emergency treatment for hemorrhage may include direct pressure to an area of an obvious bleed (see Figure 9-13) or direct pressure to the arterial pressure points on the body. For example, if blood is spurting from a wound on the lower leg, apply pressure to the femoral artery. You will note the blood flow will slow (see Figure 9-13). Call the nurse to continue treatment. Do not release pressure on the wound or pressure point until you are instructed to do so. Always apply principles of standard precautions. (See Procedure 9-5.)

SHOCK

Shock is a serious complication that may result from a decreased blood flow from the periphery of the body back to the heart and brain (decreased blood pressure). This may result from numerous causes such as hemorrhage, infection, drug reaction, myocardial infarction (heart attack), and dehydration. If the blood pressure drops too low, the brain and other vital organs are deprived of oxygen. Shock that is untreated can result in death. Notify the nurse. Position the resident flat in bed or on the floor and keep him or her warm.

Anaphylactic shock may result from an allergic reaction to drugs, food, or insect bites. The chemicals in the body set up a response; this effect may result in a local reaction such as redness, swelling, itching, and/or the formation of hives. In some persons who are extremely sensitive, the reaction may occur in the cardiovascular and respiratory systems and can lead to death. Anaphylactic shock is a medical emergency; immediately summon the nurse. Special drugs will be used to inactivate the allergic response. In the meantime, keep the resident lying flat and maintain an open airway.

STROKE

A stroke (also called a CVA (cerebrovascular accident or brain attack)) is a medical emergency that is caused by an interruption in the blood supply to the brain. Brain cells are deprived of oxygen and nourishment. Symptoms of a stroke can develop suddenly or may occur on and off for several days. These symptoms may include trouble walking, speaking or understanding, paralysis or numbness on one side of the face or body, headache, and/or problems seeing in one or both eyes. Immediate treatment is essential. The longer a stroke is untreated, the greater the chance for brain damage. If you suspect the resident is having a

PROCEDURE 9-3
One-Rescuer CPR, Adult

CVR (Compression–Ventilation Ratio Targeting Chest Compressions, Rescue Breathing)

Supplies needed:

- Disposable exam gloves
- Ventilation device

1. Gently shake or tap the resident and ask, "Are you okay?" If the resident does not respond, you must get help immediately.

2. If other personnel are available in the vicinity, call out for help. If it is not likely that others will hear your call, go immediately to the phone to call for help, according to your facility policy. Return to the resident as quickly as possible. If a second person responds to your call, advise him or her to go for help, according to facility policy. Stay with the resident and perform emergency procedures you are trained and qualified to perform.

3. Position the resident on the back with the torso on a firm surface.

4. Locate the carotid pulse on the side of the neck; palpate lightly for 5 to 10 seconds.

5. If you cannot feel the pulse, locate the "landmark" on the tip of the sternum. Move your fingers up the lower margins of the ribs. The landmark, or xiphoid process, is where the margins meet, in the center of the chest. Hold your index and middle fingers over the xiphoid process. This is a key step to prevent injury.

6. Place the heel of the opposite hand on the chest next to your fingers. Place the landmark hand on top of the other hand, interlacing the fingers. Lock your elbows.

7. Using the heels of your hands, press the sternum straight down 2 inches at a rate of 100 to 120 compressions a minute. Press only on the sternum. Avoid pressure on the ribs with your fingers. Keep your fingers interlaced and slightly elevated. Compressions should be smooth and even. Completely release pressure to allow the heart to refill with blood at the end of each compression. However, your hands must remain in contact with the chest.

8. At the end of each 30 compressions, open the airway using the head-tilt/chin-lift procedure. If dentures are loose, remove them.

9. Upon completion of four cycles of 30 compressions and two ventilations, reevaluate the resident for return of the carotid pulse. If present, monitor for spontaneous breathing. If absent, continue. If present, perform rescue breathing, using the airway adjunct, once every 5 seconds.

PROCEDURE 9-4
Positioning the Resident in the Recovery Position

1. Kneel beside the resident and straighten the legs.
2. Place the arm nearest you above the resident's head with the palm up and the elbow bent slightly.
3. Position the opposite arm across the chest.
4. Place your lower hand on the resident's thigh on the far side of the body. Pull the thigh up slightly, closer to the center of the resident's body.
5. Place your upper hand on the resident's shoulder on the opposite side of the body.
6. With one hand on the thigh and the other on the shoulder, roll the resident on the side facing you.
7. Move the resident's upper hand close to the cheek, bending the elbow. This hand should be close to the face, but not under the body. Adjust the upper body so that the hip and knee are at right angles.
8. Tilt the resident's head back slightly to keep the airway open. Now place the upper hand, palm facing down, under the cheek to maintain the head position.
9. Continue to monitor the resident closely for adequate breathing.

PROCEDURE 9-5
Hemorrhage

Gloves should be readily available throughout the facility. Apply gloves before contacting blood.

1. Call for help.
2. Find out where the bleeding area is.
3. Apply continuous, firm, direct pressure over the bleeding area with a pad or towel or whatever is available (Figure 9-12). Elevate the area (arm or leg) above the level of the heart, if possible.
4. If seepage occurs, increase the padding and the pressure. Do not remove the saturated dressings.
5. If bleeding continues, maintain firm, direct pressure over the site, continue to elevate the extremity, and apply pressure to pulse points proximal to the injury (Figure 9-13). Never use a tourniquet.
6. Keep the resident warm and quiet until help arrives.

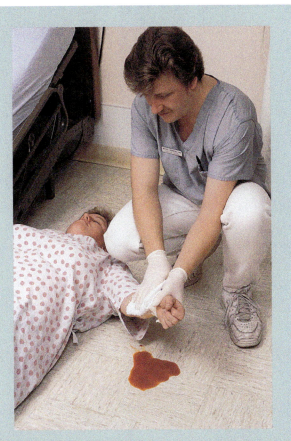

Figure 9-12 Apply continuous, firm, direct pressure over the bleeding area.

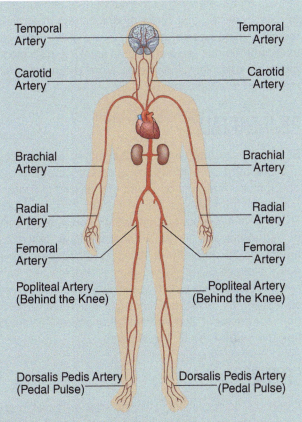

Figure 9-13 If bleeding continues, maintain direct pressure and apply pressure to pulse point proximal to the injury.

? EXERCISE 9-5

FILL IN THE BLANK

1. When a person has a rapid loss of blood, he or she _____.

MULTIPLE CHOICE
Select the one best answer.

2. The resident who is hemorrhaging will have
   (A) elevated blood pressure
   (B) ruddy complexion
   (C) weak, rapid, irregular pulse
   (D) strong, slow, regular pulse

3. A resident is bleeding from a cut on the arm. After putting on gloves, you should
   (A) lower the arm below the heart level
   (B) apply a tourniquet on the arm above the cut
   (C) allow some blood to flow before applying pressure
   (D) apply firm, direct pressure

stroke, immediately notify the nurse. It is encouraging to note, however, that fewer Americans die of strokes today because people are more aware of and attempt to control the risk factors such as smoking, high blood pressure, and high cholesterol. More extensive information on this topic can be found in Lesson 29.

RESIDENT FALLS

Since falls are one of the most common occurrences in a long-term care facility and of persons over the age of 65, all staff should be aware of the need to protect residents from wet or slippery areas (Figure 9-14). Fluids of all types can be spilled on floors, especially in bathrooms and in hallways. Lesson 8 describes measures for preventing falls. As discussed previously, prevent clutter in the resident rooms and hallways, ensure the resident is wearing proper footwear, and allow for adequate lighting. You must protect both the resident and yourself. Procedure 9-6 identifies the care of the falling resident.

SEIZURES

A seizure or convulsion involves sudden, involuntary contractions of a group of muscles. A disturbance in consciousness and changes in behavior occur. The two categories of seizures are:

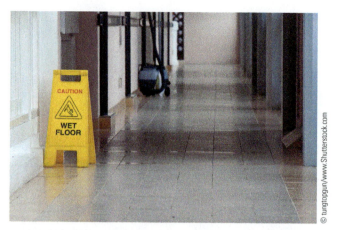

Figure 9-14 Prevent falls by being alert to wet and slippery areas.

- Partial seizure
  - The seizures begin in one part of the body. They may be considered simple (without disturbance in consciousness) or complex (with impairment of consciousness).
- Generalized seizure
  - Generalized seizures involve the entire body (Figure 9-16).

Adult-onset seizures may occur after a brain injury, along with a brain tumor, after a stroke, and along with dementia.

PROCEDURE 9-6
Care of Falling Resident

1. Keep your back straight, bend from the hips and knees, and maintain a broad base of support as you assist the falling resident.

2. Ease the resident to the floor, using your leg to let the person slide down gently to the floor. Protect the resident's head.

3. As you ease the resident to the floor, bend your knees and go down with the resident (Figure 9-15).

4. Call for help. *Do not attempt to move the resident until the nurse or physician has examined the resident and has given you instructions.*

5. Assist in returning the resident to bed or chair. Be sure you have adequate help.

6. Carry out procedure completion actions.

7. Record according to facility policy.

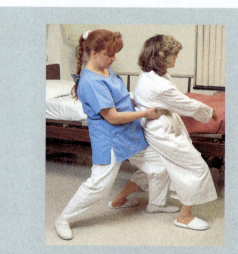

Figure 9-15 Ease the resident to the floor as you bend your knees and go down with the resident.

(A)

(B)

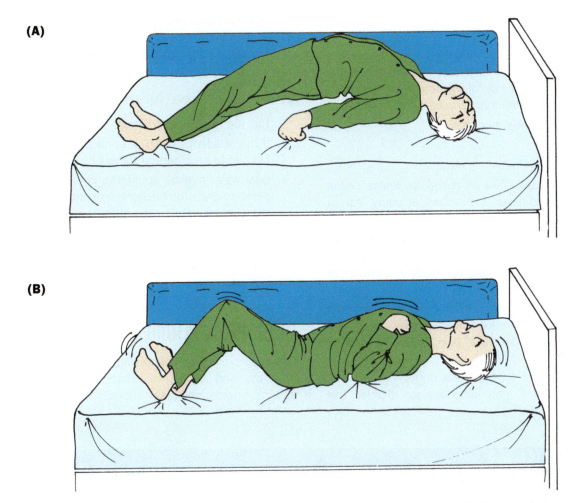

Figure 9-16 Generalized seizures involve the entire body. Note that side rails should be padded and up during a seizure. The side rails are down in the figure for clarity of the view. (A) Rigid posturing. (B) Uncontrolled movements.

Side rails on the bed may be padded if the resident may have a seizure.

Emergency Treatment for Seizures

Seizures can occur suddenly and without warning. Some people have an aura before a seizure. An aura is a sensory disturbance; the person may hear a noise, smell something, or see a certain pattern. If the resident is aware of this, he or she may have time to get to a chair or to lie down. When a seizure occurs:

1. Do not leave the resident alone. Call for help.
2. Do not restrain movements. Do not force anything into the resident's mouth. Provide privacy and keep onlookers away.
3. Protect the resident from injury. Move any objects that might cause injury.
4. Place a small pillow, folded towel, or blanket under the resident's head if the resident is on the floor.

5. Loosen clothing around the resident's head.
6. Maintain open airway. Turn the resident's head to the side, if possible.
7. Observe the seizure. Include time started and stopped and what occurred during the seizure. Most seizures stop on their own.
8. Check for breathing and pulse. Initiate appropriate actions if either is absent.
9. Incontinence is common during or after a seizure. Provide perineal care and assist the resident to apply clean clothing.
10. Allow the resident to rest.
11. After movements subside, turn the resident to the recovery position so fluid or vomitus can drain freely from mouth.
12. Comfort and reassure the resident and assist him or her in becoming reoriented.
13. Allow the resident to sleep after seizure has subsided. Position the resident on the side and observe closely while resident sleeps.

BURNS

Burns result in loss of skin integrity and may be caused by hot liquids or other substances, chemicals, or radiation. There is a high risk of infection with any burn. Burns may occur in the long-term care facility from:

- Spilling hot coffee, tea, or soup
- Hot water
- Careless use of smoking materials

Burns are classified as partial thickness or full thickness depending on the degree of injury. Partial thickness burns are:

- First-degree burns—involve only the top layer (epidermis) of skin. There is redness, temporary swelling, and pain. There is usually no permanent scarring.
- Second-degree burns—involve both epidermis and dermis. The skin color may vary from pink or red to white or tan. Blistering, pain, and some scarring occur.
- Third-degree or full-thickness burns—involve epidermis, dermis, and subcutaneous tissue. The tissue is bright red to tan and brown. There may be no pain initially because nerve endings have been destroyed. Later, pain and scarring will result.

Emergency Treatment for Burns

1. Call the nurse immediately.
2. If the resident's clothing is on fire, use a coat or blanket to smother the flames.
3. Cool water may be applied to lower the skin temperature and stop further tissue damage. Remove wet clothing. (Follow the nurse's instructions.)
4. Second-degree burns may require treatment at the hospital emergency department. Third-degree burns will probably require hospitalization for special treatment.

ORTHOPEDIC INJURIES

Orthopedic injuries include injuries to bones, joints, muscles, and ligaments. These include fractures, sprains, strains, and dislocations.

? EXERCISE 9-6

FILL IN THE BLANKS

1. A sensory disturbance experienced before a seizure is called a(an) _____.
2. The resident has sudden involuntary contractions of the muscles, which the nurse calls _____.

MULTIPLE CHOICE
Select the one best answer.

3. When assisting a falling resident
   (A) keep a narrow base of support and bend your back
   (B) ease the resident to the floor
   (C) move the resident out of the way until the nurse comes
   (D) try to get the resident back in bed

4. Adult onset seizures may occur
   (A) after brain injury
   (B) along with brain tumor
   (C) after strokes
   (D) all of these

5. When a seizure occurs
   (A) hold arms against the resident's sides
   (B) place something between the resident's teeth
   (C) move objects that might cause injury
   (D) leave the resident and get help

6. If a resident burns his hand, you should
   (A) call the nurse immediately
   (B) apply cool water
   (C) stay calm
   (D) all of these

Treatment for Orthopedic Injuries

A **fracture** is a break in a bone. If you suspect a resident has suffered a fracture:

- Stay with the resident.
- Do not attempt to move the resident.
- Call the nurse immediately.

If a fracture is suspected, the EMS will be called and the resident will be transported by ambulance to the hospital for x-rays. If a fracture is present, the physician will put a splint on the affected extremity or place the resident in traction or do surgery. (This is explained further in Lesson 28.) A cast may be applied after 48 hours.

A **sprain** is an injury to a ligament caused by sudden overstretching. A sprained ankle may occur, for example, if a person falls and turns the ankle quickly while falling. Swelling may be noted shortly afterward.

A **strain** is excessive stretching of a muscle resulting in pain and swelling of the muscle. You may strain the muscles in your back if you use incorrect lifting and moving techniques.

A **dislocation** occurs in a joint, when one bone is displaced from the other bone. This can occur in a paralyzed arm that is allowed to hang without support. The weight of the arm pulls the upper arm bone out of position in the shoulder joint. A dislocation can also be caused by improperly lifting the resident under the arms.

If you suspect that a resident has suffered a sprain, strain, or dislocation, notify the nurse at once. You may be instructed to:

- Elevate the injured extremity.
- Apply ice packs to the area. (See Lesson 21 for instructions on application of ice packs.)

After 24 hours, you may be instructed to apply warm packs to the area.

ACCIDENTAL POISONING

Immediate attention is needed if a resident is the victim of accidental poisoning. All potentially harmful substances must be kept in locked cupboards. However, a confused resident may obtain and ingest a harmful substance. If you suspect that this has happened:

- Call the nurse immediately.
- Try to determine what the resident has taken; save the container.
- The nurse may administer a substance that will cause vomiting. (Not all ingested poisons can be safely removed from the resident's body by vomiting.)
- Know where to find the telephone number for the regional poison control center.
- The resident may need to be transported to a hospital by ambulance.

FAINTING

Fainting (**syncope**) is a loss of consciousness due to temporary insufficient blood flow to the brain. The attack comes on gradually with light-headedness, perspiring, and blurred vision. Fainting can occur in otherwise healthy people and may be related to emotional shock or standing in one place for a long time. Residents experiencing these symptoms should sit down in a chair, bend forward, and lower the head between the knees, or lie down before they lose consciousness. If they faint and fall, allow them to lie still and flat unless they are in immediate danger. Recovery is usually prompt and without complications or after effects. Call for the nurse immediately. A person who has fainted should lie down and rest for several minutes. Provide reassurance and emotional support.

? EXERCISE 9-7

FILL IN THE BLANK
Select the correct term from the following list to complete each statement.

hemorrhages	fracture
automatic external defibrillator (AED)	seizures
dislocation	sprain
emergency	syncope

1. The nursing assistant should notify the nurse at once if she suspects that a resident has twisted his ankle causing a(an) _____.
2. Fainting is also called _____.

(continues)

? EXERCISE 9-7 (Continued)

3. When the resident fell, he experienced a break or _____ of the bone in the left arm.

4. The resident said that one time the shoulder and upper arm bone had been separated in a fall causing a(an) _____.

TRUE OR FALSE

Indicate whether the following statements are true (T) or false (F).

5. T F An ice pack may be applied to a sprain to reduce pain and swelling.

6. T F All potentially harmful substances must be kept in locked cupboards.

7. T F A resident in danger of fainting should be encouraged to move around to increase circulation.

8. T F If a resident faints and falls, she should be encouraged to get up as quickly as possible.

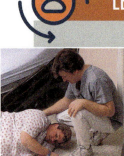

LESSON SYNTHESIS: Putting It All Together

You have just completed this lesson. Now go back and review the Clinical Focus. Try to see how the Clinical Focus relates to the concepts presented in the lesson. Then answer the following questions.

1. Mrs. Lattini is at high risk for falling. Her use of a cane is one risk factor. What observations should you make in regard to ambulation with a cane?

2. What steps can you take in an effort to prevent Mrs. Lattini from falling?

3. Describe what you would do in the event that Mrs. Lattini falls.

4. What can you do as a nursing assistant to ensure that you will know how to respond in the event of an emergency?

9 REVIEW

A. Select the one best answer for each of the following.

1. If an emergency occurs in the long-term care facility, you should

   (A) stay with the resident, if possible, and summon for help

   (B) follow instructions from the nurse

   (C) call the EMS right away

   (D) know your limitations

Signs and symptoms of cardiac arrest include

   (E) no pulse

   (F) rapid breathing

   (G) confusion

   (H) incontinence

   (I) dizziness

   (J) chest pain

2. When a resident makes an advance directive indicating that the resident does not wish to be resuscitated, the physician writes the order referred to as

(A) CPR

(B) CAB

(C) DNR

(D) EMS

3. The abdominal thrusts should be initiated when the resident

(A) is coughing

(B) suffers cardiac arrest

(C) vomits

(D) cannot speak, is not coughing, and is conscious, or clutches the throat

4. If a resident is hemorrhaging externally, you should first

(A) apply pressure directly over the wound

(B) apply pressure over the closest pressure points

(C) apply a tourniquet

(D) run for help

5. When a resident falls, you should

(A) try to hold the resident in an upright position

(B) let go of the resident immediately to avoid injuring yourself

(C) ease the resident to the floor, protecting the resident's head

(D) scream for help

6. If a resident has a seizure, you should first

(A) place something between the resident's teeth

(B) begin CPR

(C) restrain the resident's arms and legs

(D) protect the resident from injury and allow the seizure to run its course

7. If a resident suffers a burn from hot coffee, the nurse may instruct you to

(A) apply cool water to the area

(B) apply butter or some other greasy substance

(C) hold ice cubes against the area

(D) apply a warm water bottle

B. Answer each statement true (T) or false (F).

8. T F The first thing to consider in an emergency is the CABs.

9. T F Cardiopulmonary resuscitation is always administered when a resident has cardiac arrest.

10. T F If applying direct pressure to a hemorrhage is not successful, you should apply a tourniquet.

11. T F It is common for incontinence to occur during or after a seizure.

12. T F If a resident ingests a poisonous substance, you should immediately force the resident to vomit.

13. T F You should not move a resident who has fallen until the nurse has examined the resident and given instructions.

14. T F Recovery from fainting is usually quick and without complications.

15. T F When a person is in respiratory arrest, the heart may continue to beat although respirations cease.

16. T F The chain of survival refers to the immediate care given to assist a person in cardiac arrest.

17. T F The first step in the chain of survival is to use the AED.

18. T F When providing CPR, chest compressions are given at a rate of 100 per minute.

19. T F If a resident falls you must protect both the resident and yourself.

LESSON 10
INFECTION

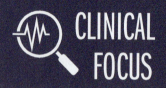

CLINICAL FOCUS

Think about the different kinds of infections a resident may present as you study this lesson.

OBJECTIVES

After studying this lesson, you should be able to:

• Define vocabulary words and terms.

• Describe how infections can be introduced to the long-term care facility.

• Discuss the causes of several important infectious diseases.

• List the ways that infectious diseases are spread.

• List the parts of the chain of infection.

• List natural body defenses against infections.

• Name five serious infectious diseases.

• Explain why residents are at risk for infections.

VOCABULARY

antibiotic (an-tih-buy-OT-ick)
antibody (AN-tih-bah-dee)
antigen (AN-ti-jen)
bacteremia (back-ter-EE-mee-ah)
carrier (KAIR-ee-er)
contagious (kon-TAY-jus)
culture and sensitivity (KUL-tyour and sen-sih-TIV-ih-tee)
flora (FLOOR-ah)

fomite (FOH-myt)
health care associated infection (HAI) (health care–infection)
hemoptysis (he-MOP-tih-sis)
hepatitis (hep-ah-TYE-tis)
human immunodeficiency virus (HIV) (HYOU-man im-MYOUN-oh-dih-fish-en-see VYE-rus)
immunity (im-MYOUN-ih-tee)
immunization (IM-myou-nigh-zay-shun)

CASE STUDY

Franklin Dwyer is 66. He is HIV positive and has a history of repeated pneumonia. He also had hepatitis A and tuberculosis in his youth. Each infection was treated aggressively with medication. He has now been diagnosed with AIDS.

immunosuppression (im-myoun-oh-suh-PREH-shun)
infection (in-FECK-shun)
inflammation (in-flah-MAY-shun)
methicillin-resistant *Staphylococcus aureus* (MRSA)
   (meth-ih-SILL-in ree-SIS-tant staff-ill-oh-KOCK-us
   AWE-ree-us)
microbe (MY-krohb)
nosocomial infection (noh-soh-KOH-mee-al
   in-FECK-shun)
opportunistic infection (op-er-TOO-nis-tick in-FECK-shun)

pathogen (PATH-oh-jen)
seropositive (see-roh-POZ-ih-tiv)
transmission (trans-MISH-un)
tubercle (TOO-ber-kul)
tuberculosis disease (too-ber-kyou-LOH-sis dih-ZEEZ)
tuberculosis infection (too-ber-kyou-LOH-sis
   in-FECK-shun)
vaccine (VACK-seen)
vancomycin-resistant enterococci (VRE) (van-koh-MY-
   sin ree-SIS-tant en-ter-oh-KOCK-sigh)

INFECTIOUS DISEASE

Infections can occur when disease-producing organisms enter the body. Infections that occur in residents who are in the care facility are called health care associated infections (HAIs); formerly these infections were referred to as nosocomial infections. Visitors, staff members, and residents can introduce infections through the spread of microbes (germs). Visitors and staff can transfer germs to residents when they cough or sneeze or even touch the resident with improperly washed hands. *This is one reason why it is so important to carry out proper handwashing techniques and to discourage visiting when infections are present.*

MICROBES

Some microbes are useful and necessary to life. These microbes are referred to as *normal flora*. For example, the lower digestive tract is filled with bacteria that help in the breakdown of food and the elimination of feces. Other microbes cause disease and are called pathogens. They are tiny forms of life that can only be seen with a microscope. Some of the most common pathogens are:

- Bacteria
- Viruses
- Fungi (yeast and molds)
- Parasites

Bacteria

There are many forms of bacteria (Figure 10-1). They can cause infections in the skin, respiratory tract, urinary tract, and bloodstream. Abscesses and strep throat are common bacterial infections.

Antibiotics are often effective against bacterial infections. However, over the years some bacteria, such as *Staphylococcus aureus*, have become resistant to most antibiotics used against them. This is a

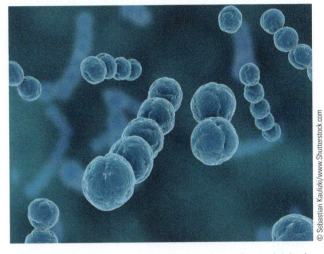

© Sebastian Kaulitzki/www.Shutterstock.com

Figure 10-1 This is the way the organisms (bacteria) look under the microscope. This organism causes scarlet fever and strep throat.

serious problem for controlling infections in all types of health care facilities. Because the microbes have become resistant to commonly used antibiotics, more expensive drugs must be used. Many of these drugs have serious side effects as compared with the previously preferred antibiotics. It is possible that these microbes will become resistant to the newer drugs in the future.

⊘N THE JOB

Only you and your conscience will ever know if you are the one who caused contamination because you did not wash your hands.

The microbes have developed resistance due to a number of factors, including inappropriate prescribing and use of the drugs. Recently, antibiotics were prescribed to treat conditions, such as viral infections. Antibiotics have no effect on the virus, but they do help control any secondary infections that may develop. If the physician suspects that the resident has a bacterial infection, it is important that a laboratory test (**culture and sensitivity**) be ordered. This test can be done on any body fluid (blood, urine, sputum) or drainage from a wound. The *culture* tells the physician the type of microbe causing the infection. The *sensitivity* tells which antibiotics are useful to treat that particular infection. An antibiotic is prescribed for a specific number of doses. It is important for the resident to take all of the medication, as prescribed, unless side effects develop. If the antibiotic is not taken for the prescribed length of time, the microbes may not be killed and the remaining microbes may develop a resistance to the drug.

Viruses

Viruses are smaller than bacteria. Viruses cause the common cold, flu, and many childhood diseases such as mumps, chickenpox, measles, and polio. Viruses also cause some forms of pneumonia, herpes simplex, herpes zoster (shingles), acquired immune deficiency syndrome (AIDS), and hepatitis. Antibiotics are not effective in controlling infections caused by viruses. Other drugs may be prescribed to control minor symptoms associated with a cold, such as a stuffy nose.

Fungi

Fungi cause skin and mucous membrane infections like yeast vaginitis, athlete's foot, ringworm, and thrush (Figure 10-2).

Parasites

Infections due to parasites are more rare but can affect the blood, lungs, and intestines when they occur.

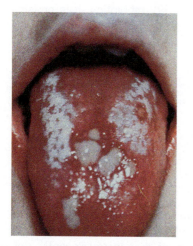

Figure 10-2 The white patches on the tongue are the result of a yeast (fungus) infection. This condition is called *thrush*.

Parasites are organisms that live within or upon another organism (the host). Examples of parasites are worms that live in the digestive tract and fleas, lice, mites, and ticks that live on the outer surface of the host.

? EXERCISE 10-1

VOCABULARY
Choose the best word to fill in each blank.

antibody
microbes
bacteremia
health care–associated carrier infections (HAIs)
infections
pathogens

1. Acquired while in the facility _____
   _____

2. Produced when microbes enter the body and cause disease _____
   _____

3. Microbes that cause disease _____
   _____

4. Germs _____

TRUE OR FALSE
Indicate whether the following statements are true (T) or false (F).

5. T F The sensitivity test tells the physician which organism is causing the infection.

6. T F Visitors and staff can transfer germs to residents by coughing or sneezing.

7. T F Parasites live within or upon another organism called the *host*.

MULTIPLE CHOICE
Select the one best answer.

8. A disease caused by a bacterium is
   (A) common cold
   (B) hepatitis
   (C) strep throat
   (D) flu

9. Viruses
   (A) can be controlled by antibiotics
   (B) are the same as bacteria
   (C) cause the common cold, flu, and many childhood diseases
   (D) are larger than bacteria

THE CHAIN OF INFECTION

Infections occur when certain conditions are met. These conditions are called the *chain of infection* (Figure 10-3) and include:

- Causative or infectious agent or microbe—pathogen germ that causes the disease. This is the statement that refers to pathogens. Non-pathogens is the word listed in the Precision exam that needs to be eliminated.
- Reservoir—human body or animals, insects, water, dirty surfaces, where the microbe can live
- Portal of exit—manner in which the microbe leaves the body (through an open wound or splatter of body fluids)
- Mode of transmission—manner in which the microbe is carried to another person. Transmission may be from person to person or from insects and animals to people.
- Portal of entry—manner in which the microbe enters another person through broken skin, respiratory tract, mucous membranes, catheters/tubes
- Susceptible host—a person who will become ill from the entry of microbes into the body

Microbes cause disease by entering the body through a portal of entry. They spread disease by leaving the body through a portal of exit and being transmitted to another person. They enter that person's body and can again cause disease.

Microbes enter and leave the body through body openings such as:

- Eyes, ears, nose, or mouth
- Breaks in the skin
- Penis, vagina, urinary meatus (bladder opening), or rectum

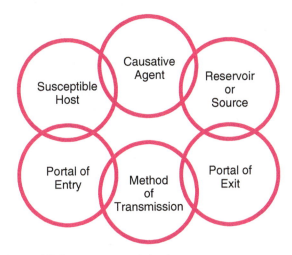

Figure 10-3 The chain of infection.

Transmission (spread) of infectious organisms may occur in one of three ways (Figure 10-4):

- Airborne transmission. Small particles remain suspended in the air and move with air currents or become trapped in dust, which is also carried in air currents. The resident breathes in the pathogens carried in this manner.
- Droplet transmission. Droplets are moist particles from coughing, sneezing, or talking. Pathogens are transmitted into the air with the droplets. Droplets usually travel only 3 feet from the source.
- Contact transmission. Direct contact occurs by touching the source of the pathogens. Indirect contact occurs when a person touches an item contaminated with pathogens, such as soiled linen or environmental surfaces. These items are known as fomites.

Not all organisms are transmitted in the same way and some organisms may be transmitted in more than one way. Figure 10-5 shows how health care providers can interrupt the chain of infection at various points and thus prevent the spread of infection.

Types of Infections

Infections can be:

- Localized (confined to one area)—such as a boil or skin abscess
- Generalized—such as pneumonia (in the lungs)
- Systemic—widespread through the bloodstream (bacteremia)

People who have pathogens in their bodies but do not show signs of disease are called carriers. Carriers can transmit diseases to others. The pathogens in their bodies are not harmful to the carriers, but they may be harmful to other people.

NORMAL BODY FLORA

Different microbes live on our body surfaces. These microbes are called the normal body flora. The flora is not the same in all body areas. For example, the organisms making up the flora of the intestinal tract are different from those of the respiratory tract. Healthy individuals live in harmony with the normal body flora. However, the balance may be disturbed by:

- Pathogenic organisms
- Normal flora organisms that become pathogenic
- Organisms from one flora that are transferred into a different body flora
- Drugs such as antibiotics that upset the normal balance of organisms within a flora, allowing one group to flourish

Airborne	Tiny microbes are carried by moisture or dust particles in air and are inhaled. Airborne microbes stay in the air longer than droplets and may be caused by:

Airborne — Tiny microbes are carried by moisture or dust particles in air and are inhaled. Airborne microbes stay in the air longer than droplets and may be caused by:
- Coughing
- Sneezing
- Talking
- Laughing
- Singing

Droplet — *Droplets spread* within approximately 3 feet (no personal contact). Droplets are larger and heavier than airborne microbes, so they cannot travel as far. Droplet nuclei are inhaled:
- Coughing
- Sneezing
- Talking
- Laughing
- Singing

Contact — *Direct contact* of health care provider with resident:
- Touching
- Toileting (urine and feces)
- Bathing
- Secretions or excretions from patient
- Rubbing
- Blood, body fluid, mucous membranes, or nonintact skin

Indirect contact of health care provider with objects used by residents:
- Clothing
- Bed linens
- Personal belongings
- Personal care equipment
- Instruments and supplies used in treatments
- Dressings
- Diagnostic equipment
- Permanent or disposable health care equipment
- Environmental surfaces such as counters, faucets, and doorknobs

Common vehicle — Spread to many people through contact with items such as:
- Food
- Water
- Medication
- Contaminated blood products

Vector-borne — Intermediate hosts such as:
- Flies
- Fleas
- Ticks
- Rats
- Mice
- Roaches

Figure 10-4 Modes of transmission of microbes.

? EXERCISE 10-2

BRIEF ANSWERS
Briefly answer the following statements.

1. Three portals of entry for pathogens into the body are:
   a. _____
   b. _____
   c. _____

TRUE OR FALSE
Indicate whether the following statements are true (T) or false (F).

2. T F Microbes may enter the body through any body opening.

3. T F The way microbes leave the body is called the *portal of entry*.

4. T F A skin abscess is a generalized infection.

(continues)

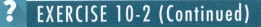

❓ EXERCISE 10-2 (Continued)

5. T F Droplet nuclei can be inhaled, transmitting disease.

6. T F Fomites are pathogens.

MULTIPLE CHOICE
Select the one best answer.

7. An example of transmission by indirect contact is
   (A) coughing   (C) having sexual contact
   (B) handling bed linens (D) touching a resident

8. Droplet transmission of infectious organisms occurs through
   (A) sneezing   (C) insects that harbor microbes
   (B) water   (D) feces

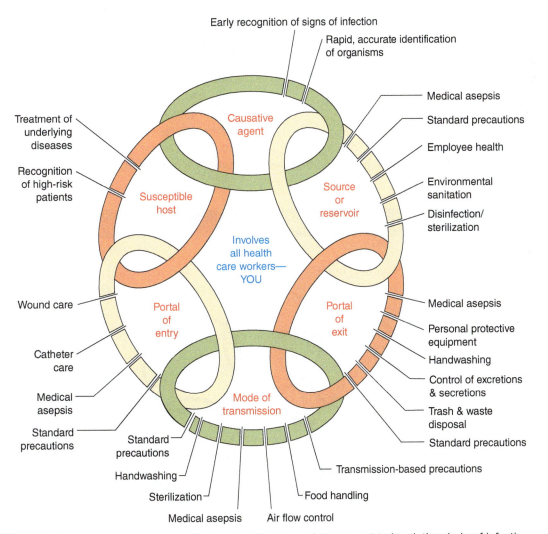

Figure 10-5 This diagram shows ways you and other health care workers can act to break the chain of infection and block the transmission of disease.

You can help avoid infections in yourself by:

- Eating a healthy diet
- Getting an adequate amount of sleep daily
- Keeping your body clean and living in a clean environment
- Avoiding unhealthy habits such as smoking, drinking alcohol, or using drugs
- Learning how to cope with stress
- Washing your hands
- Following standard precautions faithfully

NATURAL BODY DEFENSES AGAINST DISEASE

Natural body defenses that can help prevent infectious diseases include:

- Intact skin
- Tears
- Mucous membranes (the lining) of the respiratory, reproductive, and genitourinary tracts
- Hydrochloric acid in the stomach
- Hair in the nose and eyelashes
- White blood cells (leukocytes) that multiply and attempt to destroy pathogenic microbes in the body

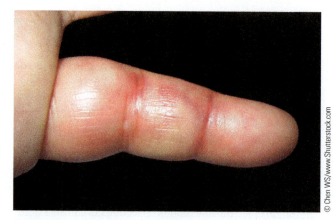

Figure 10-6 Redness, swelling, heat, pain, and loss of function are signs of the inflammatory process.

© Chen WS/www.Shutterstock.com

- Enzymes in saliva
- Antibodies that develop in the blood after a person has had an infectious disease
- **Inflammation**—a process that brings blood and white blood cells to the area of infection; a skin infection, for example, generally becomes swollen, hot, and painful, signs that inflammation is occurring (Figure 10-6).
- Temperature—an elevated temperature is believed to increase the body's ability to fight infection, unless the infection becomes too severe.

? EXERCISE 10-3

COMPLETION
Refer to the Figure below. Fill in the missing information in the chain of infection in the spaces provided.

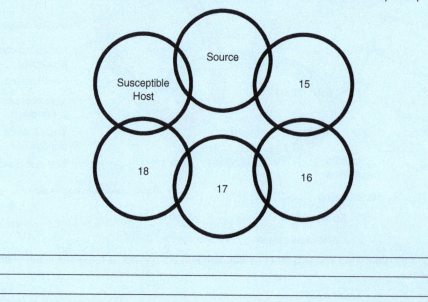

1. _____
2. _____
3. _____
4. _____

IMMUNITY

Immunity is the ability to fight off disease caused by microbes. A pathogenic microbe that enters the body is an **antigen**. In response to this, the blood develops substances called **antibodies**. These antibodies provide immunity to the disease caused by that particular antigen. For example, if an individual has antigens in the bloodstream from having had measles, he or she will form antibodies in the blood that prevent the occurrence of measles a second time.

Immunosuppression

Immunosuppression occurs when the body's immune system is inadequate and fails to respond to the challenge of infectious disease organisms that it normally would fight successfully. The individual becomes more likely to develop a variety of infections. A number of factors can lead to this condition, including:

- Diseases such as leukemia
- Advanced age
- Frailty
- Drug therapy
- Infection with human immunodeficiency virus (HIV)
- Injury or removal of the spleen
- Radiation therapy

Immunizations

Artificial defenses called **immunizations** protect against specific pathogens. Immunization is provided by **vaccines**. These are artificial or weakened antigens that help the body develop protective antibodies before the need arises. Vaccines are available to prevent most childhood diseases such

? EXERCISE 10-4

VOCABULARY
Choose the best word to fill in each blank.

antibody
artificial
flora
microbes
bacteremia
infections
pathogens

1. Weakened antigens _____
2. Germs _____
3. Protective substance produced by the body in response to an antigen _____
4. Immunization is a(an) _____ defense designed to protect against a specific disease.
5. The normal body _____ are the organisms that commonly live in a particular body area.

BRIEF ANSWERS
Briefly answer the following statements.

6. Four natural body defenses include:
   a. _____
   b. _____
   c. _____
   d. _____
7. Two vaccines commonly given to protect older people are:
   a. _____
   b. _____

as measles, rubella (German measles), mumps, polio, diphtheria, chickenpox, whooping cough, and tetanus. Pneumonia, influenza, and shingles vaccines are frequently given to elderly people. Health care workers who have direct contact with residents are advised to take hepatitis B vaccine. Federal legislation requires that employers provide this vaccine without charge to employees who are considered at risk. In general, it is advised that all health care workers receive seasonal immunizations such as influenza vaccine.

SERIOUS INFECTIONS IN HEALTH CARE FACILITIES

Serious bacterial and viral infections are increasing in health care facilities as well as in the general public. Older persons and frail people are particularly susceptible to infectious diseases, as are the very young and those with autoimmune disease or compromised (poorly functioning) immune systems.

BACTERIAL INFECTIONS

Bacteria are often the cause of serious skin, respiratory, urinary, and gastrointestinal infections in residents. If the physician suspects that a resident has a bacterial infection, a culture and sensitivity test may be ordered.

When an antibiotic is prescribed, it is important to take all the medication prescribed for the stated length of time. If the person stops taking the antibiotic too soon, some of the microbes may remain and develop a resistance to the antibiotic.

MRSA and VRE

Two groups of organisms have become resistant to two powerful antibiotics: methicillin and vancomycin. Both organisms are part of the normal flora of the human body. These organisms are:

- **Methicillin-resistant** *Staphylococcus aureus* **(MRSA)**
  Staphylococci are normally found on the skin and mucous membranes. Health care–associated-MRSA (HA-MRSA) is now found almost everywhere (endemic) in health care facilities. It can be spread by direct or indirect contact. It causes life-threatening infections involving the respiratory and urinary systems and the skin, especially

in persons with weakened immune systems. HA-MRSA is difficult to treat because the microorganisms are resistant to many antibiotic drugs. Infection control practices depend upon the type of the tissue infection. For example, standard precautions are required for a skin infection. It is important to note that these organisms can live for prolonged periods of time. They have been found to live for 7 weeks on polyester fabrics (i.e., uniforms, lab coats, bedside curtains) and up to 12 weeks on polyethylene products.

Another variant of MRSA has become a significant problem—community-acquired MRSA (CA-MRSA), which occurs in healthy people, begins as a skin boil and is spread by skin-to-skin contact. Groups such as team athletes, children in day care, and elders in senior centers, among others, may be affected. Persons who choose to get tattoos or any type of body piercings also are at risk for acquiring CA-MRSA. Figure 10-7 shows *S. aureus* organisms.

- **Vancomycin-resistant enterococci (VRE)**
  Enterococci are found in the gastrointestinal tract. They are a major cause of nosocomial infections in health care facilities. Most strains are highly resistant to many antibiotics. VRE is spread directly from the resident or caregiver to another resident. It may also be spread from contaminated surfaces or objects such as side rails or bed linens. Standard precautions are required. Newer strains are resistant to vancomycin.

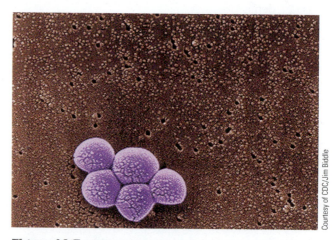

Courtesy of CDC/Jim Biddle

Figure 10-7 Methicillin-resistant *Staphylococcus aureus* (MRSA) has developed a resistance to the antibiotic of choice for treating the infection.

Other Bacterial Infective Agents

Serious infections are also caused by the following types of bacteria:

- *Streptococcus pyogenes* (*Streptococcus A*)—this pathogen is known as the "flesh-eating" bacterium. This organism is frequently involved in soft tissue destruction because it produces powerful toxins and enzymes. Without early diagnosis, treatment to remove the diseased tissue, and aggressive treatment with antibiotics, the mortality rate can be very high.

- *Pseudomonas aeruginosa*—this organism is found in water and on other environmental surfaces. It causes urinary tract infections and can be transmitted by artificial nails.

- *Escherichia coli*—bacterium commonly found in the intestinal tract where it is normally nonpathogenic. Outside the intestinal tract, however, it can be the primary cause of urinary tract infections or infections in pressure ulcers. There are many strains of *E. coli*. One strain, *E. coli O157:H7*, produces powerful toxins that can cause severe bloody diarrhea and kidney complications. The organism can live in the intestines of healthy cattle. Meat can become contaminated during the slaughtering process. The microbe is then transmitted in contaminated and undercooked meat, fruits, and vegetables that have been exposed to water and/or soils that have been polluted with feces, or by a person who has been handling tainted food. *E. coli* also has been found on cutting boards and utensils that have not been thoroughly cleaned.

- Udders of cows can become contaminated and the organisms transferred through unpasteurized milk. Thorough cooking of ground meat, drinking only pasteurized milk, and careful handwashing are important steps in controlling this foodborne disease.

- Salmonella—a group of bacteria that cause mild to life-threatening intestinal infections, including "food poisoning."

- *Mycobacterium tuberculosis*—the bacterium that causes tuberculosis.

- *Clostridium difficile* (*C. difficile* or "*C. diff*")—a bacterium that is part of the normal bowel flora but can cause serious diarrhea from inflammation of the colon in residents who have received antibiotic medications. Residents with *C. difficile* infections are placed in a private room or in a semi-private room with another resident who may have the same infection to prevent spread of the infectious disease. It is important to carry out *vigorous* handwashing

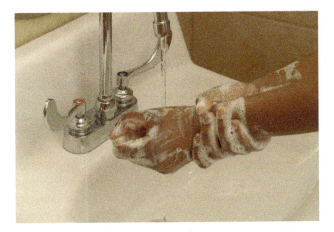

Figure 10-8 Vigorous handwashing with soap and water is required for infection control.

technique, preferably with warm water and soap as opposed to hand sanitizers because this organism forms spores that are not affected by alcohol-based products (Figure 10-8). The organisms are able to slip off the hands during rinsing with warm water and flushed down the drain. The sink can be disinfected and local sewage treatment plants kill the organism further down the line. Wear a gown and use gloves when caring for residents. (See Lesson 11.) Wash your hands again after removing the gloves. (Refer to Procedure 11-7.)

- Spores are transferred to others by persons who have touched a contaminated item or surface. The action of the spores has been likened to that of ping pong balls bouncing around in the environment. Bedrails, bed curtains, electronic rectal thermometers, bath tubs, door handles, light switches, call buttons, or anything that may have come in contact with feces or contaminated gloves can retain and shed the spores. Because the spores are so long-lived, some have been known to survive for up to one year, it is crucial to prevent cross contamination. Spores can be carried on your hands or the resident's and spread unknowingly. All furnishings and surfaces in the resident's room must be thoroughly cleansed with a 1:10 bleach solution (one of the only substances that will kill the spores). As spores will continue to spread from the wall of the intestine of the infected person for several days after the diarrhea has subsided, isolation procedures will be continued. In recent years, *C. difficile* infections have become more severe and more difficult to treat.

Tuberculosis

Before 1950 and the development of antibiotics to target tuberculosis, it was a widespread disease with a high fatality rate. The number of cases dropped over the next 30 years. However, from 1985 to 1992, the number of tuberculosis cases once more increased. The increase was due to less public effort to combat the disease and the development of forms of the organism that are resistant to the antibiotics commonly used in treatment. By 1996 the number of cases again began to decline as resistant strains were better identified, diagnostic techniques were improved, and a program of direct observation therapy was introduced. Direct observation involves delivery of the medication to the patient at home, school, or work and watching as it is taken, to ensure compliance with the prescribed drug therapy.

Today more people are at risk for infection, including those who:

- Are HIV positive
- Are infected but fail to take their medication for the full treatment period
- Live in poverty and are malnourished
- Have immigrated to the United States from countries where tuberculosis is still common
- Have inactive tuberculosis but have grown older and experience increased disability

Tuberculosis Infection

Tuberculosis infection occurs when the bacterium that causes the disease enters the body. The lungs are the most common site of involvement. The body usually responds to the infection by creating a barrier that prevents the spread of the pathogens to other parts of the body. This barrier is called a **tubercle**. As long as the tubercle remains intact and no other tuberculosis bacteria enter the body, the infection is called inactive or controlled. In this state the person is not **contagious** (capable of passing the infection to others). If the person is immunocompromised, the tubercle may not form and the person develops active tuberculosis disease (primary tuberculosis).

Tuberculosis Disease

Tuberculosis disease develops if the tubercle breaks down or more tuberculosis bacteria enter the body. The bacteria multiply, tissue damage increases, and the bacteria may spread to other parts of the body. As the disease progresses, the person will show one or more of the following signs and symptoms:

- Fatigue
- Loss of appetite and weight
- Weakness
- Elevated temperature in the afternoon and evening
- Night sweats

- Spitting up blood (**hemoptysis**)
- Coughing

The person with tuberculosis in the lungs can spread the bacteria to others through airborne droplets in respiratory secretions.

Diagnosis

The presence of tuberculosis bacteria in the body can be shown by:

- A sputum culture—grows the organisms from the person's lungs
- Chest x-rays—show the extent of the disease process in the lungs
- A positive skin test (Mantoux test)—shows the presence of antibodies to the tuberculosis organisms in the body (Figure 10-9)

Health care providers in long-term care must undergo a skin test for tuberculosis before employment. They are

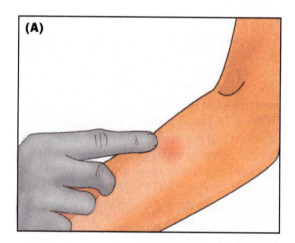

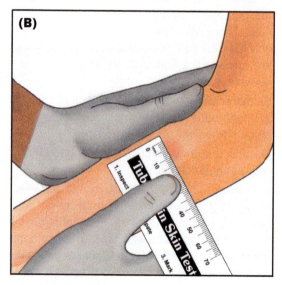

Figure 10-9 A positive Mantoux test shows redness and induration (swelling) of 10 mm (1 cm) 48 to 72 hours after the test.

then tested regularly (usually every 6 to 12 months) according to the degree of risk of exposure to ensure that they remain disease-free.

Residents usually are skin tested once a year. Because the immune response may be weaker in older persons, a two-step procedure of skin testing is recommended for those older than 50 years. If the first skin test is negative, the test is repeated in 1 to 2 weeks. The second test acts as a "booster" to the test stimulus. A negative response after the second test usually indicates the person is free from infection. If a positive reaction is noted, a chest x-ray will be ordered to determine lung involvement and appropriate treatment.

Treatment

A person with tuberculosis is treated with a selected antibiotic or combination of antibiotics. Because many disease organisms have become more resistant to specific drugs, a combination of drugs must be used to control them. Once antitubercular drug therapy starts, the resident usually becomes noncontagious (cannot spread the disease organism) within 2 to 3 weeks. The therapy, however, continues for 6 months to 2 years.

? EXERCISE 10-5

BRIEF ANSWERS

1. The letters MRSA and VRE stand for:

   M _____   V _____
   R _____   R _____
   S _____   E _____
   A _____

TRUE OR FALSE

Indicate whether the following statements are true (T) or false (F).

2. T F MRSA is a common microbe and no special precautions need to be taken.

3. T F Handwashing should be carried out before and after each resident contact.

MULTIPLE CHOICE

Select the one best answer.

4. Health care acquired MRSA
   (A) is spread by direct contact only
   (B) is easy to treat because the microorganisms respond readily to many antibiotic drugs
   (C) has a short lifespan
   (D) is found almost everywhere in health care facilities

5. *E. coli*
   (A) can be transferred through pasteurized milk
   (B) is part of normal bowel flora
   (C) can cause severe bloody diarrhea and kidney complications
   (D) can destroy tissue and blood cells

6. Vaccines that are available for protection include
   (A) mumps   (C) hepatitis B
   (B) polio   (D) all of these

7. Which of the following is not a natural body defense against infection?
   (A) elevated temperature   (C) inflammation
   (B) leukocytes   (D) antibiotics

8. An organism that causes which disease has become resistant to antibiotic therapy over the years?
   (A) mumps   (C) tuberculosis
   (B) polio   (D) valley fever

(continues)

? EXERCISE 10-5 (Continued)

9. When a person is suspected of having tuberculosis
   (A) a sputum culture may be ordered
   (B) x-ray films may be taken
   (C) skin testing may be performed
   (D) all of these

10. *C. difficile*
    (A) has a short lifespan outside the body
    (B) requires precautions of gowning and gloving
    (C) may be killed by alcohol-based products
    (D) does not require gowning or gloving

VIRAL INFECTIONS

Several viral infections are described in this section:

- Shingles (herpes zoster)
- Influenza
- Hepatitis
- AIDS

The viral infection genital herpes is covered in Lesson 27.

Shingles

Shingles (herpes zoster) occurs in people who have been infected by the virus that causes chickenpox. Although the person recovers from chickenpox, the organisms do not leave the body. These organisms remain in the body's nervous system in a nonactive state.

Years later, when the person is in a weakened condition, the organisms become active. Painful blister-like lesions develop in the skin along the paths of sensitive nerves. Eventually the lesions heal on their own. These contain infectious organisms, and contact and airborne precautions should be used.

Because chickenpox is caused by the same organism that causes shingles, infants and children who have not been immunized can get chickenpox from exposure to an adult with shingles.

A shingles vaccine has been developed. The CDC recommends the vaccine use for persons 60 years and older to prevent shingles.

Influenza

Influenza (or flu) is caused by a family of viruses. The infection can lead to serious consequences for older or frail residents. Each year new types of viruses spread rapidly by way of respiratory secretions from person to person, causing many people to become ill.

Vaccines offer some protection against influenza viruses and are often given to residents in long-term care.

Someone with the flu may experience:

- Malaise (general unwell feeling)
- Chills
- Fever
- Muscle aches and pains
- Cold-like symptoms

In addition to making the person feel ill, the viruses may lower the resident's resistance to other infectious organisms. These other organisms can cause pneumonia and other life-threatening infections. Medicines may be given that limit the effects of the viruses and antibiotics are given to combat bacterial infections that may develop. Droplet precautions should be applied.

You can help protect the residents in your care against influenza by:

- Staying healthy
- Not reporting for duty when you are ill
- Carrying out standard precautions faithfully
- Following the facility's policies regarding special precautions when a resident has a respiratory infection
- Encouraging the resident to drink fluids
- Reporting to the charge nurse when a visitor seems to be ill
- Getting an annual dose of the flu vaccine

Hepatitis

Hepatitis is an inflammation of the liver caused by several viruses, including:

- Hepatitis A virus
- Hepatitis B virus
- Hepatitis C virus
- Hepatitis D virus
- Hepatitis E virus
- Hepatitis G virus

Characteristics of these viruses are:

- Hepatitis A virus (HAV)
  - Most common
  - Transmitted by fecal-oral route
  - Vaccine available

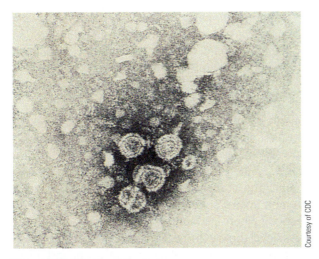

Figure 10-10 Hepatitis B virus.

- Often only minimal signs or symptoms
- Does not lead to sclerosis of the liver or chronic hepatitis
- Hepatitis B virus (HBV) (Figure 10-10)
  - Can survive many months on environmental surfaces if not appropriately disinfected
  - Most serious
  - Transmitted by way of blood, sexual secretions, and fecal-oral route
  - Vaccine available
  - Tends to cause a severe, acute infection
  - May progress to chronic infection and permanent liver damage
- Hepatitis C virus (HCV)
  - Transmitted mainly through blood and blood products, body fluids, sharing of needles by IV drug users, and sexual contact
  - May be mistaken for the flu
  - Common signs and symptoms: extreme fatigue, depression, fever, mood changes, weakness, pain, loss of appetite
  - Treated with alpha interferon; treatment is not always successful
  - Chronic hepatitis in 50% of cases
  - May cause liver cancer and liver failure
  - May be present for years before the person becomes aware if it; during this time it silently destroys the liver
  - Leading cause of need for liver transplants in the United States
- Hepatitis D virus (*delta agent hepatitis*)
  - Transmitted mainly through blood and body fluids
  - Develops only in the presence of acute hepatitis B or can cause a more severe form of hepatitis B
  - Hepatitis B vaccine can help prevent hepatitis D

- Hepatitis E
  - Transmitted by fecal-oral route; contaminated food and water
  - More common in immigrants or persons who have traveled from high-risk areas such as Asia, Africa, Middle East, or Mexico
  - Causes acute infection, like hepatitis A
- Hepatitis G
  - Transmitted through blood and blood products
  - Related to hepatitis C; may be a coinfection (occurs at the same time)
  - Usually mild course; not long lasting
  - No specific treatment (bed rest, balanced diet, avoid intake of alcohol)

The liver is a vital organ and any infection of the liver is serious. Health care workers must take hepatitis very seriously because many persons have no signs or symptoms of illness yet are able to transmit the infection to others. You can best protect yourself by:

- Using standard precautions (discussed in Lesson 11)
- Taking the vaccine, if available
- Practicing safe sex (using condoms)
- Not using illegal drugs
- Giving your full attention to the handling of sharps such as needles or razors
- Maintaining your own proper nutrition

Acquired Immune Deficiency Syndrome (AIDS)

AIDS is a viral disease. It is transmitted primarily through direct contact with the bodily secretions of an infected person. The virus that causes AIDS is the **human immunodeficiency virus (HIV)**.

The ways in which HIV is transmitted include:

- Blood to blood through:
  - Transfusion of infected blood. Note that federal regulations prohibit the use of untested and unregulated blood in the United States.
  - Treatment of hemophilia with clotting factor from infected blood
  - Needle sharing among drug users
  - Prick from a contaminated needle or sharp object
  - Unsterile instruments used for procedures such as body piercing or tattooing
  - Shaving razors and toothbrushes from infected persons
- Unprotected vaginal or anal intercourse when one partner is infected
- Infected mother to infant during:
  - Pregnancy, placental complications
  - Birth process
  - Nursing/breastfeeding

The AIDS Virus

The AIDS virus (HIV):

- Has no known cure
- Has many variants
- Does not live for long outside the body
- Is affected by common chemicals
- Depresses the body's immune system
- Makes the infected person more susceptible to infections
- Makes the infected person more likely to experience complications such as:
  - *Pneumocystis carinii* pneumonia—a serious lung infection
  - Kaposi sarcoma—a serious malignancy affecting many body organs. Figure 10-11 shows skin lesions of Kaposi sarcoma.
  - Brain involvement leading to dementia
  - Eye involvement leading to blindness
  - Tuberculosis
  - Other opportunistic infections

Incubation Period

Not everyone who comes in contact with HIV becomes infected. For those who are infected, there is always a period of time between contact and the production of detectable HIV antibody.

- During this period the virus is in infected cells but is not active in making RNA and proteins. The body does not make antibodies to the virus.
- Most people become seropositive or HIV positive (show antibodies to HIV in the bloodstream) approximately 3 months after infection. The person has HIV disease, which may progress to AIDS.

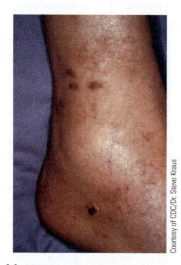

Courtesy of CDC/Dr. Steve Kraus

Figure 10-11 HIV infection predisposes the person with AIDS to develop Kaposi sarcoma. Typical cutaneous brown lesions caused by Kaposi sarcoma over the left ankle and foot.

- The asymptomatic period (when no signs and symptoms are present) following infection may last months to years. AIDS does not always develop, but the person is an HIV carrier for life.

Disease Progression

Progression of the disease process is determined by the effect of the viruses on special protective white blood cells known as CD4 cells (T cells). Over time the number of the protective white blood cells drops. As a result, the immune system of the infected person becomes more suppressed and less able to fight infection. When the number of CD4 cells drops to a critical level (below 200 cells/mm^3), the person is diagnosed with AIDS or develops one of 26 opportunistic infections.

- Symptoms of HIV infection, when they do appear, consist of:
  - Acute flu-like symptoms
  - Fever
  - Night sweats
  - Fatigue
  - Swollen lymph nodes
  - Sore throat
  - Gastrointestinal problems
  - Headache
- One-fourth to one-half of people exposed to HIV show evidence of disease within 5 to 10 years of antibody development (becoming seropositive).

Testing

Several tests have been developed to confirm the presence of antibodies to HIV (positive for HIV infection) and to confirm the presence of AIDS.

The test for antibodies is also used to check the national blood supply. When people donate blood, it is tested to be sure that it is free of HIV antibodies. This protects the people who receive blood transfusions and other blood products.

Treatment

No specific treatment is able to cure AIDS at the present time. Each opportunistic infection is treated vigorously.

- No vaccine prevents the infection from developing. However, millions of dollars are being spent on research to develop a vaccine.
- Therapy is directed toward vigorously treating each infection as it appears.
- Nutritional and other forms of preventive therapy are aimed at maintaining a person with AIDS in the best health possible.

- The drug industry continues to develop drugs that slow down the disease process or reinforce the immune system. These drugs, however, do not cure the disease. At the present time there is *no* evidence that AIDS is transmitted:
  - Through kissing, touching, or hugging an HIV-infected person
  - By eating at the same table with an infected person
  - By using the same toilet seat
  - Through insect bites

Nursing facilities are admitting more people in their thirties and forties who are seriously ill with AIDS. Many of these people have wasting or dementia (irreversible brain disease). This is stressful to the health care providers because it is easy to identify with the age group. It takes maturity to offer the support and care needed.

OTHER IMPORTANT INFECTIONS

Infection Caused by Fungi

Candida albicans (thrush) is characterized by creamy-white patches and ulcers that form on the tongue and oral mucous membranes. When the cheese-like curds are rubbed off, the underlying area appears very red and may bleed. *Candida* infections can occur in persons who are diabetics, immunosuppressed (cancer and/or AIDS), on antibiotic therapy, or on long-term tube feedings. Yeast infections of the skin may occur as the result of poor hygiene and/or moisture in dark areas (armpits, under the breasts, skin folds, and in the groin and vaginal areas).Treatment may include the use of antifungal drugs that may be taken as pills or liquids. Keep the skin clean and dry, observe for signs of infection. Always wear gloves when performing any mouth care for the resident. If the resident is able to eat food orally, the food should be bland and nonirritating until the lesions heal. (See Figure 10-2.)

Infection Caused by Parasites

Two diseases caused by parasites are becoming more common in the general public and in health facilities. Giardiasis is caused by *Giardia lamblia*, which is found in the water supplies of many communities. It causes severe diarrhea but responds to medication. Cryptosporidiosis is caused by the *Cryptosporidium* protozoa, which is found in the digestive tract of domestic animals and is transferred by contact. It causes severe diarrhea, especially in immunosuppressed people. There is no specific treatment.

External Parasites

External parasites (ectoparasites) that can live on the body are head lice and mites.

Lice (Pediculosis)

Lice are tiny, flat, wingless, parasitic insects about the size of a sesame seed. These insects live outside the body but feed on the person's blood and then inject their excrement (waste products) into the skin, thus causing intense itching of the surrounding skin. Lice can be found in the hair, on the body, and in the pubic area. These parasites are easily spread from person to person through contact with personal articles such as combs or bedding. The small eggs (nits) of lice cling to hair follicles. Contact precautions are needed. Medicated shampoos and baths are ordered and the clothing and bedding are bagged and sent to the laundry. The environment is vacuumed and then wiped with a disinfectant. At times it may be necessary to cut the hair to remove the nits. Lice can be removed by hand using a fine-toothed comb, double-sided tape, or tweezers. Your supervisor will tell you how to proceed.

Scabies

A skin disease caused by a microscopic mite is referred to as scabies (Figure 10-12). This infestation is highly contagious and spread by direct (person to person) or indirect (touching clothing or bedding that may contain the mite) contact. Health care workers and family members are susceptible to contracting scabies as well and usually undergo the same treatment regimen as the resident. Severe itching, especially at night, and a rash especially between the fingers are sometimes the only signs that a resident has contracted scabies. Figure 10-13 shows the typical rash caused by scabies. Notify the nurse immediately if you note a rash on a resident.

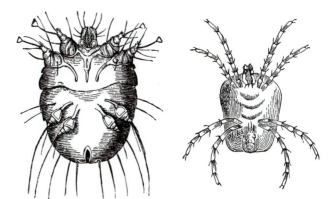

Figure 10-12 The scabies mite is microscopic and cannot be seen without a microscope.

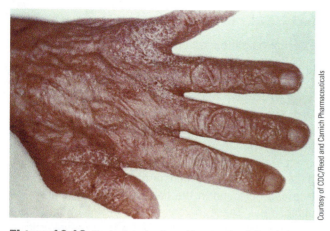

Courtesy of CDC/Reed and Carnich Pharmaceuticals

Figure 10-13 Typical rash of scabies on the legs and knees.

When caring for a resident with scabies, always wear a gown and gloves. Before the medicated lotion or cream is applied, clip the resident's nails. Do not bathe the resident before the lotion is applied or for at least 12 to 24 hours after application. Follow the specific directions of the nurse. The medication should be applied to, around, and under the fingernails, but not around the eyes or lips. If the resident's hands are washed during this time, the medication must be reapplied. All clothing and linens must be bagged separately from the rest of the facility's linens and washed separately. The room must be thoroughly cleaned as well. The mattress is to be inspected for any tears, vacuumed, and cleaned with a facility-approved disinfectant solution. Any item that cannot be cleaned must be sealed in a bag for at least 14 days; the mites cannot live without a food source for longer than this.

Contact precautions are required for 24 hours after the resident has been treated. Occasionally, a second treatment with the medicated lotion is necessary. If so, the cleaning procedure must be repeated.

WHY OLDER RESIDENTS IN LONG-TERM CARE ARE AT RISK FOR INFECTIONS

There are several reasons why older people are at risk for infections.

- Residents usually have several chronic health problems. This lowers their resistance to disease.
- Body changes caused by aging make older people more susceptible to infections. They have less ability to fight disease due to a weakened immune system.
- Residents may have colds or flu and spread the microbes to other residents.

- The skin of older persons offers less protection because it is fragile and easily broken. Any break in the skin, such as a pressure sore or skin tear, can quickly become infected.
- Poor bladder emptying and indwelling catheters increase the risk of bladder infections.
- Poor or improper incontinent care.
- Bowel-incontinent residents are at risk for infections through accidental ingestion of feces or by contact of feces with nonintact skin (skin tears, rashes, pressure sores, and ulcers).
- The ability to cough and raise secretions is reduced, so older persons have less ability to get rid of pathogens from the lungs. They also are at risk for aspiration that can lead to pneumonia.

Older residents are also more likely to develop serious complications from infections. A simple urinary tract infection can result in bacteremia (blood infection), causing the resident to be acutely ill. This can be fatal to the resident who has little ability to cope with additional health problems.

Infections may not be readily detected in older adults for the following reasons:

- Older persons are less likely to have an elevated temperature as a result of an infection.
- Older persons do not readily develop signs of inflammatory response, which may include pain, heat, and swelling at the site of the infection. These signs may be missing or delayed in older persons.
- Some older people do not feel pain as acutely as younger people. For example, they may feel no discomfort with a bladder infection.

Because of these factors, an infection may be present in the body for several days before it is detected.

GENERAL MEASURES TO PREVENT INFECTIONS

1. Assist residents to maintain an adequate fluid intake. This helps prevent urinary tract and respiratory tract infections and keeps the skin healthier.
2. Assist residents to maintain adequate nutritional intake. Report to the nurse when residents eat less or refuse food.
3. Assist residents to carry out exercise programs established by the nurse or physical therapist. Follow positioning schedules and orders for range of motion exercises and ambulation. This increases circulation, thus lowering the risk for pressure ulcers (a frequent source of infection).

Exercise improves breathing, thereby decreasing the risk of respiratory infections.

4. Encourage residents to be outdoors to enjoy the fresh air whenever possible.

5. Regularly toilet residents who need assistance. This keeps the bladder empty and assures residents that they will receive help when they need to urinate. Some residents hesitate to drink fluids for fear they will be incontinent.

6. When cleaning the perineal area of residents, be sure to wipe women from front to back. This prevents contaminating the urethra (bladder opening) with stool or vaginal excretions.

7. Perform catheter care as directed. Avoid opening the drainage system.

8. Observe residents carefully and report any unusual signs or changes, such as:
   - Changes in frequency of urination or amount of urine voided
   - Complaints of pain or burning on urination
   - Changes in character of urine
   - Coughing or respiratory problems
   - Confusion/disorientation that was not present before or that has increased
   - Drainage or discharge from any body opening or skin wound
   - Changes in skin color
   - Complaints of pain, discomfort, or nausea
   - Elevated temperature
   - Red, swollen areas on body

9. Keep residents clean and dry and promote skin integrity through the use of lotions, and proper turning and positioning (Figure 10-14).

10. Staff members who have an infectious disease should not be on duty. Caring for your own health is vital in preventing illness in residents. Friends and family of residents should be advised not to visit when they do not feel well. If you notice a visitor coughing and sneezing, or otherwise obviously sick, inform your supervisor.

11. Encourage all residents and all staff to practice good hygiene, such as proper handwashing. This is the primary means of preventing the spread of infection.

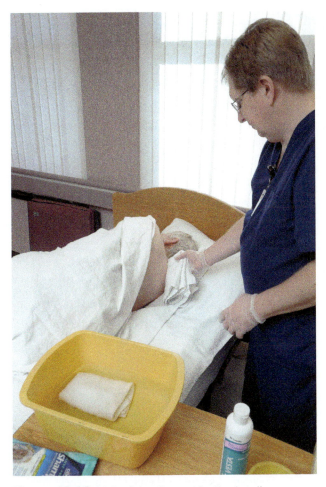

Figure 10-14 Maintaining the resident's cleanliness helps prevent infectious disease.

OUTBREAK OF INFECTIOUS DISEASE IN A LONG-TERM CARE FACILITY

An outbreak of an infection in the facility can be serious for all residents. Unless steps are taken immediately, the infection can spread rapidly. Examples of outbreaks include:

- Influenza
- Gastroenteritis
- Hepatitis
- MRSA
- Tuberculosis
- Foodborne illnesses
- Scabies (parasites that invade the skin)

Most facilities have an action plan that is used in response to an outbreak of infection. The local Public health department and the Center for Disease Control are notified of the outbreak. The Public health department will assist the facility in determining the type of outbreak and its cause. All staff are informed of the

⊘N THE JOB

Long artificial nails can accumulate organisms that cause serious infections.

? EXERCISE 10-6

COMPLETION
Select the correct term(s) from the following list.

adequate	chronic	susceptible
artificial	circulation	toileting
breathing	nutrition	inflammation
carriers	Infection	urinary

1. Residents need to maintain _____ fluid intake.

2. It is important to maintain adequate_____ so all uneaten or poorly eaten meals should be reported.

3. Exercise increases _____ and improves _____, and this decreases the risk of respiratory infections.

4. Regular _____ helps keep bladders empty and reduces the risk of _____ infections.

5. An elderly person may not feel the effects of a(an) _____ as acutely as a younger person.

6. _____ is a protective body defense mechanism.

MULTIPLE CHOICE
Select the one best answer.

7. Hepatitis A infection is
    (A) prevented with a vaccine
    (B) transmitted by fecal-oral route
    (C) very rare
    (D) transmitted by a vector

8. Hepatitis C
    (A) can lead to sclerosis of the liver and liver cancer
    (B) affects 10% of the nation's population
    (C) is transmitted through sexual secretions
    (D) is a bacterial infection

9. Someone with influenza might experience
    (A) low temperature
    (B) muscle aches and pains
    (C) a red rash
    (D) blisters around the lips

10. Nursing assistants can help safeguard residents against infection by
    (A) coming to work when they are ill
    (B) allowing ill visitors to visit
    (C) discouraging the resident from drinking fluids
    (D) staying well themselves

11. Which of the following statements about external parasites in *not* true?
    (A) They can be spread through contact with personal articles.
    (B) They include head lice and mites.
    (C) The small lice nits cling to hair follicles.
    (D) Lice cannot be removed by hand.

? EXERCISE 10-7

CLINICAL SITUATION
Answer each of the following questions.

1. You have a cold and are sneezing.
    a. Should you report for work? _____
    b. Why are the residents at risk for infection? _____

2. Mr. Kraft has a pressure ulcer on his right hip. Why is he at risk for infection? _____
    _____

3. Mrs. Curren has an upper respiratory condition. She will remain in her room away from other residents for a few days. Why is this a good idea? _____
    _____

characteristics of the disease and are trained in the precautions to be followed until the outbreak is over. Certain wings of a facility will be closed. There will be no communal dining, disposable dishes and utensils will be used, and there will be no group activities until the outbreak is resolved. If necessary, notices will be posted to advise visitors that the facility is closed to them for a specific length of time.

LESSON SYNTHESIS: Putting It All Together

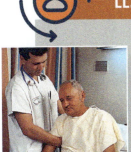

You have just completed this lesson. Now go back and review the Clinical Focus. Try to see how the Clinical Focus relates to the concepts presented in the lesson. Then answer the following questions.

1. Why should Mr. Dwyer be monitored for the possibility that his tuberculosis infection will become active again?
2. Why is Mr. Dwyer's drop in white blood cell count so important?
3. What condition did Mr. Dwyer have that might have injured his liver?
4. What effect does HIV have on Mr. Dwyer's immune system?

10 REVIEW

A. Match each term (items a–e) with the proper definition.

a. antigen
b. antibody
c. inflammation
d. pathogen
e. vaccine

1. _____ a body response to infection
2. _____ term meaning a pathogenic microbe that enters the body
3. _____ provides immunization
4. _____ develops in the body after an infection
5. _____ disease-producing microbe

B. Fill in the blanks by selecting the correct word or phrase from the list.

insects   reservoir
method of   sexual contact
transmission   sneezing
portal of entry   susceptible host
portal of exit   water

6. Complete the chain of infection by naming the parts.

(A) _____
(B) _____
(C) _____
(D) _____
(E) _____
(F) _____

7. An example of transmission by direct contact is _____.
8. An example of direct transmission is through _____.
9. A common vehicle for the transmission of microbes is _____.
10. Vectors, such as animals and _____ also transmit disease organisms.

C. Match the organism (items a–e) with the specific disease it causes.

a. *Mycobacterium tuberculosis*

b. *Candida albicans*

c. HBV

d. HIV

e. MRSA

11. _____   AIDS

12. _____   thrush

13. _____   tuberculosis

14. _____   skin and wound infections by resistant *Staphylococcus aureus*

15. _____   hepatitis

D. Select the one best answer for each of the following.

16. A person who is infected with a pathogenic organism but does not show any signs of an infection is a (an)

(A) transporter

(B) harborer

(C) infector

(D) carrier

17. White blood cells that multiply and attempt to destroy pathogens are

(A) antigens

(B) phagocytes

(C) antibodies

(D) red blood cells

18. Which of the following is not a natural body defense?

(A) antibiotic

(B) hydrochloric acid in the stomach

(C) hair in the nose

(D) tears

19. Which is an example of a local infection?

(A) pneumonia

(B) septicemia

(C) boil

(D) AIDS

20. A parasite is

(A) a type of virus

(B) an organism that lives in or on other organisms

(C) cured with antibiotics

(D) not contagious

21. When a microbe can no longer be controlled or destroyed by a drug, it is said to be

(A) difficult

(B) resistant

(C) untreatable

(D) noncompliant

22. A major reason residents are at risk for infection is

(A) they have new chronic problems

(B) aging makes them more susceptible

(C) their ability to cough is strong

(D) their skin is thicker and less likely to tear

23. Sonny, a nursing assistant, notices that the daughter of one of the residents is coughing and looks flushed. His best action is to

(A) ask the visitor to leave

(B) put a mask on the visitor

(C) put a mask on the resident

(D) refer the matter to the nurse

24. Juan is not feeling well this morning when he wakes up. He has an elevated temperature and is sneezing. He is due on duty at 1500. His best action is to

(A) call in sick

(B) go to work

(C) stay home without notifying the facility

(D) call a friend to go to work for him

25. Scabies

(A) are spread via the respiratory route

(B) can be spread person to person through contact

(C) can be controlled with a simple bath

(D) have small eggs, which burrow into the skin crevices

LESSON 11
INFECTION CONTROL

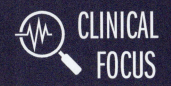

CLINICAL FOCUS

Think about ways you can prevent disease transmission and help residents avoid infections as you study this lesson.

OBJECTIVES

After studying this lesson, you should be able to:

- Define vocabulary words and terms.
- Explain the principles of medical asepsis.
- Explain the components of Standard Precautions.
- List the types of personal protective equipment (PPE).
- Describe nursing assistant actions related to Standard Precautions.
- Describe airborne precautions.
- Describe droplet precautions.
- Describe contact precautions.
- Demonstrate the following:
  Procedure 11-7   Hand Hygiene
      11-7A   Handwashing (soap and water)
      11-7B   Hand Rub (alcohol-based sanitizer)
  Procedure 11-8   Putting on (Donning) a Mask and Gloves
  Procedure 11-9   Removing (Doffing) Contaminated Gloves
  Procedure 11-10 Donning a Gown
  Procedure 11-11 Removing Contaminated Gloves, Mask, and Gown

CASE STUDY

Oscar Uritz is a resident in your care. He was transferred from home with a large, stage three pressure ulcer on his right ankle. He lost the use of his left side from an earlier stroke. He shared a room at the facility with Mr. Jules, who also had a stroke but is ambulatory. Mr. Uritz has an MRSA infection and is now in a single room on contact isolation. The nursing assistant should wear personal protective equipment when providing care for Mr. Uritz.

VOCABULARY

airborne precautions (AIR-born pree-KAW-shuns)

asepsis (ah-SEP-sis)

autoclave (AWE-toh-klayv)

biohazard (bye-oh-HAZ-ard)

communicable (kom-MYOU-nih-kah-bul)

contact precautions (KON-tact pree-KAW-shuns)

contagious (kon-TAY-jus)

contaminated (kon-TAM-ih-nay-ted)

dirty (DER-tee)

disinfection (dis-in-FECK-shun)

droplet precautions (DROP-let pree-KAW-shuns)

exposure incident (ecks-POH-zhur IN-sih-dent)

isolation (eye-soh-LAY-shun)

medical asepsis (MED-ih-kul ay-SEP-sis)

occupational exposure (ock-you-PAY-shun-al ecks-POH-zhur)

personal protective equipment (PPE) (PER-son-al proh-TECH-tiv ee-KWIP-ment)

potentially infectious material (poh-TEN-shal-lee in-FECK-shus mah-TEER-ee-al)

sharps (sharps)

Standard Precautions (STAN-dard pree-KAW-shuns)

sterile (STER-ill)

sterilization (ster-ih-lie-ZAY-shun)

work practice controls (werk PRACK-tis kon-TROLS)

In the last lesson you learned what infections are, some of their causes, and why residents are at risk for infections. This lesson introduces actions and procedures that can help prevent the transmission (spread) of infection to protect yourself, your coworkers, and those in your care.

The organisms that are causative agents for infections are microscopic, that is, unable to be seen with the naked eye. The infectious organisms do not just remain in the resident's room (doorknob, bedrail, bedside stand) but can also be found on the keyboard, telephone in the nurse's station, and on the nurse's or CNA's uniform that had touched a contaminated stethoscope. It is imperative that health care workers take precautions to prevent the spread of disease.

MEDICAL ASEPSIS

The term **asepsis** means that disease-causing pathogens and infection are not present. **Medical asepsis**, also referred to as infection control, means the methods by which cleanliness and freedom from pathogens are maintained:

- In your own personal hygiene
- With residents

- With equipment and supplies
- Throughout the facility

You will hear the terms "clean" and contaminated ("dirty") applied to equipment and supplies used in the facility. For example, the linen you take from the linen cart is "clean." After it is carried into the resident's room, it is considered to be contaminated. If it is not used, it cannot be returned to the clean linen cart but must be placed in the laundry hamper. Once linen is in the resident's room, it is exposed to the resident's pathogens. To prevent the spread of these pathogens to other residents, the linen must be laundered. Keeping each resident's equipment and supplies separate from those for other residents is part of an action called medical aseptic technique. Articles that have come into contact with known pathogens or are exposed to potential pathogens are called **dirty** or **contaminated**. Articles that are free of pathogens are considered clean or uncontaminated.

All health care workers must be very careful to prevent environmental contamination. When you are wearing gloves, after caring for a resident do not touch the bedrails, bedside curtains, doorknobs, faucets, and so on—first remove your gloves, cleanse your hands, and then carry out additional nursing activities.

Maintaining Medical Asepsis

Nursing assistant actions to maintain medical asepsis include:

1. Use appropriate hand hygiene at the correct times. (See Procedure 11-7A and B.)

2. Treat breaks in the skin immediately by washing thoroughly, cleaning with an antiseptic, and covering. Report any breaks in the skin to your supervisor.

3. Use gloves when required. Be alert for latex allergy for the resident and/or staff. Allergic reactions can range from an eczema-like rash to anaphylactic shock. The facility will supply non-latex gloves if you have an allergy to latex. Do not use latex gloves for anyone with a latex allergy.

4. Bathe or shower daily. Daily changes of clothing are necessary. Keep your hair clean and away from your face and shoulders. Keep fingernails short and clean. Do not wear rings, other than a plain wedding band. Do not wear large hoop earrings.

5. Personal hygiene for residents is maintained by following bathing schedules and giving AM and PM care as required. Change clothing daily or as needed.

6. Items used for one resident are *never* used for another resident (Figure 11-1).

7. Items such as a toothbrush, denture cup, wash basin, and emesis basin should always be placed on a separate shelf from items such as a bedpan and a urinal.

8. Disinfect personal care equipment, such as bedpans, urinals, and commodes at least once per week, according to facility policy.

9. Disinfect bathtubs and shower chairs after each use according to facility policy (Figure 11-2). Clean items used by more than one resident, such as wheelchairs, before each use. Other equipment is cleaned regularly by the housekeeping department or as indicated by facility policy.

10. Disinfect equipment, such as a stethoscope, that is used by more than one health care provider or resident before and after each use.

11. Be careful when handling bedpans and urinals after use to prevent spills and splashes. Use a cover when transporting.

12. Keep food and water supplies clean. Food trays are to remain covered until they reach their destination. Remove food dishes immediately after use. Do not place used trays on the cart until all clean trays have been delivered to residents.

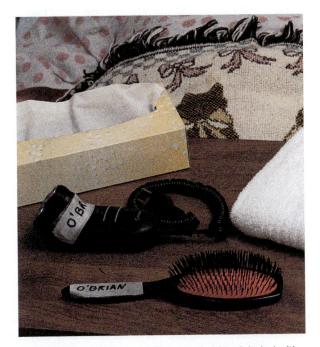

Figure 11-1 Personal care items should be labeled with the resident's name and used by that resident only.

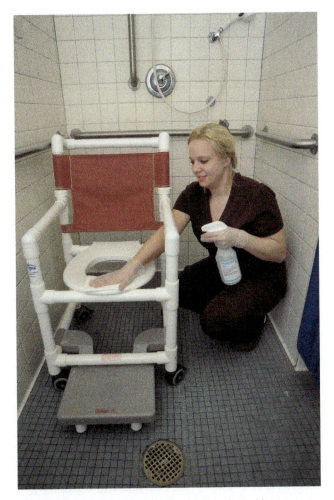

Figure 11-2 Equipment should be disinfected between uses by different residents.

13. Do not allow any resident to keep milk products or foods containing milk, such as puddings or custards, from meal trays. Bacteria multiply rapidly in these foods when they are not refrigerated.

14. Carry soiled equipment, supplies, and linens away from your uniform so that you do not spread microorganisms from resident to resident. Dispose of items according to facility policy.

15. All used disposable razors should be placed in the sharps container in the treatment room or bath/shower room.

16. The floor is heavily contaminated with pathogens. Do not use anything that has touched the floor without cleaning or sterilizing it first. If you are in doubt about whether an item is clean, do not use it. Any personal items that touch the floor should be disinfected before use. Most facilities have disinfectant wipes available for this purpose.

⊘N THE JOB

It may be tempting to take shortcuts when using precautions to prevent the spread of disease. Remember that as a caregiver you are responsible for protecting the well-being of the residents and of yourself.

17. Avoid raising dust. Vacuum cleaners, wet mops, and damp cloths are used for cleaning.

18. Do not shake linens. This scatters contaminated dust and lint. Gather or fold linens inward with the dirtiest area toward the center. Keep soiled linen hampers covered. Keep linens (even if soiled) off the floor.

19. Clean least soiled areas first and the most soiled last.

20. Keep residents' rooms as clean, bright, and dry as possible.

21. Keep work areas such as utility rooms clean. Return clean equipment to the proper storage areas after use.

HAND CARE

Many infections can be spread on the hands, so special attention must be paid to the hands, both inside and outside a health care facility. Outside the facility, wear gloves to protect your hands when tasks put you at risk for skin irritation, such as washing dishes or gardening. Use lotion to keep the skin moist and soft. Nail care is another important factor in preventing the spread of infection. Natural nail tips should be less than ¼-inch long. Long nails can hold microbes as well as cause skin damage to residents. If you wear nail polish, make sure it is smooth and not chipped to prevent areas where microbes can hide. Artificial nails have been proved to harbor microbes and increase the risk of infection. Many health care facilities do not permit caregivers to wear artificial fingernails or nail tips of any type. If you wear rings, make sure they are plain, simple bands. Rings with numerous stones and elaborate settings can hide harmful microorganisms. In addition, the stones may tear your protective gloves (Figure 11-3).

Handwashing/Hand Hygiene

The importance of hand hygiene to protect yourself and the resident cannot be overemphasized. The term *hand hygiene* refers to both handwashing with soap and warm water and antiseptic hand rubs with the use of alcohol-based hand sanitizers. In most situations, according to the Centers for Disease Control and Prevention (CDC), alcohol-based rubs are more effective in killing bacteria than soap and water (Figure 11-6). These products have been found to be less irritating than washing the hands repeatedly with soap and water and drying with paper towels. Most products contain a lotion to help protect the skin; paper towel use is unnecessary when the alcohol-based products are used.

Waterless cleansers are *never* used when caring for residents with *C. difficile* infections because they do not kill the spores. Be sure to follow the guidelines in your facility regarding the appropriate hand hygiene procedure to use for each specific type of infectious disease.

Hand hygiene is the most important procedure you will carry out to prevent and control the spread of infection. It is the foundation of all preventative techniques. (Refer to Procedure 11-7A and B.)

Hand hygiene is performed prior to and after:

- Your shift
- Caring for *each* resident
- After removing your gloves
- Your breaks and your meals
- Going to the bathroom
- Handling contaminated equipment
- Contact with blood and body fluids

If your hands are *visibly* soiled, the CDC has recommended thorough handwashing with soap and water for approximately 40 to 60 seconds (see Procedure 11-7A). The friction of rubbing the hand surfaces and crevices with soap dislodges the soil and the flowing water rinses the areas free of organisms.

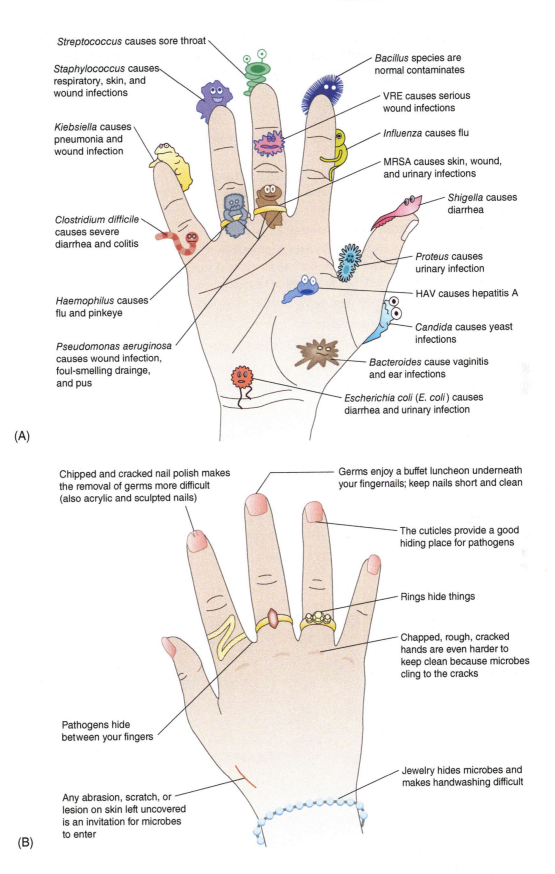

Figure 11-3 (A) Many infections are spread on the hands, so health care workers must pay close attention to good hand hygiene and eliminating areas where pathogens can hide. (B) Jewelry with many stones or complicated settings provides a hiding place for pathogens. Long fingernails, chipped nail polish, and acrylic nails also provide hiding places for microbes. Chapped, cut, cracked hands increase the risk of contracting an infection.

PROCEDURE 11-7
Hand Hygiene

A. Handwashing (soap and water)

1. Check that there is an adequate supply of soap and paper towels. A waste container lined with a plastic bag should be in the area near you.

2. Turn on the faucet with a dry paper towel held between your hand and the faucet (Figure 11-4). Adjust water to a warm temperature. Drop the towel in the waste container. Stand back from the sink so you do not contaminate your uniform.

3. Wet your hands with the fingertips pointed downward.

4. Apply soap and lather over your hands and wrists and between fingers. Use friction and interlace your fingers (Figure 11-5). Work lather over every part of your hands and to 2 inches above the wrists. Clean your fingernails by rubbing them against the palm of the other hand to force soap under the nails for:

   - 20 to 30 seconds, general washing (sing happy birthday to yourself twice)
   - 40 to 60 seconds or longer for more visible soil.

5. Rinse hands with your fingertips pointed down. Do not shake water from hands.

6. Dry hands thoroughly with a clean paper towel.

7. Turn off the faucet with another dry paper towel; drop the towel in the waste container.

8. Apply lotion to your hands.

B. Hand Rub (alcohol-based preparation)

1. Dispense the proper amount of cleanser (liquid or foam) in the palm of your hand (dime- to quarter-sized quantity depending on the product directions).

2. Rub hands together palm to palm.

3. Rub backs of hands, rub between fingers then interlace fingers palm to palm and continue rubbing.

4. Work the cleaner around the nail beds and under the fingernails.

5. Total time should take approximately 20 to 30 seconds.

6. Your hands are clean when they are dry.

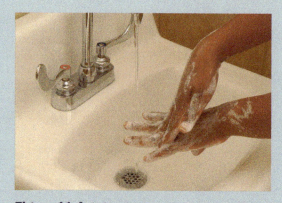

Figure 11-4 A dry, clean paper towel should be used to turn faucets on and off.

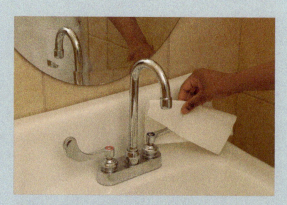

Figure 11-5 Interlace the fingers to clean between them. Keep fingers pointed down while washing and rinsing hands.

? EXERCISE 11-1

COMPLETION

Select the correct term from the following list to complete each statement.

bath   least   paper towel
clean   mouth   standard
dirty   never   waterproof
hand hygiene

1. The foundation of all medical aseptic techniques is _____.

2. Personal medical asepsis includes a daily _____.

3. Articles used for one resident should _____ be used on another.

4. Once clean linen has been carried into a resident's room, it must be considered _____.

5. If an article has even potential microbes on it, it cannot be considered_____.

6. When cleaning soiled areas, always clean the _____ soiled area first.

7. When washing hands, faucets should be turned on and off with a _____.

TRUE OR FALSE

Indicate whether the following statements are true (T) or false (F).

8. T F Medical asepsis means the absence of all microbes.

9. T F Using appropriate hand hygiene is the most important procedure you will carry out to prevent the spread of microbes.

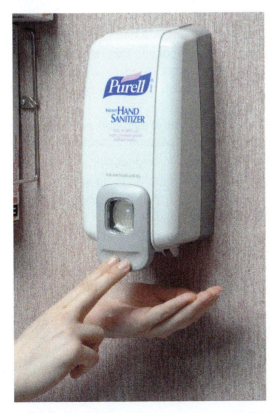

Figure 11-6 Alcohol-based hand cleaners may safely be used instead of washing at the sink unless your hands are contaminated with a protein substance.

Waterless Hand Cleaners

Alcohol-based hand cleaners are being used by an increasing number of health care facilities (Figure 11-6). The facility will have policies and procedures for using these products as well as directions for their use. Waterless cleaners are generally safe for use with routine resident care. Anytime your hands are visibly soiled, however, use traditional handwashing techniques. When using the waterless products, dispense the proper amount into the palm of your hand. The size of the portion will vary with the type of product, usually small dime- to quarter-sized quantities. Rub the cleaner onto all surfaces of the hand, between the fingers, and under and around the nails and nail beds. This process, which takes approximately 15 seconds, has been effective in reducing infections.

PROTECTING YOURSELF

As you perform your duties, you may contact **potentially infectious material**, such as blood or other body fluids that may contain pathogens (Figure 11-7). This is called **occupational exposure**.

Using proper medical asepsis technique and following Standard Precautions according to your facility

? EXERCISE 11-2

BRIEF ANSWER
Briefly answer the following statement.

1. Hands should be cleaned using appropriate hand hygiene before and after:
   a. _____
   b. _____
   c. _____
   d. _____
   e. _____
   f. _____
   g. _____
   h. _____

TRUE OR FALSE
Indicate whether the following statements are true (T) or false (F).

2. T F Waterless hand cleaners have been found to be effective in reducing infections and are appropriate for use with routine resident care.

3. T F Waterless hand sanitizers are used for *C. difficile* infections because they kill the spores.

HIV	Human Immunodeficiency Virus
HBV	Hepatitis B Virus
HCV	Hepatitis C Virus

Figure 11-7 Common bloodborne pathogens that can be transmitted from person to person through blood and body fluid contact.

policy are the best ways to limit the potential for being infected.

An **exposure incident** means that your eyes, mouth, or non-intact skin had contact with blood or other potentially infectious material. Rinse immediately with clear water. Report this at once to your supervisor and follow facility procedure.

Exposure Control

Exposure control training programs are required by OSHA. The programs must be given upon employment, yearly during employment, and whenever new tasks must be carried out that may involve exposure to bloodborne pathogens.

The training program must include information about:

- Bloodborne pathogens and their transmission
- The facility's Exposure Control Plan (where and how to obtain a copy)
- How to know which tasks may cause occupational exposure
- Use and limitations of safe work practices, engineering controls, and personal protective equipment
- Warning labels and color coding
- Who to contact and what to do in an emergency
- How to report an exposure incident, post-exposure evaluation, and follow-up
- If an exposure occurs, immediately:
  - Wash the area thoroughly
  - Report the incident to the proper authority

? EXERCISE 11-3

BRIEF ANSWER

1. Rebecca got some blood on her hands when she found her resident on the floor with a cut leg. What action should she take relating to this exposure incident?

   _____

   _____

STANDARD PRECAUTIONS

Standard Precautions (Figure 11-8) are the infection control actions used for all people receiving care, without regard for their condition or diagnosis. Standard Precautions apply to situations in which care providers may contact:

- Blood, body fluids (except perspiration), secretions, and excretions
- Mucous membranes
- Non-intact skin

Some examples of secretions and excretions are:

- Respiratory mucus (phlegm)
- Cerebrospinal fluid
- Urine
- Feces
- Vaginal secretions
- Semen
- Vomitus

This means that all health care workers follow specific procedures called work practice controls to prevent the spread of infections.

Standard Precautions stress appropriate hand hygiene and the use of personal protective equipment (PPE): gloves, gown, mask, and goggles or face shield.

TRANSMISSION-BASED PRECAUTIONS

Isolation means to separate or set apart. The purpose of isolation is to separate the resident with a communicable or contagious disease (one that is readily spread to other people) to help prevent the spread of the infectious pathogens.

For residents in isolation, the proper use of precautions, known as transmission precautions, requires extra effort by all care providers, but especially nursing assistants, and is more time consuming. The fear of infection also makes working with these precautions more stressful for the care providers. Residents in isolation and their families and other visitors also feel stress.

Psychological Aspects of Isolation

The resident in isolation fears both the disease condition requiring the isolation precautions and the practices that must be followed for these precautions to be effective. These include:

- PPE worn by all who enter the isolation unit
- Special procedures for handling waste, specimens, food, linens, and personal effects of the resident
- Restrictions on the resident's movement in the facility
- Procedures to be followed when resident is moved outside of the isolation unit
- Possible restrictions on visiting hours or number of visitors
- Need for visitors to use PPE
- Likelihood that close personal contact, such as kissing of family members, is not permitted

The resident may fear passing the infection to family and friends. If the resident does not understand the infectious process, this fear is increased. If the resident is confused, he or she may be very fearful of the PPE.

Because of the resident's fears and the possibility of decreased contact with other residents, family, and friends, the resident in isolation requires more emotional support and care. The increased time required to follow the isolation precautions, such as putting on PPE, could easily decrease the time the care providers spend with the resident at a time when the emotional attention is most needed. Nursing assistants are mindful of the resident's needs and will plan their schedules to spend the necessary time with a resident in isolation.

? EXERCISE 11-4

COMPLETION

Select the correct term from the following list to complete each statement.

clean	mouth	standard
dirty	never	waterproof

1. Actions taken with all people who are hospitalized or in long-term care facilities to prevent the transmission of infection are known as _____ precautions.

2. Gowns used as PPE must be _____.

3. When masks are worn they must cover the nose and _____.

STANDARD PRECAUTIONS

Assume that every person is potentially infected or colonized with an organism that could be transmitted in the healthcare setting.

Hand Hygiene

Avoid unnecessary touching of surfaces in close proximity to the patient.

When hands are visibly dirty, contaminated with proteinaceous material, or visibly soiled with blood or body fluids, wash hands with soap and water.

If hands are not visibly soiled, or after removing visible material with soap and water, decontaminate hands with an alcohol-based hand rub. Alternatively, hands may be washed with an antimicrobial soap and water.

Perform hand hygiene:
  Before having direct contact with patients.
  After contact with blood, body fluids or excretions, mucous membranes, nonintact skin, or wound dressings.
  After contact with a patient's intact skin (e.g., when taking a pulse or blood pressure or lifting a patient).
  If hands will be moving from a contaminated-body site to a clean-body site during patient care.
  After contact with inanimate objects (including medical equipment) in the immediate vicinity of the patient.
  After removing gloves.

Personal protective equipment (PPE)

Wear PPE when the nature of the anticipated patient interaction indicates that contact with blood or body fluids may occur.

Before leaving the patient's room or cubicle, remove and discard PPE.

Gloves

Wear gloves when contact with blood or other potentially infectious materials, mucous membranes, nonintact skin, or potentially contaminated intact skin (e.g., of a patient incontinent of stool or urine) could occur.

Remove gloves after contact with a patient and/or the surrounding environment using proper technique to prevent hand contamination. Do not wear the same pair of gloves for the care of more than one patient.

Change gloves during patient care if the hands will move from a contaminated body-site (e.g., perineal area) to a clean body-site (e.g., face).

Gowns

Wear a gown to protect skin and prevent soiling or contamination of clothing during procedures and patient-care activities when contact with blood, body fluids, secretions, or excretions is anticipated.

Wear a gown for direct patient contact if the patient has uncontained secretions or excretions.

Remove gown and perform hand hygiene before leaving the patient's environment.

Mouth, nose, eye protection

Use PPE to protect the mucous membranes of the eyes, nose and mouth during procedures and patient-care activities that are likely to generate splashes or sprays of blood, body fluids, secretions and excretions.

During aerosol-generating procedures wear one of the following: a face shield that fully covers the front and sides of the face, a mask with attached shield, or a mask and goggles.

Respiratory Hygiene/Cough Etiquette

Educate healthcare personnel to contain respiratory secretions to prevent droplet and fomite transmission of respiratory pathogens, especially during seasonal outbreaks of viral respiratory tract infections.

Offer masks to coughing patients and other symptomatic persons (e.g., persons who accompany ill patients) upon entry into the facility.

Patient-care equipment and instruments/devices

Wear PPE (e.g., gloves, gown), according to the level of anticipated contamination, when handling patient-care equipment and instruments/devices that are visibly soiled or may have been in contact with blood or body fluids.

Care of the environment

Include multi-use electronic equipment in policies and procedures for preventing contamination and for cleaning and disinfection, especially those items that are used by patients, those used during delivery of patient care, and mobile devices that are moved in and out of patient rooms frequently (e.g., daily).

Textiles and laundry

Handle used textiles and fabrics with minimum agitation to avoid contamination of air, surfaces and persons.

Figure 11-8 Standard precautions are used in the care of all residents, regardless of disease or diagnosis.

⚠ GUIDELINES FOR... STANDARD PRECAUTIONS

1. Perform hand hygiene.
   - When arriving for work and just before leaving for home
   - Immediately after touching blood, body fluids, mucous membranes, or contaminated articles, whether or not gloves are worn
   - Before putting on gloves and after taking them off
   - Before caring for a resident and after completing care for that resident
   - Before care procedures that may transfer pathogens from one part of the resident's body to another
   - Before and after personal use of the bathroom
   - Before handling food
   - Using soap provided by the facility
   - Before touching your mouth, eyes, or eyeglasses
   - Before and after touching your contact lenses
   - After touching any soiled linen, clothing, equipment, or supplies

2. Wear gloves for any contact with blood, body fluids, mucous membranes, or non-intact skin, such as when:
   - Hands are cut, scratched, or have a rash
   - Cleaning up body fluid spills
   - Cleaning potentially contaminated equipment

3. Gloves are provided in resident rooms or on supply carts.

4. Carry gloves with you so they will always be available as you need them.

5. If you have an allergy to latex gloves, follow your physician's advice. Three possible options are:
   - Change to non-latex gloves (facilities must supply them because latex allergies are not uncommon).
   - Apply a skin barrier cream to your hands before putting on latex gloves; the cream protects hands against most irritants, including latex.
   - Put on glove liners that prevent direct contact between the skin of the hands and the latex gloves.

6. Change gloves:
   - Before contacting each resident
   - Before touching non-contaminated articles or environmental surfaces
   - Between tasks with the same resident if there is contact with secretions, excretions, or infectious materials
   - When gloves become visibly soiled; *never* wash gloves and continue your task
   - Immediately before touching mucous membrane or non-intact skin
   - If gloves become torn

7. Dispose of gloves according to facility policy.

8. Wear a waterproof gown for procedures likely to produce splashes of blood or other body fluids.
   - Remove soiled gown as soon as possible and dispose of it properly according to facility policy.
   - Use appropriate hand hygiene.

9. Wear a mask and protective eyewear or face shield for procedures likely to produce splashes of blood or other moist body fluids. This is to prevent contact with pathogens by your mucous membranes.

The surgical mask covers both the nose and mouth. Masks are effective for only 30 minutes, then must be changed and hands washed. The mask is used once and discarded. When a mask is required, a new one is put on for each resident receiving care. If the mask becomes wet, a new one must be put on because the mask loses its effectiveness when moist.

10. Goggles or a face shield helps protect the mucous membranes of the eyes from splashes or sprays of blood and other body fluids. A surgical mask must be worn with goggles and with a face shield to protect the nose and mouth.

11. When using PPE, you should:
    - Know where to obtain these items in your work area.
    - Always remove the items before leaving the work area, whether it is the resident's room, an isolation unit, or the utility room.
    - Place these items in the proper container for laundering, decontamination, or disposal, according to facility policy.

⚠ GUIDELINES FOR... ENVIRONMENTAL PROCEDURES

1. Handle all resident care items so that infectious organisms will not be transferred to skin, mucous membranes, clothing, or the environment. Reusable equipment must be cleaned and decontaminated according to facility policy before it can be used with another resident. Dispose of single-use items according to facility policy.

2. Follow facility procedures for routine care and cleaning of environmental surfaces such as **beds**, bedside equipment, and other frequently touched surfaces.

3. Dispose of **sharps**—needles with syringes, razors, and other sharp items—in a puncture-resistant, leak-proof container near the point of use (Figure 11-9). The container should be labeled with the—**biohazard**—symbol (Figure 11-10) and color-coded red. Some facilities use self-sheathing needles; these must also be disposed of in the sharps container.

4. Do not recap needles or otherwise handle them before disposal.

5. Mouthpieces or resuscitator bags should be available to minimize the need for mouth-to-mouth resuscitation. You must be trained to use them.

6. Waste and soiled linen are handled as if infectious and should be placed in plastic bags and handled according to facility policy. There are separate containers for regular waste and for biohazardous waste (waste that has contacted blood or body fluids). Containers for biohazardous waste should have the biohazard symbol (see Figure 11-10) or be color-coded in red (Figure 11-11). Learn your facility policy for what is biohazardous waste and follow the guidelines.

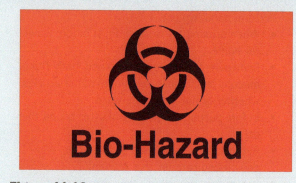

Figure 11-10 This is a universal biohazard symbol used to indicate potentially infectious waste.

7. Wipe up blood spills immediately. Disinfect the floor according to facility policy.
   - Use disposable gloves.
   - Wipe spills from the more clean area to the dirtiest area.
   - For small spills, use a 1:10 dilution of bleach or disinfectant required by facility policy. Fresh bleach solution must be made daily and dated.
   - For larger spills, use a commercial blood cleanup kit. This contains an absorbent powder that is sprinkled over the blood to absorb the spill. The blood and powder are then scooped up with the scoop provided in the kit. The material and scoop are placed in a biohazard bag for disposal (Figure 11-12).
   - Use disposable cleaning cloths.

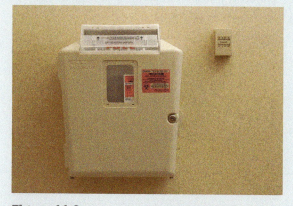

Figure 11-9 Sharps must be disposed of carefully in a safety container designed specifically for this use.

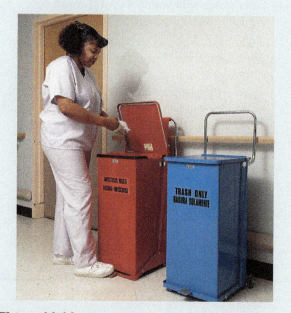

Figure 11-11 All potentially infectious materials should be disposed of in the correct waste container.

(continues)

⚠ GUIDELINES FOR... ENVIRONMENTAL PROCEDURES (Continued)

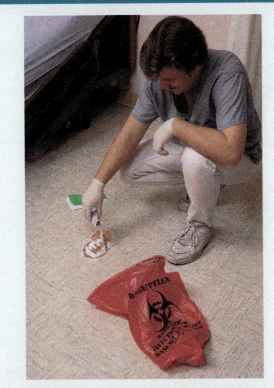

Figure 11-12 Clean all blood spills immediately using a 1:10 solution of bleach or the disinfectant approved by your facility. For larger spills, use a blood spill kit. The powder absorbs the blood quickly and can be scooped up for disposal in a biohazard bag.

8. Dispose of body fluids and contaminated articles according to facility policy. This includes the contents of:

- Urinary drainage bags
- Bedpans
- Urinals
- Emesis basins
- Ostomy bags
- Drainage receptacles from tracheal and gastric suction
- Solutions returned from vaginal douches, enemas, and bladder irrigations
- Soiled dressings
- Incontinent pads
- Vaginal pads
- Incontinent briefs
- Bedside wastebasket

9. Eating, drinking, smoking, applying cosmetics or lip balm, and handling contact lenses are prohibited in work areas where there may be exposure to infectious material.

10. Food and drink should not be kept in refrigerators, freezers, shelves, cabinets, or on countertops or bench tops where they may be exposed to blood or other materials that may be contaminated.

11. Do not pick up potentially contaminated broken glassware with your bare hands. Wear gloves and use a brush and dust pan, tongs, or forceps. Clean and disinfect properly. Discard according to facility policy.

12. Clean and dirty hampers must be separated by at least 3 feet (width of a door).

❓ EXERCISE 11-5

BRIEF ANSWER
Briefly answer the following statement.

1. List five articles that might be contaminated with body fluid that need to be carefully handled.
   a. _____
   b. _____
   c. _____
   d. _____
   e. _____

2. List the three types of transmission-based precautions.
   a. _____
   b. _____
   c. _____

(continues)

? EXERCISE 11-5 (Continued)

TRUE OR FALSE

Indicate whether the following statements are true (T) or false (F).

3. T F Food and drink may be kept in the same refrigerators as specimens.

4. T F Soiled linen from an isolation unit should be placed in a bag labeled with a biohazard label before routing to the laundry.

5. T F Guidelines for environmental procedures do not include treating waste and soiled linen as If they are clean.

Transmission-Based Isolation Precautions

Standard Precautions are used with all residents, regardless of their condition. When residents are known to have or are suspected of having an infectious disease, isolation precautions are used *in addition to* Standard Precautions. The isolation precautions used depend on the way in which the infectious pathogens are transmitted. Guidelines from the CDC indicate the specific precautions and PPE to be used based on how the disease is transmitted. The three transmission precautions are:

- Airborne precautions
- Droplet precautions
- Contact precautions

Airborne Precautions

Airborne precautions are used for diseases that are transmitted by air currents. The pathogens are suspended in the air or on dust particles in the air. They can travel a long distance from the source by natural air currents and through ventilation systems. Tuberculosis is a disease that requires airborne precautions (Figure 11-13). Figure 11-14 shows the required precautions.

- The resident must be in a private room with negative air pressure. This means that air is drawn into the room and leaves the room through a special exhaust system to the outside. Air from the room does not circulate directly into the facility. Portable

units that filter the air and create a negative pressure environment are used in facilities that do not have the special ventilation needed for airborne precautions.

- The door to the room is kept closed.
- All care providers who enter the room must wear a high-efficiency particulate air (HEPA) filter mask (Figure 11-15). The special filters in this mask protect the care provider from the very small disease-causing pathogens. A surgical mask does not provide protection. Each care provider must be fitted with a HEPA filter mask. This ensures that air entering the mask comes through the filters only. Follow all facility policies for the use of HEPA filter masks.
- A PFR95 respirator mask or N95 respirator mask are other masks that may be used in airborne precautions (Figure 11-16). They are lighter in weight and are preferred by some workers. The same precautions regarding fit and use for HEPA masks apply to these masks as well. The masks must be fit-tested by the worker each time they are worn (Figure 11-17).
- Nursing assistants should be shown the procedure for using the respirator mask and be checked or approved after this training.
- People who are not immune to measles (rubeola) or chickenpox (varicella) should not enter the room of a resident known or suspected to have either of these infections.
- If transport from the room is necessary, the resident must wear a surgical mask.

- Tuberculosis
- Varicella (chicken-pox)
- Disseminated zoster
- Rubella (measles)
- *C. difficile*

Figure 11-13 Infections requiring airborne precautions.

⊘ ON THE JOB

Keep in mind that residents of different cultures may be offended or frightened by the isolation procedures used in American health care facilities.

AIRBORNE PRECAUTIONS

(in addition to Standard Precautions)

VISITORS: Report to nurse before entering.

Use Airborne Precautions as recommended for patients known or suspected to be infected with infectious agents transmitted person-to-person by the airborne route (e.g., M. tuberculosis, measles, chickenpox, disseminated herpes zoster).

Patient placement

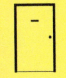

Place patients in an **AIIR** (Airborne Infection Isolation Room).
Monitor air pressure daily with visual indicators (e.g., flutter strips).

Keep door closed when not required for entry and exit.

In ambulatory settings instruct patients with a known or suspected airborne infection to wear a surgical mask and observe Respiratory Hygiene/Cough Etiquette. Once in an AIIR, the mask may be removed.

Patient transport

Limit transport and movement of patients to **medically-necessary purposes.**

If transport or movement outside an AIIR is necessary, instruct patients to **wear a surgical mask**, if possible, and observe Respiratory Hygiene/Cough Etiquette.

Hand Hygiene

Hand Hygiene according to Standard Precautions.

Personal Protective Equipment (PPE)

Wear a fit-tested NIOSH-approved **N95** or higher level respirator for respiratory protection when entering the room of a patient when the following diseases are suspected or confirmed: Listed on back.

APR

©2007 Brevis Corporation   www.brevis.com

Figure 11-14 Airborne precautions.

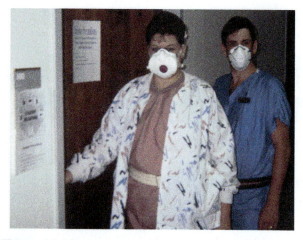

Figure 11-15 High-efficiency particulate air (HEPA) filter masks are required for care providers who work with residents placed in airborne precautions. The masks are carefully fitted to each care provider. The mask must seal around the face so that all air being breathed passes through the filters to remove the very small pathogens.

Droplet Precautions

Droplet precautions are used for diseases that can be spread by means of large droplets in the air. A person can spread droplets containing infectious pathogens by sneezing, coughing, talking, singing, or laughing. The droplets generally do not travel more than 3 feet from the source. Examples of diseases spread by droplets are listed in Figure 11-18.

Figure 11-19 shows the requirements for droplet precautions.

- If a resident cannot be placed in a private room, then residents requiring the same precautions can be placed together.
- The caregivers should wear surgical masks if they expect to be working within 3 feet of the resident. The door can be open if the bed is more than 3 feet from the door.
- If transport from the room is necessary, the resident must wear a surgical mask.

Contact Precautions

Contact precautions are used when the infectious pathogen is spread by direct or indirect contact. Direct contact occurs when the caregiver touches a contaminated area on the resident's skin or blood or body fluids containing the infectious pathogen. Indirect contact occurs when the caregiver touches items contaminated with the infectious material, such as resident's personal belongings, equipment, and supplies used in the care of the resident, contaminated linens, and so on. Principles of Standard Precautions are always used for residents who require contact precautions.

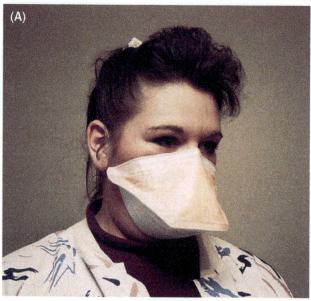

(A)

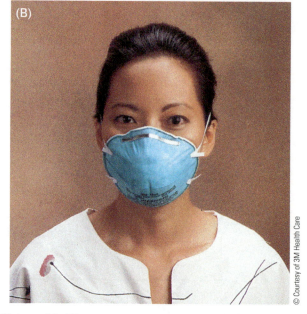

(B)

Figure 11-16 (A) The PFR95 respirator filter. (B) The N95 respirator filter.

Examples of infections requiring contact precautions are listed in Figure 11-20.

Figure 11-21 shows the requirements for contact precautions.

- The resident should be in a private room. If this is not possible, then residents requiring the same type of isolation precautions can be placed in the same room. The door can be open.
- Gloves are put on before the caregiver enters the resident's room. Gloves are changed whenever there is contact with highly contaminated matter in the room. After removing gloves, always use appropriate hand hygiene before putting on a new

© Courtesy of 3M Health Care

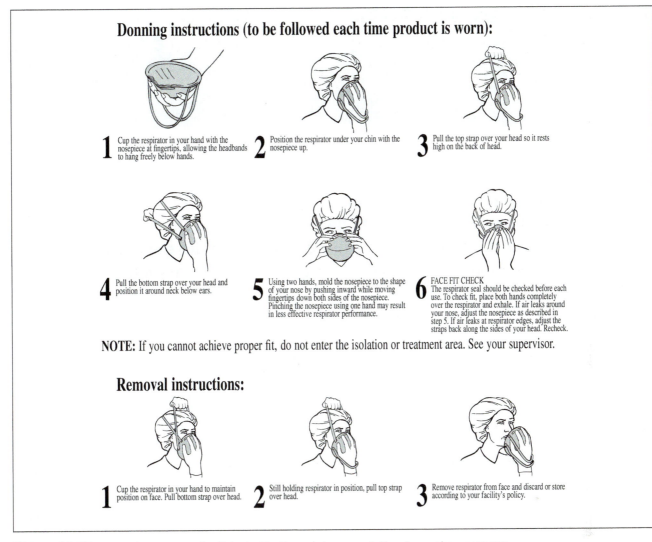

Donning instructions (to be followed each time product is worn):

1 Cup the respirator in your hand with the nosepiece at fingertips, allowing the headbands to hang freely below hands.

2 Position the respirator under your chin with the nosepiece up.

3 Pull the top strap over your head so it rests high on the back of head.

4 Pull the bottom strap over your head and position it around neck below ears.

5 Using two hands, mold the nosepiece to the shape of your nose by pushing inward while moving fingertips down both sides of the nosepiece. Pinching the nosepiece using one hand may result in less effective respirator performance.

6 FACE FIT CHECK
The respirator seal should be checked before each use. To check fit, place both hands completely over the respirator and exhale. If air leaks around your nose, adjust the nosepiece as described in step 5. If air leaks at respirator edges, adjust the straps back along the sides of your head. Recheck.

NOTE: If you cannot achieve proper fit, do not enter the isolation or treatment area. See your supervisor.

Removal instructions:

1 Cup the respirator in your hand to maintain position on face. Pull bottom strap over head.

2 Still holding respirator in position, pull top strap over head.

3 Remove respirator from face and discard or store according to your facility's policy.

Courtesy of 3M Health Care

Figure 11-17 All respirators must be fit-tested by the employee each time he or she wears one.

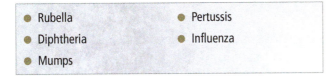

- Rubella
- Diphtheria
- Mumps
- Pertussis
- Influenza

Figure 11-18 Infections requiring droplet precautions.

pair of gloves. After care is completed, remove gloves and use appropriate hand hygiene. Use a paper towel to open the door to leave the room and discard the towel in the trash container inside the room.

- Wear a gown when entering the resident's room if your uniform may contact the resident, blood or body fluids, environmental surfaces, or other items in the room. Remove the gown before leaving the room and dispose of it according to facility policy

for biohazardous waste. Be careful not to touch environmental surfaces or other items with your uniform as you leave the room.

- Transport the resident from the room only when necessary. Continue precautions to minimize contamination of environmental surfaces, other residents, and health care personnel.

- Disposable equipment and supplies should be used where possible. Noncritical, non-disposable equipment should be used for one resident only. If equipment must be used for more than one resident, it must be cleaned and disinfected between residents.

- Revised infection control guidelines now state that some conditions, such as varicella (chickenpox), can be spread by both airborne and contact routes. In this case, both precaution signs must be posted on the room.

DROPLET PRECAUTIONS

(in addition to Standard Precautions)

STOP VISITORS: Report to nurse before entering.

Use Droplet Precautions as recommended for patients known or suspected to be infected with pathogens transmitted by respiratory droplets that are generated by a patient who is coughing, sneezing or talking.

Personal Protective Equipment (PPE)

Don a mask upon entry into the patient room or cubicle.

Hand Hygiene

Hand Hygiene according to Standard Precautions.

Patient Placement

Private room, if possible. Cohort or maintain spatial separation of 3 feet from other patients or visitors if private room is not available.

Patient transport

Limit transport and movement of patients to **medically-necessary purposes.**

If transport or movement in any healthcare setting is necessary, instruct patient to **wear a mask** and follow Respiratory Hygiene/Cough Etiquette.

No mask is required for persons transporting patients on Droplet Precautions.

DPR7

©2007 Brevis Corporation   www.brevis.com

Reprinted with permission from Brevis Corporation [www.brevis.com]

Figure 11-19 Droplet precautions.

- Chickenpox (varicella)
- Drug-resistant skin infections
- *E. coli O157:H7* + other gastrointestinal infections
- Head or body lice
- Impetigo
- Infected pressure sores or other wounds
- Infectious diarrhea caused by known pathogens
- Pseudomembranous colitis
- Scabies
- Shingles (herpes zoster)

Figure 11-20 Infections requiring contact precautions.

Preparing for Isolation

To prepare a resident room for isolation, do the following:

1. Place a card indicating the type of isolation precaution on the door to the resident's room.

2. Place an isolation cart outside the room, next to the door. Place in it quantities of PPE as needed:
   - Gowns
   - Masks
   - Gloves
   - Goggles or face shields
   - Plastic bags marked for biohazardous waste
   - Plastic bags for soiled linen

3. Line the wastepaper basket inside the room with a plastic bag labeled or color-coded for infectious waste.

4. Place a laundry hamper in the room and line it with a yellow biohazard laundry bag.

5. At the sink, check the supply of paper towels and soap. Soap should be in a wall dispenser or foot-operated dispenser.

Refer to Procedures 11-8 to 11-11 for putting on and removing PPE. Procedures 11-10 to 11-13 cover common tasks performed in the isolation unit. Procedures 11-14 and 11-15 cover transporting the resident and equipment from the isolation unit.

PROCEDURE 11-8
Putting on (Donning) a Mask and Gloves

1. Assemble equipment:
   - Mask
   - Disposable gloves in correct size
2. Use appropriate hand hygiene.
3. If gown and gloves are needed, the mask goes on first. (If a face shield is used, it is put on next.)
4. Adjust mask over nose and mouth.
5. Tie top strings of mask first, then bottom strings. If ties are elastic, slip around ears and adjust comfortably.
6. Replace mask if it becomes moist during procedures.
7. Do not reuse a mask and do not let the mask hang around your neck.
8. Pick up one glove by the cuff and place it on the other hand.
9. Repeat with glove for other hand.
10. Interlace fingers to adjust gloves on hands.
11. Remember when using gloves:
    - Use appropriate hand hygiene before and after using gloves.
    - Remove gloves if they tear or become heavily soiled. Wash hands and put on a new pair.
    - Gloves are used whenever there is the possibility of contacting body fluids, blood, secretions, or excretions with your mucous membranes or non-intact skin.
    - Change gloves between residents and wash hands.
    - Discard gloves immediately after removing in biohazard waste receptacle.

CONTACT PRECAUTIONS

(in addition to Standard Precautions)

STOP **VISITORS: Report to nurse before entering.**

Gloves
Don gloves upon entry into the room or cubicle.
Wear gloves whenever touching the patient's intact skin or surfaces and articles in close proximity to the patient.
Remove gloves before leaving patient room.

Hand Hygiene
Hand Hygiene according to Standard Precautions.

Gowns
Don gown upon entry into the room or cubicle.
Remove gown and observe hand hygiene before leaving the patient-care environment.

Patient Transport
Limit transport of patients to medically necessary purposes.
Ensure that infected or colonized areas of the patient's body are contained and covered.
Remove and dispose of contaminated PPE and perform hand hygiene prior to transporting patients on Contact Precautions.
Don clean PPE to handle the patient at the transport destination.

Patient–Care Equipment
Use disposable noncritical patient-care equipment or implement patient-dedicated use of such equipment.

Form No. **CPR7**   BREVIS CORP., 225 West 2855 South, SLC, UT 84115   © 2007 Brevis Corp.

Reprinted with permission from Brevis Corporation [www.brevis.com]

Figure 11-21 Contact precautions.

? EXERCISE 11-6

MULTIPLE CHOICE
Select the one best answer.

1. An exposure control training program must include information about
   (A) bloodborne pathogens and CPR
   (B) whom to contact if a resident dies
   (C) bloodborne pathogens and their transmission, the Faculty Exposure Control Plan, tasks that cause occupational exposure, use of safe work practices, and emergency reporting procedures
   (D) the best kind of masks to buy

2. Airborne precautions for disease do not include
   (A) using a special exhaust system to the outside
   (B) portable units that filter the air and create a negative pressure system
   (C) giving the resident an option about wearing a surgical mask
   (D) giving nursing assistants instructions for the procedure of using the respiration mask

3. Infections that require contact precautions
   (A) are not caused by indirect contact such as touching
   (B) include impetigo, chicken pox, shingles, and scabies
   (C) do not include infected pressure ulcers
   (D) cannot be transmitted by a resident's personal belongings

4. Procedures for using a mask or gloves do not include
   (A) reusing them
   (B) using appropriate hand hygiene before and after use
   (C) changing gloves between residents
   (D) removing gloves if they tear

BRIEF ANSWER
Briefly answer the following statement.

5. Four pieces of PPE used to carry out isolation precautions include:
   a. _____
   b. _____
   c. _____
   d. _____

Protective Isolation

Protective isolation is sometimes called *reverse isolation* because the resident is segregated for his or her protection from the infectious organisms of others. This technique is used when the resident has a compromised immune system or some other condition that makes him or her more susceptible to infection.

DISINFECTION AND STERILIZATION

Disinfection is the process of eliminating most harmful pathogens from equipment and instruments. A chemical called a *disinfectant* is used for this procedure.

You may be required to disinfect personal care items such as wash basins, bedpans, and urinals. You may also use disinfectants to clean wheelchairs and other furniture items. Items are usually washed before they are disinfected. The procedure for disinfecting depends on the chemicals that are used. Follow the directions of the facility for use of disinfectants. Wear disposable gloves and a gown for completing these procedures. You may also need a face shield. Wear PPE that is appropriate to the procedure.

Sterilization removes all microorganisms from an item. This process can be completed in an **autoclave**, which uses steam and pressure to kill organisms. Most facilities purchase supplies and equipment that are pre-sterilized by the manufacturer (Figure 11-27).

? EXERCISE 11-7

1. Letty has three residents in her care who are on transmission-based precautions. For each resident, check on the table the PPE she will need to perform proper technique.
   a. Mr. Smithson has tuberculosis and has been placed in airborne precautions.
   b. Mrs. Zernicki has an MRSA cellulitis of her amputated stump and has been placed in contact precautions.
   c. Mrs. Fameri has streptococcal pneumonia and has been placed in droplet precautions.

Resident	Personal Protective Equipment				
	Standard Precautions	Gloves	Gown	Mask	Goggles
a. Mr. Smithson					
b. Mrs. Zernicki					
c. Mrs. Fameri					

PROCEDURE 11-9
Removing (Doffing) Contaminated Gloves

1. Grasp cuff of one glove on the outside with the fingers of the other hand (Figure 11-22A).

2. Pull cuff of glove down, drawing it over the glove and turning the glove inside out (Figure 11-22B). Pull glove off hand.

3. Hold the glove with the still-gloved hand.

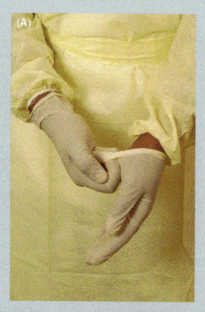

Figure 11-22A Removing contaminated gloves. With fingers of one hand, grasp glove of other hand.

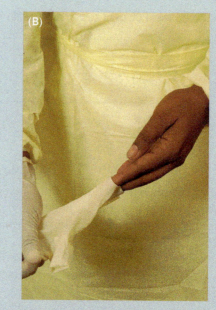

Figure 11-22B Pull glove down over the hand and the fingers and remove it. The glove is inside out with the contaminated side inside.

(continues)

PROCEDURE 11-9
Removing (Doffing) Contaminated Gloves (Continued)

4. Insert fingers of the ungloved hand under the cuff of the glove on the other hand (Figure 11-22C).

5. Pull the glove off inside out, drawing it over the first glove.

6. Drop both gloves together into the biohazardous waste receptacle.

7. Use appropriate hand hygiene. Dry with a paper towel and discard towel in proper container. Use a dry towel to turn off water faucet. Discard towel.

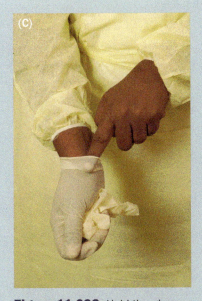

Figure 11-22C Hold the glove just removed in the gloved hand. Insert fingers of the ungloved hand inside the cuff of the other glove.

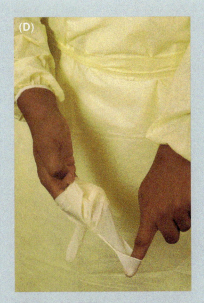

Figure 11-22D Remove glove, keep contaminated portion wadded up inside first glove.

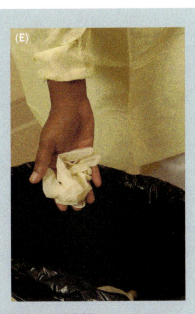

Figure 11-22E Discard gloves in appropriate waste receptacle.

PROCEDURE 11-10
Donning a Gown

To be effective, a gown should have long sleeves, be long enough to cover the uniform, and big enough to overlap in the back. Gowns should be waterproof.

1. Assemble equipment:
   - Clean gown
   - Paper towel

2. Remove wristwatch; place it on paper towel.

3. Use appropriate hand hygiene.

4. If a mask and goggles or face shield are required, put them on first.

(continues)

PROCEDURE 11-10
Donning a Gown (Continued)

5. After tying on the mask, put on the gown outside the resident's room. Put on gown by slipping arms into sleeves (Figure 11-23A).

6. Slip fingers of both hands under inside neckband and grasp ties in back. Secure neckband (Figure 11-23B).

7. Reach behind and overlap edges of gown. Secure waist ties (Figure 11-23C).

8. Take your watch into the isolation unit, leaving it on paper towel.

9. Remember when using gowns:
   - A disposable gown is worn once only and is then discarded as infectious waste.
   - A cloth reusable gown is worn once only and is then handled as contaminated linen.
   - Carry out all procedures in the unit at one time, to avoid unnecessary waste of gowns.

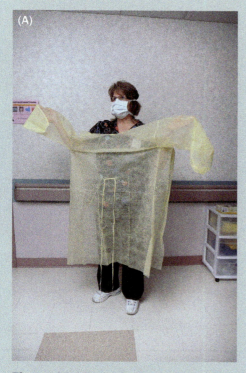

Figure 11-23A Put on the clean cover gown before entering the resident's room. After tying on the mask, put on the gown.

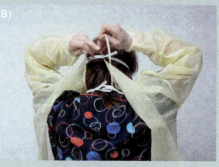

Figure 11-23B Slip fingers inside the neckband and tie gown.

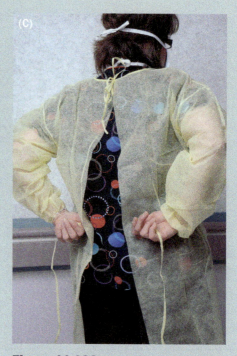

Figure 11-23C Reach behind, overlap the edges of the gown so the uniform is completely covered, and tie the waist ties.

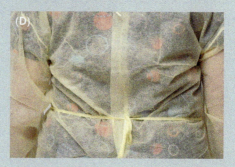

Figure 11-23D Tie the waist ties.

PROCEDURE 11-11
Removing Contaminated Gloves, Mask, and Gown

1. Assemble equipment:
    - Biohazard waste receptacle for disposable items
    - Appropriate linen hamper
    - Paper towels

2. Follow Procedure 11-9 for removing contaminated gloves.

3. Undo waist ties of gown.

4. Untie neck ties and loosen gown at shoulder (Figure 11-24A).

5. Remove mask by untying the bottom ties first (Figure 11-24B), then the top ties. Dispose of mask in appropriate waste receptacle (Figure 11-24C).

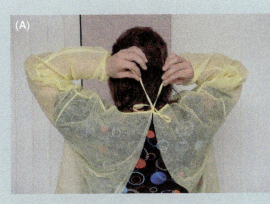

Figure 11-24A Untie neck ties of gown.

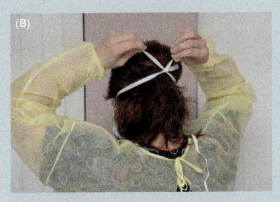

Figure 11-24B Remove mask by untying bottom ties first and then top ties.

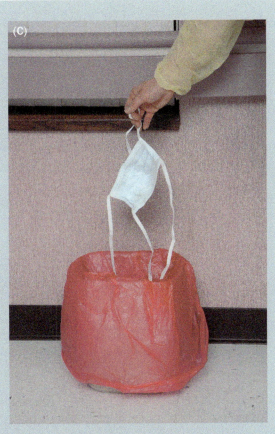

Figure 11-24C Holding mask by ties, place it in the receptacle for contaminated trash.

(continues)

PROCEDURE 11-11
Removing Contaminated Gloves, Mask, and Gown (Continued)

6. Slip finger of dominant hand inside cuff of other sleeve without touching outside of gown (Figure 11-24D).

7. Using gown-covered hand, pull the gown down over the dominant hand (Figure 11-24E) and then off both arms.

8. As the gown is removed, fold it away from the body with the contaminated side inward and then roll it up (Figure 11-24F). Dispose of gown in appropriate receptacle.

9. Use appropriate hand hygiene.

10. Remove watch from paper towel. Hold clean side of paper towel and dispose of towel to wastepaper receptacle.

11. Use clean paper towel to grasp handle to door as you leave resident's room. Discard paper towel in appropriate receptacle before you leave the unit.

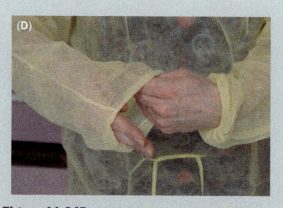

Figure 11-24D Slip fingers of one hand inside the cuff of the other hand. Pull gown down over the hand. Do not touch the outside of the gown with either hand.

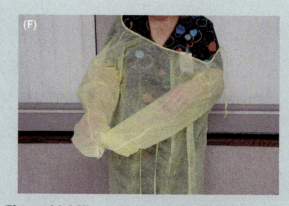

Figure 11-24F Pull the gown off your arms, being careful that your hands do not touch the outside of the gown. Hold the gown away from your uniform and roll it up with the contaminated side inside. If gown is disposable, place it in the receptacle for contaminated trash. If gown is not disposable, place it in laundry hamper for contaminated linens.

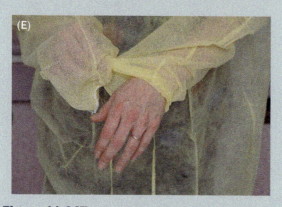

Figure 11-24E Use the gown-covered hand, pull the gown down over the other hand.

(continues)

PROCEDURE 11-11
Removing Contaminated Gloves, Mask, and Gown (Continued)

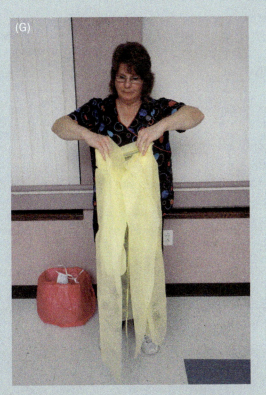

Figure 11-24G Hold the gown away from your uniform and roll it up with the contaminated side inside.

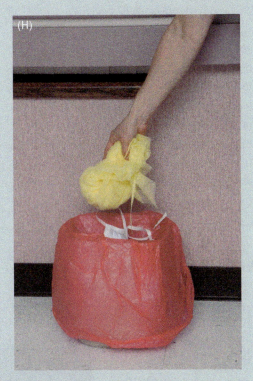

Figure 11-24H If gown is disposable, place it in the receptacle for contaminated trash. If gown is not disposable, place it in laundry hamper for contaminated linens.

PROCEDURE 11-12
Caring for Linens in Isolation Unit

1. Assemble linen required and place on chair or stand outside isolation unit.
2. Use appropriate hand hygiene.
3. Outside the isolation unit, put on PPE as required by type of transmission precautions.
4. Once inside the isolation unit, place clean linen on a chair.
5. Identify the resident and explain what you plan to do.
6. Provide privacy.
7. Allow the resident to help as much as possible.
8. Raise bed to comfortable working height.

(continues)

PROCEDURE 11-12
Caring for Linens in Isolation Unit (Continued)

9. Remove soiled linen from bed by starting at the edges and working toward the center. Roll the linen toward the center with the soiled side inside.

10. Handle soiled linen as little as possible. Pick up the linen from the bed and hold it away from your uniform and gown (if used).

11. Place soiled linen in a meltaway laundry bag (a bag that dissolves in the wash water in the laundry), or follow facility policy.

12. Place meltaway bag in laundry hamper lined with biohazard plastic bag, or follow facility policy. Bag should be labeled as biohazardous material for laundry.

13. Secure bag and route soiled linen to laundry according to facility policy.

14. If gloves are heavily contaminated from the soiled linens, remove gloves and dispose of in appropriate receptacle. Wash hands, dry, and put on a clean pair of gloves. Then remake the resident's bed with the clean linens.

15. Carry out all procedure completion actions.

You may remove your PPE after you have finished all tasks in the resident's room. Follow the instructions in Procedures 11-9 and 11-10.

NOTE: Meltaway bags are rarely used now. They have been replaced with plastic bags. If your facility uses meltaway bags, remember that they begin to disintegrate when wet linen is placed inside.

PROCEDURE 11-13
Measuring Vital Signs in Isolation Unit

NOTE: Equipment to measure vital signs in isolation should be dedicated to the resident, meaning that the equipment will remain in the room with the resident. If the equipment must be shared with other residents, it must be cleaned and disinfected before use with another resident.

1. Before entering the isolation unit:
    - Use appropriate hand hygiene.
    - Remove wristwatch and place it on a clean paper towel.
    - Put on PPE as required by the type of transmission-based precautions used.

2. Pick up the paper towel with the watch. Enter the isolation unit.

3. With the watch still on the paper towel, place it where you can see it during the procedures.

4. Identify the resident and explain what you plan to do.

5. Provide privacy.

6. Allow the resident to help as much as possible.

7. Raise bed to comfortable working height.

8. Using the equipment dedicated to the resident, measure vital signs.

9. Note the readings on a paper towel so you do not forget them.

10. Clean and store the equipment used according to facility policy.

11. Carry out all procedure completion actions.

(continues)

PROCEDURE 11-13
Measuring Vital Signs in Isolation Unit (Continued)

12. Remove and discard PPE according to facility policy.

13. Use appropriate hand hygiene and pick up watch.

14. Review your notes so you can accurately write them down when you are outside the room. If you cannot remember them, ask a coworker (who is outside the door) to write down the vital statistics that you have taken.

15. Handle only the clean side of the paper towel that held your watch and carefully pick up your towel containing the notes and discard both in the appropriate receptacle.

16. Use a paper towel to open the door and leave the isolation unit. Discard paper towel before you leave the unit.

PROCEDURE 11-14
Serving a Meal Tray in Isolation Unit

1. Before entering the isolation unit:
   - Use appropriate hand hygiene.
   - Obtain the meal tray for the resident. Check the meal card on the tray and check that the correct menu is provided.
   - Ask for the assistance of another member of the team.
   - Place the tray on the isolation cart.
   - Put on PPE as required by the type of isolation precautions used.

2. Enter the isolation room and identify the resident.

3. Explain what you plan to do.

4. Provide privacy.

5. Allow the resident to help as much as possible.

6. Raise the bed to comfortable working height.

7. Pick up the meal tray that remains in the room. Make sure the tray is clean.

8. Return to the door and open it. The team member assisting holds the meal tray while you carefully transfer items to the isolation tray.

9. Place isolation meal tray on overbed table. Prepare the resident for the meal.

10. Check the resident's identification band against the meal tray card.

11. Assist the resident with food preparation and feeding as needed.

12. When the resident finishes, note how much food and liquid have been eaten. Uneaten food (except bones) is flushed down the toilet.

13. All disposable items (bones, dishes, eating utensils, covers, plastic wrap, foil, napkins, cups, cartons) are placed in the appropriate waste receptacle.

14. Reusable dishes may be handled as follows:
    - Use a paper towel to open the door to the isolation unit.
    - Prop door open with your foot. Transfer dishes to a tray held by another assistant outside the door.
    - Assistant outside the room covers the dishes and returns the tray to the food cart.

NOTE: CDC no longer requires the use of disposable dishes on transmission-based precautions.

(continues)

PROCEDURE 11-14
Measuring Vital Signs in Isolation Unit (Continued)

15. Clean meal tray and store in the isolation unit.
16. Carry out all procedure completion actions.
17. Remove PPE and discard in the appropriate receptacle.
18. Use appropriate hand hygiene.
19. Use paper towel to open door to leave the isolation unit.

NOTE: CDC does not require this procedure.

PROCEDURE 11-15
Specimen Collection from Resident in Isolation Unit

1. Outside the isolation unit, assemble equipment:
   - Clean specimen container and cover
   - Paper towel
   - Biohazard bag for specimen container (Figure 11-25)
   - Two completed labels, one for the specimen container and one for the biohazard bag

NOTE: The biohazard bag may have a preprinted block on the bag that can be completed with the required information. In this case, a second label is not needed.

2. Place the equipment on the isolation cart while you put on PPE.
3. The biohazard bag for specimen transport remains outside the isolation unit.
4. Carry the specimen equipment into the isolation unit. Place container and cover on a paper towel.
5. Identify the resident and explain what you plan to do.
6. Provide privacy.
7. Allow the resident to help as much as possible.
8. Raise bed to comfortable working height.
9. Place specimen into container without touching the outside of the container.
10. Cover the container and apply label.
11. Clean equipment used to obtain the specimen according to facility policy.
12. Carry out all procedure completion actions.
13. Remove PPE as described in Procedures 11-9 and 11-11.

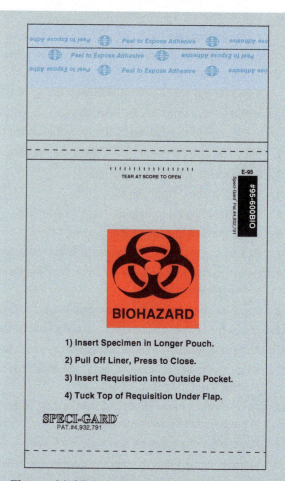

Figure 11-25 Specimens taken from residents in isolation can be transported in specimen bags marked with the biohazard symbol.

(continues)

PROCEDURE 11-15
Specimen Collection from Resident in Isolation Unit (Continued)

14. Use appropriate hand hygiene.
15. Use a paper towel to pick up specimen container. Use another paper towel to open door to leave isolation unit.
16. Outside the unit, gather the towel in your hands so the edges do not hang loosely. Place the specimen container in the biohazard transport bag, being careful not to allow the paper towel to touch the outside of the transport bag.
17. Discard the paper towels in the appropriate receptacle.
18. Follow facility policy for transport of the specimen.
19. Wash hands.

PROCEDURE 11-16
Transferring Non-disposable Equipment Outside of Isolation Unit

1. Non-disposable equipment used with a resident in transmission-based precautions may be dedicated to that resident; that is, the equipment remains in the isolation unit and is used only by that resident. Cleaning as required is done in the room by the nursing assistant or the housekeeping staff according to facility policy.
2. If the equipment must be used for other residents, it must be removed from the isolation unit and disinfected or sterilized before use with another resident.
3. Before leaving the isolation unit, clean the equipment with a disinfectant.
4. Place the equipment in a biohazard plastic bag.
5. Follow Procedure 11-11 for removing contaminated gloves, mask, and gown.
6. Pick up the bag containing the equipment and leave the isolation unit.
7. Once outside the unit, follow facility policy for disinfection or sterilization of the equipment.
8. Some equipment may be terminally (finally and completely) cleaned with disinfectant in the resident's unit when isolation is discontinued.

PROCEDURE 11-17
Transporting Resident to and from Isolation Unit

1. Use appropriate hand hygiene.
2. Assemble equipment:
   - Transport vehicle (wheelchair or stretcher)
   - Clean sheet
   - Mask for resident, if isolation precautions require it
3. Notify department to which the resident is to be transported that a resident from an isolation unit is being transported.

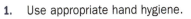

(continues)

PROCEDURE 11-17
Transporting Resident to and from Isolation Unit (Continued)

4. If the resident is to be transported by stretcher, ask for assistance in moving the resident to the stretcher. Two other care providers will be needed.

5. Cover transport vehicle with clean sheet. Do not let the sheet touch the floor.

6. Wash your hands.

7. Put on PPE as required by type of precautions being used. If other care providers are needed to move the resident onto a stretcher, they also must put on PPE.

8. Wheel transport vehicle into isolation unit.

9. Identify the resident. Explain what you plan to do.

10. Provide privacy.

11. Allow the resident to help as much as possible.

12. If the resident is to be transported by wheelchair, the bed must be in the lowest horizontal position. For transport by stretcher, raise the bed to the same height as the stretcher.

13. Assist the resident into the wheelchair or onto the stretcher.

14. Put mask on the resident, if required.

15. Wrap the resident in sheet, if required. Make sure sheet does not touch the floor.

16. Remove PPE and wash hands. Open door and take the resident out of isolation unit (Figure 11-26).

17. To return the resident to isolation unit, place wheelchair or stretcher near wall of room as you put on PPE.

18. Enter the isolation unit, unwrap the resident from sheet, and remove mask, if used.

19. Assist the resident from wheelchair or stretcher (with help of other caregivers) and return him or her to bed.

20. Carry out procedure completion actions.

21. Place sheet in laundry hamper for contaminated linens and discard mask in receptacle for biohazardous trash.

22. Remove PPE and use appropriate hand hygiene.

23. Remove transport vehicle from isolation unit. Follow facility procedure for cleaning and storing vehicle used with a resident in isolation.

24. Report completion of procedure: transport of resident in isolation to another department and back to isolation unit.

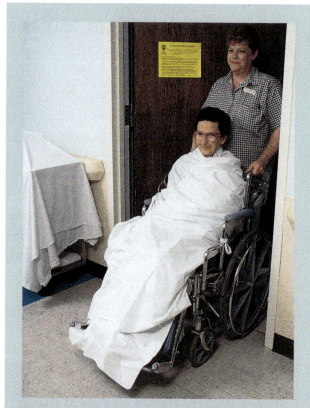

Figure 11-26 The resident is leaving her room, where contact precautions are in effect, and is being transported to another area of the facility.

? EXERCISE 11-8

MATCHING

1. item that is free of all living organisms
2. potentially hazardous waste
3. machine using steam under pressure to sterilize
4. transmissible to others
5. process used to make equipment sterile
6. easily spread to others
7. process of eliminating harmful microbes
8. articles with microbes on them
9. disease organisms are absent
10. to separate or set apart

a. asepsis
b. autoclave
c. biohazard
d. communicable
e. contagious
f. contaminated
g. disinfection
h. isolation
I. sterile
j. sterilization

STERILE PROCEDURES

Surgical asepsis is the means by which the environment is maintained free of microorganisms, both pathogens and non-pathogens. In procedures wherein surgical asepsis is used, equipment and supplies must be sterile. In other words, items used in the procedure must go through a sterilization process.

In most facilities, nursing assistants are not expected to carry out procedures requiring sterile techniques. If you are responsible for sterile procedures, you should first be given thorough training. Your responsibilities may include opening sterile packages such as gloves or other equipment to help the nurse during a procedure (Procedure 11-18).

PROCEDURE 11-18
Opening a Sterile Package

1. Use appropriate hand hygiene.
2. Assemble equipment:
   - Sterile package
3. If color code has not changed or seal does not look intact, do not consider article sterile. If you have any doubt about sterility, consider item unsterile and inform the nurse.
4. Touch only outside of package. Only sterile surfaces contact other sterile surfaces. Never reach over a sterile field.
5. Commercially prepared products will be sealed. If package is in poor condition or discolored, torn, wet, or expired use date, do not consider item sterile. Discard item.
6. Place package, fold side up, on a flat, clean surface.
7. Remove tape.
8. Unfold flap farthest away from you by grasping outer surface only between thumb and forefinger (Figure 11-27A).
9. Open right flap with right hand using same technique (Figure 11-27B).
10. Open left flap with left hand using same technique (Figure 11-27C).
11. Open final flap (nearest you) (Figure 11-27D). Touch only the outside of flap. Be careful not to stand too close. Do not allow uniform to touch flap as it is lifted free. Be sure the flaps are pulled open completely to prevent them from folding back over sterile items.

(continues)

PROCEDURE 11-18
Opening a Sterile Package (Continued)

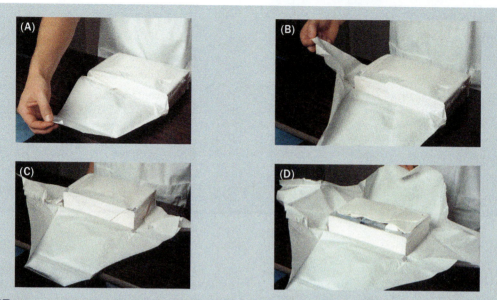

Figure 11-27 Opening a sterile package. (A) Open the top flap away from you; handle only the outside. (B) Open the right side. Do not touch the inside of the folded-over portion. (C) Open the left side, drawing the left flap to the side. (D) Without reaching over the sterile field, open the side toward you.

? EXERCISE 11-9

TRUE OR FALSE
Indicate whether the following statements are true (T) or false (F).

1. T F Complete PPE is required when working with all infected residents.
2. T F Each individual health care worker makes the decision about which protective equipment is to be used when giving care.
3. T F Disinfection is the process of eliminating harmful microbes from equipment and instruments.
4. T F Items are usually washed before they are disinfected.
5. T F When PPE is to be used, gloves are put on before the gown.
6. T F When removing a mask, untie the upper strings first.
7. T F When measuring vital signs of a resident in isolation, the wrist watch should be placed directly on the bedside table for easy viewing.
8. T F Leftover food may be returned directly to the food service cart from an isolation room.
9. T F Sterile packages should always have seals checked for security before use.
10. T F Surgical asepsis maintains an environment that is microbe free.
11. T F Surgical masks are effective for only 1 hour.
12. T F Residents of different cultures may be either offended or frightened by isolation procedures used in U.S. health care facilities.
13. T F Protective isolation is used when a resident has a compromised immune system.

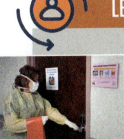

LESSON SYNTHESIS: Putting It All Together

You have just completed this lesson. Now go back and review the Clinical Focus. Try to see how the Clinical Focus relates to the concepts presented in the lesson. Then answer the following questions.

1. What kind of precautions are in use for Mr. Uritz?
2. How is MRSA spread?
3. Why is this resident in a private room?
4. When Mr. Uritz is in his room, is it necessary to keep the door shut?

11 REVIEW

A. Fill in the blanks by selecting the correct word or phrase from the list.

communicable   sterile

disinfectants   infection control

medical asepsis

1. The methods that reduce the spread of infections in health care facilities are known as _____.

2. An article is _____ when there are no living organisms present.

3. _____ are procedures to prevent the spread of infections in the work area.

4. An easily transmitted disease is called _____.

5. Chemicals that destroy pathogens on articles are called _____.

B. Answer each statement true (T) or false (F).

6. T F   Items for one resident may be used by another resident.

7. T F   Food trays should remain covered until they are delivered to the resident.

8. T F   Laundry dropped on the floor may be used as long as there is no visible dirt.

9. T F   Soiled linens may be placed on the floor until all the linen is gathered together and put in the laundry hamper.

10. T F   Hands need not be washed after gloves are removed as long as there are no tears in the gloves.

11. T F   Gloves are always used when handling bedpans and urinals.

12. T F   Occupational exposure means coming in contact with potentially infectious material as you work.

13. T F   Standard Precautions require the wearing of gloves for any contact with blood or body fluids.

14. T F   The biohazard symbol is a green square with a line through it.

15. T F   A used razor may be disposed of by dropping it in the wastebasket.

C. Select one best answer for each of the following.

16. Housing and caring for a person with an infection is known as

(A) segregation

(B) isolation

(C) sequestration

(D) separation

17. To remove PPE after caring for a resident on isolation precautions, you should

(A) remove the gown first

(B) remove the gloves first

(C) remove the mask first

(D) remove PPE in any order

18. If a nursing assistant is sensitive to latex gloves

(A) gloves need not be worn

(B) wear the latex gloves anyway

(C) ask the supervisor for non-latex gloves

(D) put powder in the gloves

19. The basic foundation of medical asepsis is

(A) hand hygiene

(B) wearing goggles

(C) wearing a mask

(D) wearing a gown

20. If there is an exposure incident, you should

(A) ignore the situation

(B) report it at once to the supervisor

(C) call the doctor

(D) tell other nursing assistants

21. Your hands were splashed with blood while the nurse changed the resident's dressing. What will you do first?

(A) Tell the nurse.

(B) Rinse your hands.

(C) Use alcohol-based hand sanitizer.

(D) Wash your hands with soap and warm water.

22. One of the following will *not* be needed to protect the CNA when caring for a resident with shingles (herpes zoster).

(A) Hand hygiene according to standard precautions.

(B) Wearing gloves when entering the room.

(C) Removing gloves after completion of care.

(D) Wearing a HEPA filter mask.

23. When washing your hands with soap and water you should:

(A) keep fingertips pointed down.

(B) keep fingertips pointed up.

(C) keep hands level with your elbows.

(D) adjust the water temperature with your bare hands.

24. You accidently drop the resident's toothbrush on the floor. What will you do?

(A) Ask the family to purchase a new toothbrush.

(B) Rinse the brush and return it to the bedside stand.

(C) Disinfect the brush with a 1:10 bleach solution.

(D) Tell the nurse.

25. After shaving the resident with a disposable razor, what is your next action?

(A) Discard the razor in the resident's wastebasket.

(B) Rinse the razor under running water and store in the bathroom.

(C) Discard the razor in the designated sharps container.

(D) Store the razor in an alcohol solution at the bedside.

26. Gloves need *not* be worn when:

(A) brushing the resident's dentures.

(B) taking the resident's pulse.

(C) emptying the urine drainage bag.

(D) giving a bedpan or urinal.

4

Characteristics of the Long-Term Care Resident

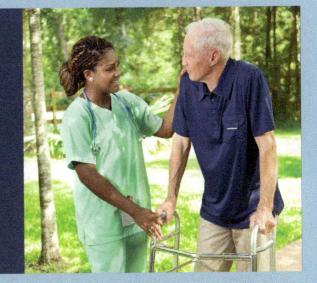

LESSON 12
THE LONG-TERM CARE RESIDENT

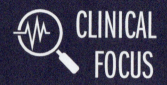

CLINICAL FOCUS

Think about how stereotypes and myths about older adults and those who live in long-term care make it difficult to recognize the uniqueness of each person as you study this lesson.

OBJECTIVES

After studying this lesson, you should be able to:

- Define vocabulary words and terms.
- Identify four physical changes that are expected to occur in normal aging.
- List five common functional changes that occur in the aging process.
- List four reasons why residents are admitted to long-term care facilities.
- List three facts about the over-65 population.
- Describe three considerations required for giving care related to the physical and functional changes of aging.
- Describe five facts to remember when caring for younger adults.
- Identify the unique needs of younger residents in long-term care facilities.
- List five procedures you can do to increase the resident's comfort.

CASE STUDY

Sam Jacobzinski, age 84, was admitted to Riverview Center in acute cardiac failure 4 years ago. There was little hope for his recovery, but Sam fooled everyone. He recovered and has been an active resident ever since. He is alert and involved in facility activities and was elected Resident Council president. Sam uses a motorized wheelchair and makes daily rounds to visit the other residents. Periodically he "overdoes it" and needs bed rest, but even then his spirit is felt throughout the facility.

VOCABULARY

chronic disease (KRON-ick dih-ZEEZ)
developmental disability (dee-vel-op-MEN-tal
  dis-ah-BILL-ah-tee)
disability (dis-ah-BILL-ah-tee)
functional changes (FUNK-shun-al CHAYN-jez)
impairment (im-PAIR-ment)
instrumental activities of daily living (IADL)
  (in-strew-MEN-tal ack-TIV-ih-tees of DAY-lee LIV-ing)

myth (mith)
self-care (functional) deficit (self-kair [FUNK-shun-al]
  DEF-ih-sit)
senescent changes (see-NESS-ent CHAYN-jez)
stereotype (STEH-ree-oh-type)
trauma (TRAW-mah)

ABOUT AGING

Some general thoughts about aging can be stated:

- Aging is progressive and universal.
- No diseases are specific to aging.
- Aging and disease are not the same thing.
- Not all functional changes from age are related to disease. Interest, personal and financial resources, family structure, genetics, attitude, and lifestyle all play a part. Elements of lifestyle that contribute to the aging process include smoking, misuse of alcohol and drugs, type of diet, and lack of exercise.
- A wider range of what is considered "normal" function exists among older people than among younger people. A greater variability occurs among older people in physical abilities, sizes, and characteristics compared to younger groups.
- All older adults are not alike. People in their sixties, seventies, eighties, and nineties are all different.

THE PROCESS OF NORMAL AGING

Aging is a natural process and is not a result of disease. The term *gerontology* means the study of aging. It is used to describe a specialty area for health care workers and other professions. The term *geriatrics* refers to the diagnosis and treatment of disorders that occur with aging. Although some changes are expected from aging, no disorders are unique to older people.

Aging is a progressive process that begins at birth and ends at death. It is a normal process experienced by all living things. During the life span, a unique person of value emerges and makes contributions to society. When older, this same person of value needs and deserves respect, support, and care. Older persons make many contributions to society.

CHANGES CAUSED BY AGING

Normal aging changes are called **senescent changes**. These changes occur in every body system, but not at any specific time or at any specific rate (Figure 12-1). Some changes are more obvious than others. Aging is both a physical and psychological process. One person may feel and act old at 60, and another may be spry at 80. Both will usually show some physical evidence of their ages. In general, with increasing age:

- The body's systems become less effective.
- This results in **functional changes;** that is, the ability to carry out activities of daily living (ADL) decreases.
- The risk of acquiring a disease and disability increases.

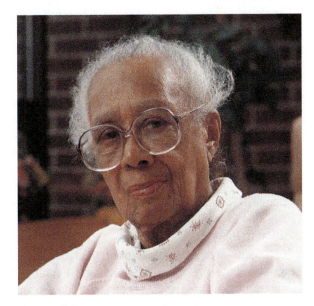

Figure 12-1 Note the many signs of aging.

Most older adults have at least one chronic health condition and many have several. Some of the most common conditions are

- Arthritis
- Hypertension
- Heart disease
- Hearing impairments
- Vision impairment
- Diabetes
- COPD
- Alzheimer's disease and other related dementias
- Osteoporosis

Normal aging changes are listed in Figure 12-2. Some of these changes are usually seen in all older adults. For example, hair begins to turn gray, the skin becomes dry, wrinkles develop, and posture changes.

Functional Changes

Functional changes may occur as people age. Consider these changes as you care for your residents.

1. Changes in the muscles and joints result in slower movements and decreased flexibility. Residents will take longer to accomplish an activity. Less flexible fingers mean that residents may need help to open and close things, to write, to dial a telephone (Figure 12-3), and to button clothing.

2. Residents have a greater risk of falling because of loss of balance when walking or moving from a sitting to a standing position. Encourage residents to use handrails and to move carefully, without haste. Exercise helps to decrease the loss in flexibility and increase bone density. Be sure that residents have the necessary aids to help them keep their mobility (Figure 12-4).

3. Changes in the urinary system may make it more difficult to empty the bladder completely. This puts the older adult at risk for bladder infections. Providing adequate fluids is important in preventing such infections. Older adults generally have to go to the bathroom more often than younger people. Provide privacy and help the residents assume a comfortable position when you help them to the toilet.

4. Changes in the intestinal tract lead to loss of muscle tone and slower peristalsis, resulting in constipation. Flatulence is more common. Provide the residents with adequate fluids and food. Help them remain physically active.

5. Visual changes mean that most older adults need to wear glasses for reading. Make sure glasses are clean and readily available. Evening hours can be hazardous because of poor lighting and shadows. Position lights for maximum illumination. Do not turn corridor lights lower in evening hours. Older adults may also be more sensitive to glare, so lights should not be shining directly into their eyes. Use indirect lighting whenever possible.

6. Hearing loss is common as people age. They may not respond as quickly because they do not hear you. They may act irritated when they hear only part of a conversation or instruction. Be patient and repeat the message using only the essential words.

7. The senses of taste and smell influence one another. Loss of appetite may occur when the ability to taste and smell decreases. Taste buds lose their sensitivity, especially for salt and sugar. As a result, older adults may use more sugar and salt in an attempt to add more flavor to foods.

8. Changes in the cardiovascular system mean older persons may tire more easily with exertion. As a result, they require more time to complete an activity. More time for resting between activities may be needed. Circulation may be impaired. Residents should be cautioned to sit with the legs uncrossed and to change positions slowly to avoid postural hypotension.

9. The sex drive in men and women may last throughout life. However, decreased estrogen production in women means there is less vaginal moisture. This may make sexual intercourse uncomfortable or painful. Men may need more time to attain an erection during sexual activity. More time may also be needed for ejaculation to occur.

The changes described here occur slowly, over many years. Because they take place so gradually, people compensate for many of these changes; that is, they learn to deal effectively with the changes.

ILLNESS AND DISABILITY

The residents are in the long-term care facility for several reasons. Many have a chronic illness or a disability. A disability occurs when there is an impairment that interferes with the individual's ability to perform the activities normal for a person of that age. A disability is present if any adult is unable to perform ADLs. An impairment is a loss or abnormality of the body structure and function. The damage to brain cells in Alzheimer's disease, for example, interferes with the

Body System	Physical Changes of Aging
Integumentary	• Hair loses color and becomes thinner • Skin dries, becomes less elastic; wrinkles develop • Increase in facial hair growth in some women • Skin is fragile and tears easily • Bruises easily (senile purpura common) • Reduced blood flow in vessels that nourish the skin results in delayed healing • Fingernails and toenails thicken • Sweat glands do not excrete perspiration as readily • Oil glands do not secrete as much oil for skin and hair • There is increased sensitivity to heat and cold • Skin discolorations (age spots) become more common • Blood supply to the feet and legs is reduced, increasing the risk of injury and ulcers, and sensations of cold • Reduced number of nerve endings
Nervous	• Tasks involving speed, balance, coordination, and fine motor activities take longer because of slowed transmission of nerve impulses • Balance and coordination problems result from deterioration in the nerve terminals that provide information to the brain about body movement and position • Temperature regulation is less effective • Deep sleep is shortened; the person awakens during the night • Brain cells are lost, but intelligence remains intact unless disease is present • Decreased number and sensitivity of nerve receptors in skin (heat, cold, pain, pressure) • Risk of injury increases because of nerve receptors in skin (heat, cold, pain, pressure) • There is decreased blood flow to the brain, which may result in mental confusion and memory loss
Sensory	• More difficult to see close objects and differentiating between color blue and green • Night vision may decrease (indoors as well as outdoors) • Cataracts (clouding of the lens of the eye) are more common • Dryness and itching of the eyes may result from decreased secretion of fluids • Side vision and depth perception diminish • Hearing diminishes in most elderly persons • Smell receptors and taste buds are less sensitive, so foods have less taste • Changes in sleep patterns • Decreased production of earwax • Decreased sensitivity to pressure and pain
Musculoskeletal	• Loss of elasticity of muscles and decrease in size of muscle mass result in reduced strength, flexibility, endurance, muscle tone, and delayed reaction time • Slower movements • Bones lose minerals, become brittle, and break more easily; arthritis and osteoporosis are common • Spine becomes less stable and flexible, increasing the risk of injury • Posture may become slumped because of weakness in back muscles • Degenerative changes in the joints result in limited movement, stiffness, and pain
Respiratory	• Lung capacity decreases as a result of muscular rigidity in the lungs • Coughing is less effective; this results in pooling of secretions and fluid in the lungs, increasing the risk of infection and choking • Shortness of breath on exertion, as a result of aging changes in the lungs • Gas exchange in the lungs is less effective, resulting in decreased oxygenation

Figure 12-2 Physical changes of aging.

(continues)

Body System	Physical Changes of Aging
Urinary	<ul><li>Kidneys decrease in size</li><li>Urine production is less efficient</li><li>Bladder capacity decreases, increasing the frequency of urination</li><li>Kidney function increases at rest, causing urination at night</li><li>Bladder muscles weaken, causing leaking of urine or inability to empty the bladder completely complete emptying of bladder becomes more difficult</li><li>Enlargement of the prostate gland in the male, causing frequency of urination, dribbling, urinary obstruction, and urinary retention</li></ul>
Digestive	<ul><li>Saliva production in the mouth decreases, causing difficulty with swallowing and digestion of starches, and increasing risk of tooth decay</li><li>Tastebuds on the tongue decrease, beginning with sweet and salt; changes in tastebuds may result in appetite changes and increase in condiment use</li><li>Loss of teeth makes food more difficult to chew</li><li>Gag reflex is less effective, increasing the risk of choking</li><li>Movement of flood into the stomach through the esophagus is slower</li><li>Food in the stomach is digested slower, so food remains there longer before moving to the small intestine</li><li>Flatulence increases</li><li>Indigestion and slower absorption of fat result from a decrease in digestive enzymes resulting in food intolerances</li><li>Food movement through the large intestine is slower, resulting in constipation</li></ul>
Cardiovascular	<ul><li>Heart rate slows, causing a slower pulse and less efficient circulation. This results in decreased energy and a slower response, causing the individual to tire easily</li><li>Blood vessels lose elasticity and develop calcium deposits, causing vessels to narrow</li><li>Blood pressure increases because of changes to the blood vessel walls</li><li>Heart rate takes longer to return to normal after exercise</li><li>Veins enlarge, causing blood vessels close to the skin surface to become more prominent</li><li>Heart may not pump as efficiently, leading to decreased cardiac output and circulation</li></ul>
Endocrine	<ul><li>Decrease in levels of estrogen, progesterone</li><li>Hot flashes, nervous feelings</li><li>Higher levels of parathormone and thyroid-stimulating hormone</li><li>Delayed release of insulin, increasing blood sugar level; incidence of diabetes increases greatly with age</li><li>Metabolism rate and body functions slow, reducing the amount of calories needed for the body to function normally. This increases the risk of overweight and obesity</li></ul>
Reproductive	*Females:*<ul><li>Fewer female hormones are produced</li><li>Ovulation and menstrual cycle cease</li><li>Vaginal walls are thinner and drier</li><li>Vagina becomes shorter and narrower</li><li>Breast tissue decreases and the muscles supporting the breasts weaken</li></ul>*Males:*<ul><li>Scrotum less firm</li><li>Prostate gland may enlarge</li><li>Hormone production decreases, decreasing size of testes and lowering sperm count</li><li>More time required for an erection</li></ul>

Figure 12-2 *(Continued)*

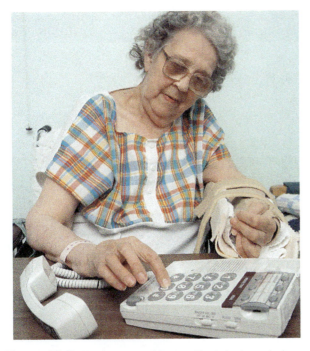

Figure 12-3 The large numbers on the telephone help the resident remain independent.

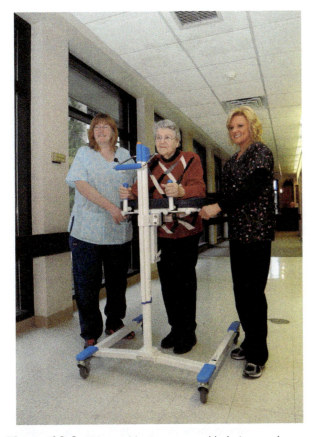

Figure 12-4 Older residents may need help to remain physically active. The walker provides support and stability, giving the resident more confidence in walking.

person's ability to perform ADLs. A disability or impairment could be the result of:

1. Chronic disease

   A **chronic disease** is one that begins slowly and is expected to continue for a long time, perhaps for life. Some chronic diseases are progressive, which means the symptoms will increase in severity as time goes on. Examples of chronic diseases are:

   - Arthritis
   - Neurologic disorders such as multiple sclerosis, Parkinson's disease (Figure 12-5), Huntington's disease, Alzheimer's disease and other related dementias, epilepsy, or migraines
   - Heart or lung disease
   - Diabetes
   - Cancer
   - Illnesses with acute onset that have chronic after-effects, such as stroke

2. Trauma

   Trauma refers to injuries received in an accident. These accidents may result in brain injuries, spinal cord injuries, multi-organ damage, or amputation of one or more extremities. The injuries may prevent the individual from being independent.

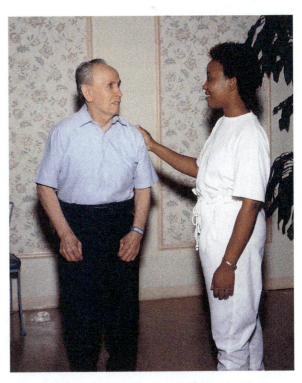

Figure 12-5 Note the typical bent posture in this front view of a resident with Parkinson's disease.

? EXERCISE 12-1

TRUE OR FALSE

Determine whether the following changes are normal changes in aging by answering true (T) or false (F).

1. T F Hair gets thinner.

2. T F Skin gets more moisture.

3. T F Temperature regulation is more effective.

4. T F Risk of injury increases from decreased ability to feel pressure and temperature changes.

5. T F Night vision increases.

6. T F Side vision decreases.

7. T F Spine becomes less stable.

8. T F Muscles lose elasticity.

9. T F Lung capacity decreases.

10. T F Coughing is less effective.

11. T F Aging is a process that results from disease alone.

12. T F Gerontology refers to the study of aging.

MULTIPLE CHOICE

Select the one best answer.

13. Some ideas of aging include
    (A) some diseases are specific to aging
    (B) aging and disease are the same thing
    (C) as people age, not all functional changes are related to disease
    (D) all older adults are alike

14. An example of a chronic disease is
    (A) arthritis   (C) spinal cord injury
    (B) amputation   (D) none of these

15. Aging is a progressive process beginning at
    (A) birth   (C) 65 years
    (B) 21 years   (D) 85 years

---

3. Developmental disabilities

    A **developmental disability** is a permanent condition that is present at birth or occurs before the age of 21. Developmental disabilities limit the ability to care for oneself in an independent way (Figure 12-6). Cerebral palsy is an example of a developmental disability. This topic is discussed further in Lesson 31.

4. Acquired immune deficiency syndrome (AIDS)

    An increasing number of persons with AIDS are being cared for in long-term care facilities. This disease makes the individuals more susceptible to other infections and diseases. Admission generally occurs when the person is in the terminal stages of disease and needs continual care.

5. Many long-term care facilities have residents with cancer. Sometimes they are receiving treatments specific for the cancer (chemotherapy or radiation). Other residents may be in the terminal stage of the illness.

6. A growing number of residents in long-term care are admitted directly from hospitals for additional care after surgery or illness or for rehabilitation after fractures or strokes. These residents generally stay for a short time, with stays ranging from several weeks to several months. The goal is to return these residents to their homes or to another facility where more independent living is possible. In many facilities, these residents are cared for in the subacute care unit (see Lesson 33).

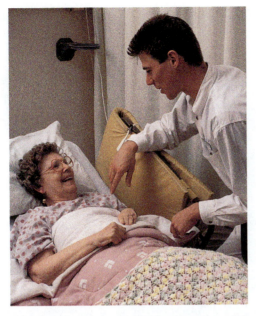

Figure 12-6 This woman has had a developmental disability since birth.

Most residents in long-term care facilities are women because women have a longer life expectancy than men. The older a person gets, the greater the chance that a chronic illness will develop. Most residents have multiple health problems. A resident may be admitted because of a stroke, but also have diabetes and a heart problem. Because of the health problems, residents have self-care (functional) deficits. This means they are unable to care for themselves in one or more areas of ADLs (Figure 12-7). The ADLs include:

- Personal grooming and hygiene
- Bathing
- Dressing and undressing
- Eating
- Toileting
- Mobility

? EXERCISE 12-2

Select the correct term from the following list to complete each statement.

chronic	impairment
developmental disability	myth
disability	senescent
functional change	stereotypes
functional (self-care)	trauma
IADL	natural

1. An illness that continues for a long time is called _____.

2. _____ refers to injuries received in an accident.

3. A (An) _____ occurs when an adult is unable to perform the activities of daily living.

4. A self-care deficit may also be called a (an) _____ deficit.

5. A (An) _____ is a loss or abnormality of body structure or function.

6. Normal changes are also called _____ changes.

7. _____ is the changing ability to carry out activities of daily living (ADL) independently.

8. A (An) _____ is a permanent condition that is present at birth or occurs before the age of 21.

9. Aging is a (an) _____ process.

MULTIPLE CHOICE
Select the one best answer.

10. Residents may be admitted for a short period to long-term facilities for
    (A) acquired immune deficiency syndrome (AIDS)
    (B) terminal cancer
    (C) fracture rehabilitation
    (D) Alzheimer's disease

11. A developmental disability
    (A) is a temporary condition
    (B) limits the ability of one to care for oneself
    (C) occurs following a stroke
    (D) promotes independence

There are also **instrumental activities of daily living (IADLs)** (Figure 12-8). The IADLs include activities such as:

- Managing a household
- Managing money
- Driving a car

? **EXERCISE 12-3**

COMPLETION

Complete the chart to indicate which activity is an ADL and which is an Instrumental activity of daily living (IADL).

1. Managing a household
2. Bathing
3. Dressing and undressing
4. Managing money
5. Eating
6. Toileting
7. Mobility
8. Driving a car

ADL	IADL

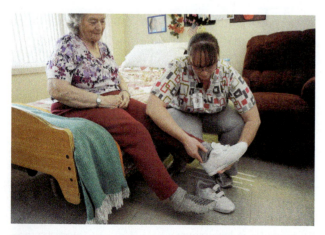

Figure 12-7 This resident needs assistance in completing her ADL.

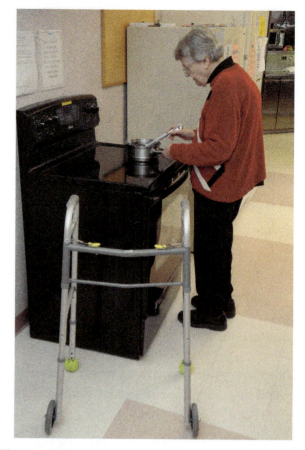

Figure 12-8 Cooking is an example of an IADL.

STEREOTYPES AND MYTHS

Stereotypes of people are rigid ideas about people as a group. A stereotype may partly be true, or it may be true for some people, but all members of a group are never totally alike. For example, many older people are hearing impaired, but not all of them. Beliefs of this kind that are not even partly true are **myths**.

Imagine someone asking you to describe a cat if you had only seen two small, black, short-haired cats in your life. You would undoubtedly say that cats are small, black, and short-haired. As you know, this does not even begin to describe all the different cats throughout the world. Describing all cats with one narrow set of characteristics establishes a stereotype for cats; it is only partly true. It is easy to form stereotypes, because limited experience tends to make us think that everyone in a certain group has the same characteristics as the few people we know in that group.

The Dangers of Stereotyping

Stereotypes about older persons are limiting to both the people who believe them and to the older persons themselves. This is true for several reasons.

- *Stereotyping does not consider the uniqueness of the individual.* Although they have certain characteristics in common, the older members of society have developed from their own special life experiences. This makes each person different, in some ways, from all others.

- *Stereotyping may make people devalue themselves because they see themselves as a reflection of what others think.* If people are treated with respect, they feel respectable and behave in respectable ways. If people are viewed as helpless and unable to make their own decisions, some may lose confidence in their ability to handle their own affairs and become increasingly dependent on others.

CLINICAL FOCUS

Think of Sam, the resident described in the Clinical Focus. Does Sam meet any stereotyped ideas that you may have had before you took this course? Think about what your ideas about aging were before this course and now.

It is unwise and unfair to take stereotypes at face value. It is especially important for those who work in long-term care facilities to realize that the people in their care are not representative of all people in the age group.

You can help residents by:

- Resisting the temptation to stereotype
- Accepting them as individuals
- Giving them as much control over their lives as possible
- Supporting their efforts to remain as independent as possible
- Treating all residents with respect and courtesy

Myths

A *myth* is an untruth that some people believe. It is a myth that age alone causes the diseases that are often associated with older residents. Although many older residents have cancer, heart disease, diabetes, or strokes, younger people also have these conditions.

Another myth is that age alone determines the value of the contributions a person can make to society. Many people make their most valuable contributions to society in their later years. Civic groups and charities could not survive without the involvement of older people (Figure 12-9).

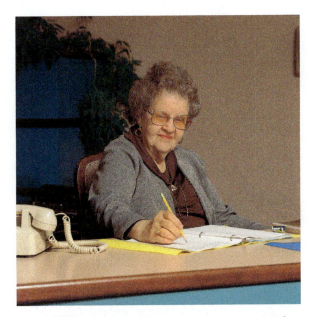

Figure 12-9 Age alone does not determine a person's abilities or activities.

Commonly Held Beliefs

- *As people age, they experience the same characteristic changes in the structure and function of their bodies.* This stereotype is partly true. Aging is usually shown by graying of the hair, diminished eyesight, and slower reaction times. The rate and type of changes due to aging are different for different people. In general, the functioning of the body is slowed but is still adequate to meet the needs of the older lifestyle.

- *Older people are incompetent and unable to make correct judgments and decisions.* This is a myth. Sensory losses occur with aging, but most older people remain mentally sound until they die. They manage their own affairs, can learn new skills, and process new information (Figure 12-10).

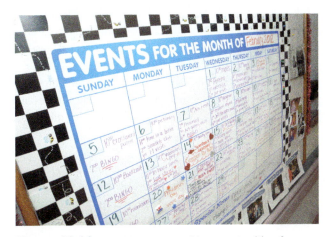

Figure 12-10 Activities can provide opportunities for acquiring new skills and information.

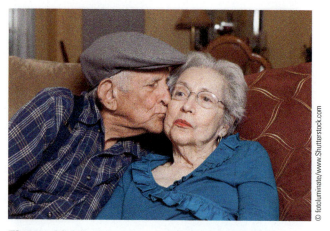

Figure 12-11 Older persons have the same emotional needs as younger people.

- *Older people are unhappy, without focus in their lives, and have little interest in sex.* In general, the older population is no less and no more content with life than younger people. They fill their lives with activities suitable to their needs. Their views of life in later years are usually a reflection of the attitudes they had in younger years. They are still sexual beings and can express sexual feelings and fulfill sexual needs (Figure 12-11).

- *Old people are sent to nursing homes because society does not want to be bothered with them.* Compared to the general population, a small number of people over 65 years live in long-term care facilities. The percentage increases with age. For persons aged 64 to 74 years, only 1% live in these facilities. This number increases to 4% for persons 75 to 84 years and to 18% for persons over 85 years. Admission to a long-term care facility is often a difficult decision for the individual and the family. The decision is usually based on the fact that the person needs the type of care available only in the long-term care facility.

- *Being "old" is determined solely by the number of years a person has lived.* This is not necessarily true. The term *old* is subjective and relative and has a great deal to do with a person's outlook on life. To a child 5 years old, someone of 35 years is old. See Figure 12-12A and B.

Myths pertaining to the physical and mental abilities of older adults persist. Caring for older persons may be time consuming. Before assuming that the older person cannot do something because of physical or mental changes related to aging, first test the person's abilities. Be patient and encourage independence for each person according to his or her capabilities.

? EXERCISE 12-4

MATCHING
Determine the reason each resident is in a long-term care facility based on the medical diagnosis. Place the appropriate letter in the space provided.

REASON FOR LONG-TERM CARE

1. _____ Ms. Sacco	Multiple sclerosis	a. trauma
2. _____ Mrs. Byron	Head injury after an auto accident	b. chronic disease
3. _____ Mrs. Lyon	Alzheimer's disease	c. developmental disabilities
4. _____ Mrs. Mata	Stroke	d. immunodeficiency disease
5. _____ Mr. Narvaez	Chronic lung disease (emphysema)	
6. _____ Mr. Versacksca	Congestive heart failure	
7. _____ Mr. Saivedra	Bilateral leg amputation	
8. _____ Mr. Liu	AIDS	
9. _____ Mrs. Massey	Arthritis	
10. _____ Mrs. Rosenberg	Cerebral palsy	
11. _____ Mrs. Nasser	Parkinson's disease	
12. _____ Mrs. Byrne	Huntington's disease	

? EXERCISE 12-5

TRUE OR FALSE

Indicate whether the following statements are true (T) or false (F).

1. T F Being old is sufficient reason to be admitted to a long-term care facility.
2. T F AIDS is an example of a developmental disability.
3. T F The elderly make little contribution to the welfare of society.
4. T F Today, people can expect to live into their 70s and 80s.
5. T F The older a person becomes, the greater the likelihood that he or she will develop a chronic disability.
6. T F Gerontology refers to the study of aging.
7. T F All ethnic groups think about aging in the same way.
8. T F Feelings of nausea cause distress.
9. T F Symptoms of brain disorders include confusion and disorientation.
10. T F "Goose pimples" are a symptom of an elevated temperature.
11. T F Men have a longer life expectancy than women.
12. T F Older people are incompetent and cannot make correct judgments.
13. T F Not all people experience the same characteristic changes in the structure and function of their bodies.
14. T F In general, society has little concern or caring about the elderly.

? EXERCISE 12-6

COMPLETION

Select the correct term(s) from the following list to complete each statement.

biased	diseases	rigid
birth	infections	valuable
childhood	myths	85
development	natural	65
stereotypes		

1. _____ are rigid, biased ideas.

2. The average age of residents in most long-term care facilities is approximately _____ years.

3. Stereotypes are _____ and _____ ideas about people as a group.

4. Stereotypes that are not true are called _____.

5. A developmental disability is a permanent condition that is present at _____ or that occurs during _____.

6. Immunodeficiency diseases make a person more susceptible to other _____ and _____.

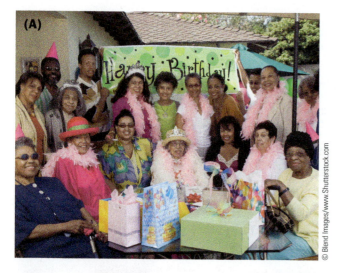

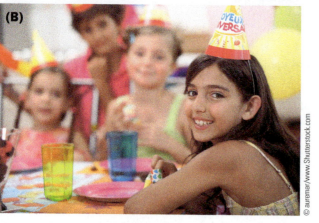

Figure 12-12 Celebrating one's eightieth birthday (A) is as much fun as celebrating one's eighth (B) when health is good.

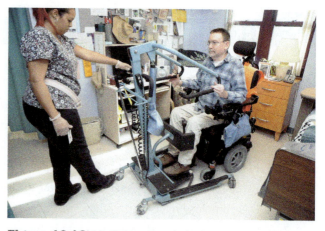

Figure 12-13 Multiple sclerosis is an example of a chronic disease that may affect a younger person.

THE YOUNGER RESIDENT IN THE LONG-TERM CARE FACILITY

You may care for younger people in the long-term care facility. These young people may be there because of surgery, injuries from accidents, birth defects, or disease. Common reasons for admission are:

- Traumatic brain injuries
- Spinal cord injuries
- Developmental disabilities
- Chronic diseases (Figure 12-13)
- AIDS
- Orthopedic or other types of surgery

The health care team must recognize that although the needs of all humans are the same, regardless of age, the ways in which individuals meet these needs may vary with age.

Young residents have the same needs as other persons their age. Their natural development has often been interrupted during a critical stage of life. Some of them may have been unable to complete their education, to experience a career, to marry, or to have children. Others may have a spouse and young children at home. It is often difficult for these residents to adapt to and accept the change in their lifestyle.

Adjustment to a long-term care facility may be more difficult for the younger resident. Young people have had fewer years in which to accumulate the resources for dealing with crises. Their lives have been interrupted and they still have more years of living ahead of them. Because of improved medical technology, young persons with a chronic disease or disability can expect to live almost as long as they would have without the disease or disability.

- Privacy for all residents is essential. For younger people, privacy is necessary to allow them opportunities to think things through and to daydream (which is normal if not used to excess).

- Assist the activities department in providing activities that are appropriate to the resident's age and interests. It is good for them to participate in some activities with older people, but the total program should include activities just for younger residents. If there are not enough younger residents to form a group, then one-to-one activities may be necessary.

- As a caregiver, you may find yourself identifying with younger residents. For example, you may begin to treat a resident your own age as a personal friend. If you are a parent, you may think of a younger resident as your child. It is important that you be aware of this possibility. It is appropriate to have empathy for all residents, but at the same time you need to remember the distinction between caregiver and friend and caregiver and parent.

- Keep in mind that visitors of younger residents may be more boisterous than those of your older residents. Young residents may exhibit unacceptable

⚠ GUIDELINES FOR... CARING FOR YOUNGER RESIDENTS

Remember when caring for younger residents that:

1. Many younger residents may be your peers. You will need to learn how to have empathy (putting yourself in the other person's place) without becoming emotionally involved to the extent that you cannot remain objective.

2. They may be frustrated and angry because their lives have been interrupted; they may never have the opportunity to marry, have a family, or earn a living.

3. Sexual feelings are at the most intense level during young adulthood. These feelings do not decrease just because the person is in a long-term care facility. Residents may act out these feelings. Discuss these situations with the nurse so that you are prepared to handle them. Like all residents,

they need to have privacy and an opportunity for intimacy with a companion, whether a spouse or "significant other."

4. If the young resident has children, try to provide a place where the family can visit together without interruption.

5. Socialization with other people of the same age is essential to the continuing development of the individual. Younger residents may not wish to be constantly with the older residents. If there are several younger residents in a facility, they may enjoy age-related activities together.

6. Emotional problems such as depression may be present in residents of any age. These problems must be addressed by the interdisciplinary health care team.

behavior just as they might if they were home. For example, friends may try to bring in alcoholic beverages or smoking materials to a resident who is not of legal drinking age. You need to report this to your supervisor so that appropriate action can be taken.

Opportunities for continuing education may be provided. Vocational training may be a part of the care plan for some younger residents.

🌐 BUILDING CULTURAL AWARENESS

The aging process is thought of differently by different cultural groups. Think of racial and ethnic persons you have known and whether their treatment of older adults differed from that in this country.

❓ EXERCISE 12-7

TRUE OR FALSE
Indicate whether the following statements are true (T) or false (F).

1. T F It is not good for younger residents to participate in some activities with older people.
2. T F As a caregiver, you may find yourself identifying with younger residents.
3. T F A common reason younger people are residents in a long-term care facility Is traumatic brain injury.
4. T F In addition to the specific health needs of a young person in a long-term care facility, their level of psychosocial development has to be considered.

CLINICAL SITUATION
Read the following situations and answer the questions.

Peter Driscoll was irritable, depressed, and often unpleasant. He was only 20 years old when his motorcycle ran into a van that caused severe head injuries, leaving his right side paralyzed. His injuries interfered with his thought processes, and his plans to become a lawyer had to be changed. His girlfriend visited him often at first but now she seldom visits. Explain why adjustment to the long-term care facility is especially difficult for this younger resident.

_____

_____

COMFORT, REST, AND SLEEP

Comfort, rest, and sleep are physical needs. If these needs are not met, the resident may suffer complications. *Comfort* refers to the absence of mental and emotional distress and physical pain. Rest and sleep are not usually possible when discomfort is present. Comfort is not possible when rest and sleep are insufficient.

Comfort

A level of comfort is necessary for healing and human survival. A lack of comfort may result from either internal or external factors. Internal factors include:

- Pain
- Nausea
- Hunger and thirst
- Elevated temperature
- Anxiety
- Confusion and disorientation
- Agitation
- Anger

External causes of discomfort include environmental factors:

- Temperature
- Ventilation
- Noise
- Lighting
- Unpleasant odors
- Appropriate furnishings

When all internal and external factors are in balance, comfort is present and rest and sleep are possible. As a nursing assistant, you can do much to increase the comfort of the residents.

Procedures for Internal Factors

- Observe the resident carefully for signs of discomfort (see Lesson 6). Report these signs to the nurse immediately. Remember that persons of other cultures may express their feelings of pain differently than you might expect.
- Feelings of nausea create distress. Try to avoid these feelings by eliminating unpleasant odors and sights from the environment, especially during meals. Report nausea to the nurse, because medication may be needed to control the nausea and prevent vomiting.
- Hunger pains are unpleasant and can also cause nausea. For complaints of hunger, provide a small snack that follows the resident's dietary orders.
- Thirst may be due to inadequate fluid intake and is also a symptom of some medical conditions such as diabetes. Make sure the resident always has fresh water at the bedside (unless ordered otherwise) and offer water frequently to those who need assistance.
- An elevated temperature causes restlessness. As the temperature goes up, the resident feels chilly and may have "goose pimples." You may need to provide another blanket for warmth. Feeling "hot" occurs as the temperature reaches its peak and the resident becomes restless. You may need to remove the extra covers. After the temperature begins to fall, the resident perspires. To increase comfort, you may need to give a sponge bath, assist the resident to change clothes, and put clean linens on the bed.
- Anxiety is a reaction to stressful situations. It is noted by excessive activity such as pacing or thrashing about in bed. Persons in long-term care facilities may be worried about families and finances as well as their medical conditions.
- Confusion and disorientation are symptoms of brain disorders and may be temporary or permanent. A resident may be aware that he is confused or disoriented and also know that he is unable to change the situation. The resident then feels very stressed and anxious.

Lessons 13, 20, and 30 provide more information on these topics. It is usually easier to control the external factors that can lead to discomfort and restlessness. Refer to Lesson 16 for environmental factors.

Procedures for Rest and Sleep

Rest and sleep are essential for good health. As a caregiver, you can do much to help the resident fulfill these needs. Performing these tasks at certain times (such as at bedtime) can increase comfort:

- A bath and backrub can help the resident feel refreshed, relaxed, and comfortable. (See Lesson 16.)
- Fresh linens on the bed, free from wrinkles, increase comfort.
- Provide a snack and non-caffeinated beverage if the resident is hungry or thirsty if approved by the nurse.

- Provide a quiet, well-ventilated, odor-free room with a comfortable temperature.
- Assist the resident to a position of comfort. (See Lesson 22.)
- Assist the resident to empty the bowel and bladder as necessary.

- Inquire as to whether the resident has any habits that help to induce sleep, such as listening to soft music, having a nightlight on, wearing socks to bed, using two pillows, or the use of aromatherapy.

You will find that a resident who is physically, mentally, and emotionally comfortable is a satisfied resident.

? EXERCISE 12-8

MULTIPLE CHOICE
Select the one best answer.

1. Which of these statements about comfort is true?
   - (A) Comfort can be affected negatively only from internal factors.
   - (B) External factors that can cause discomfort are pain, nausea, and anxiety.
   - (C) When internal and external factors are in balance, comfort is present and rest and sleep are possible.
   - (D) Comfort refers to the absence of physical pain.

2. Which task does not increase residents' comfort?
   - (A) Providing fresh bed linens
   - (B) Providing a bath and backrub
   - (C) Educating them about your grandmother's proven tricks to get to sleep
   - (D) Assisting them to empty their bowels or bladders as necessary

---

LESSON SYNTHESIS: Putting It All Together

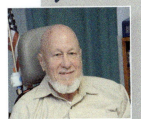

You have just completed this lesson. Now go back and review the Clinical Focus. Try to see how the Clinical Focus relates to the concepts presented in the lesson. Then answer the following questions.

1. How does Sam indicate his desire to stay an active participant in life?

2. How does Sam compare with the common stereotypes and myths about aging?

3. What situations might lead to a younger person's entering a long-term care facility?

4. What needs do nursing assistants have to meet that are the same for older and younger residents in long-term care? What needs must nursing assistants meet that are different for older and younger residents?

12 REVIEW

A. Select the one best answer for each of the following.

1. Residents are admitted to long-term care facilities because they

(A) are old

(B) need health care

(C) have no loved ones

(D) have no other place to live

2. A chronic disease

(A) results from an injury

(B) comes on suddenly and is usually cured

(C) is a form of cancer

(D) begins slowly and is expected to continue for a long time

3. The need to receive long-term health care because of trauma may be due to

(A) spinal cord injury

(B) heart attack

(C) stroke

(D) dementia

4. The aging process begins

(A) during middle age

(B) after age 65 years

(C) at birth

(D) at age 21

5. Instrumental activities of daily living (IADL) include

(A) bathing

(B) toileting

(C) eating

(D) household management

6. Many older persons

(A) are unable to learn

(B) have no interest in sexuality

(C) have sensory losses

(D) are incontinent

7. One of the following factors may *not* lead to a greater incidence of falls among residents

(A) loss of balance

(B) less flexible muscles and joints

(C) increased energy

(D) poor vision

8. Older persons are at greater risk for falls because

(A) they tend to be constipated

(B) of decreased flexibility

(C) of decreased appetite

(D) of increased sensitivity to cold

9. Older persons are more likely to suffer skin injuries because

(A) fingernails grow longer

(B) wrinkles develop

(C) the skin becomes drier and more fragile

(D) fluid intake is inadequate

10. Changes in the urinary system mean older persons need to

(A) void more often

(B) empty the bladder less often

(C) limit liquid intake

(D) eat more fiber

11. Changes in the cardiovascular system mean that when you care for the older adult, you should remember to

(A) encourage vigorous exercise

(B) allow more rest time between activities

(C) have residents breathe deeply before exercise

(D) continue exercise even if fatigue develops

12. Older adults may add more sugar and salt to their food than younger people because

(A) the food served has no flavor

(B) they are fussy eaters

(C) taste buds are less sensitive

(D) they cannot see as well

13. A resident's comfort may be increased by

(A) providing adequate room ventilation

(B) hunger

(C) pain

(D) not disturbing the resident to remove wrinkles from bed linens

14. A resident may be assisted to sleep by

(A) watching a science fiction movie

(B) reading the newspaper

(C) having a backrub

(D) having a cup of regular coffee

15. If a resident appears to be having pain, you should first

(A) tell him to think of something else to distract his mind

(B) tell him to take deep breaths until the pain subsides

(C) report the pain to the nurse

(D) give him pain medication

B. Match each term with the correct definition.

a. injury received in accident

b. permanent condition present at birth or occurs during childhood

c. one that begins slowly and is expected to last a long time

d. loss or abnormality of the structure or function

e. inability to perform activities normal for one's age

f. an untruth that some people believe

g. rigid ideas about a group of people

16. _____   impairment

17. _____   disability

18. _____   trauma

19. _____   chronic disease

20. _____   developmental disability

21. _____   myth

22. _____   stereotype

C. Answer each statement true (T) or false (F).

23. T F A developmental disability is always present at birth.

24. T F Parkinson's disease is an example of a chronic illness.

25. T F The inability to feed oneself is an example of a self-care deficit.

26. T F There are more men over age 65 than women over age 65.

27. T F The over-65 population is the fastest growing age group.

28. T F Stereotypes are true generalizations about specific types of groups.

D. Indicate which of the following is myth (M) and which is stereotype (S) regarding residents of advanced age.

29. S M Age alone causes diseases.

30. S M All older people have gray/white hair.

31. S M Only people who are young are of value to society.

32. S M Elderly people are always more peaceful.

33. S M Eyesight diminishes in all older people.

34. S M All older people are unable to manage their own affairs.

35. S M All older people have little interest in sex.

36. S M Reaction time is prolonged in all older adults.

37. S M Being old is only determined by the number of years lived.

38. S M All older people have less energy.

39. S M All older people live in poverty.

40. S M All older people are self-confident.

THE PSYCHOSOCIAL ASPECTS OF AGING

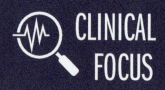

CLINICAL FOCUS

Think about how you can assist residents in meeting their psychosocial needs as you study this lesson.

OBJECTIVES

After studying this lesson, you should be able to:

• Define vocabulary words and terms.

• Identify the needs common to all human beings.

• Describe the developmental tasks of older adults.

• List the ways in which you can help residents feel safe and secure.

• List the ways in which you can help residents fulfill psychosocial needs.

• Describe how you can assist a resident to maintain sexuality.

• Discuss the challenges to adjustment faced by residents.

• Identify signs of stress reaction.

• Describe actions to take when residents display unusual behaviors.

VOCABULARY

amulet (AM-you-let)
compensation (kom-pen-SAY-shun)
defense mechanism (dee-FENS MECK-ah-niz-em)
demanding behavior (dee-MAN-deeng bee-HAY-vyour)
denial (dih-NIGH-al)

decline (dee-TER-ee-or-ayt)
developmental tasks (dee-vel-op-MEN-tal tasks)
manipulative behavior (mah-NIP-you-lah-tiv bee-HAY-vyour)

CASE STUDY

Mr. Warner, age 87, has been a resident of your facility for 2 years since his wife of 51 years died. During that time you have come to know him well. He uses a wheelchair but his mind is still very clear. He confides to you one morning that he really misses "having a woman" and wishes that he had a way to relieve his sexual tension. The staff is sensitive to his needs.

masturbation (mass-tur-BAY-shun)
personality (per-son-AL-ih-tee)
projection (proh-JECK-shun)
rapport (rah-POHR)

rationalization (rash-un-al-ih-ZAY-shun)
self-esteem (self-es-TEEM)
suppression (suh-PRESH-un)
talisman (TAL-iz-man)

BASIC HUMAN NEEDS

Basic human needs are the things and activities required by all persons to successfully and satisfactorily live their lives and realize their full potential as human beings. The needs are the same for all people at all ages, although individuals' abilities to meet these needs may vary widely.

Cultural backgrounds influence the way in which individuals fulfill these basic needs. *Culture* refers to those customs and practices that are common to groups of people, including beliefs, habits, health practices, expressions of spirituality, and ways of celebrating. These cultural patterns are part of the uniqueness of each individual and must be considered when providing for the person's care.

Abraham Maslow and Eric Erikson are two leaders in the field of human behavior. They helped us understand basic human needs and how people go about satisfying these needs.

Maslow's Hierarchy of Needs

Maslow originally proposed five steps in the continuum of needs: physical needs, safety and security needs, love and belonging needs, self-esteem needs, and self-actualization (accomplishment) needs. He later expanded the hierarchy to seven levels to include the growth needs of knowing, understanding, exploring, and appreciating symmetry, order, and beauty; and the ability to help others find self-fulfillment and realize their potential. This step he called *transcendence*.

The five original steps of the hierarchy help us understand the basic needs that must be met (Figure 13-1). Within the five original steps, Maslow described the basic needs as:

- Physical (physiological) needs (food and water)
- Security and safety needs
- Psychosocial needs (being part of a family or group)

Maslow believed that the order in which needs are satisfied is based on their importance to survival. Physical or physiological needs must be satisfied first. Safety and security needs are next in importance to survival. Only after these needs are satisfied can the psychosocial needs (emotional) be considered.

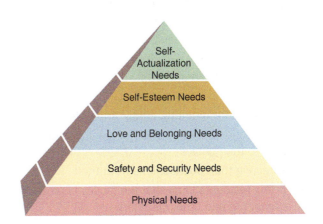

Figure 13-1 Maslow's Hierarchy of Needs. People meet needs in order of their importance to survival. Physical needs must be satisfied first.

? EXERCISE 13-1

TRUE OR FALSE
Indicate whether the following statements are true (T) or false (F).

1. T F Maslow described safety and security as basic human needs.
2. T F The basic need that must be satisfied first is the psychosocial need.
3. T F Psychosocial needs must be met before physical needs are met.

Physical Needs (Physiological)

The most basic human needs relate to the physical functioning of our bodies. These needs must be met to maintain life:

- Oxygen
- Water
- Food
- Sleep/rest

⊘ ON THE JOB

Health care workers often excel at giving physical care but neglect the psychosocial needs of residents.

- Activity
- Elimination
- Sexuality

Safety and Security Needs

Residents who do not feel safe will experience anxiety and fear. Living in a state of fear prevents an individual from achieving psychosocial well-being. You can help residents feel safe by:

- Being dependable and trustworthy
- Being kind and considerate
- Providing care promptly, gently, and safely
- Helping the residents maintain a lifestyle structured to their choice
- Protecting their possessions from theft
- Letting residents know that the facility is protected against fire and other disasters
- Providing for privacy

Psychosocial Needs

The psychosocial needs of the older persons are the same as those at any age. There is a need to:

- Love and be loved
- Be treated with respect and dignity
- Feel needed
- Feel important as an individual
- Feel appreciated

When residents first enter a long-term care facility, they often feel depressed and frightened. They are in a strange environment and they fear that they will lose all privacy and control of their own lives.

Their self-esteem is threatened. Each person has in his or her own mind an idea of how they appear and wish to appear to others. This idea of self is referred to as self-esteem and must be protected. How residents respond to a threat to their self-esteem depends on how the resident has handled such threats previously and how those who are caring for the resident understand and respond to these feelings.

Some residents react to a threat of self-esteem with an aggressive response and complaints about all levels of care. Others may become quiet, withdrawn, and depressed. The nursing assistant must be aware of the residents' underlying feelings. Remain open and receptive and do not take personal offense at things the resident may say or do in frustration.

You can help residents meet their psychosocial needs if you:

- Treat each resident as an individual with specific characteristics and needs.

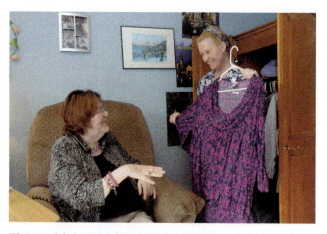

Figure 13-2 Assist the resident whenever necessary, but encourage her to make her own decisions.

- Give the resident choices whenever possible (Figure 13-2).
- Honor the residents' identities. Call residents by the names they choose. Allow them to reflect their identity by the way they dress, the way they arrange their rooms, and the activities they choose.
- Allow residents to do as much as possible for themselves. Encourage their independence to the level their conditions permit.
- Respect the residents' rights.

Personality

The way each resident satisfies psychosocial needs depends on personality. Personality is the sum of the ways we react to the events in our lives. Personality is gradually formed through life experiences.

Erikson suggests that as we mature from infancy to old age, we pass through several developmental stages. During each stage, certain tasks must be accomplished. These are called developmental tasks (Figure 13-3).

The developmental tasks specific to older adults are just as important as those for younger people. They include the need to:

- Adjust to decreased abilities such as physical limitations caused by the aging process
- Integrate life experiences through reminiscing
- Accept the onset of chronic illness
- Accept one's place in the community structure
- Adapt to possible changes in social and financial security
- Recognize and accept that life is limited
- Act as a role model for others

Physical Stage	Year of Occurrence	Tasks to Be Mastered
Oral-sensory	Birth–1 year (infant)	To learn to trust (Trust)
Muscular-anal	1–3 years (toddler)	To recognize self as an independent being from mother (Autonomy)
Locomotor	3–5 years (preschool years)	To recognize self as a family member (Initiative)
Latency	6–11 years (school-age years)	To demonstrate physical and mental skills/abilities (Industry)
Adolescence	12–18 years	To develop a sense of individuality as a sexual human being (Identity)
Young adulthood	19–35 years	To establish intimate personal relationships with a mate (Intimacy)
Adulthood	35–50 years	To live a satisfying and productive life (Generativity)
Maturity	50+ years	To review life's events and examine how they have influenced the development of a unique individual (Ego integrity)

Figure 13-3 Erikson's tasks of personality development from infancy through old age.

? EXERCISE 13-2

BRIEF ANSWERS

Select the correct term(s) from the following list to complete each statement. Some terms may be used more than once; some are not used at all.

articles	fantasizing	religious	sleeplessness
choices	identity	residents	slower
choose	independent	respect	space
individual	restlessness	themselves	wish
decreased	loss	rights	

1. You can help residents meet psychosocial needs if you:
   a. Treat each person as a(an) _____.
   b. Give residents the opportunity to make _____ about their lifestyle.
   c. Permit residents to arrange their rooms as they _____.
   d. Encourage residents to _____ the activities in which they wish to participate.
   e. Allow residents to do as much as possible for _____.
   f. Encourage residents to be as _____ as possible.
   g. Abide by all the residents' _____.
   h. Honor a resident's _____ by calling him or her by name.
   i. _____ a resident's desire for periods of privacy.
   j. Allow residents to _____ their own clothing.
   k. Support residents as they express their _____ beliefs.

Nursing assistants can play an important role in helping residents accomplish the developmental tasks by:

- Allowing residents to talk about their experiences and feelings
- Creating an atmosphere of acceptance where the residents are not judged

If these stages are interrupted and not completed because of illness, the individual may display behavior that is inappropriate for the age and the culture we live in.

CULTURAL INFLUENCES

The residents you care for may come from different cultures. More complete care is given if nursing assistants are sensitive to the cultural influences on a resident's behavior. People from the same culture usually share similar values, customs, clothing, and food preferences.

Even the cause of illness is influenced by cultural beliefs. Many European Americans share in the belief that illness is punishment for sins and self-abuse. Many African Americans believe that illness is caused by spirits and demons and is punishment from God. Cultural values and customs are passed from generation to generation and are the foundation for accepted behavior. Cultural influences play an important role in how a person views and reacts to illness. For example, it is a common cultural practice in Asian American cultures to seek care from traditional healers. The healer reestablishes the balance between the negative (*yin*) energy that is believed to be the cause of illness and the positive (*yang*) energy of health.

Each culture may have its own belief system and religious faith. Belief systems influence choices in various cultures. For example, some Native American people create elaborate sand paintings to diagnose and treat illness. Hispanic Americans may treat illness with prayer, wearing of medals, and consumption of special food. An understanding of some of the major belief systems will help you assist your residents meet their needs. Remember that you are caring for an individual within a cultural framework. Within the framework of each belief system, there are individual differences in depth of belief and extent of practice.

SPIRITUALITY

Spirituality is the part of a person that gives a sense of wholeness by fulfilling the human need to feel connected with the world and to a power greater than self. Spirituality and religion (an organized system of belief) are products of the individual's cultural background and experience. Spiritual values form the guiding principles that people may use to determine right or wrong.

Facing death, coping with loss, and accepting life as it really is are all spiritual tasks for older people.

A person's spiritual feelings play an important part in helping him or her through crises and stress periods. Spiritual feelings are personal, are expressed in different ways, and may or may not be associated with a specific religion (Figure 13-4).

RELIGION

Religion is not the same as spirituality, although spiritual people are frequently religious. Religion is a formal system that includes rituals and ceremonial acts that are an outward expression of faith. Many religions have objects of special significance, ranging from **amulets** (protective charms), **talismans** (engraved stones, rings, or other objects to ward off evil), copper or silver bracelets, and religious medals, to holy books such as the Bible, Koran, and Torah. You must be careful to handle

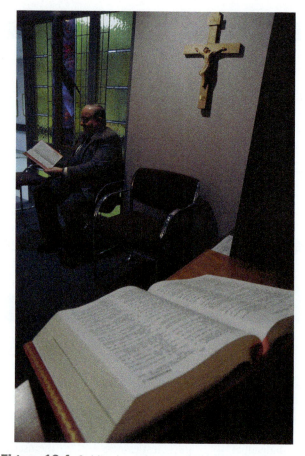

Figure 13-4 Spiritual needs must be respected and supported.

all items having religious significance with respect and to protect them from damage or loss.

Residents may wish to talk to you about their beliefs or may need help in carrying out certain practices or rituals. Be open to discussions with the resident even if you do not share the same beliefs. The nursing assistant supports the resident's spirituality and religious practices by:

- Being a willing listener
- Respecting the resident's without judgment belief system
- Never trying to convert the resident to your belief system
- Respecting religious symbols
- Not interrupting during religious rituals
- Reading aloud resident's favorite passages from religious books such as the Bible, Talmud, Koran, or Book of Mormon, for example
- Providing privacy during prayers and meditation and when clergy visits
- Being sensitive at all times to information that residents share with you about their cultural beliefs and practices

? EXERCISE 13-3

MULTIPLE CHOICE
Select the one best answer.

1. The most basic human needs relate to the functioning of our bodies and include:
   (A) security and safety
   (B) food, water, rest, and sexuality
   (C) food, water, oxygen, rest, activity, elimination, and sexuality
   (D) sexuality

2. Which of the following statements about self-esteem is true?
   (A) All residents who react to a self-esteem threat do so with aggressive behavior.
   (B) Nursing assistants should politely ignore residents who show signs of threatened self-esteem.
   (C) Self-esteem means feeling as if you are the best.
   (D) How residents respond to self-esteem threats depends on how they handled the threat previously and how caregivers appreciate these feelings.

3. Which of the following statements about cultural influence is not true?
   (A) Many European Americans believe that illness is punishment for sins and self-abuse.
   (B) All individuals within the framework of a cultural belief system share the same depth of belief and extent of practice.
   (C) Common in Asian American culture is the practice of seeking care from traditional healers.
   (D) Many African Americans believe that illness is caused by demons and spirits.

4. Cultural values are
   (A) of no value once one grows old
   (B) the foundation for accepted behavior
   (C) ideas formed by one individual
   (D) all of these

5. An example of a spiritual task for all elderly is
   (A) deciding what to wear
   (B) ignoring current situations
   (C) facing death
   (D) getting along with a roommate

6. Some religious articles treasured by residents include
   (A) amulets
   (B) talismans
   (C) Bibles
   (D) all of these

SEXUALITY AND INTIMACY

Sexuality is a lifelong characteristic that defines the maleness or femaleness of each person. This definition may be different for each person. All individuals are sexual beings.

Being old or disabled does not decrease human sexuality. However, our society tends to define sexuality as youth, beauty, and physical agility. Applying this definition, older people would not be considered sexual beings.

The human person within the aging body does not change. Although the hair is gray, the skin is wrinkled, and the body not so agile, the person inside still has the basic human need to love and to be loved. When this need is not met, self-esteem decreases. (Self-esteem is how one feels about oneself.) With low self-esteem, human beings do not feel good about themselves.

As people age it becomes more difficult to share love. Relationships that provided love, affection, and friendship may be lost through death or geographic distance. In addition, not all people understand that older persons are still interested in and capable of sexual expression and experience. Some caregivers ignore these needs or pretend they do not exist. Others feel that there is something wrong or childish about residents who want to express their sexuality.

Sexual Expression

Sexual expression may take many forms. Sexual intercourse, genital and non-genital caressing, tender communications, **masturbation** (self-stimulation), and mental imaging (fantasizing) are examples of ways that people satisfy their sexual needs.

Sexual Intercourse

Sexual intercourse is desired and can be achieved by many older couples. Before sexual intercourse actually occurs, there is an excitement phase. This phase is brought about by sexual thoughts or physical caressing. Erection occurs as the tissues of the penis fill with blood and the penis becomes firm and enlarged. During this phase, the vagina becomes moist. The excitement reaches a plateau of arousal and is then followed by orgasm (climax) and a release of sexual tension.

- In the woman, the sexual sensations are centered in the vagina, uterus, rectum, and clitoris.
- In the man, they are associated with ejaculation (release of semen).
- Orgasm for both men and women is a series of pleasurable muscular contractions that are strong initially and gradually slow and stop.

Men must wait a while before repeating intercourse, but women may experience another orgasm very soon if stimulated adequately.

Sexual intercourse has psychological and physical benefits because it meets sexual needs and is good physical exercise. Even those with severe physical limitations can have successful sexual experiences.

Self-Stimulation

Masturbation is the act of stimulating oneself sexually. Many men and women find this sexual outlet satisfying. It is a common way of gaining comfort when stressed and when other sexual opportunities are not available.

You may feel uncomfortable when you notice such an activity, but you must remember that the appropriate response is to:

- Treat the situation calmly
- Draw the curtains to provide privacy or move the resident to a more private area
- Not criticize or make fun of the resident

Helping Residents Express Their Sexuality

Health care providers now recognize that older adults have sexual needs and that satisfying these needs often has beneficial results. Many facilities are revising their procedures to allow couples living in the facility to express their sexuality without fear of interruption by staff or other residents. Some facilities now provide a secure area where a spouse living outside the facility can have a sexual relationship with the spouse living in the facility in privacy and without fear of embarrassment.

Nursing Assistant Actions

Nursing assistants can help residents maintain their sexuality. First, however, you must think honestly about your own sexuality and your attitude regarding

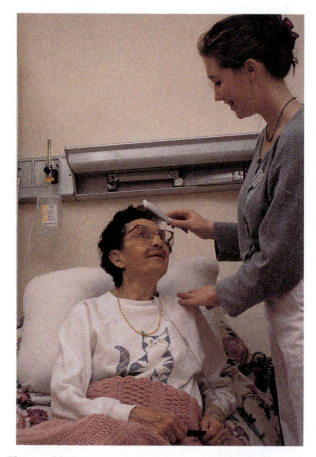

Figure 13-5 Sincere compliments assure residents that they are still worthy of respect.

the sexuality of the older people in your care. These feelings may influence your actions. You can help residents if you:

1. Help them to maintain their appearance and look their best. Give sincere compliments to residents about their appearance. This assures them of their attractiveness (Figure 13-5).

2. Use touch frequently. Touch is the only sense that does not usually diminish with aging and yet it is the sense most likely to be neglected and deprived. Remember, however, to use touch according to the cultural preferences of the resident. Some cultures consider the casual touch of a nonfamily member or member of the opposite sex to be improper. This is especially true in the Islamic culture.

3. Support friendships among residents (Figure 13-6). Treat all relationships with dignity and respect.

4. Residents who are mentally competent have the right to do in private whatever is pleasing to them both unless there are medical reasons to prevent it.

5. Always knock before entering a room. If you accidentally interrupt sexual activity, leave the room and quietly shut the door.

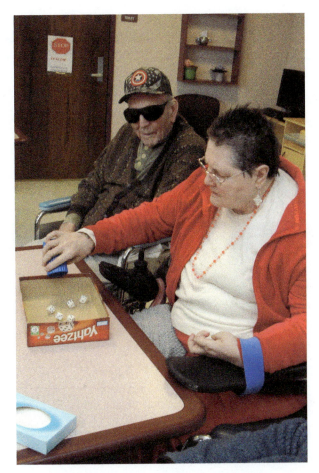

Figure 13-6 Support friendship among residents.

6. Provide privacy for residents and visiting mates. They have a need to talk and to hold each other. Some couples may wish to continue a sexual relationship.

7. Provide privacy for a resident who is masturbating.

8. Protect the rights of residents who do not want to be involved in sexual activity.

The health care staff is responsible for protecting residents who are mentally incompetent or physically unable to protect themselves from sexual advances. Care providers, visitors, and other residents cannot be allowed to sexually abuse residents. Report any observations of potential sexual abuse to your supervisor immediately.

MAJOR CHALLENGES TO ADJUSTMENTS

Each phase of life brings with it challenges to be met and adjustments to be made. The challenges that develop personality often come as the result of a major life crisis. Three crises older people are likely to experience are:

- Loss of a loved one (spouse or companion)
- Living with illness and disability
- Loss of independence

For many people, these events occur in close succession, and the stress can be overwhelming.

? EXERCISE 13-4

APPROPRIATE ACTIONS

Answer the following statements about nursing assistants' actions to encourage residents to maintain their sexuality with A for appropriate or I for inappropriate. If the action is inappropriate, write the appropriate action in the space provided.

1. _____ Call attention to the fact that the resident spilled some lunch.

   _____

2. _____ Touch a resident's hand often.

   _____

3. _____ Encourage residents to make friends with other residents.

   _____

4. _____ Prevent mentally competent residents from privately caressing one another.

   _____

5. _____ Provide privacy for visiting spouses.

   _____

6. _____ Walk into rooms without knocking first.

   _____

(*continues*)

❓ EXERCISE 13-4 (Continued)

7. _____ Separate embracing couples when one is not competent or willing.
_____

8. _____ Provide situations that encourage residents to talk to each other.
_____

9. _____ Leave a resident in soiled clothing because the resident dribbles urine.
_____

❓ EXERCISE 13-5

CLINICAL SITUATION
Read the following situations and answer the questions or indicate an appropriate nursing assistant response.

1. The nursing assistant knocks on the door, but when the door is opened, Mrs. Carnover and her husband are seen embracing in bed.
_____
_____
_____

2. As she enters the room, Rhonda notices Mrs. Burton, alone, rubbing her genitals. What action should Rhonda take?
_____
_____
_____

3. Jeff notices that Bill often tries to touch Amelia. Amelia is disoriented and becomes upset. What action would Jeff take?
_____
_____
_____

Loss of a Loved One

A person who loses a loved one faces major psychological adjustments. This is a time of great uncertainty at any age. It is particularly difficult when one is old, with failing health and limited resources. Many important decisions about the future must be made at a time when loneliness, confusion, and grief are at a peak.

When a spouse dies, the surviving spouse may sense a loss of identity or place in social situations. If able, he or she will eventually adjust to a new life alone. Although family and friends can help in the process, it is the individual who must face the loss and make the adjustment.

Sometimes a pet is a beloved member of the family to an elderly person. The loss of the pet through death can also require major psychological adjustments similar to those experienced when a human family member dies. Most facilities do not allow personal pets, however pet visits are frequently encouraged. The person who leaves a pet behind to enter a long-term care facility also feels a great sense of loss as well as guilt about leaving the pet. The separation is painful for the resident.

Having someone to confide in can help the older person work through the grief and adjustment period. The nursing assistant who has good rapport (sympathetic and understanding relationship) with the resident can help fill this role (Figure 13-7).

Giving the resident the opportunity to talk about lost loved ones helps to put feelings and memories into a proper perspective. Working through feelings gives the resident a sense of strength and better understanding of himself.

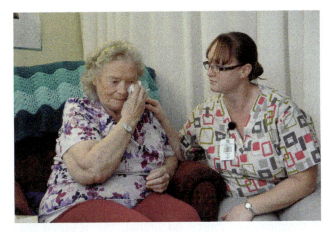

Figure 13-7 The nursing assistant can help residents work through a period of grieving.

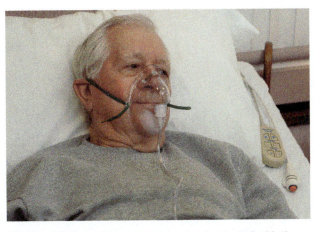

Figure 13-8 Residents may become frustrated with the changes occurring in their lives.

Chronic Illness

Many older people must adjust to the changes caused by aging and the problems associated with a chronic illness.

Some people try to deny these changes. They become angry when they realize they cannot control the changes going on in their bodies. Over time, most people adjust to and accept their limitations. Eventually they accept that life does not go on forever and that death is inevitable.

Loss of Independence

The third crisis involves the loss of independence that comes with the move to a long-term care facility. Dependency is natural for a child but not for a mature adult. The emotional distress before admission is high. Making the decision to enter a long-term care facility is never easy for the family or the person involved. It may require separation from loved ones, personal possessions, and pets. A person's sense of independence is threatened just by knowing that this type of care and support is necessary.

The anxiety and stress levels may be even higher once the person is admitted to the facility. New surroundings, new people, a room shared with another resident, and new procedures and rules now define the resident's world. Feelings of fear and frustration grow as the resident comes to know the degree to which independence is sacrificed (Figure 13-8). The calm manner, caring attitude, and patience of the nursing assistant are vital factors in helping the new resident adjust to life in the facility.

USING DEFENSE (COPING) MECHANISMS

Making positive psychological adjustments in later life depends to a large extent on how well the developmental tasks of earlier life periods were mastered and how the personality was formed. The ways of adjusting that a person used successfully through life become part of the person's **defense** (or coping) **mechanisms**.

Residents will react to situations using defense mechanisms that worked for them in the past. Residents may use defense mechanisms to protect their self-esteem. The use of defense mechanisms is harmful only when they become the major way of dealing with stressful situations. If this occurs, a mental health professional may counsel the resident. Here are some definitions for common defense mechanisms:

1. **Suppression:** refusing to recognize a painful thought, memory, feeling, or impulse. A person who has been abused, for example, may refuse to admit the memory of the abuse.

2. **Projection:** attributing one's own unacceptable feelings, thoughts, and actions to others. For example, a resident may tell you the bed is wet because you did not bring the bedpan on time. The resident is blaming you rather than admitting that she is incontinent (Figure 13-9).

3. **Denial:** pretending that a problem does not exist. For example, a resident is in denial when he or she talks about going home but there is little realistic chance that this will occur. This is different from similar expressions in dementia.

4. **Rationalization:** giving false but believable reasons for a situation. A resident may be rationalizing

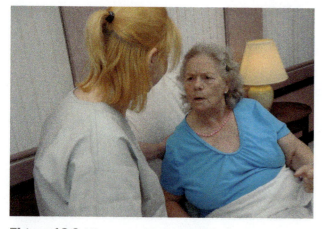

Figure 13-9 When a resident blames a nursing assistant for her own actions, it is a demonstration of projection.

when he or she tells you that he or she must stay in bed all day because there was too much noise to sleep the night before.

5. **Compensation:** making up for a situation in some other way. A woman who received much satisfaction from caring for a husband and children may compensate for this loss by caring for and protecting other residents.

MEETING RESIDENTS' PSYCHOSOCIAL NEEDS

It is important to see each resident as a whole person. The psychological needs of each resident must be recognized and met. Unmet psychological needs have a great effect on physical needs and status. For example, if psychological needs go unmet, the resident may become depressed and refuse to cooperate in therapy. Such a refusal may start a physical and emotional decline that rules out any chance of the resident returning home and could lead to death.

Nursing assistants can do much to help the residents meet their needs. If the residents' rights are respected at all times, you will be helping the residents to fulfill their psychosocial needs.

? EXERCISE 13-6

BRIEF ANSWERS
Select the correct term(s) from the following list to complete each statement. Some terms may be used more than once; some are not used at all.

agitation	depression	manipulative behavior	sag
articles	fantasizing	religious	sleeplessness
choices	identity	residents	slower
choose	independent	respect	space
chronic complaining	individual	restlessness	themselves
decreased	loss	rights	wish
delayed	lubrication	routines	withdrawal
demanding behavior	maladaptive behavior	behavior	safety

1. It is easier for new residents to make a successful emotional adjustment if the nursing assistant:
   a. meets physical and _____ needs first
   b. introduces other _____ and staff members
   c. explains the facility _____
   d. encourages the resident to display personal _____
   e. helps the resident learn the area of his or her personal _____

2. Six signs that a resident is experiencing stress include
   a. _____   d. _____
   b. _____   e. _____
   c. _____   f. _____

3. Unusual behaviors indicating that residents cannot handle their stress are
   a. _____
   b. _____
   c. _____

1. Remember that emotional needs cannot be fulfilled unless the residents' physical and safety needs are first met.
2. New residents must adjust to living in the long-term care facility. Help them to:
   - Develop trust in staff members
   - Meet other residents
   - Adapt to the routine of the facility
   - Adjust to having less personal space. You must respect the space that is theirs
   - Adjust to the loss of a home and many personal belongings
   - Use their own personal possessions, such as clothing or books
   - Display family photos and mementos
   - Find activities that have meaning and contribute to the resident's sense of self-worth
3. Always give residents the opportunity to be as independent as possible. Allow choices whenever possible.
4. Attend to the residents' comfort. Report complaints of pain or signs of anxiety immediately.
5. Explain procedures and routines to residents; notify your supervisor if the resident does not understand procedures and routines.
6. Listen carefully to everything residents say.
7. Recognize that each resident is an individual with likes and dislikes.
8. Answer signal lights promptly.
9. Treat all residents as adults.
10. Help residents feel loved and accepted by:
    - Accepting each resident in a nonjudgmental manner
    - Using touch appropriately to indicate your acceptance of the person
11. Help residents feel positive self-esteem and respect from others by:
    - Calling them by the names/titles of their choice
    - Learning about them, their families, and their histories
12. Unless they choose not to, residents should have the opportunity to contribute to facility life. These activities must be voluntary and written into the care plan so no violation of the resident's rights occurs. Activities may include:
    - Visiting other residents who may have no family and few visitors
    - Sharing their knowledge of a hobby with other residents
    - Working on the facility newsletter
    - Creating items for a facility craft sale
    - Delivering mail to other residents
    - Stuffing envelopes for mailings
    - Caring for nursing home pets such as birds or fish
    - Serving on the Residents' Council
    - Playing the piano or leading singing groups
    - Leading current events groups

STRESS REACTIONS

When defense mechanisms are inadequate, stress reactions develop and can take several forms. Examples are:

- Chronic complaining without reason
- Agitation
- Restlessness
- Sleeplessness
- Depression
- Withdrawal
- Aggression

Some residents may just give up and begin to **decline** physically and mentally. This means their condition weakens. Others may become combative in an attempt to assert themselves and their frustration grows.

REACTIVE BEHAVIORS

Residents display reactive behaviors when they are not able to meet their psychosocial needs. They are frustrated by their lack of control and use these behaviors in an attempt to satisfy the unfulfilled needs and to ease anxieties. Some reactive behaviors include:

- Demanding behavior—expressing excessive wants or needs
- Manipulative behavior—directing the actions of others for one's own purposes
- Maladaptive behavior—abnormal responses

Demanding Behavior

Demanding behavior occurs when residents make unreasonable requests for service, special meals, or special treatment. For example, a resident may ask to be repositioned every 10 to 15 minutes.

Try to learn and appreciate the factors that are causing the behavior. Demands and complaints are often due to the residents' feelings about their loss of control over their lives. Give the residents as much personal control as possible and offer choices.

Listen to the resident and be sensitive to body language. The resident may feel more secure if caregiving is consistent, with all staff members completing procedures in a consistent manner. Try to talk with the resident at times other than when care is needed. Do not take the resident's behavior personally. Rarely is a resident angry with you, but rather with the situation over which they have little control.

Family members may exhibit similar demanding behaviors when they are concerned about the well-being of the resident. As with the resident, determine the cause of the demanding behavior. It may be that family members feel a sense of guilt because their parent or sibling must receive care in a long-term care facility rather than at home. Do not try to handle the situation yourself; alert the nurse, who will be able to work with the family members.

Manipulative Behavior

Residents who develop devious methods to get staff members to do what residents want them to do are using manipulative behavior.

Residents may become manipulative in an attempt to control their lives. They may try to develop a special relationship with you. If the resident with manipulative behavior compliments you, accept the compliment graciously and in a matter-of-fact manner. Do not allow the compliments to influence your judgment or cause you to show favoritism to the resident. The resident with manipulative behavior may voice criticisms of other staff members to you. Avoid agreeing with critical comments. If the resident persists in the comments, tactfully tell the resident to talk to the nurse or social worker about the problems.

Do not falsely label a resident as manipulative. Compliments may be sincere and the resident may have real problems with another staff member. Relay concerns to the nurse if the behavior becomes a pattern.

All staff members should treat the resident in a consistent manner. Develop a sense of trust with the resident. Do not make promises you cannot keep; respond to requests promptly.

It is possible for family members to display manipulative behaviors as well as the resident. Discuss your concerns with the nurse; do not attempt to handle these situations on your own. It may take a team approach to work with the resident and family.

Maladaptive Behaviors

Maladaptive behaviors are abnormal behaviors. These behaviors may be noted when a resident is unable to function smoothly with staff, other residents, and perhaps family. Depression and disorientation are examples of maladaptive behaviors. These situations require assessment and planning by members of the interdisciplinary team. Interventions by a mental health professional or psychiatrist are often necessary. However, you can also help residents with maladaptive behaviors.

Aggression

Aggression may be expressed either physically or verbally. Physical aggression may be forceful and involve biting, hitting, pinching, scratching, or kicking. Verbal aggression may include swearing or threatening. These reactions may be triggered by anger or fear and possibly by a dementia-related disorder. Aggression also may be triggered by medical conditions such as a high fever or possibly an adverse reaction to a medication. Take all threats seriously but protect both the resident and yourself from physical harm. Always inform the resident what you are going to do before you carry out a procedure. Be calm as you approach the resident and speak in low tones. Do not touch the resident to avoid further aggressive outbursts. If the aggressive behavior occurs in a public space such as the dining room or lobby, move the aggressive resident when it is safe to do so. Seek help if necessary. Always inform the nurse of the situation.

Passive aggressiveness is another form of aggression that may occur when a resident feels they are unable or unwilling to carry out the expectations of another person (Figure 13-10). For example, the resident agrees that she should eat her meals in the dining room but at the last minute finds a way to avoid going and eats in her room. She says she is "too sick" or "is not dressed appropriately."

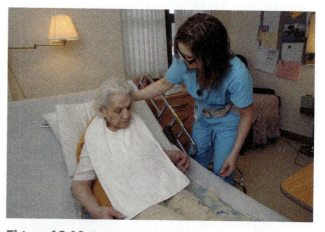

Figure 13-10 Passive aggression may occur when the resident feels unable or unwilling to carry out the expectations of the nursing assistant.

Depression

Depression is a serious condition that requires professional treatment. If you are caring for any residents who are suffering from depression:

1. Stress the resident's worth and assist him or her in using available support systems.
2. Do not pity the resident. This validates depressed feelings.
3. Make sure the resident has eyeglasses and hearing aids if these are needed. Residents who cannot see or hear well may not interact successfully with others. This often causes the resident to withdraw.
4. Provide the resident with activities that help him think beyond himself.
5. Avoid tiring activities.
6. Use simple language and speak slowly.
7. Encourage and assist the resident to participate in activities involving physical exercise.
8. Monitor intake, elimination, and sleep patterns. Depression may cause major changes in these functions.
9. Monitor skin condition. Depression often results in less movement, increasing the risk for skin breakdown.
10. Be a good listener.

Be alert for the potential for suicide. Watch for and report:

- A change in response or mood
- Withdrawal or secretiveness
- Sudden loss of a support system
- Refusal of medications, food, fluids, or nursing care
- Sudden interest or disinterest in religion
- Attempts to obtain scissors, knives, or other dangerous objects
- Statements about "ending it all," "killing myself," or "nothing to live for"
- An inability to complete simple tasks without a physical reason
- Deep preoccupation with something that they cannot explain

Disorientation

Residents who are disoriented do not know one or all of the following:

- The time of day, day of the week, month, year
- Where they are: facility, city, state
- Who they are

This is discussed in more detail in Lesson 29.

? EXERCISE 13-7

Match the resident's behavior with the action it communicates.

Resident Behavior Indicates

1. _____ becomes very secretive
2. _____ cannot recall own name
3. _____ says "I have nothing to live for"
4. _____ cries
5. _____ tells you "You are the best nursing assistant I have ever met"
6. _____ insists that mail be delivered to him or her first before other residents
7. _____ refuses all food and water
8. _____ criticizes many other staff members
9. _____ attempts to hide a knife from the dinner tray
10. _____ has been attending religious services regularly but suddenly loses interest
11. _____ tells you that you are the only person the resident can depend on
12. _____ shows less interest in visiting with other residents; prefers to remain in a corner alone
13. _____ cannot complete simple tasks without a physical reason
14. _____ does not understand why everyone is decorating a pine tree with paper circles in the dayroom
15. _____ insists that clothes be hung in a specific way

a. depression behavior
b. potential suicidal behavior
c. disorientation behavior
d. manipulative behavior
e. demanding behavior

? EXERCISE 13-8

CLINICAL SITUATION

Read the following situations and answer the questions or indicate an appropriate nursing assistant response.

1. The staff recognizes that Mrs. Franklin is depressed. Her first response to the nursing assistant is that "No one really cares."

   _____

   _____

2. Later in the day, Mrs. Franklin tells the nursing assistant, "I might as well end it all and kill myself."

   _____

   _____

3. The staff knows that Mr. Smith has poor self-esteem. The nursing assistant wants to help Mr. Smith feel better about himself.

   _____

   _____

   _____

LESSON SYNTHESIS: Putting It All Together

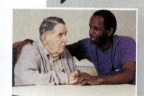

You have just completed this lesson. Now go back and review the Clinical Focus. Try to see how the Clinical Focus relates to the concepts presented in this lesson. Then answer the following questions.

1. What factors make it more difficult for the resident in long-term care to meet sexual and psychological needs?

2. How does the attitude of the staff help or hinder the expression and satisfaction of psychosocial needs of residents?

3. What ways do residents have to indicate that their needs are not being met? Do they always act directly?

4. What losses do you think Mr. Warner has suffered that have contributed to his level of stress? Are these stresses common to many older residents in long-term care?

13 REVIEW

A. Fill in the blanks by selecting the correct word from the list.

deterioration   self-esteem

personality   sexuality

masturbation

1. The sum of the ways we react to the events in our lives: _____

2. A lifelong characteristic that describes the maleness or femaleness of a person: _____

3. Gradual weakening of physical and mental abilities: _____

4. Feelings about oneself: _____

5. Self-stimulation for sexual pleasure: _____

B. Select the one best answer for each of the following.

6. A resident who uses her call bell repeatedly even though she frequently does not require immediate attention is showing

(A) loss of independence

(B) manipulative behavior

(C) demanding behavior

(D) depression

7. When caring for a resident who is depressed, the nursing assistant should

(A) show pity

(B) engage the resident in many activities to produce fatigue so the resident will sleep

(C) stress the resident's problems so he understands you care

(D) use simple language and speak slowly

8. According to Maslow, which human needs must be met first?

(A) psychological needs

(B) social needs

(C) security needs

(D) physical needs

9. Helping the residents maintain a lifestyle structured to their choices helps meet the residents'

(A) psychological needs

(B) social needs

(C) security needs

(D) physical needs

10. A nursing assistant helps residents meet psychological needs by

(A) selecting the residents' clothing

(B) making sure the door is always open during care

(C) protecting residents' possessions from theft

(D) calling residents by the names of their choice

11. Which of the following is a physical need?

(A) to be treated with kindness

(B) to be loved

(C) elimination

(D) to feel needed

12. Spirituality

(A) is an organized system of beliefs

(B) gives an individual a sense of wholeness

(C) is a type of religion

(D) is present at birth

13. The nursing assistant can promote self-esteem in a resident by

(A) being respectful and touching the resident as little as possible

(B) ignoring what the resident says because older persons tend to ramble

(C) giving sincere compliments

(D) insisting that residents contribute by serving on the Residents' Council

14. A resident is withdrawn and secretive and has suddenly shown an interest in religion. You report this to the nurse because you suspect the resident is

(A) manipulative

(B) demanding

(C) angry

(D) depressed

15. The resident has been attempting to hit and kick the staff anytime they approach him. What is the best approach prior to carrying out a task for the resident?

(A) restrain him

(B) talk to him in a calm voice

(C) ignore him

(D) ask the family to help

16. Adam Walenski has been calling out and yelling obscenities, sometimes in English and sometimes in Polish, his native language. What is the *first* step in helping to manage this problem?

(A) attempt to determine the cause

(B) ask the nurse to sedate him

(C) distract him with other activities

(D) isolate him

17. Ming Tsau agrees to go to the dining room for a group activity. When you plan to take her to the Sing-A-Long, she refuses because she has a headache. From reading her care plan, you note this happens frequently. You are aware that this is a sign of:

(A) depression

(B) passive aggression

(C) withdrawal

(D) rationalization

18. According to Erickson, the tasks to be mastered in maturity include:

(A) learning to trust

(B) develop a sense of individuality

(C) establish intimate personal relationships

(D) examine how life events influence the individual

19. One of the following behaviors is *not* typical of the resident who is depressed.

(A) refusing to eat lunch

(B) sudden interest in religion

(C) offering to deliver mail to other residents

(D) stating, "I have nothing to live for"

C. Match each defense mechanism (items a–d) with the correct example.

a. projection

b. denial

c. compensation

d. rationalization

20. _____ Mr. Brooks spills a glass of water and explains that it happened because the glass was too close to the edge of the overbed table.

21. _____ Miss Alcott wants to stay in her room because, she says, the other residents do not like her.

22. _____ Mrs. Jones spends most of her time out of bed helping other residents, even when they do not want or need the help.

23. _____ When the nursing assistant tries to talk to Miss Anderson about her incontinence (she had wet the bed the night before), Miss Anderson says, in a tone of injured innocence, "Why, I don't know what on earth you are talking about!"

24. _____ Mr. Ramirez tells everyone how much his family loves him and that they would visit him more often if they lived closer. You know that his family lives in the same town as the facility and that they have transportation.

D. Clinical Situation

Mr. Williams is 85 and confined to a wheelchair. He has been a resident in your facility for years. He came to the facility after his wife of 50 years died. He never tires of describing how happy they were. Recently the staff has noticed that he has occasionally been masturbating alone in his room. Answer the following questions by circling yes (Y) or no (N).

25. Y N Are Mr. Williams' actions abnormal for a man his age?

26. Y N Should the staff try to stop his actions?

27. Y N Do you think Mr. Williams is trying to meet a basic human need?

28. Y N If Mr. Williams acted this way in front of others, would you leave him in their presence?

29. Y N Will masturbating cause Mr. Williams harm?

ALTERNATIVE AND CULTURALLY BASED HEALTH BEHAVIORS

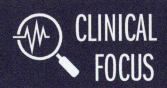

CLINICAL FOCUS

Think about how your knowledge of alternate health practices can be supportive of residents' right to individual choice as you study this lesson.

OBJECTIVES

After studying this lesson, you should be able to:

- Define vocabulary words and terms.
- Identify the steps of the scientific (Western) approach to health care.
- Define alternative therapy.
- Explain, in simple terms, six common alternative therapies.
- Identify five adjunctive therapies.
- State the value to the nursing assistant of an understanding of alternative practices.
- Name six major cultural groups in the United States.
- Describe the way major cultures differ in their need for personal space and their health beliefs and practices.
- List ways nursing assistants can develop knowledge and sensitivity about cultures other than their own.

VOCABULARY

acupressure (ak-you-PRESH-ur)
acupuncture (AK-you-punk-tjer)
adjunctive (complementary) therapy (ADD-junk-tihv THER-ah-pee)
alternative therapy (all-TURN-uh-tihv THER-ah-pee)

Ayurveda (eye-ur-VEE-duh)
Chinese medicine (chy-NEEZ MED-ih-sin)
chiropractic (ky-row-PRAK-tik)
cultural heritage (KUL-cher-alHER-i-tig)
ethnicity (eth-NIS-i-te)

CASE STUDY

Millicent Milburn is 67 years old and is in the early stage of Alzheimer's disease and has moderate high blood pressure. She spent many years in India where her husband was stationed. There are times when she states her strong reliance on the alternative health practice of Ayurveda.

folk medicine (fohk MED-ih-sin)
herbal (erb-BALL)
holistic (hoh-LISS-tik)
homeopathy (HOH-mee-oh-path-ee)
naturopathic medicine (nayt-jer-oh-PATH-ik MED-ih-sin)
protocol (PROH-tuh-kahl)

race (RAS)
reiki (RA-kee)
sensitive (SEN-si-tiv)
spiritual healing (SPIH-riht-joo-ul HEEL-ing)
spirituality (SPIH-riht-joo-ul- ih-tee)
tai chi (TIE CHEE)

SCIENTIFIC (WESTERN) APPROACH TO HEALTH CARE

The prevalent approach to health care practices in the United States is based on biomedical principles (natural science related to physical life processes). A great deal of emphasis and value are placed on the technical aspects of care. The technique follows a specific pattern, including:

- Gathering information through
  - Assessment of body systems
  - Identifying signs and symptoms
  - Carrying out laboratory tests such as cultures, blood tests, and body scans
- Establishing a diagnosis by comparing gathered data against known disease or injury status
- Prescribing treatment following a **protocol** (plan of treatment) designed to treat symptoms and correct the underlying disease pathology, including:
  - Medication
  - Surgery
  - Radiation

ALTERNATIVE AND ADJUNCTIVE THERAPIES

Alternative therapies are nontraditional health practices (compared to the Western approach to health care) used alone or in combination with scientific techniques. The use of alternative therapies is believed to lead a person to a healthier lifestyle, maintain health, improve a health problem, or increase the effectiveness of a treatment.

Alternative health practices focus on and stress a **holistic** (applying to the whole) approach to treatment and care. Holism is a philosophy that recognizes the interaction and interrelationship of the person with his environment. The term *holistic* also may be used to describe alternative treatment modalities. In the broadest definition of holistic medicine, conventional and alternative therapies would be combined to treat the person as a whole (Figure 14-1). For example, emotional stress can have a negative effect on the physical immune system of an individual, making that person more susceptible to disease.

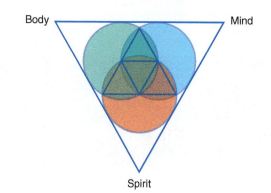

Figure 14-1 Holistic care looks at the resident as a person. Practitioners believe mind, body, and spirit must be balanced for health and wellness.

Culture and cultural values often influence a person's belief in and acceptance and use of alternative therapies. The most common alternative therapies (Figure 14-2) include:

- Acupressure
- Acupuncture
- Aromatherapy
- Ayurveda
- Balneotherapy (hydrotherapy)
- Biofeedback
- Chinese medicine
- Chiropractic
- Folk medicine
- Homeopathy
- Naturopathic medicine
- Reflexology
- Reiki

In addition to the alternative therapies described in this figure, there are many other **adjunctive (complementary) therapies** that people try and in which they have faith. These therapies include:

- Light therapy
- Magnetic therapy
- Spiritual healing or spirituality
- Tai chi
- Touch therapy

- **Ayurveda**—Natural system developed in India that focuses on prevention of disease and return to optimum health through exercise, herbal remedies, minerals, massage, and nutritional counseling, according to an individual's specific body type.
- **Chinese medicine** (traditional)—Emphasizes herbal remedies, acupuncture, acupressure, tai chi, cupping, and bleeding.
- **Chiropractic**—Treatments related to aligning the neuromuscular segments of the spinal column through manipulation, exercise, and lifestyle changes.
- **Folk medicine**—Culturally based; emphasizes traditional remedies passed from one generation to the next.
- **Homeopathy**—Employs plant, animal, and mineral substances to encourage the immune system to accelerate healing and strengthen the individual's own body to achieve the healing process.
- **Naturopathic medicine**—Employs fasting, special diets, and supportive approaches to assist the healing process.

Figure 14-2 Common alternative therapies.

Figure 14-3 provides a description of some of these therapies.

Cultural values greatly influence a person's choice of alternative practices or remedies and his or her willingness to share this information with health care workers. The resident may fear that others may not be open to or understand her beliefs. It is very important to listen carefully to residents, without making value judgments, as they discuss their personal health practices with you.

Acupressure

Acupressure is similar in practice to acupuncture, but no needles are involved. Practitioners use their hands, elbows, or feet to apply pressure to specific points along the body's "meridians." Meridians are channels that carry life energy throughout the body. Studies show acupressure might decrease nausea for chemotherapy patients and reduce anxiety in people scheduled for surgery.

Acupuncture

Though most people think of needles when describing **acupuncture**, the term actually describes an array of procedures that stimulates specific points on the body. Some studies find acupuncture helpful for chronic pain and depression.

Aromotherapy

Aromatherapy uses essential oils (concentrated extracts from the roots, leaves, seeds, or blossoms of plants) to promote healing. The oils can be inhaled, massaged into the skin, or taken orally. Each oil has a specific purpose: inflammation, infections, relaxation, headaches, pain reduction, anxiety, and depression.

Ayurveda

Ayurveda is a holistic approach to alternative health maintenance. It is an ancient philosophy that originated in India and has been practiced for more than 3,000 years. The translation of *ayurveda* means "knowledge of life." This system is based on the belief that disease is due to an imbalance in a person's consciousness. Practices include lifestyle interventions (diet and exercise), natural remedies (herbal treatments), and regaining a balance between the body, mind, and the environment. The process begins with an internal purification process, in combination with a special diet, herbal remedies, massage therapy, yoga, and meditation. It is commonly used to treat high blood pressure, reduce high cholesterol, and reduce stress.

Balneotherapy (Hydrotherapy)

Balneotherapy involves the use of water for therapeutic purposes and it dates back to 1700 B.C. It's based on the idea that water benefits the skin and might treat a range of conditions from acne to pain, swelling, anxiety with the use of mudpacks, douches, and wraps.

Biofeedback

Biofeedback techniques allow people to control bodily processes that normally happen involuntarily—such as heart rate, blood pressure, muscle tension, and skin temperature—in order to improve conditions such as high blood pressure, headaches, and chronic pain. Patients work with a biofeedback therapist to learn relaxation techniques and mental exercises. Electrodes are attached to the skin to measure bodily states. Researchers aren't sure how or why biofeedback works, but a lot of studies suggest it does work.

Chinese Medicine

Chinese medicine is an ancient holistic-based practice that has been passed down through many generations. The basic concept of Chinese medicine is that there is a universal energy or vital life force that surges through the body. The energy is called *qi* or *chi* (pronounced "chee") and travels along specific pathways called meridians. When qi runs freely there is health, but when qi is blocked, illness and pain result.

- Acupressure—Pressure applied with the finger or a ball-pointed instrument to acupuncture points. Similar to acupuncture but noninvasive.

- Acupuncture—Ancient practice that involves the insertion of needles in specific areas of the skin to influence body functions. Sometimes heat (moxibustion) or electrical stimulation us used in conjunction with the needle placement (Figure 14-4).

- Aromatherapy—Essential oils are used to stimulate the person's sense of smell, which in turn sends messages to the brain. It is commonly used to promote relaxation, relieve pain and nausea, and boost the immune system.

- Biofeedback—Uses machines to assist the person in becoming aware of changes in body functions. The person then retrains their own mind to control or alter his or her own physiology.

- Body work—Includes chiropractic in addition to other hands-on massage techniques such as foot reflexology, lymphatic massage, Rolfing, and Swedish massage.

- Electromagnetic therapy—Treatment is based on correcting imbalances in the electrical and magnetic fields that are believed to exist in the body. Different forms of electrical energy are used to correct imbalances. Some examples of electromagnetic approaches to treatment include the TENS (transcutaneous electrical nerve stimulation) unit to relieve pain or the defibrillator to start the heart.

- Herbal therapy—Herbs are widely used throughout the world for their medicinal effects. Examples include those herbs used in food products, as well as medications made from the plants. It is important to use herbal products under the supervision of a trained practitioner because some are very strong and can be toxic (Figure 14-5).

- Hypnotherapy—The person becomes more open to the power of suggestion while in an altered state of consciousness. This therapy can be used to treat pain, anxiety, depression, and insomnia.

- Light therapy—Exposure to controlled light is used to influence and regulate the daily biologic (circadian) functions of the body. In addition to treating mood and sleep disorders, jet lag, and depression, blue light therapy has been used to treat jaundice in newborns and ultraviolet light has been used to treat psoriasis.

- Massage—Therapy is provided by licensed massage therapists. Massage stimulates and improves circulation, providing relaxation and pain relief. The therapy increases feelings of well-being and reduces stress and fatigue. It is believed that massage can stimulate the immune system to fight disease.

- Nutrition therapy—The person's diet is evaluated to ensure that it contains optimal nutrition for health, wellness, and healing. Vitamins, minerals, and nutritional supplements may be added according the person's needs. Calcium may be added to prevent osteoporosis; vitamin C may be added to promote tissue healing.

- **Spiritual healing**—Individual, alone or with help, attempts to reach a unity with a higher power. This may be achieved through prayer alone or in combination with meditation or other religious rituals.

- Tai chi—Slow, graceful, and precise body movements combined with breathing techniques that are believed to improve posture, spiritual and mental clarity, and improve the life energy flow (qi) within the body.

- Therapeutic touch—Not to be confused with touching a resident in a caring manner, therapeutic touch involves using the hands to exchange energy and stimulate healing. The hands do not touch the person's body (Figure 14-6). The goal of the therapy is to restore an unbalanced energy field and align the mind, body, and spirit for good health. This procedure has been used to treat chronic pain, anxiety, and high blood pressure.

- Yoga—Union between the mind and the body. This practice involves a combination of breath control, posture, relaxation, and meditation to improve lung function and circulation, decrease pain, and reduce anxiety.

Figure 14-3 Common complementary (adjunctive) therapies.

Yin and yang must be balanced or disharmony occurs. The Chinese medicine practitioner looks for a pattern of disharmony and then attempts to correct it through one or more of the following:

- Herbal remedies—use of selected roots, stems, seeds, flowers, and leaves. Some eliminate toxins, some redistribute the life force (qi), and some strengthen specific organs or the body as a whole.

- Qigong—a series of slow stretches, breathing exercises, meditation, and visualization designed to balance the flow of qi.

- Tai chi—a noncombative series of gentle exercises and meditation designed to unite body and spirit and to improve muscle tone.

- Tui ma—a traditional therapy combining acupuncture and chiropractic.

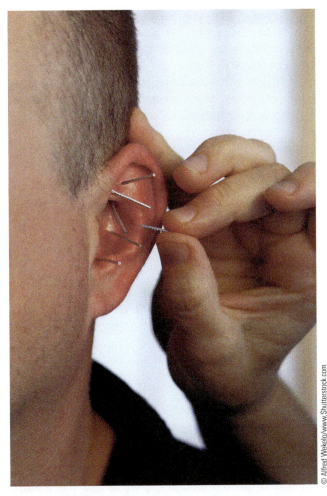

Figure 14-4 Acupuncture is used to treat many different conditions by correcting energy imbalances throughout the body. The needles are left in place from 5 to 20 minutes.

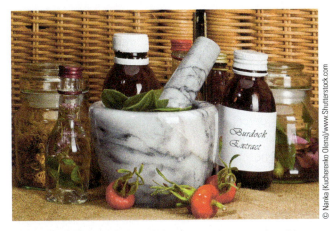

Figure 14-5 Herbs are potent natural substances with medicinal properties.

Japanese Influence

Reiki is a Japanese term meaning universal energy. The treatment modality is becoming increasingly popular in the United States. It does not require that

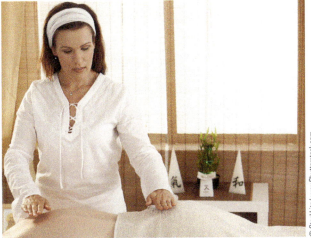

Figure 14-6 Therapeutic touch imparts healing energy from the practitioner's hands to the client's body. The therapeutic touch practitioner does not touch the client.

the practitioner or the participant follow any spiritual or faith system; it is not a religious belief. According to the National Institutes of Health's National Center for Complementary and Alternative Medicine, Reiki is defined as energy medicine. It is similar to the Chinese *chi*, but focuses on positive energy rather than disharmony within the body. Traditional medicine focuses on altering or eliminating the disease process through the use of drugs, surgical interventions, or radiation and other modalities. Reiki, however, can be used in healthy persons as well as those who may be ill. It focuses on the connection between the positive healing energy that is thought to be present in the environment and channeling that energy to the recipient's own energy. In the area of pain management, Reiki is becoming recognized as a valuable tool for persons in hospice care as well as in palliative care, during chemotherapy, and even during surgical procedures.

The treatment consists of the practitioner placing the hands on or slightly above the recipient for approximately 2 to 5 minutes so that the transfer of energy moves from the practitioner to the recipient. Recipients and practitioners both report a variety of sensations during the sessions. These sensations include warmth, relaxation, tingling, and sleepiness. Each session can last up to 45 minutes depending upon the recipient's needs.

Chiropractic

The **chiropractic** system considers the spine the core of human health. The condition of the spinal column is viewed as a critical factor in a person's well-being. It is also considered a key to maintaining the health of the nervous system. Chiropractic also teaches that a body that is functioning correctly will cure itself.

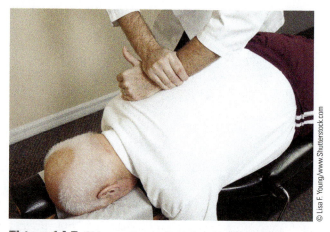

Figure 14-7 Chiropractors adjust the position of the spinal vertebrae through manipulation and massage.

Poor posture or trauma cause misalignment of the vertebrae, resulting in pressure on the spinal nerves. Diminished function and illness may result from this pressure.

Chiropractic treatment seeks to restore the proper flow of nerve impulses to and from the spinal column. Chiropractors adjust the position of the spinal vertebrae through manipulation and massage (Figure 14-7).

Folk Medicine

Folk medicine is culturally based and is usually conducted in the individual's own home under the guidance of a "healer" or family member. The treatment choices, which have been passed down from generation to generation, include remedies that have been found effective. Often these remedies are derived from plants and flowers. There is a strong holistic emphasis and prevention is stressed.

Homeopathy

Homeopathy remains one of the most controversial areas of alternative therapy.

Believers in homeopathy see signs and symptoms as the way the body heals itself. Therefore, symptoms are encouraged to be fully expressed, not suppressed. Plants, roots, and mineral substances are given to promote signs and symptoms rather than suppress them. These substances are given in minute doses in the belief that the immune system will be stimulated to fight disease.

Naturopathic Medicine

Naturopathy is a holistic approach that focuses on wellness. Emphasis is placed on prevention and self-care. Naturopathic practitioners look at the cause of illness, rather than only treating symptoms. They also cooperate closely with the physician and other health care providers for medical diagnosis and treatment when necessary.

Naturopathic medicine emphasizes the healing power of nature. Much emphasis is placed on teaching and helping individuals understand their illnesses and assume responsibility for management of their conditions. The naturopathic physician uses dietetics, with stress on nutrition and nutritional supplements for natural hygiene. There is not a large body of scientific evidence proving that the naturopathic approach is really effective.

Osteopathy

The osteopathic practitioner, Doctor of Osteopathy (D.O.), completes a program of study that is similar to that of a medical doctor (M.D.). In addition, the D.O. receives additional training on osteopathic manipulative treatment that is similar to chiropractic adjustment. This manipulative treatment is used in combination with regular medical treatment.

Reflexology

Reflexology involves applying pressure to specific areas on the feet, hands, or ears. The theory is these points correspond to different body organs and systems. Millions of people around the world use the therapy to complement conventional treatments for conditions including anxiety, cancer, diabetes, kidney function, and asthma.

Spirituality

Spirituality and religion are also components of nontraditional health care practices. For many people, spirituality and religion are the same; they are not. Spirituality is something that acts like an umbrella to help define:

- Our perceptions of our place in the universe (Figure 14-8)
- A higher power (if any)
- Our responsibilities to others
- Our beliefs and fears about living and dying

Religion is an organized system of belief in a deity (higher power). Both religion and spirituality are products of a person's cultural background and experience. Spiritual values and religious beliefs form the rules of what a person considers right or wrong. The key to caring for residents' spiritual needs is to respect each resident as an individual and appreciate that no two persons are alike. For some persons, spirituality is enmeshed in their religious beliefs; for others, it is a

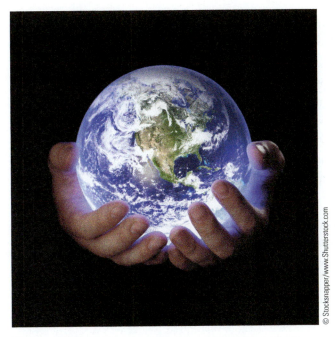

Figure 14-8 Spirituality defines our perceptions of our place in the universe and our responsibilities to others.

spirit leading to greater harmony and balance in their lives. Spirituality is a blending of physical, mental, and emotional aspects of one's self.

Nursing assistants must use care to avoid making judgments about residents' spiritual, religious, ethnic, and cultural beliefs and practices. Although these beliefs are considered to be a private concern, the need for caring is fundamental when serious health problems and life-altering situations occur. Listen to what the residents tell you and be supportive of their individual needs. If necessary, inform the nurse or the social worker of the resident's concerns. It may be necessary to seek assistance, interventions, or referrals from others to help the resident. The lifting of an emotional burden can bring a great sense of relief to the resident.

CULTURAL COMPETENCE

The United States is a nation made up people from a variety of countries. Our ancestors were among the first immigrants to this country. These persons brought aspects of their cultural heritage with them, their beliefs and customs as well as their language. The United States has been referred to as a "melting pot" of nationalities and cultures. The earliest immigrants came primarily from northern European countries and Scandinavia. In addition to the Native American population, these people have shaped the United States into a diverse mix of people. Today, immigration continues to impact the United States. The rich cultural heritage of these persons must be respected.

Health care workers need to be culturally competent and sensitive to the values and beliefs, hygiene and health care practices, and the varied religions of persons from other cultures. You must accept and respect the cultural differences among people. You must learn to adapt your care to meet the cultural needs of the individual resident. In addition, health

---

? EXERCISE 14-1

VOCABULARY EXERCISE
Select the correct term from the following list to complete each statement.

Ayurveda	folk medicine
Chinese medicine	homeopathy
chiropractic	neuropathic medicine

1. _____ emphasizes herbal remedies, acupuncture, acupressure, tai chi, cupping, and bleeding.

2. The adjunctive therapy that employs fasting, special diets, and supportive approaches is _____.

3. _____ uses exercise, herbal remedies, minerals, massage, and nutritional counseling, according to specific body type.

4. Treatments to align the neuromuscular segments of the spinal column are _____.

5. The therapy that uses the traditional remedies passed from one generation to the next is

_____.

6. _____ employs plant, animal, and mineral substances to encourage the immune system to accelerate healing.

? EXERCISE 14-2

TRUE OR FALSE

Indicate whether the following statements are true (T) or false (F).

1. T F Acupressure refers to the practice of inserting fine needles in specific areas of the skin to influence body functions.
2. T F Biofeedback uses machines to assist the person to become aware of changes in body functions.
3. T F Bodywork includes hands-on massage techniques such as foot reflexology and rolfing.
4. T F Electromagnetic therapy attempts to reduce pain through reaching a unity with a higher power.
5. T F Therapeutic touch is used to restore an unbalanced energy field.
6. T F Light therapy is used to regulate daily circadian functions of the body.
7. T F Tai chi is an aggressive martial art that improves muscle tone and eliminates free radicals.
8. T F Chiropractic treatment maintains that the spinal column is a key to maintaining the health of the nervous system.
9. T F The practice of Ayurveda originated in India and is over 3,000 years old.

care workers must be careful to avoid stereotyping beliefs about varied cultural groups. Stereotypes are rigid beliefs based on generalizations, not facts (Table 14-1).

Cultural customs and traditions influence the way that people react. A person's sense of identity is based on a combination of cultural heritage, race, and ethnicity. Race classifies people by shared physical characteristics such as skin color, facial features, hair texture, and bone structure. Ethnicity refers to special groups of persons within a culture who share certain characteristics such as customs, language, and national origin. Cultural differences among ethnic groups include such factors as family organization, traditions, religions, personal space requirements, communication (language variations), and beliefs about health, illness, and health care practices. Table 14-1 illustrates the interpretation of nonverbal communication and personal space among different cultural groups.

Culture	Nonverbal Communication
American (U.S.)	Personal space 18 to 36 inches. Eye contact is acceptable. Lack of eye contact may be interpreted as lack of self-esteem or not telling the truth.
African American	Eye contact is acceptable; close personal space.
American Indian	See Native American.
Arab American	Women usually avoid eye contact with males and others whom they do not know well. Close personal space. Male health care workers may be prohibited from touching some or all parts of the female body.
Asian	Eye contact is acceptable; close personal space, but avoid touching.
Brazilian	Lack of eye contact is viewed by some as a sign of respect. Close personal space.
Cambodian	Eye contact is acceptable; close personal space.
Chinese American	Avoid eye contact with authority figures as a sign of respect; will make eye contact with family and friends. Distant personal space.
Columbian	May avoid eye contact in presence of an authority figure. Close personal space.
Cuban	Eye contact expected during conversation. Close personal space with friends and family.

Table 14-1 Cultural Interpretation of Nonverbal Communication and Personal Space

(continues)

Culture	Nonverbal Communication
Ethiopian	Avoid eye contact with those perceived to be in authority. Close personal space with family and friends.
European	Eye contact acceptable; distant personal space.
Filipino	May avoid eye contact with authority figures. Close personal space.
Gypsy (Romany)	Facial expressions reflect mood. Close personal space with family members. Generally avoid contact with non-Gypsies. Also avoid surfaces considered unclean (areas that lower body has touched).
Haitian	Avoid eye contact with those perceived to be in authority.
Hmong	Avoid prolonged eye contact, which is considered rude.
Iranian	Make eye contact only with equals and close family and friends. Close personal space.
Japanese American	Little eye contact. Touching may be considered offensive.
Korean	Little direct eye contact. Touching is considered offensive. Although Koreans maintain close personal space with family, invading their personal space is a sign of disrespect.
Mexican American	Avoid eye contact with those perceived to be in authority. Some may believe touch by strangers is disrespectful or offensive.
Native American	Eye contact avoided as a sign of respect. Distant personal space is considered respectful. May converse in very low tones; listen attentively. It is considered impolite to say "Huh?" or give any indication the conversation was not heard.
Puerto Rican	Personal space varies with age group; generally closer with younger women, more distant with older women.
Russian	Close personal space with family and friends. Direct eye contact acceptable during conversation. Avoid smiling and handshaking; may be interpreted as disrespectful and arrogant.
South Asian	May consider direct eye contact with older individuals offensive or rude. Close personal space with family members.
Vietnamese	Avoid eye contact with those perceived to be in authority. Distant personal space.
West Indian	Eye contact is avoided. Distant personal space.

Table 14-1 (Continued)

As health care workers who give holistic care to the residents, it important to develop cultural sensitivity. The nursing assistant can do this by:

- Reviewing your own belief systems
- Considering how your own culture influences your behavior
- Viewing residents as individuals within a culture
- Recognizing that residents are a combination of heritage, culture, and community
- Understanding that culture influences how people behave and interact with others
- Remembering that personal space needs, eye contact, and ways of communicating are often culturally related
- Recognizing that some cultures have beliefs about health, wellness, and illness that may be different from your own and may be deeply ingrained
- Being willing to modify your care according to the resident's cultural background and practices
- Not stereotyping members of a cultural group to behave in exactly the same manner

- Caring for religious articles with respect
- Trying to learn about the practices, beliefs, and cultural heritage of the persons who are most likely to be your residents
- Politely asking residents about practices that are unfamiliar
- Attending staff development classes or in-service education programs designed to promote cultural sensitivity
- Do not overlook the resident's nonverbal communication. You may miss important information the resident is conveying.

IMPORTANCE FOR THE NURSING ASSISTANT

Despite changes in living arrangements, people often continue to use health practices they found helpful in the past. Therefore, the nursing assistant must be prepared to understand alternative health practices and be open to residents as they share these practices. Faith in the alternative practices often alters the willingness of the resident to follow the care plan. Remember that many of the alternative practices are accepted and used in conjunction with conventional Western therapy. It is important that you:

- Continue to learn about alternative practices to better understand and support the residents

- Make sure the supervising nurse is aware of any practices that residents are employing
- Accept practices that residents wish to share with you
- Be supportive of practices that are not harmful to current therapy.

? EXERCISE 14-3

MULTIPLE CHOICE
Select the one best answer.

1. Which of the following statements about Western therapy is not true?
    (A) It establishes a diagnosis by comparing gathered data against known disease or injury status.
    (B) It prescribes treatment designed to correct the underlying disease pathology.
    (C) It gathers information from an assessment of body systems, identifying signs and systems, and carrying out various laboratory tests.
    (D) It is based on natural science and touch therapy.

2. Which statement best explains the difference between Western therapy and alternative therapy?
    (A) Western therapy emphasizes technical aspects of care.
    (B) Western therapy follows biomedical principles while alternative therapy stresses a holistic approach to treatment and care.
    (C) Alternative therapy does not prescribe treatment following a protocol.
    (D) Western therapy uses surgery; alternative therapy does not.

3. Which of the following statements best describes alternative therapies?
    (A) The holistic approach of alternative therapies focuses on particular parts of the individual.
    (B) Holistic care recognizes the interaction and interrelationship of the person with his or her environment.
    (C) Alternative therapies are not influenced by cultural values.
    (D) Alternative therapies do not stress a holistic approach.

4. Ayurveda
    (A) originated in China
    (B) is based on the individual's spiritual beliefs
    (C) is based on the belief that disease is due to an imbalance in a person's consciousness
    (D) encourages the use of food and herbs with free radicals

5. Chinese medicine
    (A) emphasizes the blockage of chi to promote health
    (B) tries to look for a pattern of disharmony and then attempts to correct it
    (C) relies only on herbal remedies to restore balance
    (D) does not believe in using acupuncture

6. Which of the following statements about folk medicine is not true?
    (A) Folk medicine is culturally based.
    (B) Remedies are derived from plants and flowers.
    (C) Remedies are learned under the guidance of a "healer" and passed from one generation to another.
    (D) A problem with folk medicine is that it is not holistic.

7. Reiki
    (A) focuses on disharmony in the body
    (B) refers to universal energy
    (C) can only be used in people who are ill
    (D) energy is transferred from recipient to practitioner

(continues)

? EXERCISE 14-3 (Continued)

8. Homeopathy
    (A) remedies are given in large doses to stimulate the immune system
    (B) believes that it is important to fully express symptoms of illness
    (C) believes signs and systems should be suppressed
    (D) is not controversial because it uses plants, roots, and natural remedies

9. Which of the following statements about nursing assistants' understanding of alternative therapies is not true?
    (A) Nursing assistants must realize that many of these practices are used along with conventional therapy.
    (B) Nursing assistants should encourage residents to work with conventional therapy instead of alternative therapy.
    (C) Nursing assistants should tell the supervising nurse of any practice a resident uses.
    (D) Nursing assistants should learn as much as possible about alternative therapies.

10. Which of the following statements about cultural sensitivity is not true?
    (A) We should be willing to modify our care to fit cultural backgrounds.
    (B) Lack of eye contact always means people don't like you.
    (C) It is important to think about how our own culture influences our behavior.
    (D) We need to treat religious articles with respect.

LESSON SYNTHESIS: Putting It All Together

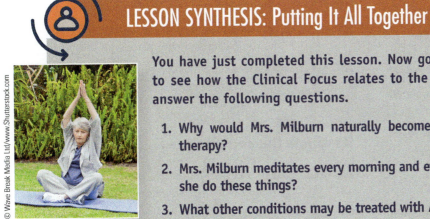

You have just completed this lesson. Now go back and review the Clinical Focus. Try to see how the Clinical Focus relates to the concepts presented in the lesson. Then answer the following questions.

1. Why would Mrs. Milburn naturally become interested in Ayurveda as an alternative therapy?

2. Mrs. Milburn meditates every morning and every evening and practices yoga. Why would she do these things?

3. What other conditions may be treated with Ayurveda?

© Wave Break Media Ltd/www.Shutterstock.com

14 REVIEW

A. Select the one best answer for each of the following.

1. Biomedical principles include all but which one of these?

    (A) assessment

    (B) praying to a higher power

    (C) identifying signs and symptoms

    (D) carrying out laboratory tests

2. Culturally based traditional remedies passed from generation to generation best describes:

    (A) folk medicine

    (B) naturopathic medicine

    (C) biofeedback

    (D) hydrotherapy

3. Residents who use oils from plants and flowers for restorative effects practice the adjunctive therapy known as

(A) hydrotherapy

(B) aromatherapy

(C) acupressure

(D) biofeedback

4. The insertion of fine needles in specific areas of the skin to influence body function is known as

(A) biofeedback

(B) acupressure

(C) tai chi

(D) acupuncture

B. Answer each statement true (T) or false (F).

5. T F Today, homeopathic therapy remains one of the least controversial areas of alternative therapy.

6. T F Herbal products should be used under the supervision of a trained practitioner.

7. T F Naturopathy emphasizes helping the individual assume responsibility for personal health.

8. T F Chiropractors may perform manipulation to properly align the spine.

9. T F Cultural values are an important aspect of alternative therapies.

10. T F People can learn to become aware when their blood pressure is rising and then to voluntarily lower their blood pressure.

11. T F Folk medicine is based on biomedical principles.

12. T F Cupping and bleeding are techniques used in traditional Chinese medicine.

13. T F Chiropractors believe that light therapy and herbal medicine are the best ways to treat illness.

14. T F Ayurveda is an ancient system to prevent disease and help people return to wellness.

C. Match the term for each adjunctive therapy with its description.

a. acupressure

b. hypnotherapy

c. massage therapy

d. biofeedback

e. yoga

f. tai chi

15. _____ Uses machines to assist a person in becoming aware of changes.

16. _____ Uses slow, graceful body movement to improve the flow of qi.

17. _____ Increases feelings of well-being; reduces stress and fatigue.

18. _____ May relieve pain and speed healing by increasing blood flow.

19. _____ Noninvasive; may apply a ball-pointed instrument to selected places on the body.

20. _____ Improves lung function and circulation through breath control, posture, relaxation, and meditation.

D. Circle the correct answer.

21. Rigid, biased ideas about people are called _____. (stereotypes) (characteristics)

22. Classification by shared physical characteristics is based on _____. (ethnicity) (race)

23. The way a group of people views the world and the group's traditions are the basis for a _____. (race) (culture)

24. Caucasians prefer to stand and speak from about _____ apart. (18 inches) (4 feet)

25. The Asian resident looks down and says little when you speak. This is _____ in his culture. (rude) (respectful)

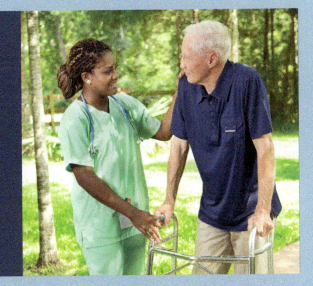

5

Meeting the Residents' Basic Needs

LESSON 15
CARE OF THE RESIDENTS' ENVIRONMENT

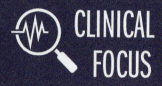

CLINICAL FOCUS

Think about how controlling the environment for the resident contributes to the resident's sense of well-being and comfort as you study this lesson.

OBJECTIVES

After studying this lesson, you should be able to:

• Define vocabulary words and terms.

• State three components of the resident's environment.

• Name four ways in which a safe, comfortable, and pleasant environment can be maintained for the resident.

• Describe two actions to be taken at the beginning and end of each resident care procedure.

• Demonstrate the following:

  Procedure 15-19 Unoccupied Bed: Changing Linens

  Procedure 15-20 Occupied Bed: Changing Linens

VOCABULARY

draw sheet (draw sheet)
environment (en-VIRE-on-ment)
mitered corner (MY-terd KOR-ner)
occupied bedmaking (OCK-you-pyed BED-may-king)

procedure (proh-SEE-djur)
square corner (skwair KOR-ner)
unoccupied bedmaking (un-OCK-you-pyed BED-may-king)

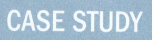

CASE STUDY

Mabel Campbell is a resident who is 96 and constantly complains of feeling cold. She has congestive heart failure, non–insulin-dependent diabetes mellitus, and chronic respiratory infections. She shares a room with another resident whose grandchildren visit and the noise bothers her. She reads but requires extra lighting. On warm days, she likes to sit on the enclosed patio.

RESIDENT ENVIRONMENT

The resident's **environment** is the surroundings in which the resident lives. Anything that is part of the environment affects the resident's sense of comfort, happiness, and security. The environment includes:

- Physical surroundings
- People who interact with the resident
- Quality of care given
- General atmosphere of the facility and staff

Nursing assistants have a responsibility for maintaining a safe, clean, and pleasant environment for the residents (Figure 15-1).

The resident's sense of well-being is a reflection of how the resident believes he or she is being treated. Residents respond positively when they are treated with respect, are viewed as people with value, are encouraged to exercise some control over their lives, and experience some personal independence. Negative feelings result when residents feel neglected, unimportant, unworthy, and powerless. A warm and friendly atmosphere promotes the well-being of both residents and health care providers.

⊘N THE JOB

Residents who are more independent may have many items in their rooms, causing a cluttered environment. It may be difficult to maintain a safe, orderly room for these residents.

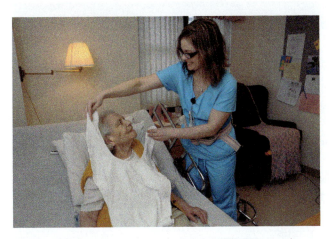

Figure 15-1 The nursing assistant contributes greatly to the friendly and comfortable atmosphere that creates a pleasant environment.

❓ EXERCISE 15-1

TRUE OR FALSE
Indicate whether the following statements are true (T) or false (F).

1. T F The resident's environment is the surroundings in which the resident now lives.

2. T F When people feel neglected and unimportant, the atmosphere is unfulfilling.

3. T F A nursing assistant has tremendous power to influence the atmosphere in which the resident lives.

4. T F It may be easier to maintain a safe, orderly room for residents who are more independent and have many items in their room.

PERSONAL SPACE

Personal space is the area immediately around a person's body. The boundaries of personal space are viewed differently by different cultures and by individuals within a culture. Refer to Lesson 14.

For a resident in a long-term care facility, personal space is often extended to include personal articles and the room in which the resident lives (Figure 15-2). You can show respect for a resident's personal space by:

- Making sure a resident's personal articles are not placed in another resident's area when a room is shared.
- Allowing the resident to arrange personal possessions as desired as long as safety is not an issue. Do not rearrange the resident's personal

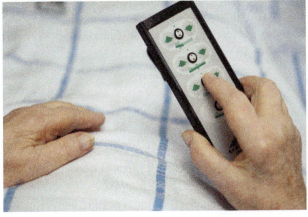

Figure 15-2 Electric control of the bed positions is used in many facilities.

© kaarsten/www.Shutterstock.com

possessions without permission. Residents are encouraged to keep a favorite chair or chest, as space permits. Moving these items can upset the resident. Because the residents become used to the placement of furniture in the room, moving furniture may cause accidental injury.

- Treating personal belongings with respect. Residents are encouraged to keep blankets, spreads, pillows, plants, photos, and mementos of family and their lives before their admission to the facility. These reminders help residents make the transition to living in the facility.
- Being sensitive to the clues the resident gives you about how the resident views personal space
- Knocking before entering the room
- Speaking before drawing back a privacy curtain
- Closing privacy curtains before carrying out procedures
- Explaining procedures and asking permission before starting the procedure
- Being patient with residents and treating each as a person of value

The unit equipment includes:

- Bed
- Privacy curtain
- Bedside table
- Closet space
- Call or signal cord/lights
- Bathroom equipment
- Overbed table
- Chair
- Sink and running water

Note that residents are not usually allowed to keep certain items in their rooms because these items are a safety hazard. Items that are not permitted vary from state to state. Some of these items include:

- Uncovered food
- Perishable food
- Matches and lighters
- Razor
- Knife
- Medications
- Cigarettes
- Alcohol

Check the facility regulations for items residents are not allowed to keep in their rooms.

RESIDENT UNIT

The resident's immediate environment is the unit or room where the resident lives. This room is often shared with another resident. The most important item in the room for the resident's comfort is the bed. Although many residents can be dressed and up for the day, some residents must remain in bed. The comfort and safety of the bed are important considerations for all residents.

Beds

The typical bed is adjustable and can be raised to make giving care easier. At the end of care, the bed

---

? EXERCISE 15-2

FILL IN THE BLANKS

Select the correct term from the following list to complete each statement.

permission	area
boundaries	knock
respect	personal space

1. _____ is the area immediately around a person's body, including the resident's room, living area, and personal articles.

2. Not all cultures view the _____ of personal space in the same way.

3. When residents share a room, personal articles of one resident should not be placed in the other resident's _____.

4. Carefully handling personal pictures and mementos demonstrates _____.

5. Before entering a resident's room when the door is closed, the nursing assistant should always _____.

6. Personal articles should not be rearranged without _____.

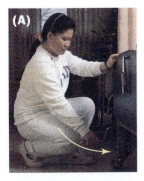 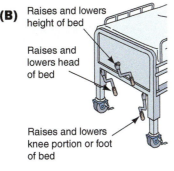

Raises and lowers height of bed

Raises and lowers head of bed

Raises and lowers knee portion or foot of bed

Figure 15-3 (A) For safety, fold the gatch handles under the bed when not in use. (B) Gatch handles.

is lowered to make it easier and safer for residents to get into and out of the bed. The back and foot of the bed can be raised to different positions for comfort and therapeutic reasons. Beds may be provided with adjustable quarter rails. Unless needed for positioning, most facilities do not use the side rails, because they are restrictive and restraining.

Electric control of the bed positions is used in many facilities (Figure 15-2), but some manually, crank-operated beds may still be used. If the bed has cranks to change positions, be sure the cranks are returned to the nonuse position so that no one will be injured by hitting them (Figure 15-3A and B). The wheels of the bed should be locked to prevent the bed from rolling. If the bed has large wheels, they should be turned inward to prevent tripping over them.

Call Signal/Lights

Each bed is equipped with a call signal. This may be a simple cord with a pushbutton or a more elaborate panel that is attached to the side rail (Figure 15-4A and B). When the resident signals, a light is activated both over the door to the room and at the nurses' station. Make sure that the resident knows how to use the system. A special system is found in the bathing area and bathroom. This signal is an emergency signal, which rings loudly and has a flashing red light. This signal indicates the need for immediate help and must be answered at once. Make sure that residents can always reach their call signals. If the resident is up in a chair, make sure the call light is within easy reach. Residents who have limited use of the hands may need a call signal that can be activated by lighter touch of the hand or fist. (See Figure 15-4B.) For example, a resident who is paralyzed on the left side should have the signal readily available on the right side.

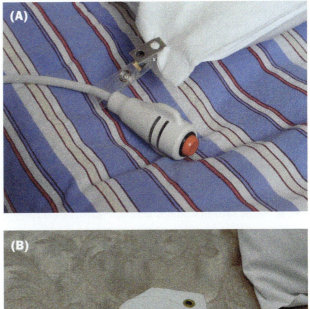

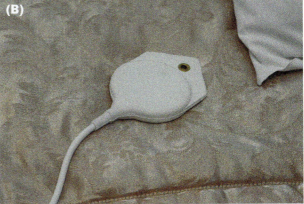

Figure 15-4 (A) Signal light button; (B) adaptive signal light button for limited mobility.

EXTENDED RESIDENT ENVIRONMENT

All facility employees are responsible for ensuring that safety, physical comfort, and a spirit of well-being are maintained throughout the extended resident environment, which includes the:

- Dining room
- Bathing area
- Activity area
- Therapy rooms
- Lounges
- Lobby

To achieve these conditions, the following factors must be managed:

- Cleanliness and order
- Adequate air circulation
- Proper temperature
- Adequate lighting
- Noise control
- Odor control

? EXERCISE 15-3

FILL IN THE BLANKS
Select the correct term from the following list to complete each statement.

matches	side rails
call light	crank-operated, electric control

1. _____ are protective devices attached to beds that can be lowered or raised for resident safety.

2. _____ or _____ are types of adjustable beds.

3. A _____ when used, activates a light over the resident's door and at the nurses' station.

4. Most facilities do not permit residents to keep _____ in their units.

TRUE OR FALSE
Indicate whether the following statements are true (T) or false (F).

5. T F All bed cranks should be returned to the nonuse position after use.

6. T F Unit equipment includes bed, privacy curtain, bathroom equipment, medications, and chair.

7. T F A resident only needs their call light when in bed.

Cleanliness and Order

Dust and dirt, crumbs from food, and dirty dishes and glasses are contaminated by microbes that can contribute to the spread of disease. Food left in the residents' rooms may attract insects such as cockroaches and ants. The food can also cause unpleasant odors. Remove all dishes as soon as the resident finishes a meal or nourishment. Clean up any spills and crumbs immediately. Remember that residents are not usually allowed to store food in their rooms. Some facilities permit candy in the room if it is sealed or in a closed container. Perishable food should be labeled with the resident's name and the date and stored in the refrigerator.

The routine cleaning of the windows, bathroom, and floor is the responsibility of housekeeping, but the nursing department is expected to keep the rest of the environment safe and orderly.

Disposable items such as latex gloves and paper products should be disposed of in the proper receptacle in the dirty utility rooms. Reusable equipment must be cleaned and disinfected or sterilized before being used with another resident. Reusable equipment, such as bed cradles, basins, or commodes, is usually very expensive and should be properly handled in the following manner:

- Wear gloves and follow standard aseptic procedure.
- Rinse article with cold water; never use hot, because heat tends to cause blood and body tissues to harden on the article.

- Wash with warm, soapy water.
- Dry carefully.
- Check carefully for breakage or defects. Report defects if found.
- Disinfect or sterilize according to facility policy.
- Return article to proper storage area.

Clutter is a safety hazard and often is disturbing to the older adult. Return all equipment to its proper place as soon as you finish using it. Move equipment carefully to avoid hitting walls and furniture.

Adequate Air Circulation (Ventilation)

Everyone feels refreshed when fresh, clean air is available. Most facilities have central controls to manage ventilation. Some facilities have controls in each resident room so ventilation can be controlled to meet individual needs.

Circulating air may produce drafts. Blankets, screens, and curtains are used to control the flow of air to meet the residents' comfort needs.

Temperature Control

Older adults often prefer warmer temperatures than do younger people. The facility temperature is usually controlled at 70° to 72°F. A resident may use a lap robe, sweater, or shawl for comfort and to protect dignity when wearing a dress (Figure 15-5).

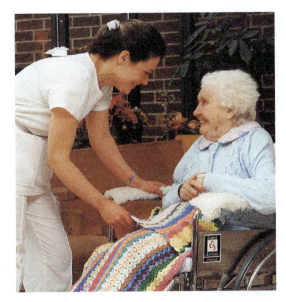

Figure 15-5 A lap robe provides comfort and protects the resident's dignity if she is wearing a dress.

Adequate Lighting

Make sure there is adequate lighting for resident and staff safety. This is especially important at dusk and during the night. The light level can be controlled by adjusting the overbed light, any lamps that may be in the room, and the room light (Figure 15-6). The overbed light usually has more than one level of brightness. The cord for controlling the overbed light should be within reach of the resident whenever the resident is in bed or sitting near the bed. A nightlight near the floor will not disturb the resident at night and is an added safety feature. Lights must be left on in the hallways and on stairways at night. Bright sunlight can be controlled using curtains and shades.

Noise Control

Loud noises can be disturbing. Older adults are often more sensitive to noise and find a noisy environment upsetting. Noisy equipment, banging trays, loud radios or televisions, ringing telephones, squeaking wheels, and loud or excited voices all add to the noise level in the facility. Health care providers can make the environment more pleasant by controlling noise when they work (Figure 15-7).

Odor Control

Odors can be a problem in a long-term care facility unless everyone makes an effort to control them. Odors should be eliminated, not covered up. Residents who

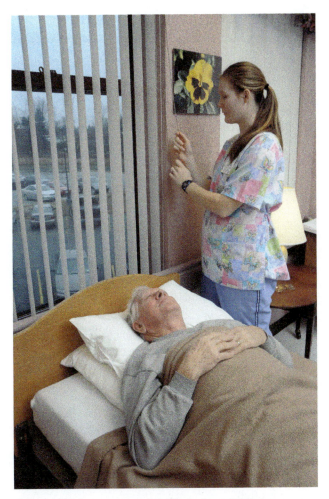

Figure 15-6 The best lighting is indirect lighting.

are incontinent must be cared for immediately. Soiled pads, garments, and linens must be placed in covered containers and handled according to facility policy.

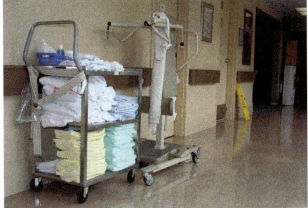

Figure 15-7 Handle equipment carefully to control noise. Position equipment according to facility policy to prevent clutter.

© Hannamariah/www.shutterstock.com

⚠ GUIDELINES FOR... ENSURING A SAFE AND COMFORTABLE ENVIRONMENT

The nursing assistant makes important contributions to maintaining a safe and comfortable resident environment.

Follow all infection control guidelines and use standard precautions for the care of all residents.

CLEANLINESS

1. Remove dishes immediately after use and clean up crumbs and spills.

2. Check that the resident is not storing food in the room. If food is permitted, check that it is marked with a date and wrapped or in a closed container.

3. Clean overbed table after use; use disinfectant, if necessary.

4. If the floor is soiled with blood or body fluids, call housekeeping for immediate cleanup, or follow facility policy.

5. Pick up resident clothing and place in laundry hamper if soiled or hang in closet.

6. Each time you enter the room, check it for cleanliness and order, paying special attention to clutter that may cause accidents.

7. Provide a bag for used tissues and change it often.

8. Empty wastebaskets if full and reline with a plastic bag (this is usually done by housekeeping, but a basket may become full before the scheduled change).

9. Try to keep dresser and table tops uncluttered, but remember that the resident has the right to display personal items and to expect that they will not be disturbed. Ask permission to clean around them when necessary.

NOISE

1. Exercise care in using and moving equipment to keep the noise level down.

2. Speak in a conversational tone of voice. Call out to other staff members only if the resident has had an incident, you cannot leave the resident, you cannot reach the call button, and you need assistance; otherwise, walk to another staff member to talk.

3. Keep radio and television volumes at a reasonable level on a station selected by the resident.

4. Close the door to the resident's room, and tell the resident why you are doing so, if cleaning or construction is under way in the hallway or a nearby room.

ODOR

1. Control odors by caring for incontinent residents immediately.

2. Follow facility policy for handling of clothing and bed linens soiled by feces, urine, vomitus, respiratory secretions, wound drainage, or food spills.

3. Empty bed pans, urinals, and commodes promptly. Clean and disinfect after each use or according to facility policy.

OTHER ENVIRONMENTAL CONCERNS

1. Be aware of residents' needs for ventilation and air circulation, temperature control, and adequate lighting; assist the resident as necessary to ensure comfort.

2. Check that all equipment used by the resident is in good repair and safe to use.

3. Be sensitive to residents' wishes relating to cultural preferences and accommodate them as much as possible without violating facility policy.

Bedpans, urinals, commodes, and emesis basins should be emptied, cleaned, and disinfected immediately after use, or as dictated by facility policy. Utility rooms and dining areas must be cleaned regularly.

Nursing assistants have a major responsibility for influencing the environment in which the residents live. Each day you will care for the residents' belongings and ensure that the resident unit and other areas are safe and clean.

CRITICAL PROCEDURE ACTIONS

Caring for residents safely means you must perform tasks in a manner specified by facility policy. Such tasks are called procedures. As you continue your study, you will learn the procedures for many nursing assistant tasks. You have already learned several emergency care and infection control procedures, including hand hygiene. The procedures that follow give you step-by-step directions for performing tasks that involve personal care of residents.

? EXERCISE 15-4

TRUE OR FALSE

Indicate whether the following statements are true (T) or false (F).

1. T F An older person may frequently complain of feeling too warm.

2. T F A temperature between 60° and 65°F is most comfortable for the elderly person.

3. T F Residents are encouraged to stay up and dressed as much as possible.

4. T F A unit may be clean, but if the resident does not feel of value, the environment is unacceptable.

5. T F Inadequate lighting may cause an accident.

6. T F Keeping personal care equipment stored properly is not a suitable activity for a nursing assistant.

7. T F The nursing assistant who spills urine on the floor can safely leave it until housekeeping can clean it up.

8. T F Speaking to residents in a loud excited voice is a good thing to do because it keeps residents stimulated.

9. T F Odors should be eliminated, not just covered up.

10. T F A personal lock box is used to keep medications away from residents.

Certain steps must be done before you perform the actual resident care procedure. These steps are called *beginning procedure actions*. When the resident care procedure is completed, another series of steps, called *procedure completion actions*, must be done (Figure 15-8).

BEDMAKING

You will learn two basic methods of making the resident's bed:

- **Unoccupied bedmaking** (when the resident is not in the bed)—see Procedure 15-19

Beginning Procedure Actions	Rationale
1. Assemble equipment needed and take to resident's room.	1. Improves the efficiency of the procedure. Means you do not have to leave the resident.
2. Knock on the resident's door and identify yourself by name and title.	2. Respects the resident's right to privacy. Notifies the resident who is giving care.
3. Wait for permission to enter.	3. Ensures that you are caring for the correct resident.
4. Identify the resident by checking the identification bracelet (if this is used).	4. Respects the resident's right to privacy. Shows hospitality to visitors by advising them where to wait.
5. Ask visitors to leave the room and advise where they may wait.	5. Informs the resident of what is going to be done and what is expected. Gives the resident an opportunity to get information about the procedure and the extent of resident participation.
6. Explain what you are going to do and how the resident can assist. Answer questions about the procedure.	6. Applies the principles of Standard Precautions. Prevents the spread of microorganisms.
7. Use appropriate hand hygiene.	7. Respects the resident's right to privacy. All three should be closed even if the resident is alone in the room.
8. Provide privacy by closing the door, privacy curtain, and window curtain.	8. Applies the principles of Standard Precautions. Protects the care provider and resident from transmission of pathogens.
9. Apply gloves if contact with blood, moist body fluids, secretions, excretions, or nonintact skin is likely.	9. Applies the principles of Standard Precautions. Protects your uniform from contamination with bloodborne pathogens.

Figure 15-8 Beginning procedure actions and procedure completion actions.

(continues)

10. Apply a gown if your uniform will have substantial contact with linen or other articles contaminated with blood, moist body fluids (except sweat), secretions, or excretions.

11. Apply a gown, mask, and eye protection if splashing of blood or moist body fluids is likely.

12. Raise the bed to a comfortable working height. Make sure wheels are locked.

13. Lower the side rail on the side where you are working, if side rails are used for positioning by the resident.

10. Applies the principles of Standard Precautions. Protects the care provider's mucous membranes, uniform, and skin from accidental splashing of bloodborne pathogens.

11. Prevents back strain and injury caused by bending at the waist.

12. Provides an obstacle-free area in which to work.

Procedure Completion Actions	Rationale
1. Check to make sure the resident is in good alignment.	1. All body systems function better when the body is correctly aligned. The resident is more comfortable when the body is in good alignment.
2. Raise the side rail, if clinically indicated.	2. Resident's right to a safe environment. Prevents accidents and injuries.
3. Remove gloves. Wash hands.	3. Prevents contamination of environmental surfaces from the gloves.
4. Remove other personal protective equipment, if worn, and discard according to facility policy.	4. Prevents unnecessary environmental contamination from used gloves and protective equipment.
5. Use appropriate hand hygiene.	5. Applies the principles of standard precautions. Prevents the spread of microorganisms.
6. Return the bed to the lowest horizontal position.	6. Resident's right to a safe environment. Prevents accidents and injuries.
7. Open the privacy and window curtains.	7. Privacy is no longer necessary unless preferred by the resident.
8. Leave the resident in a position of comfort and safety with the call signal and needed personal items within reach.	8. Prevents accidents and injuries. Ensures that help is available. Eliminates the need to call or reach for needed personal items.
9. Use appropriate hand hygiene.	9. Although the hands were washed previously, they have contacted the resident and other items in the room. Wash them again before leaving to prevent potential transfer of microorganisms to areas outside the resident's unit.
10. Inform visitors that they may return to the room.	10. Provides courtesy to visitors and resident.
11. Report completion of the procedure and any abnormalities or other observations.	11. Inform the nurse that your assigned task has been completed so further resident care can be planned and you can be reassigned to other duties. Notifies the nurse of abnormalities and changes in the resident's condition for further assessment.
12. Document the procedure and your observations.	12. Ongoing progress and care given are documented. Provides a legal record. Provides a record of what has been done, for other members of the interdisciplinary team.

Figure 15-8 (Continued)

- **Occupied bedmaking** (when the resident is in the bed)—see Procedure 15-20

The following linens are used to make the resident's bed:

- Sheets, top and bottom (the bottom sheet may be contoured or have elastic edges to fit over the edges of the mattress)
- Pillowcases, usually two although more may be required if several pillows are used to position and support the resident in bed
- **Draw sheet** or lift sheet, a small sheet or a regular top sheet folded in half and placed sideways across the bed to cover the area between the resident's upper back and thighs
  - The sides of the draw sheet may or may not be tucked under the mattress.
  - The draw sheet can be changed frequently without changing the rest of the bed linen if the bottom sheet is not soiled.

- The draw sheet can be used to lift the resident to change position in bed (in this case, the edges of the draw sheet would not be tucked under the mattress).
- Bed protectors are made of cotton ideally. These incontinence pads are superior to the disposable type because they tend to wick the moisture away from the skin. Protectors that are made from plastic and paper fibers can cause irritation to the resident's skin.
- Blanket
- Spread (when the resident is out of bed, the spread is usually placed on the bed and covers the pillows)

Bed linens that are not soiled by blood, body fluids, body secretions or excretions, or spilled food are changed according to a schedule set by the facility. All soiled linens are changed immediately.

⚠ GUIDELINES FOR... HANDLING LINENS AND MAKING THE BED

HANDLING LINENS

1. Use appropriate hand hygiene and use gloves as required; other personal protective equipment may be required.
2. Laundry hampers placed in the hallway should be at least three feet from clean linen carts.
3. The clean linen cart is always covered; replace covers after removing required linen.
4. Take only the linens you need into the resident's room.
5. Linens that touch the floor are considered dirty and placed in the laundry hamper; they are not used.
6. Avoid contact between the linens and your uniform (for both clean and soiled linens).
7. Unused linen is never returned to the clean linen cart; it is placed in the laundry hamper.
8. As soiled linen is removed from the bed, keep the soiled areas on the inside and fold or roll the linen toward the center.
9. Never shake soiled bed linens, because microbes will be released into the air.
10. Soiled linen is never placed on environmental surfaces in the room, such as overbed table, chair, or floor; soiled linens are placed in the appropriate laundry hamper (follow facility policy).
11. Fill laundry hampers no more than two-thirds full.

12. Many facilities do not permit laundry hampers or barrels to be taken into the resident's room. Soiled linen may be placed in a plastic bag or a pillowcase in the room. Make a cuff at the top of the bag or open end of the pillowcase and place the cuff over the back of the chair. When the bag or case is two-thirds full, secure the top and place it in the hamper in the hallway.
13. If disposable underpads or briefs are used, soiled ones should be discarded in a plastic bag and into the biohazard container per agency protocol.
14. Laundry hampers or barrels are returned to utility room after use, or as directed by facility policy.

MAKING THE BED

1. Use proper body mechanics at all times to prevent back injury.
2. Work on one side of the bed at a time to complete removing soiled linen and placing clean linen (see Procedures 15-19 and 15-20). Always work from head of bed to foot of bed.
3. Make sure the bottom sheet and underpads, cotton or disposable, (if used), are smooth and unwrinkled (wrinkles in bed linens can lead to skin breakdown, especially for residents who remain in bed).
4. Follow the care plan for the positioning of the head and foot of the bed, the number of pillows to be used, and the need for pillows for positioning.

PROCEDURE 15-19
Unoccupied Bed |
Changing Linens

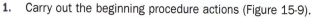

OBRA

1. Carry out the beginning procedure actions (Figure 15-9).

2. Assemble equipment:

    ▪ Disposable gloves (if linens are soiled with blood or body fluids, secretions, or excretions)

    ▪ Pillowcases

    ▪ Spread

    ▪ Blankets, as needed

    ▪ Two large sheets (90 × 109) (substitute one fitted, if used)

    ▪ Cotton bed protectors or disposable underpads, for selected residents

    ▪ Laundry hamper (Figure 15-10)

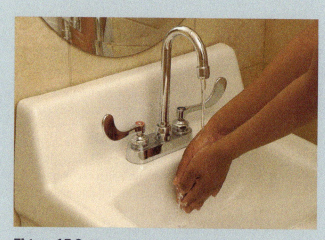

Figure 15-9 Remember to start and end each procedure by using appropriate hand hygiene.

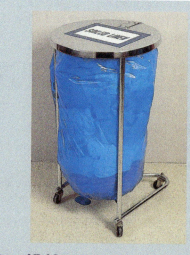

Figure 15-10 If facility policy permits, take a laundry hamper or barrel into the room with you.

3. Lock bed wheels so the bed will not roll and place chair at the side of the bed.

4. Raise bed to comfortable working height.

5. Arrange linens on chair in order in which they are to be used. Make a cuff at the top of a plastic bag or pillowcase. Place the cuff over the back of the chair and use the bag or case for the disposal of soiled linen.

6. Remove soiled linen as follows:

    ▪ Loosen the bedding on one side of the bed by lifting the edge of the mattress with one hand and drawing the linens out with the other.

    ▪ Remove the pillow from the bed. Grasp pillow with one hand. Using the other hand, gather the pillowcase and pull it back over the pillow so it is inside out. Place pillow on chair and put pillowcase in bag for soiled linen.

    ▪ If the bedspread is clean and to be reused, fold it lengthwise by bringing the far edge toward the near edge. Fold it once more from the center lengthwise. Then fold the spread from top to bottom and place it over the back of the chair.

NOTE: If the bedspread is soiled, it must be handled as the sheets are handled.

    ▪ Gather the top sheet by folding the edges inward so that the dirtiest side is on the inside. Place sheet in bag.

    ▪ Gather up the underpads (if used) by folding the dirtiest side inward. Place in bag.

(continues)

PROCEDURE 15-19
Unoccupied Bed |
Changing Linens (Continued)

- Repeat process with the bottom sheet. Before putting the linen in the hamper or pillowcase, remember to check it for items such as dentures, eyeglasses, hearing aids, equipment, supplies, syringes, and so on. Remove the items and follow facility policy for cleaning, disinfection, storage, or disposal. Mattresses have a plasticized top for protection against soiling. If the top of the mattress is wet from the linens, wipe dry using a disinfectant. Secure top of plastic bag or pillowcase and place in hamper in hallway. Remove gloves and dispose of properly. Wash hands, dry, and put on fresh gloves, if required.

7. Position mattress to head of bed by grasping handles on mattress side.

8. Work from one side of the bed until that side is completed, and then go to the other side of the bed.

9. Place bottom sheet lengthwise on mattress with fold at center of bed. Be sure the smooth side (hem side) is up and the narrow hem is even with the foot of the mattress (Figure 15-11A). See Figure 15-11B if a fitted bottom sheet is used.

10. Tuck 12 to 18 inches of sheet smoothly over the top of the mattress if using a flat sheet.

11. Make a mitered (Figure 15-12) or square corner.

12. Tuck in the sheet on one side, keeping it straight. Work from the head to the foot of the bed. If a fitted sheet is used, adjust it over the head and bottom ends of the mattress.

13. Unfold the top sheet and place wrong side up, top hem even with the upper edge of the mattress, and center fold on the center of the bed. Tuck in sheet at the bottom of the bed, as shown in Figure 15-13.

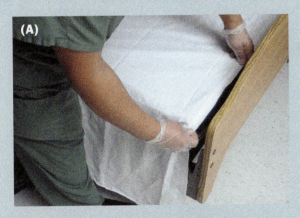

Figure 15-11A Place flat bottom sheet even with the end of mattress at foot of bed.

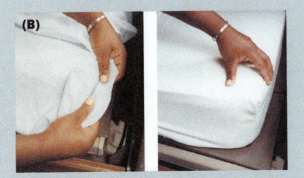

Figure 15-11B If a fitted bottom sheet is used, fit it properly and smoothly around the corner of the mattress.

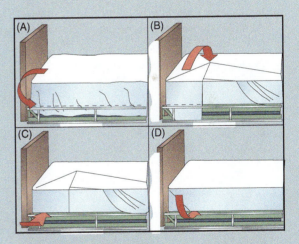

Figure 15-12 Making a mitered corner. (A) The sheet is hanging loose at the side of the bed. (B) Pick up the sheet about 12 inches from the head of the bed to form a triangle. Pull back toward the bed to smooth the sheet and lay triangle on the bed. (C) Tuck in sheet at head of bed. (D) Pick up triangle and place other hand at edge of bed near head to hold edge of sheet in place. Bring triangle over edge of mattress and tuck smoothly under mattress. Tuck in the rest of the sheet along the side of the mattress. Make sure sheet is smooth.

(continues)

PROCEDURE 15-19
Unoccupied Bed |
Changing Linens (Continued)

14. Spread blanket over the top sheet and foot of mattress. Keep blanket centered.

15. Tuck top sheet and blanket under mattress at the foot of the bed as far as the center only and make a mitered or square corner (Figure 15-14).

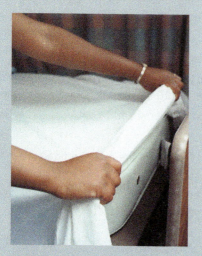

Figure 15-13A Gather about 12 to 18 inches of the top sheet at bottom of bed.

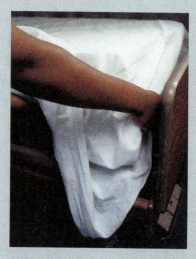

Figure 15-13B Face foot of bed and lift mattress with near hand.

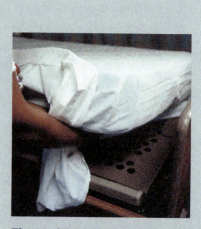

Figure 15-13C Using other hand, bring sheet smoothly over end of mattress.

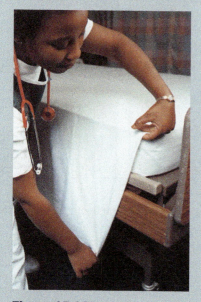

Figure 15-14A Make the square (box) corner following the steps of Figure 15-12A–C. Then, holding the corner with one hand, grasp the bottom of the sheet and pull it straight down until fold is even with the edge of the mattress.

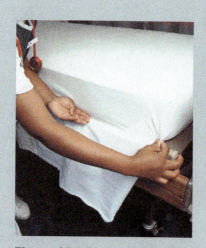

Figure 15-14B Holding the square corner in place, tuck sheet under mattress.

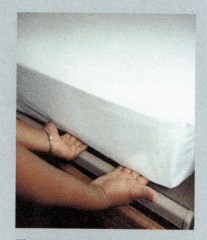

Figure 15-14C Finished square corner should look like this.

(continues)

PROCEDURE 15-19
Unoccupied Bed |
Changing Linens (Continued)

16. Place spread with top hem even with head of mattress.

17. Unfold to foot of bed.

18. Tuck spread under mattress at the foot of one side of bed (Figure 15-15) and make mitered or square corner.

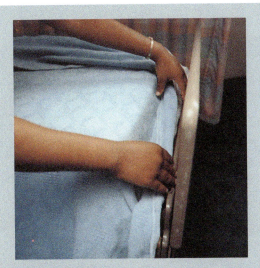

Figure 15-15A Gather top sheet and spread together and smooth evenly over end of mattress.

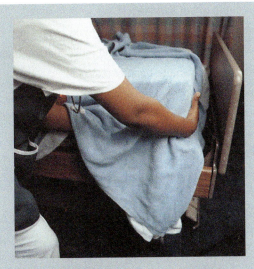

Figure 15-15B Tuck sheet and spread under mattress together.

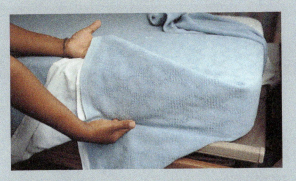

Figure 15-15C Continue as in the procedure for a mitered corner.

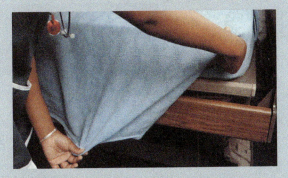

Figure 15-15D Slide finger to end to make a smooth edge.

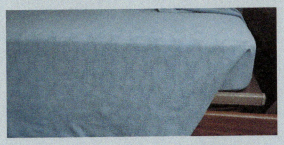

Figure 15-15E The completed top bedding. The procedure is repeated on the other side.

(continues)

PROCEDURE 15-19
Unoccupied Bed |
Changing Linens (Continued)

19. Go to other side of bed and fanfold the top sheet, blanket, and spread to the center of the bed to work with lower sheets and pad.

20. Tuck bottom sheet under head of mattress and make mitered or square corner. Working from top to bottom, smooth out all wrinkles and tighten sheet as much as possible, or adjust fitted bottom sheet smoothly and securely around mattress corners.

21. Tuck in top sheet and blanket.

22. Fold top sheet back over blanket, making an 8-inch cuff.

23. Tuck in spread at foot of bed and make a mitered or square corner.

24. Bring top of spread to head of mattress.

25. Insert pillow in pillowcase properly. Be sure corners of pillows are in corners of pillowcases.

26. Place pillow at head of bed with open end away from the door.

27. Spread is brought up to cover pillow.

28. Lower bed to lowest horizontal position.

29. Replace bedside table parallel to bed. Place chair in assigned location. Place overbed table over the foot of the bed opposite the chair.

30. Use appropriate hand hygiene.

31. Perform procedure completion actions.

32. Report completion of task.

PROCEDURE 15-20
Occupied Bed |
Changing Linens

 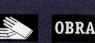

1. Carry out each beginning procedure action.

2. Assemble equipment:
   - Disposable gloves (if linens are soiled with blood, body fluids, secretions, or excretions; gown is required if there may be contact between your uniform and soiled linens)
   - Cotton bed protectors or disposable underpads, for selected residents
   - Two pillowcases
   - Two large sheets (or one large sheet and one fitted sheet)
   - Spread
   - Laundry hamper

3. Place bedside chair at the foot of the bed.

4. Arrange bed linen on chair in the order in which it is to be used.

5. The bed should be flat with wheels locked, unless otherwise indicated. Raise to working horizontal height with side rails in "up" position.

6. If bed linens are soiled with blood or body fluids, wash hands and put on disposable gloves.

7. Loosen the linens on one side by lifting the edge of the mattress with one hand and drawing bedclothes out with the other.

(continues)

PROCEDURE 15-20
Occupied Bed |
Changing Linens (Continued)

8. Adjust mattress to head of bed. If resident's condition permits, have resident bend knees, grasp side rails or headboard of bed with hands, and pull on frame as you draw mattress to the top or have another person help from the opposite side.

9. Remove covers, except for top sheet, one at a time. Fold to bottom and pick up in center. Place over the back of chair.

10. Place a clean sheet over top sheet. Have the resident hold the top edge of the clean sheet, if possible. If not, tuck the sheet beneath the resident's shoulder.

11. Slide out the soiled top sheet, from top to bottom. Place in hamper.

12. Ask the resident to roll toward you and assist if necessary. Move one pillow with the resident. Pull up side rail for safety.

13. Go to the other side of the bed. Fanfold the bed protector, if used, and the bottom sheet close to the resident (Figure 15-17).

14. Place a clean bottom sheet on the bed so that the narrow hem comes to the edge of the mattress at the foot and the lengthwise center fold of the sheet is at the center of the bed.

15. Tuck top of clean bottom sheet under the head of the mattress.

16. Make a mitered or square corner. Tuck side of bottom sheet under mattress, working toward the foot of the bed.

17. Position clean draw sheet if used. Tuck it under the mattress. If used, place protective underpad on top of draw sheet.

18. Ask the resident to roll toward you and assist as needed. Move the pillow with the resident.

19. Raise side rail for safety.

20. Go to the other side of the bed. Remove soiled linen by rolling the edges inward.

21. Keep soiled linen away from your uniform, and place in hamper, plastic bag, or pillowcase.

22. Change gloves or remove gloves and perform hand hygiene before handling clean linens.

23. Complete the bed as for an unoccupied bed. Some residents prefer not to have the blanket, top sheet, or spread tucked in.

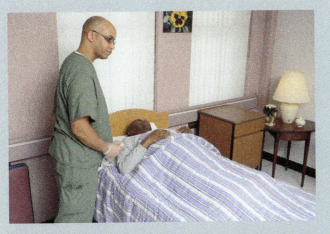

Figure 15-16 Wash hands and put on disposable gloves if linens are soiled with blood or body fluids.

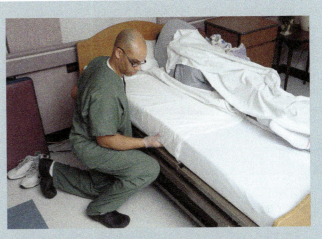

Figure 15-17 Note that the bottom linen is flat and the resident is positioned on the far side of the bed.

(continues)

PROCEDURE 15-20
Occupied Bed |
Changing Linens (Continued)

24. Turn resident on back. Place clean case on pillow. Replace pillow. If other pillows are used for positioning, change pillowcases each time bed linens are changed, or according to facility policy.

25. Remove and dispose of gloves (if used) according to facility policy. Use appropriate hand hygiene.

26. Adjust bed position for the resident's comfort.

27. Be sure side rails are lowered unless use is clinically indicated. Lower bed to lowest horizontal position.

28. Replace bedside table and chair.

29. Make sure call signal and fresh water are within reach of resident.

30. Carry out each procedure completion action.

31. Report completion of task.

Low Beds

Low beds are commonly used in long-term care facilities to prevent falls for residents who are at risk (Figure 15-18). The bed frame is usually 4 to 6 inches from the floor, topped by the mattress. Large sanitizable foam pads may be placed on the floor next to the bed to prevent further injury in case the resident falls from the bed.

Even though the bed is helpful for the resident, it may be more difficult for you to change the bed linens. If the bed has a high-low feature, use this when necessary, but always return the bed to its low position after you have completed your tasks. If the bed is stationary, in order to prevent back injuries the nursing assistant must use good body mechanics when caring for residents or making the low bed. Kneel on the floor mat, if possible. Always use your leg muscles when lifting and turning the resident; avoid bending at the waist and using the muscles of your back. Use a transfer belt and a mechanical lift if possible to get the person into and out of the bed. Remember that the floor mat can create a hazard that could cause the nursing assistant or a family member to trip and fall. Use caution when walking around the room. When it is

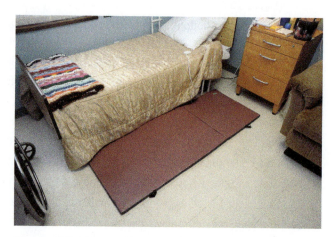

Figure 15-18 Low beds may be used for residents who are at risk for falls. Organize the bedmaking procedure carefully to avoid injury to your back.

dark, leave a night light on or turn on the overhead light to prevent injury to personnel.

The bed-making procedure for low beds is the same as that described earlier in this lesson. Think through the procedure carefully before you begin because you may be making the bed while you are in a kneeling position.

? EXERCISE 15-5

VOCABULARY EXERCISE
Select the correct term from the following list to complete each statement.

call light	side rail
square corner	center

(continues)

? EXERCISE 15-5 (Continued)

underpad   disinfectant
mitered corner   unoccupied

1. _____ type of bed linen corners made on an angle

2. _____ type of bed linen corners made with straight boxed edges

3. _____ disposable pads placed under incontinent residents

4. Linens should be removed from the bed with the dirtiest area toward the _____.

5. Plasticized mattresses that are soiled should be wiped with a(an) _____.

? EXERCISE 15-6

APPROPRIATE ACTIONS

Answer the following statements about nursing assistants' actions with A for appropriate or I for inappropriate. If the action is inappropriate, write the appropriate action in the space provided.

1. _____ In the long-term care facility, soiled linen needs to be changed at least once a week.
   _____

2. _____ Side rails are made for each bed and therefore do not need to be checked for security once in place.
   _____

3. _____ Leave bed wheels unlocked as you make the bed because it is easier to move the bed as you step around it.
   _____

4. _____ Make the entire unoccupied bed bottom first to see that there are no wrinkles in the linen.
   _____

5. _____ If you are making a stationary low bed it will be necessary to make the bed while positioned on your knees.
   _____

6. _____ Loosen bedding without shaking the linen.
   _____

7. _____ Tuck the pillow under your neck as you remove the soiled pillow case.
   _____

8. _____ Gather and remove dirty linen by rolling it up.
   _____

9. _____ Tuck the top sheet and blanket in together.
   _____

10. _____ If the linens are soiled with blood or body fluids, you must wear gloves.
    _____

11. _____ When making an occupied bed, keep the bed at its lowest horizontal height.
    _____

12. _____ When making an occupied bed, make each side of the bottom first before making the top.
    _____

13. _____ Rinse reusable items with hot, soapy water.
    _____

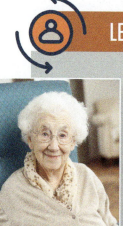

LESSON SYNTHESIS: Putting It All Together

You have just completed this lesson. Now go back and review the Clinical Focus. Try to see how the Clinical Focus relates to the concepts presented in the lesson. Then answer the following questions.

1. What actions could you take to increase Mabel Campbell's comfort when the grandchildren of her roommates visit?

2. How should the environment be adjusted to increase safety during evening hours?

3. How can you help Mrs. Campbell to be comfortable when she is sitting on the patio area and the sun is shining in?

4. How does a well-made bed, properly positioned, contribute to the safety and well-being of the resident?

15 REVIEW

A. Match each term (items a–e) with the proper definition.

a. side rails

b. underpad

c. environment

d. mitered corner

e. unoccupied bed

1. _____   water-proof bed protector

2. _____   bed without a resident

3. _____   sheet tucked in at a 45-degree angle

4. _____   safety feature on beds that can be regarded as a restraint

5. _____   surroundings in which the resident lives

B. Select the one best answer for each of the following.

6. Most facilities regulate the room temperature to approximately

(A) 60 to 62°F

(B) 64 to 66°F

(C) 70 to 72°F

(D) 78 to 80°F

7. A positive atmosphere is created when

(A) radios play loudly

(B) residents are treated with respect

(C) odors are covered up

(D) equipment is out of place

8. Which of the following is not usually permitted to be stored in the resident's room?

(A) uncovered food

(B) books

(C) radio

(D) pictures

9. To ensure privacy, you should

(A) arrange the resident's belongings to please yourself

(B) enter rooms without knocking

(C) close curtains around the bed before carrying out procedures

(D) leave curtains open around a resident receiving care if only her roommate is present

10. Underpads

(A) are half-sheets

(B) reduce pressure

(C) can be easily changed when soiled

(D) are also called fitted sheets

C. Answer each statement true (T) or false (F).

11. T F Adjustable beds provide for resident comfort and therapeutic positioning.

12. T F Bed linens are completely changed every day even if they are not soiled.

13. T F Disposable underpads made from plastic and paper fibers may cause skin irritation for the resident.

14. T F When making an unoccupied bed, make one side completely before going to the opposite side.

15. T F It is important that the bottom sheet be smooth.

16. T F When making a bed, linens should be arranged on a chair in the order in which they are to be used.

17. T F The mattress should be positioned to the top of the bed before clean linen is applied.

18. T F If the linen is soiled with blood, the nursing assistant should wear gloves when making the bed.

19. T F When changing the bed, soiled linens should be placed on the floor.

20. T F If clinically indicated, side rails should be checked for security when up in place.

21. T F If a crank is left protruding, it can cause an injury.

22. T F Beds should be raised to a comfortable working height before linens are changed.

23. T F The nursing assistant is responsible for maintaining a safe and comfortable environment for the resident.

24. T F Side rails must be up and secured for all residents, regardless of condition.

25. T F When stripping soiled linen from a bed, the linens should always be gathered so the dirtiest part is inside.

LESSON 16
CARING FOR THE RESIDENTS' PERSONAL HYGIENE

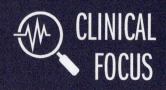

CLINICAL FOCUS

Think about ways you can assist residents in meeting their personal hygiene needs as you study this lesson.

OBJECTIVES

After studying this lesson, you should be able to:

- Define vocabulary words and terms.
- Name the parts and functions of the integumentary system.
- Review changes in the integument due to aging.
- Describe common skin conditions affecting the long-term care resident.
- Identify factors that contribute to skin breakdown.
- List actions that prevent skin breakdown.
- Explain the use of comfort and positioning devices.
- Demonstrate the following:
  - Procedure 16-21   Backrub
  - Procedure 16-22   Bed Bath Using Basin and Water
  - Procedure 16-23   Bed Bath Using a Rinse-Free Cleanser and Moisturizer
  - Procedure 16-24   Tub Bath or Shower
  - Procedure 16-25   Partial Bath
  - Procedure 16-26   Female Perineal Care
  - Procedure 16-27   Male Perineal Care
  - Procedure 16-28   Daily Hair Care

CASE STUDY

Mary Mandell is one of your residents, who is a charming lady, full of stories about growing up on an Oklahoma cattle ranch. She is right-handed. A stroke 2 years ago left her paralyzed on the right side. She is up in a wheelchair most of the day, and a small reddened area has developed over her sacrum.

VOCABULARY

axilla (ack-SILL-ah)
bridging (BRIJ-ing)
caries (KAIR-eez)
constricting (kon-STRICK-ting)
cuticle (KYOU-tih-kul)
decubiti (dee-KYOU-bih-tie)
dermis (DER-mis)
dilating (DIE-lay-ting)
dry sterile dressing (DSD) (dri STER-ill DRESS-ing)
epidermis (ep-ih-DER-mis)
friction (FRICK-shun)
genitalia (jen-ih-TAIL-ee-ah)
halitosis (hal-ih-TOH-sis)
integumentary system (in-teg-you-MEN-tair-ee SIS-tem)

keratosis (ker-a-TO-sis)
lesion (LEE-zhun)
oil gland (oil gland)
oral hygiene (OR-al HIGH-jeen)
perineal care (pair-ih-NEE-al kair)
pore (por)
pressure ulcer (PRESH-zhur UL-sir)
pubic (PYOU-bick)
receptor (ree-SEP-tor)
senile lentigines (SEE-nile len-TIJ-ih-nees)
shearing (SHEER-ing)
skin tear (skin tair)
subcutaneous tissue (sub-kyou-TAY-nee-us TISH-you)
sweat gland (swet gland)

The **integumentary system** consists of the skin, oil and sweat glands of the skin, hair, nails, teeth, and the environmental sense organs. The teeth are formed from the tissues of the integument (body shell) but also make a major contribution to the digestive system.

The outermost layers of the skin make up the **epidermis** (Figure 16-1). Under the epidermis is the **dermis**, and under the dermis is the **subcutaneous tissue** that attaches the skin to the muscles.

EPIDERMIS

The epidermis consists of dead outer cells that are constantly shed as new cells move upward from the dermis. There are no blood vessels in the epidermis, so injury to this level does not produce bleeding. Nerve endings reach into this outer covering. The nerves form sense organs that keep us in contact with changes

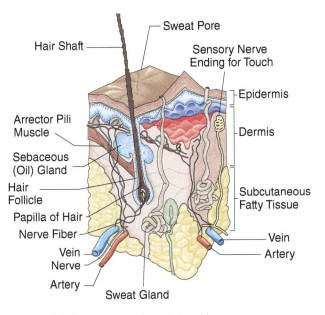

Figure 16-1   Cross-section of the skin.

in the environment. Nerve endings called receptors receive information about temperature, pressure, and pain.

DERMIS

The dermis contains blood vessels, nerve fibers, and two kinds of glands:

- Sweat glands
- Oil glands
- Hair follicles

Sweat Glands

Sweat glands are widely spread over the body, with the greatest concentration on the palms of the hands, the soles of the feet, and the forehead.

The sweat glands produce perspiration that reaches the skin surface through tubes or ducts that end in openings called pores. Heat from deep in the body is brought to the skin by blood vessels. At the skin surface, the perspiration and the heat are lost through the pores to the air. The heat of the body is controlled by changes in the size of the blood vessels in the skin.

- Dilating (enlarging) blood vessels bring more heat to the body surface.
- Constricting (narrowing) blood vessels bring less heat to the body surface.

Oil Glands

Oil glands lubricate and keep flexible the hairs found in the skin. Hair covers almost all the body surfaces except for the palms of the hands and the soles of the feet.

Hair Follicles

The hair follicle regulates hair growth.

SKIN FUNCTIONS

The skin has many functions that are critical to the well-being of the body:

- Protection—forms a continuous membranous covering and regulates body temperature
- Storage—stores fat and vitamins
- Elimination—loses water, salts, and heat through perspiration
- Sensory perceptions—contains nerve endings that keep us aware of environmental changes

? EXERCISE 16-1

COMPLETION

Identify the areas indicated in the diagram by writing in the names of the structures shown in the accompanying figure in the space provided.

1. _____
2. _____
3. _____
4. _____
5. _____

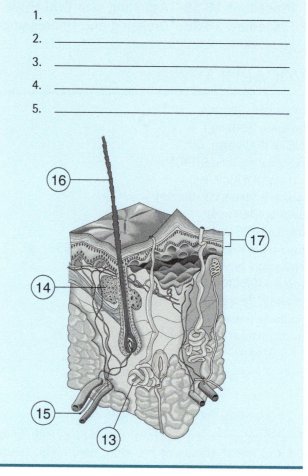

SKIN CHANGES CAUSED BY AGING

Common Changes in the Aging Skin

As people age, changes occur in the integumentary system (Figure 16-2). These changes include:

- Sweat glands decrease in activity and number.
- Loss of elasticity and fatty tissue causes wrinkling. The eyelids tend to droop.
- The skin becomes drier as oil gland secretions decrease, and it becomes thin like tissue paper.
- Areas of pigmentation seem more pronounced. In light-skinned people, the skin becomes more sallow or yellow and less pink. Skin tags and moles are more common.

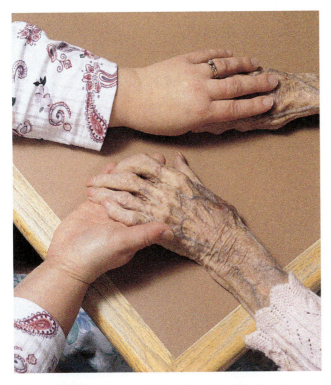

Figure 16-2   Look carefully at the skin of the hands of the nursing assistant and the resident. Note the aging changes in the skin of the resident.

- The hair loses its color, becoming first gray and then white. Less oil causes the hair to become drier and duller. The amount of hair, especially in men, diminishes.
- Nails on both fingers and toes thicken, becoming more brittle and likely to split. They also may become yellow due to **keratosis** (thickened, horny-like growth).
- Peripheral blood vessels weaken. These are more easily seen under the thinned epidermis. Small hemorrhages occur due to the weakness of the blood vessels. Peripheral circulation to the skin decreases so that general skin nutrition is less satisfactory.

Injury and Healing

The skin is exposed to the environment and is constantly in danger of trauma and infection. The skin of the older adult is fragile because of aging changes. Injuries to the skin of older adults are slower to heal. Compared to younger people, the skin receives less blood flow and, as a result, fewer nutrients to help the healing process.

Caution is always required when caring for older persons to prevent injury to the skin. Bathing, dressing, positioning, and bed making (occupied bed) are all situations in which older persons may experience skin injuries if the nursing assistant is not careful. Use care when transferring residents from the bed and wheelchair as these transfers may lead to injury.

SKIN LESIONS

Changes in the structure of the skin are called **lesions**. The lesions may be caused by the aging process, disease, trauma, or wear. It is the nursing assistant's responsibility to observe the residents carefully. Observations about the condition of the skin and changes in the skin are important. Any changes noted should be reported immediately and described accurately. The following types of lesions are discussed: skin cancer, senile lentigines, skin breakdown, and pressure ulcers.

Skin Cancer

Cancers of the skin are fairly common in the older individual. Be sure to report any changes you note in the size or shape of a wart or mole or indications of inflammation (redness) around the area of a wart or mole. Skin cancer can also appear as an area of darkened pigmentation in the skin. Skin that has been exposed to the sun for long periods of time over the years is susceptible to skin cancer. The earlier any changes noted are reported, the earlier treatment can begin.

Senile Lentigines

Areas of skin pigmentation seem to become more pronounced with advancing years. **Senile lentigines** (Figure 16-3) are sometimes called liver spots although they are not related to liver function. They are thought to be a response to environmental exposure. They appear as yellowish or brownish spots on exposed skin surfaces.

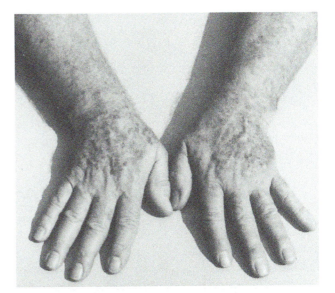

Figure 16-3   Senile lentigines.

A professional evaluation may be needed to determine if a lesion is a relatively harmless senile lentigine or an early indication of skin cancer.

Skin Breakdown

Friction, shearing, pressure, poor nutrition, and moisture are common causes of skin breakdown. **Friction** occurs when the skin moves against a firm or rough surface, including bed linens, wheelchair parts, a crutch or brace, or tubing, such as a nasogastric tube or urinary catheter (Figure 16-4). Friction also occurs when parts of the body rub together, for example, ankles or knees rubbing against each other. The rubbing action may cause skin abrasions that can lead to deeper tissue injury.

Shearing occurs when the skin moves in one direction while the structures under the skin, such as the bones, remain fixed or move in the opposite direction. This can happen when residents are dragged rather than lifted up in bed, when positions are changed, or when residents slide down in bed or in a wheelchair (Figure 16-5). Blood vessels become twisted and stretched, causing the tissues being served to lose essential oxygen and nutrients, leading to breakdown. In addition, shearing may cause actual tears in fragile skin. These **skin tears** are painful, a portal of entry for infectious pathogens, and commonly lead to further breakdown, which may be difficult to heal.

When pressure is put on tissues for a long time, skin breakdown can occur. The tissues are usually trapped between a bony prominence such as the heel, hip bone, or sacrum and the source of the pressure. The pressure causes the collapse of tiny blood vessels.

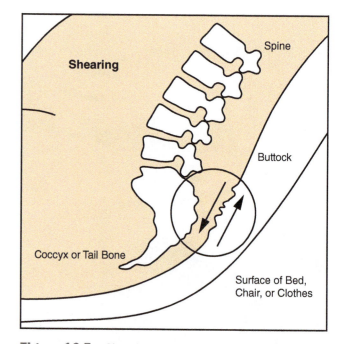

Figure 16-5   Shearing can occur when the resident's position is poorly supported. As the resident slides down in bed or in a chair, the skeleton remains stationary but the skin slips, causing tension both on the skin and on the underlying blood vessels, leading to tissue damage.

Skin surfaces receiving less nourishment through the damaged vessels quickly break down, sometimes in as little as 15 minutes of constant, uninterrupted pressure.

⊘ON THE JOB

Residents often slip from proper alignment after you have positioned them properly. Check frequently to make sure correct position is maintained.

Pressure Ulcers

Skin breakdown may progress to the formation of deep, painful lesions called **pressure ulcers** (also known as **decubiti**). They are a serious problem, especially for older adults. Residents are assessed by the interdisciplinary team for the probability of developing pressure ulcers. A care plan is developed with specific actions to prevent the formation of pressure ulcers. In some facilities, this activity is performed by a nurse who is specially trained in skin and wound care. Pressure ulcers can form in as little as 15 minutes and after 2 hours of pressure, may be difficult to ever heal, depending on the health of the resident.

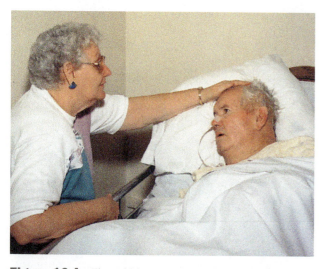

Figure 16-4   The rubbing of nasal catheters, nasogastric tubes, or urinary catheters can cause skin breakdown.

Factors Leading to Breakdown

Pressure ulcers can frequently be prevented by conscientious care and attention. Nursing assistants must be alert to the factors that contribute to their formation, including:

- Being older
- Being bedridden
- Having fragile skin
- Impaired circulation due to chronic disease such as diabetes or vascular disease
- Impaired circulation due to pressure
- Prolonged contact with moisture
- Prolonged contact with excretions/secretions
- Poor nutrition and debilitation

- Dehydration
- Shearing forces and friction
- Immobility
- Incontinence (fecal or urinary)

Signs of Tissue Breakdown

Tissue breakdown is described and classified in four stages. Unless action is taken, the damage is progressive and sometimes irreversible (Figure 16-6).

1. Stage one: The intact skin surface shows redness or blue-gray discoloration over a pressure point, which does not disappear after 30 minutes when the pressure is removed (Figure 16-6). In darker-skinned persons, the area may seem drier, and when applying pressure it may become darker or

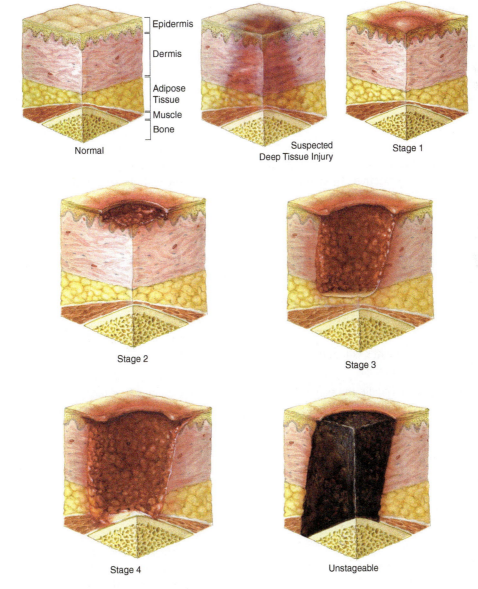

Figure 16-6   Pressure ulcer stages.

purplish in color, and feel warm to the touch. This is an early warning sign to take preventive action.

2. Stage two: The reddened skin is broken and may be accompanied by an abrasion, blisters, or a shallow crater (Figure 16-6). The epidermis alone or the dermis may be involved. The area around the site is reddened; the area looks like an abrasion. A stage two ulcer is easily treatable.

3. Stage three: All layers of skin are broken down. The ulcer extends to the deeper subcutaneous tissues and a deep crater is formed (Figure 16-6). Some stage three ulcers are difficult to heal; and may have a bad odor. It may take up to 1 year to heal completely and there is risk of infection.

4. Stage four: The ulcer extends to the deeper tissues, into the muscle, and sometimes to the ligaments, bones, and joints. At this stage, residents experience fluid loss and are at great risk for infection (Figure 16-6). Treatment involves extensive medical and sometimes surgical therapy.

5. Unstageable: If you cannot see the base of the ulcer, it cannot be staged.

Actions to Take When Breakdown Occurs

It is easier to prevent skin breakdown than to treat the results. It is also more cost-effective. Residents with existing skin breakdown may be admitted to the long-term care facility from home or another health care facility. At other times, despite careful preventive care, skin breakdown occurs. In these situations, the nursing assistant actions include:

- Performing the actions listed in the guidelines to prevent further breakdown
- Following the care plan exactly
- Reporting indications of infection, such as fever, odor, drainage, bleeding, and changes in size
- Keeping the area around the breakdown clean and dry
- Assisting with whirlpool baths, if ordered, to keep the area clean

The nurse or physician may perform other procedures to care for areas of skin breakdown. For example:

- The area may be covered with a **dry sterile dressing (DSD)**. Holding a DSD in place without causing additional injury is not easy. The skin of older adults may be sensitive to regular tape. In this case, silk tape, paper tape, cellophane tape, or other hypoallergenic tape may be used. To prevent injury when removing the tape before a dressing change, a saline solution is applied to loosen the tape.
- Residents may be placed on alternating-pressure mattresses or pressure-reducing mattresses or beds.
- In some facilities, the open lesions are packed loosely with gauze soaked in a wound gel. The gel keeps the lesions moist, breaks down dead cells, and promotes healing.

⚠ GUIDELINES FOR... PREVENTING SKIN BREAKDOWN

Nursing assistant actions are vital in identifying potential causes of breakdown and taking steps to eliminate or minimize them.

1. Carefully inspect the resident's skin during care and report findings to the nurse.

2. Bathe resident regularly. Handle the skin gently and use a mild cleansing agent. Avoid hot water and do not scrub the skin. Dry thoroughly by patting the skin with the towel. Closely inspect potential pressure or friction areas.

3. Immediately remove feces, urine, or moisture of any kind, including perspiration, from the resident's skin. Prolonged contact is irritating to the skin. Keep the skin clean and dry. Use barrier protection ointments as directed.

4. Use underpads or briefs that absorb moisture, to help keep the resident dry.

5. Use lotion on dry skin areas but do not use on broken skin. Pat lotion on skin gently; do not rub vigorously.

6. Encourage good nutrition and adequate fluid intake.

7. Change the position of a bed-bound resident at least every 2 hours to reduce pressure in any one area. Some residents may need repositioning more often than others. The care plan for each resident must be followed carefully. The turning schedule will be posted in the care plan and in the room. Figure 16-7 shows an example of the sequence of turns.

8. Keep bed linens wrinkle-free and free of crumbs (food or powder).

9. Encourage residents sitting in geri-chairs or wheelchairs to raise themselves or change position to relieve pressure every 15 minutes. This is referred to as "off-loading." If the resident is

(continues)

⚠ GUIDELINES FOR... PREVENTING SKIN BREAKDOWN (Continued)

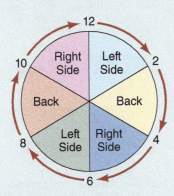

Figure 16-7 Example of a turning schedule with a position change every 2 hours.

not able to do so, assist the resident in repositioning at least every hour.

10. Check for improperly fitted or worn braces, shoes, and restraints that may rub the skin.

11. Check nasogastric tubes and urinary catheters to be sure they are positioned so they do not irritate the skin. Keep nasal and urinary openings clean and free of drainage. These areas must be checked frequently and carefully.

12. Do passive range of motion exercises twice daily or as directed by the nursing supervisor.

13. Use a bed protector to help move dependent residents in bed. Some residents may be able to help reposition themselves in bed by using a trapeze. Do not drag the resident over the bed linens to avoid shearing and friction. *Shearing* occurs when the skin moves in one direction while the underlying bony structures moves in another direction;

the skin rubbing against the surface of the sheets may cause *friction* and damage the skin.

14. Do not elevate the head of the bed too high. This may cause shearing of tissues as the resident slides down in bed. An elevation of no more than 30 degrees is recommended for residents who are at risk for pressure ulcers.

15. Separate body areas that are likely to rub together, especially over bony prominences, by using pillows or foam wedges, according to the care plan. Prevent irritation under fat folds or between skin surfaces that touch such as under the breasts, between the toes, or between fleshy thighs. Separate the skin surfaces with a layer of clothing, if possible.

16. For residents sitting in wheelchairs, use foam, gel, or air cushions to reduce pressure on buttocks and sacrum.

17. For residents in bed, relieve pressure on heels by floating the heels off the bed by using a pillow properly placed beneath the ankles. Heels should not touch the pillow.

18. Use special pressure-reducing mattresses or alternating-pressure mattresses for residents in bed.

19. Report signs of infection, such as fever, odor, drainage, inflammation, pain, or bleeding to the nurse.

20. OBRA and The Joint Commission (TJC) require that the health care team develop an individualized care plan to prevent pressure ulcers in residents at risk.

❓ EXERCISE 16-2

BRIEF ANSWERS

1. List five general nursing assistant actions that support wound healing.

    a. _____
    _____

    b. _____
    _____

    c. _____
    _____

    d. _____
    _____

    e. _____
    _____

- The area may be protected and kept moist by using special dressings. They have a clear plastic covering that permits air to reach the tissues as well as keeping them moist to promote healing. The dressing must extend beyond the wound edge. It is held in place with a frame of either paper or silk tape. The dressing must be changed every 3 to 5 days unless there is leakage, or according to facility policy.

- The wounds may be cleaned by the nurse or physician with saline solution and debrided (dead tissue removed) using instruments and proteolytic enzymes.

- Antiseptic sprays, antibiotic ointments, barrier creams, and dressings are used to prevent skin breakdown and control infection. Any creams or ointments that contain medications must be administered only by the medication or treatment nurse.

- Wound VAC (vacuum-assisted closure) or negative pressure wound therapy (NPWT) is a system that promotes healing at the wound site through the use of special patented dressings and a vacuum system that helps to remove any infectious material and promote healing.

- Surgery may be needed to close the ulcerated area in severe cases.

Residents are encouraged to participate to whatever extent is possible in their own care. Attentive nursing care is essential in preventing skin breakdown. Remember that it is far easier to prevent pressure ulcers than to heal them.

Blood Circulation to Tissues

Ensuring adequate circulation to tissues is a major factor in preventing skin breakdown. This can be accomplished by:

- Positioning the resident properly, avoiding pressure on bony prominences
- Using mechanical aids

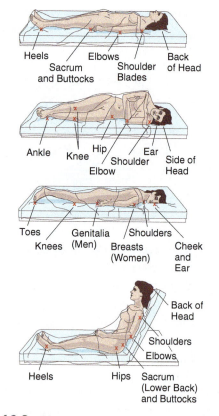

Figure 16-8   Most common sites for skin breakdown.

- Providing gentle backrubs
- Performing active or passive range of motion exercises
- The most common sites for skin breakdown are shown in Figure 16-8.

Positioning

Five basic in-bed positions are used to relieve pressure as the resident's condition permits. Each position must be supported for comfort. The nursing assistant must remember that not all residents can assume the full range of positions, because of disabilities such as arthritis,

---

? EXERCISE 16-3

MATCHING

1.   Match the characteristics of each stage of tissue breakdown and the appropriate nursing assistant actions.

ACTIONS STAGE CHARACTERISTICS

a.   _____ an early warning sign to take preventive action

b.   _____ difficult to heal at this stage of skin surface over pressure point

c.   _____ very treatable at this stage

d.   _____ fluid loss and great risk of infection

I redness—blue-gray discoloration

II red skin—blisterlike lesion

III subcutaneous tissue breakdown

IV breakdown involves deeper tissues (muscles and bones)

contractures, or breathing limitations. Residents who sit in geri-chairs or wheelchairs for long periods of time must also change position to relieve pressure.

Residents with special problems require extra care when they are positioned in bed. For example:

- Be sure the resident can breathe properly.
- Remember that a fractured hip is never rotated over the unaffected leg.
- If the resident had a stroke, elevate the weak arm to reduce edema.
- Always maintain proper body alignment.
- The resident with a recent stroke is turned on the unaffected side.

The five basic positions residents assume in bed are:

- Supine position (back-lying)
- Prone position (lying on back)

- Lateral position (side-lying)
- Sims or semi-prone position
- Fowler's position (semi-sitting)
- These positions are described fully and illustrated in Lesson 22 on restorative care.

Mechanical Aids

Mechanical aids are used to reduce pressure. Examples are:

- Sheepskin pads (or artificial sheepskin)
- Foam pads, pillows, and wedges
- Protectors for areas such as heels and elbows (Figures 16-9 and 16-10) that are subject to friction as the resident moves in bed
- Bed cradles (foot cradles)

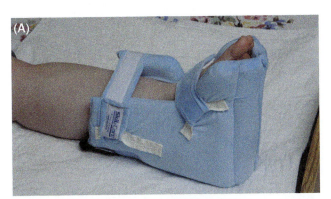

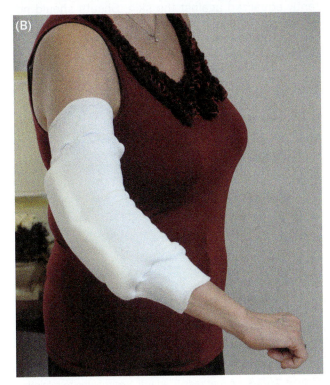

Figure 16-9   (A) Heel protector, (B) elbow protector.

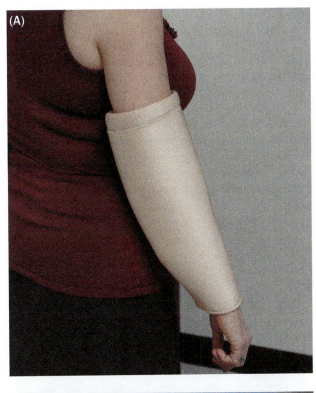

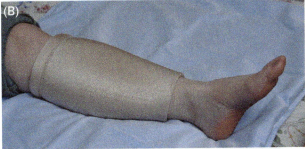

Figure 16-10   (A) Skin sleeves offer excellent skin protection against skin tears and bruises. (B) Leg protectors are also available.

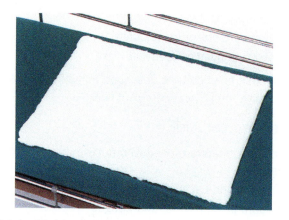

Figure 16-11   A soft, synthetic fleece pad takes pressure off the back.
Courtesy of J. T. Posey Company, Arcadia, CA

- Alternating pressure mattresses
- Flotation mattresses
- Pillows
- Gel-filled mattresses

Sheepskin Pads (or Artificial Sheepskin)
These absorb moisture and reduce friction when placed under the resident (Figure 16-11).

Foam Pads and Pillows
These are used to bridge areas to reduce pressure. Watch residents for signs of disorientation that might be caused by the feeling of weightlessness. Adequate fluid intake to prevent urinary stasis must be provided and conscientious range of motion exercises must be carried out. Rubber or hard doughnut-shaped pads are not effective and rarely used. Although they shield the affected areas, they create pressure by their own shape.

Bed (Foot) Cradles
These devices can lift the weight of bedding but must be carefully positioned and may be padded, because injury can occur if the resident strikes them (Figure 16-12).

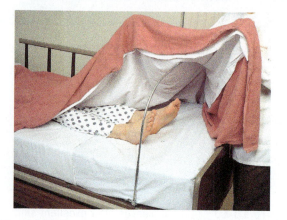

Figure 16-12   A bed cradle keeps the sheet and blanket from putting pressure on the feet.

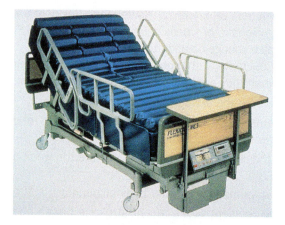

Figure 16-13   Alternating air pressure mattress overlay. Alternating air pressure in the mattress cells changes pressure points against the resident's skin and gently massages the skin.
Courtesy of Hill-Rom, Charlestown, SC

Alternating-Pressure Mattress (Air Mattress)
This type of mattress (Figure 16-13) is used in some facilities. Air pressure is reduced in a different area of the mattress on an alternating basis. The pressure alteration reduces pressure against the body so that no skin area is continuously subjected to pressure.

Flotation Mattress
This mattress (Figure 16-14) is a water bed with controlled temperature. The weight of the resident's body displaces water to the extent that pressure is consistently equalized against the skin. Sheets should not be tucked tightly over the flotation mattress because this will restrict the function of the mattress.

Special Equipment
Specialized beds or over lays are available for residents who need continuous pressure relief. One type of bed is the Clinitron bed (Figure 16-15). It is filled with a

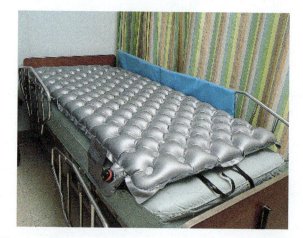

Figure 16-14   A mattress filled with water helps to minimize pressure points on the body.

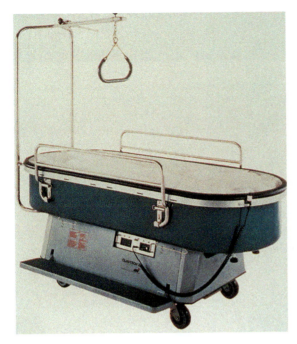

Figure 16-15   Clinitron® air-fluidized mattress.
Courtesy of Hill-Rom, Batesville, IN

sandlike material. Warm, dry air circulates through the material to maintain an even temperature and support the body evenly.

Gel-Filled Mattress

The gel in this type of mattress has a consistency similar to body fat. It allows for a more equal distribution of body weight by conforming to the body contours.

Pillows

Pillows are used in a technique called **bridging**. In bridging, body parts are supported by pillows in such a way that spaces are left to relieve pressure on specific areas.

Each of these aids reduces pressure, but nothing can take the place of nursing observation and care.

BACKRUB

Regular back care is given after the bath. It may also be given after use of the bedpan or after changing a resident's position. When performed properly, with long, smooth, gentle strokes, it stimulates the resident's circulation and aids in preventing skin breakdown. It is also soothing and refreshing and provides positive human contact. (See Procedure 16-21.)

BATHING RESIDENTS

A complete bath two or three times a week will maintain cleanliness. Too frequent bathing can lead to skin dryness and itching. Many facilities require a

---

? EXERCISE 16-4

BRIEF ANSWERS

1. Refer to the figures below. Using both figures, draw a circle around at least eight areas at risk for the development of pressure ulcers.

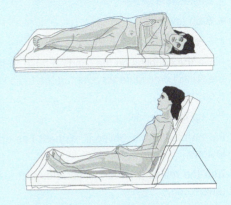

2. Briefly explain why the areas you have circled are most prone to breakdown.

_____

_____

3. List six mechanical aids that might be used to reduce pressure.

a. _____

_____

b. _____

_____

c. _____

_____

d. _____

_____

e. _____

_____

f. _____

_____

---

daily partial bath. Incontinent residents are bathed as often as necessary.

Bathing may be performed as:

- Complete bed bath
- Partial bed bath
- Perineal care
- Tub bath
- Shower bath
- Whirlpool bath
- Therapeutic

PROCEDURE 16-21
Backrub

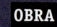 OBRA

1. Carry out each beginning procedure action.
2. Assemble equipment:
   - Disposable gloves
   - Bath towel
   - Soap and lotion
3. Place the supplies on the overbed table. Follow the facility procedure for covering the table with a barrier.
4. Put up far side rail.
5. Put on disposable gloves if resident has open lesions.
6. Turn the resident on his or her side with back toward you.
7. Expose and wash back, dry carefully. This step is not necessary if backrub is given after a bath.

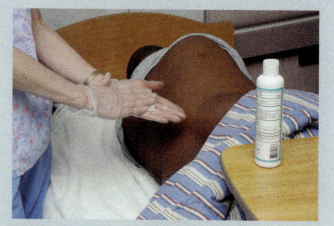

Figure 16-16 Warm lotion between your hands.

8. Pour a small amount of lotion into one hand; warm the lotion between your hands (Figure 16-16).
9. Apply to skin and rub with gentle but firm strokes. Give special attention to all bony prominences (Figure 16-17).
10. Begin at base of spine:
    - With long, soothing strokes rub up the center of back, around the shoulders, and down sides of back and buttocks (Figure 16-18, left).

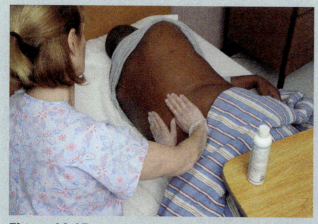

Figure 16-17 Use long, smooth strokes as you apply the lotion.

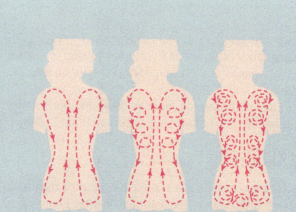

Figure 16-18 Strokes to be used during the backrub.

- Repeat previous step four times, using long, soothing upward strokes and circular motion on downstroke (Figure 16-18, middle).
- Repeat, but on downward stroke rub in small circular motions with palm of hand. Include areas over coccyx (over base of spine) (Figure 16-18, right).
- Repeat long, soothing strokes on muscles for 3 to 5 minutes (Figure 16-18, left).

(continues)

PROCEDURE 16-21
Backrub (Continued)

- Dry area well.
- If redness on pressure areas is noted, report to nurse. Straighten and tighten bottom sheet and bed protector (if used).

11. Change resident's gown if needed.
12. Replace equipment.
13. Carry out each procedure completion action.

? EXERCISE 16-5

BRIEF ANSWERS

1. Refer to the figures below and draw each type of stroke specified.

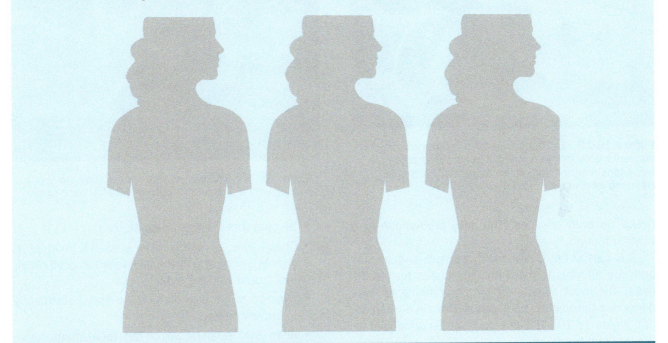

⊘N THE JOB

The odor of a facility reveals much about how carefully personal care is being provided for the residents.

During bathing, special attention should be given to skin areas that touch, including:

- Between the legs
- Under the arms
- Under the breasts
- Under the scrotum
- Between the buttocks
- Around the anus
- For obese people, under folds of skin or fat
- Between the toes

Gently sponge and thoroughly pat these areas dry. Rubbing areas dry will cause chafing which can result in bleeding. Follow facility policy for the use of powder. Apply powder sparingly so that it does not

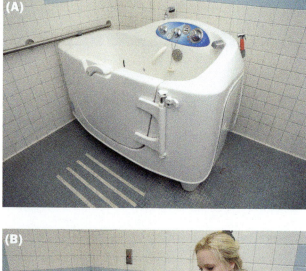

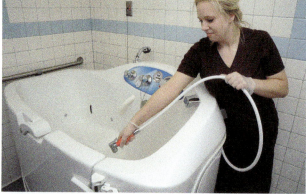

Figure 16-19   (A) This tub water circulates around the resident's body to give a mild therapeutic massage that helps tone muscles and relieve tension. (B) It is also cleansed after use.

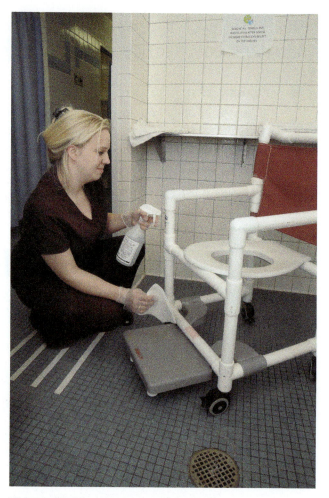

Figure 16-20   The shower and shower chair are cleansed with a disinfectant before and after each use.

"cake" in body crevices. This may predispose to a yeast infection.

A partial bath, bed bath, and tub and shower bath are all ways to meet resident needs for cleanliness. The most stimulating form of bathing for residents is a therapeutic bath that is given in a whirlpool tub (Figure 16-19). The whirlpool bath is beneficial for the resident because:

1. The temperature of the water can be regulated to an optimum 97°F.
2. The movement of the water stimulates circulation.
3. Being surrounded by warm circulating water is relaxing and invigorating.

Safety Issues

General safety issues must be considered when giving a tub or shower bath:

- The tub or shower must be clean before and after use (Figure 16-20).

- Be sure that there is adequate help.
- Check that all safety aids such as hand rails, shower seats, and hydraulic lifts are in good repair and proper working order.
- Wipe up all water spilled on the floor immediately to prevent falls.
- Keep the temperature of the room comfortable and the area free of drafts.
- Wear gloves if there may be contact with open lesions, body fluids, mucous membranes, or the perineum.
- Observe the skin for any changes or irregularities. Do not disturb or injure any warts or moles. Report anything unusual.
- Protect the resident from fatigue by transporting the resident to and from the tub room and carrying out the bathing procedure as efficiently as possible.
- Use good body mechanics to protect yourself and the resident.

- Use a bath thermometer to be sure the temperature of the water is correct. If a bath thermometer is not available, test the water with your wrist or elbow. (See Procedures 16-22 to 16-24.)

Waterless Bed Bathing

Some facilities use a bathing system that uses a rinse-free cleanser and moisturizer rather than the usual basin

PROCEDURE 16-22
Bed Bath Using Basin and Water

OBRA

1. Carry out each beginning procedure action.
2. Assemble equipment (Figure 16-21).
   - Disposable gloves (for perineal care)
   - Bed linen
   - Bath blanket
   - Laundry bag or hamper
   - Bath basin
   - Bath thermometer, if used
   - Soap and soap dish
   - Washcloth
   - Face towel
   - Two bath towels
   - Facility gown or the resident's clothes
   - Lotion
   - Equipment for oral hygiene
   - Nail brush, emery board, and orangewood stick (if available)
   - Brush and comb
   - Bedpan and cover or urinal

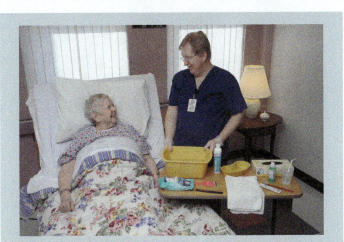

Figure 16-21 Assemble equipment for bed bath.

3. Close the door and windows to prevent chilling the resident.
4. Close privacy curtain.
5. Put towels and linen on chair in order of use.
6. Place laundry hamper so that it is convenient.
7. Offer bedpan or urinal. Put on gloves if resident wants to use bedpan or urinal. Empty and clean before proceeding with bath. Return to storage. Remove gloves and discard according to facility policy. Perform hand hygiene.
8. Put on disposable gloves (if facility requires or resident has open lesions).
9. Lower the back of bed and side rails on side you are working. Be sure opposite side is up.
10. Loosen top bedclothes. If blanket is to be reused, remove it from bed, fold it, and place it over the back of the chair. Otherwise, place bath blanket over top bedclothes and remove top bedclothes by sliding them out from under the bath blanket. Place in laundry hamper.
11. Leave one pillow under resident's head. Place other pillow on chair.
12. Remove resident's nightwear or clothing and place in laundry hamper.
13. Fill bath basin two-thirds full with water at 105–110°F or according to agency policy. Use a bath thermometer if available or test water on your wrist or with your elbow. The water should feel comfortably warm.
14. Assist resident to move to the side of the bed nearest you.

(continues)

PROCEDURE 16-22
Bed Bath Using Basin and Water (Continued)

15.　Fold face towel over upper edge of bath blanket to keep blanket dry.

16.　Form a mitten by holding washcloth around hand (Figure 16-22). Wet washcloth; wash eyes, using separate corners of cloth for each eye. Do not use soap near eyes.

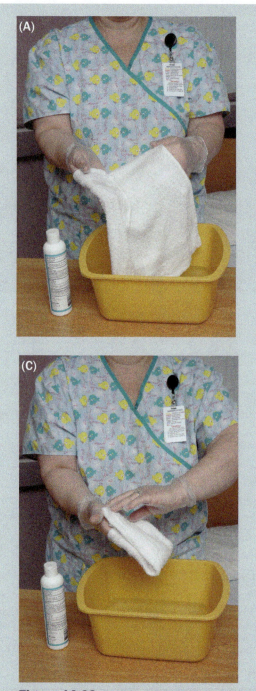
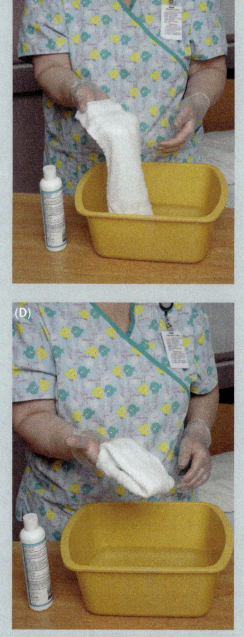

Figure 16-22 To make bath mitt, wrap the washcloth around one hand (A). Then bring the free-end back over palm (B) and tuck in the end (C). Thumb is free to hold washcloth in place (D). *Note:* If gloves are used in the procedure, make the bath mitt over the glove.

PROCEDURE 16-22
Bed Bath Using Basin and Water (Continued)

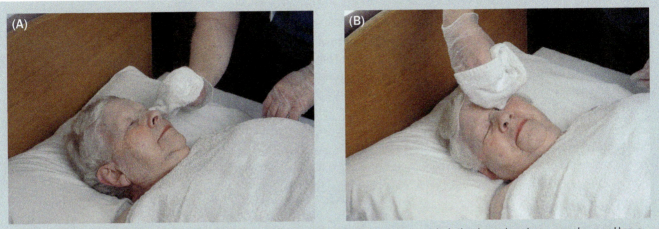

Figure 16-23 Wash face carefully, doing eyes separately. Do not use soap on washcloth when cleaning around eyes. Use a different area of wash cloth for each stroke.

17. Rinse washcloth and apply soap if resident desires. Squeeze out excess water.

18. Wash and rinse resident's face, ears, and neck (Figure 16-23). Use towel to pat dry.

19. Expose resident's far arm. Protect bed with bath towel placed under arm. Wash, rinse, and dry arm and hand. Make sure to pat, and not rub, the skin surfaces until they are thoroughly dry. Be sure **axilla** (armpit) is clean and dry. Apply deodorant if resident agrees. Repeat for other arm.

20. If necessary, care for hands and nails as follows:

    a. Place each hand in basin and soak for 10 minutes before proceeding with nail care to prevent damage to skin and cuticles. While hand is soaking in basin, wash each hand carefully.

    b. Rinse and dry. Push back cuticle (base of fingernails) gently with towel while wiping the fingers. Be sure to dry the areas between the fingers.

    c. Clean under nails with orangewood stick and shape with emery board. Be careful not to file nails too close. If resident is diabetic, inform the nurse if nail care is needed.

21. Discard used bath water and refill basin two-thirds full with water at 105°F.

22. Put bath towel over resident's chest, and then fold blanket to waist. Under towel, wash with soap, rinse, and dry chest. Rinse and dry under breasts of female resident. Wash carefully to avoid irritating skin.

23. Fold bath blanket down to **pubic** area. Wash with soap, rinse, and dry abdomen. Replace bath blanket over abdomen and chest. Slide towel out from under bath blanket.

24. Ask resident to flex far knee if possible. Fold bath blanket up to expose thigh, leg, and foot. Protect bed with bath towel, and put bath basin on towel. Place resident's foot in basin (Figure 16-24). Wash and rinse leg and foot. When moving leg, support leg properly.

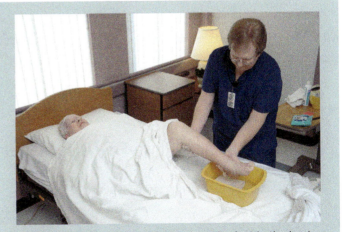

Figure 16-24 Support leg and place the foot in the basin.

(continues)

PROCEDURE 16-22
Bed Bath Using Basin and Water (Continued)

25. Lift leg and move basin to other side of bed. Dry leg and foot. Dry well between toes.

26. Repeat for other leg and foot. Take basin from bed before drying leg and foot.

27. Care for toenails as necessary. File nails straight across. Do not round edges. Do not push back the cuticle because it is easily injured and infected. Apply lotion to feet of resident with dry skin, except between toes. Observe toenails carefully so that you can report condition of nails to nurse. If resident is diabetic, inform nurse if toenail care is needed. Many facilities contract with a podiatrist who cares for toenails and feet of diabetics.

28. Discard used bath water and refill basin two-thirds full with water at 105–110°F. Several water changes are suggested in this procedure, but you may need to change water more often.

29. Help resident to turn on side away from you and to move toward center of bed. Place towel lengthwise next to resident's back. Wash, rinse, and dry neck, back, and buttocks. Use long, firm strokes when washing back.

30. A backrub is usually given at this time. (See Procedure 16-21.)

31. Help resident turn on back.

32. Place towel under buttocks and upper legs. Place washcloth, soap, basin, and bath towel within convenient reach of resident. Instruct resident to wash **genitalia**, assisting if necessary. (You must assume responsibility for this procedure if resident has difficulty. Residents often are reluctant to acknowledge the need for help. Wear gloves when assisting.) When assisting a female resident, always wash from front to back, drying carefully. When assisting a male resident, carefully wash and dry penis, scrotum, and groin area. If male is uncircumcised, gently push foreskin back and carefully wash and dry penis. Then gently pull foreskin down when you are finished. Ask the resident to turn to the side so that you can wash, rinse, and dry the buttocks and anal area. Remove gloves (if used) and discard according to facility policy. Perform hand hygiene.

33. Carry out range of motion exercises as ordered.

34. Cover pillow with towel and comb or brush hair. Oral hygiene is usually given at this time. (See Procedures later in this lesson.)

35. Place used towels and washcloth in hamper.

36. Provide clean gown or clothing.

37. Clean and replace equipment, according to facility policy.

38. Change bed linen, following occupied bed procedure. Put soiled linen in laundry hamper.

39. Remove and discard disposable gloves according to facility policy. Perform hand hygiene.

40. Raise side rails if used for positioning.

41. Carry out each procedure completion action.

NOTE: It may be easier to do the nail care following completion of the bath. See Items 20 and 27.

PROCEDURE 16-23
Bed Bath Using a Rinse-Free Cleanser and Moisturizer

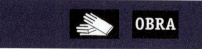

1. Carry out each beginning procedure action.

2. Assemble equipment:
   - Waterless bathing product
   - Towel

(continues)

PROCEDURE 16-23
Bed Bath Using a Rinse-Free Cleanser and Moisturizer (Continued)

(Use a package of eight washcloths for a full bath or a four-pack for a partial bath. Packages may be resealed and dated if you do not use the whole pack. Do not use a previously opened package after 72 hours or if the cloths are dry.)

3. Follow steps 3 through 12 of the regular bed bath procedure (Procedure 16-22).

4. Open pack of cloths. Extract one, make a mitt, and cleanse resident's face and neck (solution can safely be used around the eyes).

5. Place towel over resident's chest. Fold blanket down to waist and cleanse chest. Be sure area under breasts is carefully cleaned.

6. Fold bath blanket down to pubic area and wash abdomen. Replace bath blanket over abdomen and chest. Remove towel by sliding it out from under the bath blanket. Dispose of washing cloth per facility policy.

7. Uncover resident's far arm. Protect bed with bath towel placed under arm. Use a new cloth and wash arm and hand. Be sure axilla is clean. Apply deodorant if resident desires. Dispose of used cloth. Using another new cloth, repeat for near arm and hand.

8. Care for hands and nails as needed.

9. Ask resident to flex far knee, if possible. Fold bath blanket up to expose thigh, leg, and foot. Protect bed with bath towel. Use a new cloth and cleanse thigh, leg, and foot. Be sure area between toes is left dry. Care for toenails as needed. Remove bath towel. Cover with bath blanket.

10. Repeat with near thigh, leg, and foot.

11. Help resident move to the center of the bed and turn on side away from you. Place a bath towel lengthwise next to resident's back. Use a new cloth to cleanse neck and back, clean buttocks and rear perineal area. Dispose of cloth per facility policy. A backrub is usually given at this time. Remove towel.

12. Assist resident to turn on back. Place towel under buttocks and upper legs. Hand resident a new cloth to cleanse the perineum. Assist as necessary.

13. Complete nursing care following steps 33 through 41 of the regular bed bath.

PROCEDURE 16-24
Tub Bath or Shower

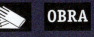 **OBRA**

1. Carry out each beginning procedure action.

2. Assemble equipment:
    - Disposable gloves
    - Soap
    - Washcloth
    - Two to three bath towels
    - Bath blanket
    - Resident's gown, robe, and slippers, or clothing
    - Bath thermometer, if used
    - Chair or stool
    - Bath mat

3. Take the supplies to the bathroom and prepare it for resident. Make sure tub is clean.

(continues)

PROCEDURE 16-24
Tub Bath or Shower (Continued)

4. Fill tub one-third full with water at 105°F or adjust shower flow. Use your elbow to test the water temperature. The water should feel comfortably warm. Assist resident to bathroom and toilet resident if needed. Assist resident with robe and slippers or clothing.

5. Help resident undress. Give resident a towel to wrap around midriff. Cover resident with bath blanket when going to and from bath or shower.

6. Assist resident into tub or shower. For resident's safety, the bottom of the tub and the shower floor are covered with a nonskid surface. In addition, a tub chair or a shower chair can be provided so the resident can sit safely while bathing. If using a tub lift chair, make sure safety straps are secure.

7. Put on disposable gloves if there are open lesions.

8. Wash the body in the same order as with the bed bath. Observe skin for signs of redness or breaks. If resident's condition permits, allow resident to assist as much as possible in the procedure. Give resident the choice of washing genitalia. If you assist with this part of the procedure, put on gloves. On completion, remove gloves and discard according to facility policy. Perform hand hygiene.

9. If resident shows any signs of weakness, remove plug and let water drain out, or turn off shower. Allow resident to rest until feeling better before making any attempt to assist him or her out of tub or shower. Keep resident covered with bath towel to avoid chilling.

10. If resident wants a shampoo and you have permission to do so:
    - Ask resident to hold washcloth over eyes.
    - Pour small amount of water on hair (enough to wet hair thoroughly).
    - Use a small amount of shampoo to lather hair.
    - Massage scalp gently.
    - Rinse hair with warm water.
    - Repeat lathering, massaging, and rinsing, if necessary.
    - Towel dry hair.

11. Hold bath blanket around resident when he or she is stepping out of tub or shower. A resident may choose to remove wet towel under bath blanket.

12. Assist resident to dry, apply deodorant, put on clean gown or clothing, and return to unit.

13. Put on gloves and clean bathtub. Remove gloves and discard according to facility policy. Perform hand hygiene. Put supplies away.

14. Carry out each procedure completion action.

---

of water and soap and a rinsing procedure (Figure 16-25). The solution-saturated cloths (eight per package) are heated in the microwave oven. After use, the skin does not require drying. The procedure is similar to that of the bed bath, with cleansing performed in the same order:

- Face, neck, and chest
- Far arm and hand
- Near arm and hand
- Far leg and foot
- Near leg and foot
- Back
- Buttocks
- Perineum

Advantages of the system include:

- Less fatigue for the resident
- Refreshing and cleansing without soap
- Less friction, because the drying step is eliminated

The following precautions are taken to prevent injury to the resident:

- Monitor temperature of the cleansing cloths carefully.

- Do not heat in the microwave for more than 1 minute.
- Discard cleansing cloths 72 hours after opening the package or immediately if they are dry.
- Label should be peeled open without completely removing it before heating the package.
- Cloths are for individual use only.
- Discard used washcloths in a plastic trash bag or according to facility policy. Do not flush the cloths down the toilet.

Partial Bath

A partial bath is cleaning of the face, hands, axillae, under the breasts of females, skin folds, buttocks, and genitalia. It is very refreshing. Many residents can help with the bath process and, whenever possible, should be encouraged to do so. (See Procedure 16-25.)

Therapeutic Bath

A therapeutic bath is one in which a specific substance is added to the water to treat a problem such as a rash. Follow the care plan's directions for the type of therapeutic bath you are giving.

Perineal Care (Peri-Care)

Perineal care is the cleaning of the genital area between the resident's legs. Keeping this area clean is

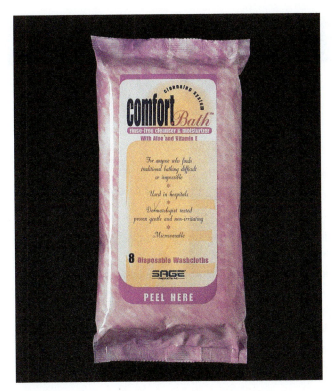

Figure 16-25 Package containing eight cleansing washcloths. Washcloths may be warmed in microwave or warmer. One cloth is used for each of the following body areas: (1) face, neck, and chest; (2) right arm; (3) left arm; (4) perineum; (5) right leg; (6) left leg; (7) back; and (8) buttocks.
Courtesy of Sage Products, Inc.

PROCEDURE 16-25
Partial Bath

OBRA

1. Carry out each beginning procedure action.
2. Assemble equipment:
   - Disposable gloves
   - Bed linen
   - Bath blanket
   - Bath thermometer, if used
   - Soap and soap dish
   - Washcloth
   - Face towel
   - Bath towel
   - Gown and robe or clothing
   - Laundry bag or hamper
   - Bath basin
   - Lotion
   - Equipment for oral hygiene

(continues)

PROCEDURE 16-25
Partial Bath (Continued)

  OBRA

- Nail brush, orangewood stick, and emery board
- Brush, comb, and deodorant
- Bedpan or urinal and cover
- Paper towels or bed protector

3. Close the door and any windows to prevent chilling resident.

4. Put towels and linen on chair, in order of use. Place laundry hamper so that it is convenient.

5. Put on disposable gloves.

6. Offer bedpan or urinal. Empty and clean before proceeding with bath. Remove gloves and discard according to facility policy. Perform hand hygiene and put on pair of new gloves.

7. Elevate head of bed, if permitted to a comfortable position if resident is assisting. Lower head of bed if nursing assistant is performing the bath.

8. Loosen top bedclothes. Remove and fold blanket and spread and place over back of chair. Place bath blanket over top sheet and remove sheet by sliding it out from under bath blanket.

9. Leave one pillow under resident's head. Place other pillow on chair.

10. Assist resident to remove gown or clothing. Place gown in laundry hamper. Wrap bath blanket around resident.

11. Place paper towels or bed protector on overbed table.

12. Fill bath basin two-thirds full with water at 105–110°F and place on overbed table.

13. Push overbed table comfortably close to resident.

14. Place towels, washcloth, and soap on overbed table within easy reach.

15. Instruct resident to wash as much as he or she is able and that you will return to complete the bath.

16. Place call light within easy reach. Ask resident to signal when ready.

17. Remove gloves and discard according to facility policy. Perform hand hygiene and leave unit.

18. Perform hand hygiene and return to unit when resident signals. Put on a new pair of gloves.

19. Change bath water. Bathe those areas the resident could not reach. Make sure the face, hands, axilla, buttocks, anal area, back, and genitalia are washed and dried.

20. Give a backrub with lotion.

21. Assist the resident in applying deodorant and fresh gown or clothing.

22. Cover pillow with towel and comb or brush hair. Assist with oral hygiene if needed.

23. Clean and replace equipment according to facility policy.

24. Change bed linen, following occupied bed procedure. Discard soiled linen in laundry hamper.

25. Remove and dispose of gloves according to facility policy.

26. Carry out each procedure completion action.

? EXERCISE 16-6

COMPLETION

Select the correct term(s) from the following list to complete each statement. Some words may be used more than once.

clean	irritating	temperature
cleanser	privacy	therapeutic

(continued)

? EXERCISE 16-6 (Continued)

constant	routine	1°F
dignity	safety	110°F
help	safety	aids

1. Beginning procedure actions ensure _____, _____, and _____ of the resident and caregiver.

2. Each beginning procedure action and each procedure completion action should become a _____ part of the care given.

3. Before and after giving a bath be sure the tub is _____.

4. Always be sure there is adequate _____ when giving a bath.

5. Check all _____ such as handrails to be sure they are in proper working order before giving a bath.

6. Always provide _____ when giving personal care such as a bath.

7. Keep the _____ of the room and water comfortable during the bathing procedure.

8. Using too much soap is unwise because it may be very _____.

9. The best temperature for bath water is _____.

10. Cleansing cloths should never be heated over _____ minute.

11. 11. Waterless bed bathing uses a rinse-free _____ and moisturizer.

12. A _____ bath has a specific substance added to the water to treat some problem.

13. List six types of bathing procedures and describe their differences.

    a. _____
       _____

    b. _____
       _____

    c. _____
       _____

    d. _____
       _____

    e. _____
       _____

    f. _____
       _____

especially important when residents are unable to control bladder and bowels. Excreta (urine or feces) left on the skin is unpleasant and uncomfortable. If left unattended, it can lead to skin breakdown.

Perineal care, sometimes referred to as peri-care, may be performed as part of general bathing or as a separate procedure as needed. (See Procedures 16-26 and 16-27.)

PROCEDURE 16-26
Female Perineal Care

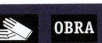 OBRA

1. Carry out each beginning procedure action.

2. Assemble equipment:

    ■ Disposable gloves

    ■ Bath blanket or topsheet

(continues)

PROCEDURE 16-26
Female Perineal Care (Continued)

- Bedpan and cover
- Soap
- Basin with warm water (105–110°F)
- Bath thermometer, if used
- Bed protector
- Washcloth and towel

3. Lower side rail on side where you will be working. Be sure opposite side rail is up and secure.

4. Remove bedspread and blanket. Fold and place on back of chair.

5. Resident is to be on back. Cover resident with bath blanket and fanfold sheet to foot of bed.

6. Put on disposable gloves.

7. Ask resident to raise hips while you place bed protector underneath resident.

8. Offer bedpan to resident. If used and resident is on intake and output, record amount. Then empty and clean the bedpan before continuing with the procedure. Remove gloves and discard according to facility policy. Perform hand hygiene and put on a new pair of gloves.

9. Position bath blanket so only the area between the legs is exposed.

10. Ask resident to separate her legs andx flex knees. *Note:* If resident is unable to spread legs and flex knees, turn the resident on her side with legs flexed. This position provides easy access to the perineal area.

11. Wet washcloth, make mitt, and apply a small amount of liquid soap. *Note:* Heavy soap application may be difficult to rinse off completely. Soap residue is irritating.

12. Use one gloved hand to stabilize and separate the vulva (Figure 16-26). With the other gloved hand, proceed as follows.

    a. Bring soaped washcloth in one downward stroke over urethra.

    b. Using a different part of the washcloth, bring the soaped washcloth in one downward stroke along the far side of the outer labia to perineum.

    c. Do not place used washcloths back in basin of water; place in the hamper. Use a new washcloth to rinse the perineum.

    d. Repeat steps b and c, washing the inner far labia.

    e. Repeat steps b and c, washing inner near labia.

    f. With gloved hands, separate labia. Rinse inner part of vulva to perineum. Repeat steps a through e.

    g. Pat area dry with towel.

13. Turn resident away from you. Flex upper leg slightly if permitted.

14. Make a mitt, wet, and apply soap lightly.

15. Expose anal area. Wash area, stroking from perineum to coccyx (front to back) (Figure 16-27).

16. Rinse well in the same manner.

17. Dry carefully.

18. Return resident to back.

Figure 16-26 Spread the vulva with one hand. With the washcloth in the other hand, start at the front and stroke downward along the outer labia.

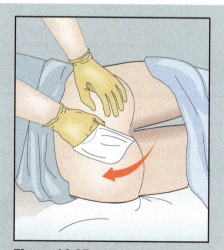

Figure 16-27 With one hand, lift up on the buttocks to expose the rectal area. Wipe from the perineum back toward the anus.

(continues)

PROCEDURE 16-26
Female Perineal Care (Continued)

19. Remove and dispose of bed protector according to facility policy.
20. Remove and dispose of gloves according to facility policy. Perform hand hygiene.
21. Cover resident with sheet.
22. Gloves should be removed after touching the perineum before touching the resident, bedding, or other items.
23. Remove, fold, and place bath blanket according to facility policy.
24. Replace top covers, tuck under mattress, and make mitered corners. (Resident may prefer that the top covers not be tucked in.)
25. Put up side rail if used for positioning.
26. Put on gloves. Empty water, clean equipment, and dispose of or store, according to facility policy.
27. Remove gloves and discard according to facility policy. Perform hand hygiene.
28. Carry out each procedure completion action.

NOTE: If your facility uses a Peri-wash solution for perineal care, follow facility protocol to carry out the procedure.

PROCEDURE 16-27
Male Perineal Care

OBRA

1. Carry out each beginning procedure action.
2. Assemble equipment:
   - Disposable gloves
   - Bath blanket
   - Bath thermometer, if used
   - Urinal and cover
   - Soap, washcloth, and towel
   - Plastic bag, laundry bag, or hamper
   - Bed protector or bath towel
   - Ordered solution (if other than water)
3. Fill basin with warm water at approximately 105–110°F.
4. Lower side rail and position bed protector (or towel) under resident's buttocks.
5. Fanfold blanket and spread to foot of bed.
6. Cover resident with bath blanket and fanfold sheet to foot of bed.
7. Put on disposable gloves.
8. Offer bedpan or urinal. If used and resident is on intake and output, record amount. Then empty and clean the bedpan or urinal before continuing with the procedure. Remove gloves and discard according to facility policy. Perform hand hygiene and put on a new pair of gloves.
9. Have resident flex and separate knees. *Note:* If the resident is unable to spread legs and flex knees, the perineal area can be washed with the resident on the side with legs flexed. This position provides easy access to the perineal area.
10. Draw bath blanket upward to expose perineal area only.
11. Make a mitt with washcloth and apply a small amount of soap. *Note:* Heavy soap application may be difficult to rinse off completely. Soap residue is irritating.

(continues)

PROCEDURE 16-27
Male Perineal Care (Continued)

12. Grasp penis gently with one hand and wash. Begin at the meatus and wash in a circular motion toward the base of the penis (Figure 16-28).

13. If resident is not circumcised, draw foreskin back (Figure 16-29). Be sure entire penis is washed. Rinse thoroughly. If uncircumcised, do not over-dry the penis to prevent skin tears when pulling the foreskin back into place.

14. Wash scrotum. Lift scrotum and wash perineum.

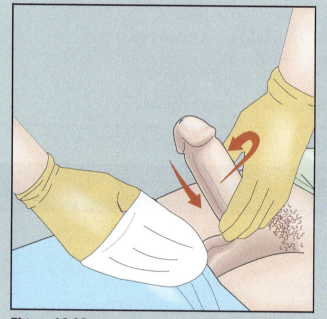

Figure 16-28 Grasp the penis gently with one hand. With the other hand, wipe in a circular motion from the glans (head) down to the base of the penis.

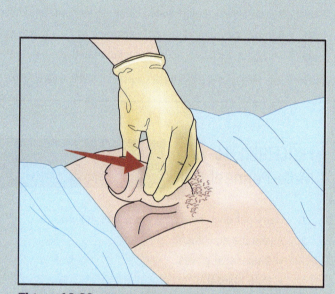

Figure 16-29 If the resident is not circumcised, gently push the foreskin back so the glans can be washed. Once the penis is washed and dried, the foreskin is returned to its normal position.

15. With a new washcloth, remake mitt, and rinse area just washed.

16. Pat dry washed area with towel. Reposition foreskin if necessary.

17. Turn resident away from you. Flex upper leg slightly if permitted.

18. Make a mitt, wet, and apply soap lightly.

19. Expose anal area. Wash area, stroking from perineum to coccyx.

20. Rinse well in the same manner.

21. Pat dry carefully.

22. Return resident to back.

23. Remove and dispose of bed protector according to facility policy.

24. Remove gloves. Perform hand hygiene.

25. Cover resident with sheet.

26. Remove blanket and place in hamper.

27. Replace top covers, tuck under mattress and make mitered corners. (Resident may prefer that the top covers not be tucked in.)

(continues)

PROCEDURE 16-27
Male Perineal Care (Continued)

28. Put up side rail if used for positioning.

29. Put on gloves. Empty water, clean equipment, and dispose of or store, according to facility policy.

30. Remove gloves and discard according to facility policy. Perform hand hygiene.

31. Carry out each procedure completion action.

HAIR CARE

Neat, attractively arranged hair contributes to a feeling of being well groomed. Daily hair care is part of the morning care but should be done whenever it is needed to keep the resident groomed. Residents should be encouraged to take care of their hair and choose the style they prefer.

In many facilities, barbers and beauticians visit once a week to cut, wash, and style the hair of residents who desire the service. Often there is a charge for the service. Normally the residents are prescheduled for their hair care. Some residents may have standing appointments every week or every 2 weeks. The nursing assistant should know which residents have hair appointments. The hair would not be washed just before the appointment.

Hair types will vary for the residents. Some persons may have thin, fine hair; others may have coarse, wiry, or curly hair. Some persons may wear their hair in tiny braids, "cornrows," whereas other may choose to wear traditional braid, and others may wear dreadlocks.

A number of special hair-care products are available. Be sure to use the appropriate product for each resident. Some will require oil-based shampoos and conditioners. African American and Asian residents may use specialized products due to the nature of their hair types. Ask the family which products are to be used. Occasionally, medicated hair products are used. Check the care plan carefully to note the appropriate product for the resident.

The hair should be combed and/or brushed each morning. Combing does require different techniques depending upon the hair type. A regular comb and brush may be used on "normal" or thin, fine hair, whereas a wide-toothed comb is easier to use on coarse, wiry, or curly hair. First section the hair, loosen the tangles by working from the end of the hair up to the scalp on each section until all tangles are removed (see Figure 16-30). Proceed to style the hair according to the resident's wishes. If the hair is long, braiding will prevent further tangling.

If the resident wears cornrows or dreadlocks, the hair may be washed without removing the braids. Never

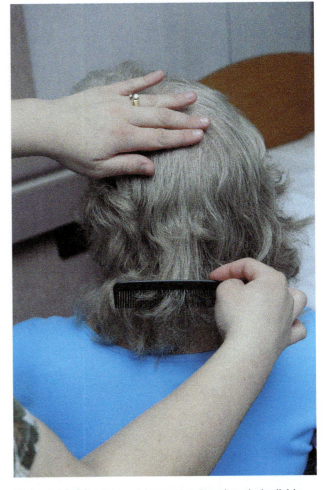

Figure 16-30 To remove tangles from long hair, divide the hair into sections. Work with one section at a time. Hold hair near the scalp to reduce pulling and start combing at the ends of the hair, working toward the scalp.

remove the cornrows or dreadlocks without the resident's or family's permission.

Some residents prefer to have their hair washed in the tub or shower. Be sure you have specific instructions. When assisting with a shampoo in the tub or shower, you must:

- Protect the resident's eyes with a washcloth
- Towel dry the hair thoroughly

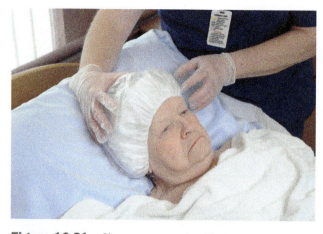

Figure 16-31   Shampoo caps simplify the hairwashing procedure for bedfast residents. The products leave the hair feeling clean and tangles are reduced.

If the resident must remain in bed and a shampoo is ordered, it can be given using a shampoo cap (Figure 16-31) or a shampoo tray. Shampoo caps are comfortable for the resident and easy to use. Warm the cap in the microwave for 30 seconds or less or in the product warmer. Place the cap on the resident's head; rub gently for 1 to 2 minutes for short hair and 4 to 5 minutes for longer hair. Then remove the cap and gently towel dry and comb the hair. Shampoo caps do not leave a residue like some dry shampoo products.

Some residents may not be able to afford the cost of shampoo caps. Most facilities have shampoo trays that can be taken to the bedside. Assemble all equipment.

- Waterproof bed protector
- Shampoo tray
- Water pitcher
- Towels and washcloth
- Shampoo and conditioner
- Basin to catch shampoo runoff

Move the resident to the side of the bed. Protect the bed and the mattress from water.

Place a shampoo tray under the resident's head so that the water drains into a basin on a chair at the bedside (see Figure 16-32). Fill a pitcher with warm water (105–110°F). Wet the hair, apply shampoo, and cleanse the hair. Rinse thoroughly to remove all shampoo residues (it may require more than one rinsing). You may need to empty the "catch" basin several times during the procedure. Proceed to towel dry and then blow dry the hair if needed. Style as preferred by the resident. Be sure there are no puddles of water on the floor to prevent falls.

When caring for the hair of an African American resident, it is important to be aware of the special needs

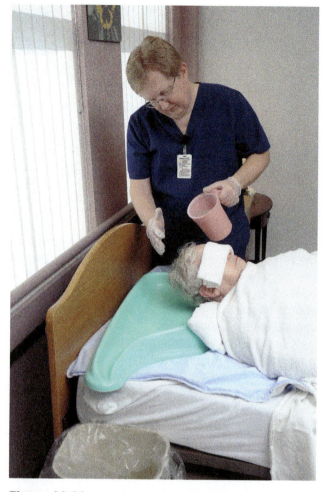

Figure 16-32   A shampoo tray is used to shampoo a resident in bed. The tray is directed to the side of the bed so water drains in a collecting dish.

related to their hair care. If possible, ask the family what hair product the resident has used at home; special products or adaptations may be needed. Avoid using products recommended for whites. These products remove too much oil from the hair and cause it to become brittle. If a shampoo designed for "black hair" is not available, use baby shampoo. Shampooing should be done no more than once a week and possibly every 2 weeks; refer to the care plan for instructions for each resident. Gently towel dry the hair after shampooing, and use a wide-tooth comb to remove tangles and snarls (see Figure 16-30). If the resident does not have a product referred to as hair "grease," apply baby oil to the scalp and gently work it through the hair with a soft brush. Remove any excess oil or grease by rubbing the hair with a dry towel. The hair should appear shiny.

If the resident's hair is braided, make sure that rubber bands are not used to secure the ends of the braids; use a hair tie or a barrette to secure the ends of the hair. If a rubber band *must* be used, liberally grease or oil the band.

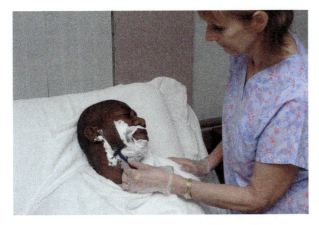

Figure 16-33 Shaving is part of the daily routine for most men.

FACIAL HAIR

Men feel better groomed when they are shaved regularly (Figure 16-33). This procedure is usually done during the morning care. For safety, use an electric razor or rotary razor. Refer to Figure 16-34 for safety considerations for shaving. Razors should never be shared between residents so it may be necessary to ask family members to provide one. Used disposable razors should be placed in the appropriate sharps container after use.

Older women have an increase in the growth and coarseness of hairs on the chin and upper lip. Many women find this distressing. Tweezers can be used to remove some of the hairs, but a more permanent method is to have the hairs removed professionally with an electric needle. Some women may require a shave. In some facilities nursing assistants are not permitted to shave women residents. Be sure to check the policy of your facility.

HAND AND FINGERNAIL CARE

Fingernails are routinely cleaned during the morning care. Use a soft brush and orangewood stick to gently clean under the nails. Fingernail care can also be carried

- Wear disposable gloves.
- Use the resident's own shaving equipment if possible. Otherwise, use disposable, one-use safety razors.
- If the resident is receiving anticoagulants, a special procedure may be required. For example, an electric razor provides the greatest safety. Check with your supervisor for the proper procedure.
- If oxygen is being given, it may be possible to discontinue it during this procedure. Consult the nurse and follow facility policy.

Figure 16-34 Special shaving precautions.

out as a separate procedure. Soak the hands in warm soapy water. Creams can be used to soften the cuticles, which can then be gently pushed back with a towel. When cutting the fingernails, follow the curve of the finger and then file any rough edges. Be careful not to injure the corners of the fingers when cutting the nails.

Some facilities do not permit nursing assistants to perform nail care on diabetic residents.

FOOT AND TOENAIL CARE

Residents should be given routine foot care, including bathing, massage of the feet, and attention to the toenails. Proceed carefully:

- Pat feet dry carefully after soaking in warm water.
- Give special attention to drying between the toes.
- Carefully inspect the feet and apply lotion to dry areas. Pat, rather than rub, lotion on skin. Do not apply lotion between toes. Use towel to wipe off excess lotion.
- Check the resident's toenails. If the nails are thick or curved and need trimming, inform the nurse.
- Report shoes that are too tight due to edema (swelling of the feet) or too loose due to weight loss; both situations may lead to a safety risk, falls.

PROCEDURE 16-28
Daily Hair Care

OBRA

1. Carry out each beginning procedure action.

2. Assemble equipment:
   - Towel
   - Comb and brush

3. Ask resident to move to the side of bed nearest you, or resident may sit in chair if permitted. If a resident is sitting up, put a towel around her shoulders.

4. Cover pillow with towel.

(continues)

PROCEDURE 16-28
Daily Hair Care (Continued)

5. Remove eyeglasses and store safely.

6. Part or section hair and comb with one hand between scalp and end of hair.

7. Brush or comb carefully and thoroughly.

8. Have resident turn so hair on back of head may be combed and brushed. If hair is snarled, work section by section to unsnarl hair, beginning near ends and working toward scalp. Check scalp carefully for breaks in the skin or any abnormalities.

9. Complete brushing or combing and arrange attractively. Braid long hair to prevent repeated snarling, or style hair according to resident's preference.

10. Clean and replace equipment according to facility policy.

11. Carry out each procedure completion action.

PROCEDURE 16-29
Shaving Male Resident

OBRA

1. Carry out each beginning procedure action.

2. Assemble equipment:

    - Disposable gloves

    - Electric shaver or safety razor

    - Shaving lather or preshave lotion for electric razor

    - Basin of water (105–110°F)

    - Face towels

    - Mirror

    - Washcloth

    - Aftershave lotion

        Ask nurse about oxygen removal, if electric razor is being used

3. Put on gloves.

4. Raise the head of the bed. Place equipment on overbed table and make sure there is adequate lighting.

5. Place one face towel across resident's chest and one under head.

6. Moisten face and apply lather (or preshave lotion).

7. Starting in front of ear:

    a. Hold skin taut and bring razor down over cheek toward chin (Figure 16-35).

    b. Repeat until lather on cheek is removed and area has been shaved. Rinse razor frequently.

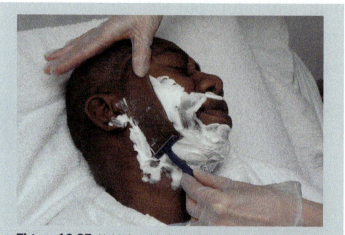

Figure 16-35 Hold the skin taut with one hand. Using short strokes, bring razor down over cheek toward chin. Start near the ear. Rinse the razor often in basin.

(continues)

PROCEDURE 16-29
Shaving Male Resident (Continued)

    c. Repeat on other cheek.

    d. Use firm short strokes. Shave in direction of hair growth.

    e. Rinse razor frequently.

8. Lather neck area and stroke up toward the chin. Rinse and repeat until all lather is removed.

9. Wash face and neck and dry thoroughly.

10. Apply aftershave lotion if desired.

11. If the skin is nicked, apply pressure directly over the area and then apply an antiseptic and an adhesive bandage. Report incident to nurse.

12. Clean and replace equipment. Dispose of razor according to facility policy. Remove head of electric razor. Use razor brush to remove clippings. Disinfect and store. Store according to facility policy. Remove and dispose of gloves according to facility policy.

13. Carry out each procedure completion action.

PROCEDURE 16-30
Hand and Fingernail Care

 OBRA

NOTE: Check with nurse and nursing care plan to learn if this procedure is permitted for the resident or if it is to be modified because of the resident's condition.

    This procedure can be carried out independently or can be modified and added to the bath procedure.

1. Carry out each beginning procedure action.

2. Assemble equipment:

- Basin with water at 105–110°F
- Bath thermometer, if used
- Soap
- Bath towel and washcloth
- Lotion
- Paper towels or bed protector
- Nail clippers
- Nail file
- Orangewood stick
- Nail polish (optional)

3. Elevate head of bed, if permitted, and adjust the overbed table in front of resident. If resident is allowed out of bed, assist to transfer to a chair and position overbed table waist-high across lap.

4. Place paper towels or bed protector on overbed table.

5. Fill basin with warm water at approximately 105–110°F using bath thermometer to test temperature. Place basin on overbed table.

6. Use a soft brush or orangewood stick to clean under nails.

7. Instruct resident to put hands in basin and soak for approximately 10 minutes. Place towel over basin to help retain heat. Add warm water if necessary. Remember to remove resident's hands if you need to add more warm water.

(continues)

PROCEDURE 16-30
Hand and Fingernail Care (Continued)

8. Perform hand hygiene. Push resident's cuticles back gently with washcloth. (A cream may be used to soften the cuticles first.)

9. Pat hands dry with towel.

10. Use nail clippers to cut resident's fingernails straight across. Do not cut below tips of fingers. Keep nail cuts on protector to be discarded.

11. Shape and smooth resident's fingernails with nail file. Apply polish to nails if resident desires.

12. Pour small amount of lotion in your palms and gently smooth on resident's hands.

13. Empty basin of water. Gather equipment, clean, and store according to facility policy.

14. Return overbed table to foot of bed. If resident has been sitting up for the procedure, assist into bed.

15. Carry out each procedure completion action.

In some facilities, only the RN is allowed to cut toenails. A podiatrist provides this service for residents with poor circulation or diabetes. The podiatrist may do toenail care for all residents in some facilities.

Part of good foot care includes being sure that the resident's shoes fit well and are securely laced so that they offer optimum support.

NOTE: Be sure to check with the nurse and the nursing care plan to learn if this procedure is permitted for the resident. In some cases, this procedure may be modified according to the resident's condition.

PROCEDURE 16-31
Foot and Toenail Care

 OBRA

1. Carry out each beginning procedure action.

2. Assemble equipment:
   - Basin
   - Soap
   - Bath mat, if available
   - Bath thermometer, if used
   - Lotion
   - Nail brush
   - Disposable bed protector
   - Paper towels/towel
   - Bath towel and washcloth
   - Orangewood stick

3. If permitted, assist resident out of bed and into chair.

4. Place bath mat, towel, bed protector, or paper towels on floor in front of resident. Fill basin with warm water (105–110°F). Put basin on barrier.

5. Remove slippers and allow resident to place feet in water. Cover with bath towel to help retain heat.

6. Soak feet approximately 10 minutes. Add warm water as necessary. Lift feet from water while warm water is being added.

7. At end of soak period, wash feet with soap.

(continues)

PROCEDURE 16-31
Foot and Toenail Care (Continued)

8. Rinse and pat dry. Note any abnormalities such as corns or calluses.

9. Remove basin, covering feet with towel.

10. Use orangewood stick to gently clean toenails. If nails are long and need to be cut, report this fact to the nurse. Follow facility policy.

11. Pour lotion into palms of hands. Hold hands together to warm lotion and apply gently to feet. Do not apply lotion between toes. Wipe off excess lotion using a towel.

12. Assist resident with socks or stockings and shoes if ambulatory. Otherwise, return resident to bed.

13. Make resident comfortable.

14. Gather equipment, clean, and store according to facility policy. Leave unit neat.

15. Carry out each procedure completion action.

? EXERCISE 16-7

Select the correct term(s) from the following list to complete each statement. Some words may be used more than once.

antiseptic	electric	lotion
chin	feet	nurse
directly	fit	short
downward	frequently	support
drying	gloves	warm water

FOOT CARE

1. Routine foot care includes:

   a. Soaking in _____

   b. Giving special attention to _____ between toes

   c. Carefully inspecting _____ and applying _____ to dry areas

   d. Checking the resident's toenails and reporting condition to the _____

   e. Ensuring that shoes or slippers _____ well and offer optimum _____

FACIAL HAIR CARE

2. When shaving you should:

   a. Wear _____.

   b. Use firm _____, _____ strokes when shaving the face.

   c. Rinse the razor _____.

   d. Stroke toward the _____ when shaving the neck.

   e. Not use a(an) _____ razor when the resident is receiving oxygen.

3. If a resident is nicked during shaving, you should:

   a. Apply pressure _____.

   b. Apply a(an) _____.

   c. Report incident to _____.

ORAL HYGIENE

Older persons need good oral hygiene just as much as younger people. Regular cleansing by brushing (Figure 16-36) and flossing should be carried out routinely three times daily when the resident has any teeth of his or her own. Residents should be encouraged to do as much for themselves to maintain independence. Visits by a dentist can help maintain existing dental function. Older people can develop dental caries (cavities) just as readily as younger people. Regular cleaning helps make the breath fresh and eliminates halitosis (bad breath). Improved appetite can also result. (See Procedures 16-32 and 16-33.)

Dentures

Many residents wear dentures. Care of dentures includes:

- Cleaning dentures daily under cool running water
- Storing dentures in a safe place when out of the resident's mouth
- In addition, you will care for the resident by:
- Cleaning and checking the resident's mouth daily for signs of irritation
- Checking resident's lips for cracking and dryness
- Applying creams or petroleum jelly to lips for excessive dryness. Remember to avoid petroleum jelly products if the resident is using oxygen.

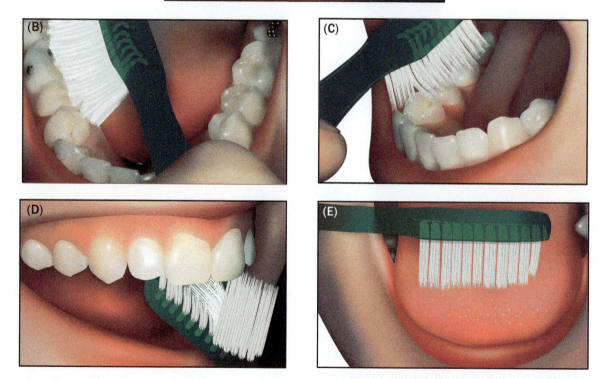

Figure 16-36 (A) Place the head of the toothbrush beside the teeth, with the bristle tips at a 45 degree angle against the gumline. Move the brush in a circular motion (half-a-tooth wide) using a gentle scrubbing motion. Brush the outer surfaces of each tooth, upper and lower, keeping the bristles angled against the gumline. (B) Use the same method on the inside surfaces of all teeth, still using circular motion. (C) Scrub the chewing surfaces of the teeth with a light, circular motion. (D) To clean the inside surfaces of the front teeth, tilt the brush vertically and make several gentle circular strokes with the "toe" (the front part) of the brush. (E) Brushing the resident's tongue will help freshen breath and clean the mouth by removing bacteria.

PROCEDURE 16-32
Assisting Resident to Brush Teeth

 OBRA

1. Carry out each beginning procedure action.

2. Assemble equipment:

    - Disposable gloves
    - Emesis basin
    - Toothbrush
    - Toothpaste
    - Glass of cool water
    - Mouthwash (if permitted)
    - Hand towel
    - Bed protector
    - Dental floss

3. Elevate head of bed. Help resident into comfortable position.

4. Lower side rails and position overbed table across resident's lap.

5. Cover table with protector and place equipment on table.

6. Place towel across resident's chest.

7. Be prepared to help as resident brushes and flosses teeth. Use gloves if you do assist (Figure 16-37).

8. After resident has brushed teeth, push overbed table to foot of bed.

9. Gather equipment, clean, and store according to facility policy. Place soiled linen in proper receptacle.

10. Remove disposable gloves, if used, and discard gloves according to facility policy.

11. Lower head of bed. Help resident to assume comfortable position and adjust bedding.

12. Raise side rails if used for positioning.

13. Carry out each procedure completion action.

Figure 16-37 Assemble equipment to brush teeth.

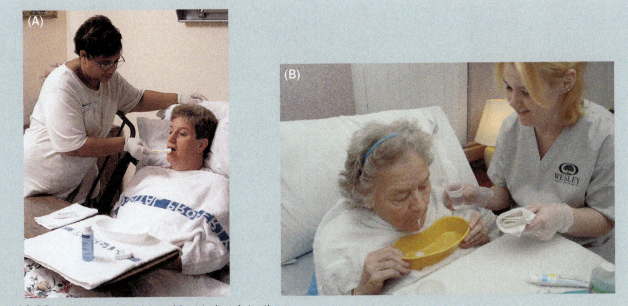

Figure 16-38 If necessary, assist resident to brush teeth.

PROCEDURE 16-33
Cleaning and Flossing Resident's Teeth

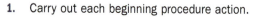

OBRA

1. Carry out each beginning procedure action.

2. Assemble equipment:
   - Disposable gloves
   - Emesis basin
   - Toothbrush
   - Toothpaste
   - Glass of cool water
   - Mouthwash (if permitted)
   - Hand towel
   - Bed protector
   - Dental floss

3. Elevate head of bed. Help resident into a comfortable position.

4. Lower side rails and position overbed table across resident's lap.

5. Place protector on overbed table and arrange equipment on table.

6. Place towel across resident's chest.

7. Put on disposable gloves.

8. Place a small (pea size) amount of toothpaste on moistened toothbrush.

9. Clean all surfaces of each tooth. Use a circular motion working from gumline to tip of tooth. In addition, brush roof of mouth and tongue.

10. Have resident rinse mouth with water or mouthwash into emesis basin.

11. Select a piece of dental floss about 12 inches long. Wrap ends of dental floss around middle fingers, leaving center area free (Figure 16-39).

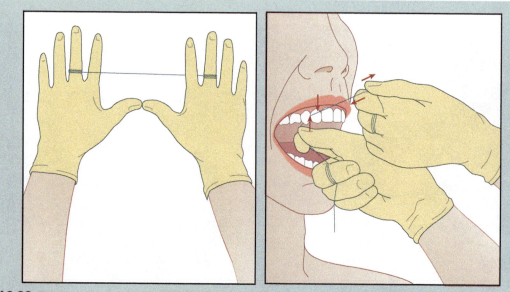

Figure 16-39 Floss is wrapped around the middle fingers (left). The proper method of using the floss is to clean between the teeth (right).

(continues)

PROCEDURE 16-33
Cleaning and Flossing Resident's Teeth (Continued)

12. Ask resident to open his or her mouth. Gently insert floss between each tooth down to, but not into, gumline.
13. Ask resident to rinse mouth with water or mouthwash using emesis basin.
14. Pat resident's face dry with towel.
15. Push overbed table to the foot of bed.
16. Gather equipment, clean, and store according to facility policy. Place soiled linen in proper receptacle.
17. Remove and discard gloves according to facility policy.
18. Position resident comfortably. Be sure that water and call light are close at hand.
19. Raise and secure side rails, if used for positioning.
20. Carry out each procedure completion action.

Many residents have partial plates, which are removable but attached by small metal clips. Partial plates should be given the same care as full dentures.

Dentures should be stored in a labeled denture cup inside the bedside stand when not in use.

Some residents prefer storing dentures dry, but most prefer to store dentures in a special solution. If in doubt, store dentures in water when out of the mouth to keep them moist and prevent cracking. (See Procedure 16-34.)

PROCEDURE 16-34
Caring for Dentures

OBRA

1. Carry out each beginning procedure action.
2. Assemble equipment:
   - Disposable gloves
   - Tissues
   - Emesis basin
   - Brush
   - Toothpaste and/or denture cleanser
   - Mouthwash, if permitted
   - Gauze squares
   - Applicators
   - Denture cup
3. Apply disposable gloves.
4. Allow resident to clean dentures if he or she is able to do so. If resident cannot, give tissue to resident and ask him or her to remove dentures. Assist if necessary.
   a. To remove upper dentures: Using a 2 × 2-inch gauze square, grasp dentures firmly from the side of the mouth, ease downward and then forward, and remove from the mouth.
   b. To remove lower dentures: Using a 2 × 2-inch gauze square, grasp dentures firmly, ease upward and then outward, and remove from the mouth.
5. Place dentures in a denture cup or emesis basin padded with gauze squares or paper towel or according to facility policy. Take to bathroom or utility room.
6. Place a paper towel or washcloth in the bottom of the basin to protect the dentures. Add a small amount of cool water.

(continues)

PROCEDURE 16-34
Caring for Dentures (Continued)

7. Dentures may be soaked in a solution with a cleansing tablet before brushing, if necessary as per product instructions.

8. After adequate soaking, put toothpaste or tooth powder on brush. Hold dentures in palm of hand and brush until all surfaces are clean (Figure 16-40).

9. Rinse dentures thoroughly under cool or warm running water. Never use hot water. Rinse denture cup.

10. Fill denture cup ½ full with cool water and cover with lid, unless instructed otherwise.

11. Place dentures in cup and take them to bedside.

12. Place a towel over pillow and gown for protection. Assist resident to rinse mouth with mouthwash, if permitted. Otherwise use water. Hold mouth open gently with wooden tongue depressor. Clean gums and tongue with applicators moistened with mouthwash or water or use foam Toothettes®.

13. Use 2 × 2-inch gauze to hand wet dentures to resident. Insert if necessary. Upper denture should be inserted first moving denture in and up; lower denture is inserted in and down.

14. Clean and replace equipment and dispose of oral swabs according to facility policy.

15. Remove and dispose of gloves according to facility policy.

16. Carry out each procedure completion action.

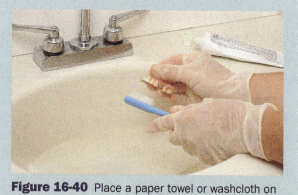

Figure 16-40 Place a paper towel or washcloth on the bottom of the sink and partially fill the sink with water. Place toothpaste or denture cleaning paste on the brush and hold the dentures over the sink while you brush them clean. Rinse with warm water. Never use hot water on dentures.

Special Oral Hygiene

Residents who are unconscious still require oral hygiene. Toothettes®, a commercially prepared sponge swab, may be used to give oral care. If this type of product is not available in your facility, wrap gauze sponges securely around a tongue depressor, dip in a solution of half water and half mouthwash, squeezing out any excess moisture against the side of the cup, and proceed to cleanse the mouth (tongue and gums), always turning their head to the side. Use care to prevent aspiration; the gag reflex may be reduced in the unconscious resident. Routine oral hygiene can however reduce the incidence of pneumonia. It is also important to refrain from inserting dentures in the mouth of an unconscious resident because these too may be aspirated. Special oral hygiene is indicated for the resident who may be taking anticoagulant drug therapy. Use a soft toothbrush to prevent irritation and bleeding of the gums. Because the resident cannot participate, the staff must carry out this procedure for the resident. (See Procedure 16-35.)

PROCEDURE 16-35
Assisting with Oral Hygiene for the Unconscious Resident

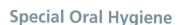 OBRA

1. Carry out each beginning procedure action.

2. Assemble equipment:
   - Disposable gloves
   - Emesis basin
   - Bath towel

(continues)

PROCEDURE 16-35
Assisting with Oral Hygiene for the Unconscious Resident (Continued)

- Plastic bag
- Disposable cup with water and/or mouthwash
- Tissues
- Water-based lubricant for lips
- Toothettes® or oral swabs
- Applicators

3. Put on disposable gloves.

4. Cover pillow and gown with towel and turn resident's head to one side. Place emesis basin under resident's chin.

5. Gently pull down on chin to open mouth and gently separate teeth with padded tongue depressor.

6. Using Toothettes® moistened with a mixture of ½ mouthwash (15 mL) and ½ water (15 mL), wipe gums, teeth, tongue, inside and roof of mouth (Figure 16-41).

7. Repeat procedure as necessary/remove any excess solution with a dry oral swab.

8. Discard used swabs in plastic bag.

9. Using clean applicators, apply lubricant to lips. Place used applicators in plastic bag.

10. Clean and replace equipment.

11. Remove and discard gloves according to facility policy.

12. Carry out each procedure completion action.

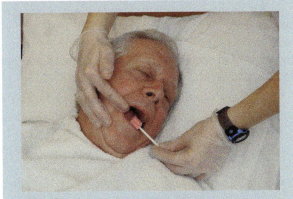

Figure 16-41 Using commercially prepared swabs (like Toothettes®), wipe gums, teeth, and tongue.

? EXERCISE 16-8

MOUTH CARE
Select the correct term(s) from the following list to complete each statement.

outward   floss   special
basin   forward upward
downward   hot

1. Residents need to brush and _____ their natural teeth.

2. When caring for dentures, always pad a denture cup with gauze and never use _____ water.

3. Protect dentures when cleaning by filling a _____ with water.

4. When removing upper dentures, using a 232-inch gauze square, grasp between thumb and forefinger and ease _____ and _____.

5. Remove lower dentures by grasping between thumb and forefinger and easing _____ and _____.

6. Residents who are unconscious require _____ oral hygiene.

DRESSING RESIDENT

Residents are encouraged to wear their own clothes because it contributes to their sense of identity. If residents are not confined to bed, they dress after morning care every day.

Some residents will be able to dress themselves with assistance; those who are totally dependent will have to be dressed by the staff. It is part of your responsibility to see that the clothing is clean and neat and in good repair. You should remember to:

- Whenever possible, allow the resident to choose their own clothing. The clothing should be lightweight but provide adequate warmth. Do not offer too many choices because that may confuse the resident. Clothing should be seasonal and in good repair.
- Encourage resident to participate in the dressing or undressing procedure, to the extent of the resident's ability. Some residents may require adaptive clothing.

The resident who requires complete help is easiest to dress in bed. Residents who can help themselves may wish to sit in a chair with clothing placed nearby. You can help by:

- Arranging the clothing in the order that it will be put on.
- Being prepared to assist with shoes and stockings, even for residents who can do much themselves. Bending over to adjust shoes and stockings can result in dizziness and loss of balance.
- Putting clothing on the affected or weakest side first if the resident has difficulty moving one side or is paralyzed.
- Removing clothing from unaffected or strongest side first if the resident has difficulty moving one side or is paralyzed.

PROCEDURE 16-36
Dressing and Undressing Resident

OBRA

1. Carry out each beginning procedure action.
2. Select appropriate clothing and arrange in order of application. Encourage resident to participate in selection.
3. Cover resident with bath blanket and fanfold top bedclothes to foot of bed.
4. Elevate head of bed to sitting position.
5. Assist resident to comfortable sitting position.
6. Remove night clothing, keeping resident covered with bath blanket. Remove from strong side first and then from affected side. Place in laundry hamper.
7. If the resident wears a bra, slip straps over resident's hands (affected side first), move straps up arms, and position on shoulders. Adjust breasts in cups of bra. Then hook bra in back (assist resident to lean forward so bra can be fastened).
8. For an undershirt, or any garment that slips on over the head:
    a. Gather undershirt and place it over the resident's head.
    b. Grasp resident's hand (affected side first) and guide it through the arm hole by reaching into the arm hole from the outside.
    c. Repeat procedure with opposite arm.
    d. Assist resident to lean forward, and adjust undershirt so it is smooth over upper body.
9. Alternate procedure for slipover garments:

NOTE: Garment must be large enough or made of stretchy fabric for this procedure.

    a. Place garment front side down on resident's lap with bottom opening facing the resident.
    b. Put resident's hands into bottom of garment and, one at a time (affected side first), into the sleeve holes.
    c. Pull the sleeves up as far as possible on the resident's arms and pull hands through at wrist if it is a long-sleeved garment. The garment should now be high on the resident's chest.
    d. Gather up the back of the garment with your hand and slip the garment over the resident's head.
    e. Smooth the garment down and position it comfortably about the resident's body. Adjust sleeves and shoulders as needed.

(continues)

PROCEDURE 16-36
Dressing and Undressing Resident (Continued)

10. Shirts or dresses that fasten in the front:
    a. Insert your hand through sleeve of garment and grasp hand of resident (affected side first), drawing sleeve over your hand and resident's.
    b. Adjust sleeve at shoulder.
    c. Assist resident to sit forward. Arrange clothing across back.
    d. Gather sleeve on opposite side by slipping your hand in from the outside.
    e. Grasp resident's wrist and pull sleeve of garment over your hand and resident's hand. Draw upward and adjust at shoulder.
    f. Button, zip, or snap garment.

11. Underwear or slacks:
    a. Facing foot of bed, gather resident's underwear from waist to leg hole.
    b. Slip underwear over one foot at a time (affected side first). Pull underwear up legs as high as possible.
    c. Assist resident to raise buttocks and draw garment over buttocks and up to waist. If resident cannot raise buttocks, assist resident to roll first to one side as you pull up the garment and then the other side. Adjust garment until it is comfortable.
    d. Fasten garment if required.

NOTE: A variety of disposable incontinence products are available for use by the resident. Follow agency protocols related to use of these products (see Figure 16-42).

12. Socks or knee-high (or thigh-high) stockings:
    a. Roll sock or stocking with heel in back and place over toes; start with weak side first.
    b. Draw sock up over foot and adjust until smooth. Pull stockings smoothly up to knee or thigh.
    c. Repeat for other foot.

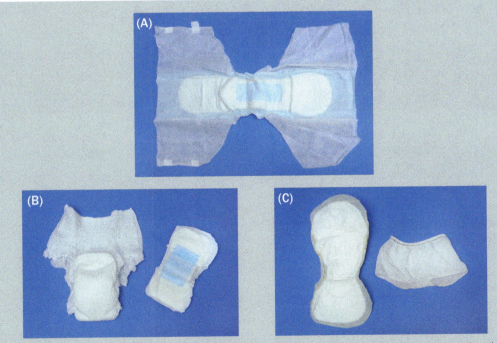

Figure 16-42 Disposable garment protectors. (A) and (B) Complete incontinence brief; (C) pant liner and undergarment.

(continues)

PROCEDURE 16-36
Dressing and Undressing Resident (Continued)

13. Pantyhose:

    a. Gather pantyhose and adjust over toes and feet (affected side first). Draw up legs as high as possible.

    b. Draw over hips as described in step 11c. Adjust until comfortable at waist.

14. Shoes:

    a. Slip shoe on, using shoe horn if necessary; start with side first.

    b. Be sure shoe is fastened securely (Velcro tabs or ties). If the shoes tie, be sure that ends of shoelaces do not drag on the floor. The shoes should be fastened tight enough to prevent them from slipping off the resident's feet but not so tight that circulation is impaired.

    c. Shoes should have rubber soles for better traction. Leather soles slide easily on tile and linoleum floors.

NOTE: Adaptive devices are available to assist the resident with dressing. See Lesson 22 for examples of these devices.

15. To undress, reverse order of steps.

16. Carry out each procedure completion action.

LESSON SYNTHESIS: Putting It All Together

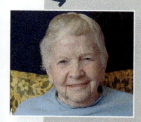

You have just completed this lesson. Now go back and review the Clinical Focus. Try to see how the Clinical Focus relates to the concepts presented in the lesson. Then answer the following questions.

1. Do older persons really care about how they look? What relationship does appearance have to self-esteem?

2. What danger does Mary Mandell face because of sitting in a wheelchair for so many hours?

3. What evidence is there to concern the staff and what steps must be taken?

4. How can the nursing assistant help Mary Mandell feel that she still has some control over her personal hygiene?

16 REVIEW

A. Match each term (items a–e) with the proper definition.

a. caries   d. dentures

b. pressure ulcer   e. skin tears

c. lesions

1. _____ skin breakdown due to prolonged pressure over bony prominences

2. _____ artificial teeth

3. _____ changes in skin structure

4. _____ small breaks in the skin

5. _____ dental cavities

B. Brief answers

6. Name five factors that contribute to skin breakdown.

7. List three ways you can encourage adequate circulation to tissues.

8. Briefly describe each of the four stages of pressure ulcer development.

9. Name five basic positions that are routinely used to ensure that pressure is not prolonged on any body part.

10. List five ways to relieve pressure on body parts.

C. Fill in the blanks by selecting the correct word or phrase from the list.

dentures	senile lentigines
diabetes	skin tears
friction	strong
oral hygiene	turning schedule
pressure ulcers	weak
sacrum	

11. Liver spots are more properly called _____.

12. Small breaks that occur in fragile skin are called _____.

13. When body parts rub together, _____ results, which may cause tissue damage.

14. Skin breakdown may progress to the formation of deep, painful lesions called _____.

15. For residents who are confined to bed, a _____ is followed to relieve pressure on body parts.

16. One of the most common sites for skin breakdown is the _____.

17. Generally, nursing assistants are not allowed to perform nail care, especially toenail care, on residents with _____.

18. The process of cleaning teeth, the tongue, and the inside of the mouth is called _____.

19. Artificial teeth are known as _____.

20. When dressing a resident with a weakness on one side due to a stroke or other condition, clothing is applied to the _____ side first. Clothing is removed from the _____ side first.

D. Select the one best answer for each of the following.

21. Which of the following is not a function of the skin?

(A) perception of sensations

(B) regulation of body temperature

(C) protection of structures under the skin

(D) production of insulin

22. Which of the following is a characteristic of the aging skin?

(A) skin glands produce more oil

(B) fingernails and toenails thin

(C) sweat glands increase activity

(D) circulation to the skin decreases

23. Shearing of tissues is most likely to occur when the resident

(A) is resting on her abdomen

(B) is positioned with the head of the bed elevated

(C) is walking around

(D) is resting flat on her back in bed

24. Select the best position for the resident considering the condition given.

(A) Position the resident with respiratory problems flat in bed.

(B) Position the resident who has had a recent stroke by turning her on the affected side.

(C) Position the resident who has had a recent stroke by turning her on the unaffected side.

(D) Position the resident who has a fractured hip by rotating her over the unaffected leg.

25. When the resident's hair is tangled, begin brushing at

(A) the ends of the hair.

(B) the forehead and brush to the ends.

(C) the nape of the neck, forward.

(D) the sides near the ears.

E. Clinical Experience

26. Janine was assisting Mrs. Docker with her tub bath when Mrs. Docker said she felt dizzy. What action should Janine take?

27. Carl is giving foot care to Mr. Dobrinski. The toenails are long and thick. What action should Carl take?

28. Chris is shaving Mr. Gates, who moves suddenly. The razor makes a small nick in the skin. How should Chris handle this situation?

29. Mrs. Marks has long curly hair that frequently tangles. How can Holly, her nursing assistant, care for Mrs. Marks' hair during morning care to reduce the amount of tangles?

30. Mrs. Gonzales has very thin, fragile skin. How can Jean, her nursing assistant, try to prevent skin tears?

MEETING THE RESIDENTS' NUTRITIONAL NEEDS

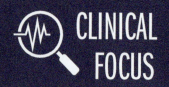

CLINICAL FOCUS

Think about how food is processed by the body and how you can help residents meet their nutritional needs as you study this lesson.

OBJECTIVES

After studying this lesson, you should be able to:

- Define vocabulary words and terms.
- Identify the parts and function of the gastrointestinal system.
- Review changes in the digestive system as they relate to the aging process.
- Name the six classes of nutrients.
- List the functions of each class of nutrients.
- Name the five food groups.
- List four diets commonly provided in long-term care facilities.
- Name six therapeutic diets ordered in long-term care facilities.
- Demonstrate how to measure intake correctly using the metric system.
- State ways the nursing assistant can promote adequate nutrition.
- Explain how to assist the resident who can feed herself or himself.
- Explain how to feed the dependent resident.
- List alternate ways of delivering nutrition.
- Briefly describe seven gastrointestinal disorders.
- Demonstrate the following:
  Procedure 17-37 Measuring and Recording Fluid Intake
  Procedure 17-38 Assisting the Resident Who Can Feed Self
  Procedure 17-39 Feeding the Dependent Resident

CASE STUDY

Mrs. Hartley, a Christian Scientist, is 92 and almost blind. Although she can make out light and dark, everything is blurred and shadowy. She has a cold and wants to rest in bed instead of going to the dining room to eat. Nursing assistants are serving trays and assisting residents to eat. Mrs. Hartley has dentures and an order for a soft diet. The nursing assistant serving trays notes that Mrs. Hartley seems listless and her skin is dry.

VOCABULARY

anus (AY-nus)
carbohydrate (kar-boh-HIGH-drayt)
colon (KOH-lon)
constipation (kon-stih-PAY-shun)
cubic centimeter (cc) (KYOU-bick SEN-tih-mee-ter)
defecation (def-eh-KAY-shun)
dehydration (dee-high-DRAY-shun)
digestion (die-JEST-shun)
diverticuli (die-ver-TICK-you-lie)
diverticulitis (die-ver-tick-you-LIE-tis)
duodenum (dew-oh-DEE-num)
dyspepsia (dis-PEP-see-ah)
dysphagia (dis-FAY-jee-ah)
edema (ee-DEE-mah)
electrolytes (ee-LECK-troh-lights)
enzymes (EN-zighms)
esophagus (eh-SOF-ah-gus)
fats (fats)
feces (FEE-cees)
fiber (FYE-ber)
flatulence (FLAT-you-lens)
gastritis (gas-TRY-tis)
gastrointestinal system (gas-troh-in-TES-tih-nal SIS-tum)
gastrostomy (G) tube (gas-TROS-toh-mee toob)
hemorrhoids (HEM-oh-royds)

hernia (HER-nee-ah)
hiatal hernia (high-AY-tal HER-nee-ah)
high density (high DEN-sih-tee)
homeostasis (hoh-mee-oh-STAY-sis)
hyperalimentation (high-per-al-ih-men-TAY-shun)
ileum (ILL-ee-um)
inguinal hernia (ING-gwih-nal HER-nee-ah)
intake and output (I&O) (IN-tayk and OUT-put)
jejunum (jeh-JOO-num)
metric system (MET-rick SIS-tum)
milliliter (mL) (MILL-ih-lee-ter)
mineral (MIN-er-al)
nasogastric (NG) tube (nay-zoh-GAS-trick toob)
obesity (oh-BEES-ih-tee)
peristalsis (per-i-STAL-sis)
pharynx (FAR-inks)
protein (PROH-teen)
regularity (reg-you-LAIR-ih-tee)
rupture (RUP-chur)
therapeutic (ther-ah-PYOU-tick)
total parenteral nutrition (TPN) (TOH-tal pah-REN-ter-al new-TRISH-un)
USDA
vitamin (VYE-tah-min)
water (WOT-er)

THE DIGESTIVE SYSTEM

The digestive system processes the foods eaten, releasing simple nutrients that are needed by the body. There are six nutrients: vitamins, minerals, water, fats, proteins, and carbohydrates. The nutrients pass through the wall of the intestine into the bloodstream; they are carried in the blood to where they are used by the body cells.

Chemicals (enzymes) help break down or digest the food, and the non-digestible portion of what is eaten is eliminated from the body as solid waste called feces. This process is called a bowel movement (BM) or defecation.

The digestive system (Figure 17-1) is also called the gastrointestinal system. It is a tube about 30 feet long, stretching from the mouth to the end opening called the anus. The walls of the tube are made of smooth muscle and the entire tract is lined with mucous membrane. The digestive system consists of the true digestive organs:

- Mouth (Figure 17-2)
- Pharynx
- Esophagus
- Stomach
- Small intestine
- Large intestine

The true digestive organs receive the help of other organs in breaking food into simpler substances. These organs are called *accessory organs* and include the:

- Tongue
- Salivary glands
- Teeth
- Liver
- Pancreas
- Gallbladder

The liver produces bile, which is stored in the gallbladder. The pancreas produces digestive enzymes as well as the hormones insulin and glucagon. The tongue and teeth mechanically break down the food and direct it toward the rest of the tract.

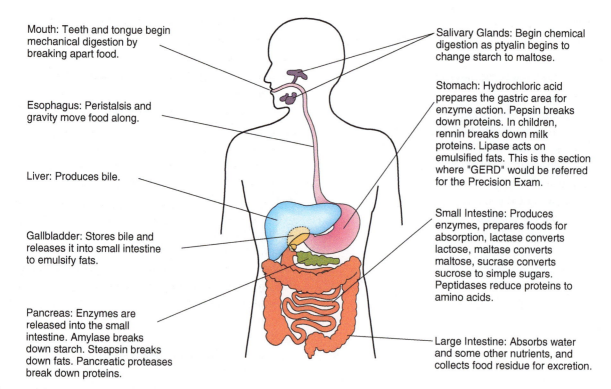

Mouth: Teeth and tongue begin mechanical digestion by breaking apart food.

Esophagus: Peristalsis and gravity move food along.

Liver: Produces bile.

Gallbladder: Stores bile and releases it into small intestine to emulsify fats.

Pancreas: Enzymes are released into the small intestine. Amylase breaks down starch. Steapsin breaks down fats. Pancreatic proteases break down proteins.

Salivary Glands: Begin chemical digestion as ptyalin begins to change starch to maltose.

Stomach: Hydrochloric acid prepares the gastric area for enzyme action. Pepsin breaks down proteins. In children, rennin breaks down milk proteins. Lipase acts on emulsified fats. This is the section where "GERD" would be referred for the Precision Exam.

Small Intestine: Produces enzymes, prepares foods for absorption, lactase converts lactose, maltase converts maltose, sucrase converts sucrose to simple sugars. Peptidases reduce proteins to amino acids.

Large Intestine: Absorbs water and some other nutrients, and collects food residue for excretion.

Figure 17-1 The gastrointestinal system.

THE DIGESTIVE PROCESS

The process of **digestion** is both mechanical and chemical. Foods are broken up and moved along the tract by rhythmic muscular contractions called **peristalsis**. At the same time, digestive enzymes and bile are mixed with the food. The digestive enzymes from the stomach, pancreas, and small intestine (see Figure 17-1), together with bile, chemically break the foods into simple nutrients:

- Proteins are changed to amino acids.
- Carbohydrates are changed to simple sugars like glucose.
- Fats are changed to fatty acids and glycerol.

The undigestible portion of food is moved along in the intestines and finally excreted from the body as feces.

Mouth

Digestion begins in the mouth. The teeth and tongue break the food into smaller pieces, mix it with saliva, and form a rounded mass of food. The food is swallowed into the pharynx and moves down the esophagus into the stomach.

The tongue is a skeletal muscle covered with taste buds. It:

- Pushes the food between the teeth
- Propels the food backward to aid swallowing
- Assists in speech

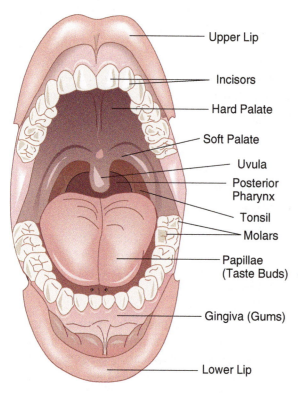

Upper Lip

Incisors

Hard Palate

Soft Palate

Uvula

Posterior Pharynx

Tonsil

Molars

Papillae (Taste Buds)

Gingiva (Gums)

Lower Lip

Figure 17-2 The mouth.

Salivary glands secrete saliva, which contains an enzyme, salivary amylase, to start carbohydrate digestion. Saliva:

- Moistens food for easier swallowing
- Amounts to about 1½ quarts daily in the average adult. The amount of fluid varies with the person and may be altered by specific health problems. Teeth mechanically break up the food. These:
- Number 32 in the adult
- May be replaced by dentures when lost
- The pharynx is a common passageway for:
  - Food to the esophagus
  - Air to the trachea

The gag reflex normally occurs if food begins to go into the trachea instead of the esophagus. This causes coughing and clearing of the airway.

Stomach

The stomach begins protein digestion by the action of the enzyme pepsin and hydrochloric acid (HCl). It:

- Holds the food about 4 hours
- Churns and mixes the gastric juice with the food to form a liquid

Small Intestine

The small intestine is about 20 feet long and is coiled in the abdominal cavity. It is divided into three parts:

- Duodenum
- Jejunum
- Ileum

The small intestine is attached by the duodenum to the stomach and by the ileum to the large intestine.

The small intestine produces a fluid containing digestive enzymes and receives:

- Food from the stomach
- Bile from the liver and gallbladder to begin fat breakdown
- Pancreatic fluid from the pancreas, which completes the breakdown of:
  - Proteins to amino acids
  - Carbohydrates to simple sugar (glucose)
  - Fats to fatty acids and glycerol

Most of the digestion and absorption of nutrients occur in the small intestine. Figure 17-3 shows the functions of the basic nutrients and the forms in which they are used in the body.

As food moves slowly through the small intestine, the simple nutrients pass through the wall of the intestine and into the bloodstream, where they are carried to the liver for more action before being used by the body cells.

Once released from foods, the following nutrients can be absorbed directly:

- Water
- Vitamins
- Minerals

Large Intestine

The large intestine is called the colon. It extends from the end of the small intestine to the rectum, which ends in the anus. It is not as long as the small intestine. Its main purpose is to carry the unused food out of the body, but some vitamins and water are absorbed through the colon walls. A muscle holds the anus closed and can be voluntarily relaxed to permit defecation.

Nutrient	Form Used	Function
Carbohydrates	Glucose	Provide fuel and energy for body
Proteins	Amino acids	Build and repair tissues
Fats	Fatty acids, glycerol	Supply energy and heat; needed to benefit from fat-soluble vitamins
Water	Water	Needed to carry on body chemistry
Vitamins	Fat-soluble—A, D, K, E, water-soluble—B, C	Needed for normal functioning of the body
Minerals	Calcium, phosphorus, potassium, sodium, and traces of others	Important in formation of body tissues and regulating body chemistry

Figure 17-3 Basic nutrients and their functions.

? EXERCISE 17-1

SCIENCE PRINCIPLES

Write the names of the organs of the digestive tract shown in the figure below. Be sure the names are spelled correctly. Select the terms from the list provided.

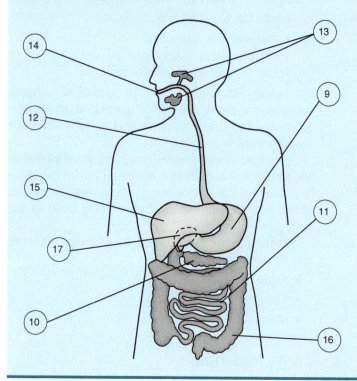

esophagus	pancreas
gallbladder	salivary gland
large intestine	small intestine
liver	stomach
mouth (teeth and tongue)	

1. _____
2. _____
3. _____
4. _____
5. _____
6. _____
7. _____
8. _____
9. _____

? EXERCISE 17-2

Complete the chart to show the end products of digestion.

1. Carbohydrates ⟶ (acted on by enzymes) ⟶ _____

2. Proteins ⟶ (acted on by enzymes) ⟶ _____

3. Fats - ⟶ (acted on by enzymes) ⟶ _____

AGING CHANGES

As the body ages, some changes take place in the digestive process.

- The flow of gastric secretions and enzymes is somewhat decreased.
- The muscular walls of the tract lose some tone and strength so that movement along the tract is slower.

- The gag reflex that prevents food from slipping into the trachea is not as active, so choking is possible.
- Absorption of nutrients is slower.

Figure 17-4 is a summary of the changes in the digestive process that are the result of aging. Some older persons find they may not tolerate foods they previously enjoyed.

? EXERCISE 17-3

amino acids
carbohydrates
chemically
constipation and flatulence more common
decreased taste buds
electrolytes
fats
fatty acids
feces

fewer enzymes
food tolerated less well
gag reflex less active
glucose
homeostasis
hydrochloric acid
less saliva
minerals
peristalsis

protein
saliva
slower absorption
small intestine
vitamins
water
32
2,000

1. Digestive enzymes break down foods _____.

2. Rhythmic muscular waves that move the food along the digestive tract are called _____.

3. Salivary glands secrete _____.

4. Nondigestible portions of foods are eliminated as _____.

5. The adult teeth number _____.

6. An acid found in the stomach is called _____.

7. _____ are essential to the chemical functioning of the body.

8. The nutrients absorbed from the colon are some _____ and _____.

9. Movement of nutrients (absorption) from the intestinal tract into the bloodstream primarily occurs through the wall of the _____.

10. The balance of body functions that depends on many body activities is called _____.

11. List seven digestive changes associated with the aging process.

   a. _____   e. _____
   b. _____   f. _____
   c. _____   g. _____
   d. _____

? EXERCISE 17-4

1. The six classes of nutrients needed by the body are:

   a. _____
   b. _____
   c. _____
   d. _____
   e. _____
   f. _____

- Decreased number and function of taste buds causing increased desire for salty and sweet flavors
- Reduced digestive enzymes and secretions
- Thirst mechanism altered
- Thicker saliva
- Tongue more sensitive
- Movement of food not as efficient
- More flatulence (gas production)
- Less effective gag reflex
- Poorer tolerance of some foods
- Faulty absorption of nutrients
- Decreased chewing/poor dentures/gum diseases
- Weaker muscular walls
- Decreased total body water
- Constipation (difficult defecation) more common

Figure 17-4 Changes in the digestive system caused by aging.

NUTRIENTS

Nutrients provide us with essential materials to:

- Build and repair tissues
- Perform body functions
- Provide energy for the work the body does

It takes energy to perform activities such as walking or getting in and out of bed. Even when a person is quiet and inactive, energy is needed for the heart to beat and for the kidneys to produce urine. These are examples of vital body activities that sustain life.

Energy is supplied by the nutrients in the foods we eat. The amount of energy from nutrients is measured in units of heat called *calories*. When not enough nutrients are eaten, the body gradually uses up its stored supply and becomes depleted; loss of weight and illness follow.

Classes of Nutrients

There are six classes of nutrients. Many foods contain more than one nutrient. The basic nutrients are:

- Carbohydrates
- Fats
- Proteins
- Vitamins
- Minerals
- Water

Carbohydrates are the primary source of immediate body energy and are classified into two categories: simple and complex. One gram of carbohydrates provides 4 calories of energy. Many foods contain this nutrient. Fruits, vegetables, breads, cereal, and pasta products are good sources. Carbohydrate foods supply the body with fiber. Fiber helps maintain regularity (bowel activity).

Fats provide energy and are found in both plant and animal foods. One gram of fat provides 9 calories of energy. Fat maintains skin, hair, cushions vital organs, and provides insulation to the body. Sources of fats include butter, meat, nuts, egg yolks, and vegetable oils.

Proteins are essential for tissue building and repair as well as a healthy immune system. One gram of protein provides 4 calories. Foods rich in protein include meats, fish, poultry, eggs, beans, nuts, and lentils.

Vitamins and minerals regulate body processes. The 13 different kinds of vitamins are represented by letters. Vitamins A, D, K, and E are fat-soluble and are found in fatty foods as well as in fruits and vegetables. Vitamins B and C are water-soluble and are found in fruits, vegetables, and whole-grain products. Minerals are not a source of energy and are obtained through a varied diet. The minerals include sodium, potassium, calcium, and iron and are involved in many body functions.

Water is essential to life. Most of our body weight (60–70%) is made up of water. Each person needs to take in about 2½ quarts (2½ liters or 2,500 milliliters [mL]) of water in some form daily. (In certain circumstances, under a doctor's order, water intake may be limited.) Water is consumed in drinks such as plain water, tea, coffee, and other beverages. Water is also taken in with foods such as fruits and vegetables that have high water content and helps to control our body temperature and carries nutrients and waste products from our cells.

ELECTROLYTE BALANCE

Electrolytes are minerals that are essential to the chemical functioning of the body. The electrolytes in the body fluids must be balanced for proper functioning. You may be familiar with electrolytes as solid substances, such as sodium chloride (table salt) and sodium bicarbonate, an antacid used to relieve indigestion.

In the body fluids, the electrolytes break apart to form ions that take part in the body's chemical reaction. Two important electrolytes are:

- Sodium
- Potassium

The homeostasis (balance) of body functions depends on many body activities. The endocrine, cardiovascular, and renal systems play an important role in the process.

When there is an electrolyte imbalance in the body, many problems—sometimes serious—can occur.

Two common problems are:

- Increased levels of sodium in the blood. The sodium causes body tissues to hold fluid, resulting in swelling or edema. This is often seen in the feet and legs of older residents (Figure 17-5). Fluid may also accumulate in the lungs, causing respiratory distress.

- Decreased levels of potassium in the blood. This leads to a slower heart rate, feelings of weakness, and a lack of interest in surroundings.

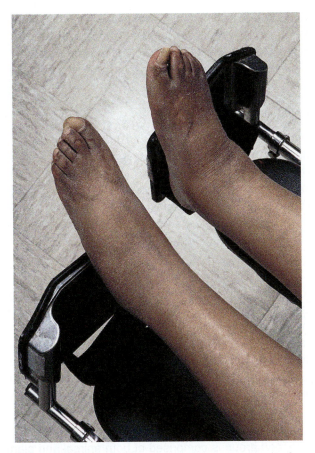

Figure 17-5 Edema of the feet and legs as a result of electrolyte imbalance.

- Swelling of hands, face, feet, and/or legs
- Respiratory distress
- Slower than normal pulse rate
- Lack of interest in surroundings
- Feelings of weakness
- Intake and output (if ordered)

Figure 17-6 Observations to be reported for the resident with electrolyte imbalance.

Figure 17-6 lists observations to report for residents with electrolyte imbalance.

THE 2015–2020 DIETARY GUIDELINES FOR AMERICANS

The *2015–2020 Dietary Guidelines for Americans* (2015DGAC) were developed by the Dietary Guidelines Advisory Committee, a group of scientists appointed by the secretaries of the Department of Health and

Human Services and the United States Department of Agriculture (USDA). The guidelines are reviewed and revised every 5 years, as necessary. Primary use of these guidelines is to provide information for the American general public, health care providers, nutritionists, and nutrition educators to develop nutrition-related educational programs.

The DGAC Report for 2015 is different from previous reports. It is addressed to the American public, the majority Americans are obese and at the same time undernourished in several nutrients. It encourages people to make personal choices that result in an eating pattern that is nutrient dense and calorie balanced. Americans generally eat too few fruits, vegetable, high-fiber whole grains, seafood, and low-fat milk and milk products and consume too much added sugar, solid fats, refined grains, and sodium. The research indicated that added sugars and solid fats (SoFAS) comprise approximately 35% of the American diet. An increased intake of dietary potassium is encouraged to help offset the effects of increased sodium on blood pressure. It is hoped that the diet recommendations in the Report will provide a flexible approach that incorporates a wide range of food preferences and meet individual tastes.

Based on the latest scientific evidence, the 2015 DGAC provides information that can lead to a healthy lifestyle for the general public age 2 and beyond. It includes information about choosing a nutritious, plant-based diet, maintaining a healthy weight, getting adequate exercise, and avoiding foodborne illness by keeping foods safe, improving school lunch programs, and reducing children's exposure to allergens (in food and in the environment). In addition, there is emphasis on increasing the number of smoke-free laws, reducing the use of cancer-causing tanning beds, and in getting more people covered by health insurance. Many of these changes will require new state regulations to aid with enforcement. The federal government hopes that people will relate to the 2015 goals and will take responsibility in making healthy choices in diet and lifestyle changes for this generation and coming generations.

MyPyramid evolved from the 2005 DGAC. It was developed to help individuals implement the recommendations contained in the guidelines. In 2010, the food pyramid was reconfigured and the *MyPlate* icon (Figure 17-7) was designed to simplify the nutritional information in order to make it easier for Americans to formulate good food choices. The 2015–2020 Dietary guidelines for Americans emphasize the importance of creating a healthy eating

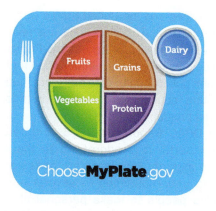

Balancing Calories
- Enjoy your food, but eat less.
- Avoid oversized portions.

Foods to Increase
- Make half your plate fruits and vegetables.
- Make at least half your grains whole grains.
- Switch to fat-free or low-fat (1%) milk.

Foods to Reduce
- Compare sodium in foods like soup, bread, and frozen meals – and choose the foods with lower numbers.
- Drink water instead of sugary drinks.

Figure 17-7 *MyPlate* food guide.

© Courtesy of the USDA.

pattern to maintain health and reduce the risk of disease. The health messages in the 2015 DGAC are simple and easy to understand. Examples of the messages include:

- *Balancing Calories:* Enjoy your food but eat less; avoid oversized portions.

- *Foods to Increase:* Make half your plate fruits and vegetables; make that least half your grains whole grains, and switch to fat-free or low-fat (1%) milk.

- *Foods to Reduce:* Compare sodium in foods like soup, bread, and frozen meals and choose food with lower numbers; drink water instead of sugary drinks.

Food Groups

The food groups are represented on the *MyPlate* icon by various colors on the placemat showing (see Figure 17-7) a segmented plate and glass. The Fruit group is red, the Vegetable group is green, the Grain group is tan, the Protein group is purple, and the Dairy group is represented by the color blue. The new icon stresses the importance of a plant-based diet.

The Fruit Group (Red Segment)

This group provides nutrients such as potassium, vitamin C, and dietary fiber, and folate. Most fruits are low in sodium, calories, fat, and contain no cholesterol. The fruits may be fresh, canned, frozen, or dried. They may be eaten whole, cut-up, or pureed (preferable to juicing). A serving size of fruit should be approximately the size of a tennis ball.

The Vegetable Group (Green Segment)

The vegetable group also is an important source of vitamins and minerals and most are low in calories. Vegetables should be bright in color, red, orange, or dark green. These, too, may be fresh frozen, canned, steamed, and baked. Beans such as garbanzo, black, kidney, and pinto beans are included in this category, but also are considered to be a plant-based protein.

The Grain Group (Tan Segment)

Foods made from wheat, rice, oats, cornmeal, barley, or other cereal grains are contained in this group. Grains may be served in a variety of ways: breads, crackers, pasta, breakfast cereals including oatmeal, grits, tortillas, and popcorn. Grains are usually classified as whole or refined grains. When choosing the grain to eat, at least one-half should be the whole-grain variety.

The Protein Group (Purple Segment)

This food group is comprised of both animal and plant sources of protein. Meats, poultry, seafood, and eggs are animal sources. Plant sources include beans, peas, nuts, seeds, and soy products such as tofu and "veggie burgers." Animal protein should be lean and low fat; fat can be trimmed from the meats, drained following cooking, and skin should be removed from poultry. Nuts and seeds are concentrated sources of protein. For example, ½ ounce of loose nuts or 1 tablespoon of peanut butter is equivalent to 1 ounce of protein. A variety of protein sources should be chosen in the meal plan, including seafood twice a week.

The Dairy Group (Blue Circle)

Milk, cheese, yogurt, and fortified soy milk are included in the Dairy group. These foods provide a rich source of calcium, vitamin D, and protein. It is important to choose low-fat varieties: skim or low-fat (1%) milk, low-fat or reduced fat cheese, substitute yogurt for sour cream, and limit the use of sweet dairy foods (frozen yogurt, ice cream, flavored milks, and puddings) that may add empty sugar calories.

Salt/Sodium (Cautions)

Most Americans have acquired a taste for salt. Salt (sodium chloride) plays a role in helping in causing

10 tips

Nutrition
Education Series

choose MyPlate

10 **tips** to a great plate

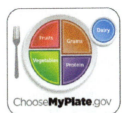

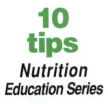

Making food choices for a healthy lifestyle can be as simple as using these 10 Tips.
Use the ideas in this list to *balance your calories*, to choose foods to *eat more often*, and to cut back on foods to *eat less often*.

1 balance calories
Find out how many calories YOU need for a day as a first step in managing your weight. Go to www.ChooseMyPlate.gov to find your calorie level. Being physically active also helps you balance calories.

2 enjoy your food, but eat less
Take the time to fully enjoy your food as you eat it. Eating too fast or when your attention is elsewhere may lead to eating too many calories. Pay attention to hunger and fullness cues before, during, and after meals. Use them to recognize when to eat and when you've had enough.

3 avoid oversized portions
Use a smaller plate, bowl, and glass. Portion out foods before you eat. When eating out, choose a smaller size option, share a dish, or take home part of your meal.

4 foods to eat more often
Eat more vegetables, fruits, whole grains, and fat-free or 1% milk and dairy products. These foods have the nutrients you need for health—including potassium, calcium, vitamin D, and fiber. Make them the basis for meals and snacks.

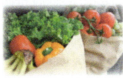

5 make half your plate fruits and vegetables
Choose red, orange, and dark-green vegetables like tomatoes, sweet potatoes, and broccoli, along with other vegetables for your meals. Add fruit to meals as part of main or side dishes or as dessert.

6 switch to fat-free or low-fat (1%) milk
They have the same amount of calcium and other essential nutrients as whole milk, but fewer calories and less saturated fat.

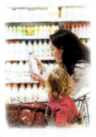

7 make half your grains whole grains
To eat more whole grains, substitute a whole-grain product for a refined product—such as eating whole-wheat bread instead of white bread or brown rice instead of white rice.

8 foods to eat less often
Cut back on foods high in solid fats, added sugars, and salt. They include cakes, cookies, ice cream, candies, sweetened drinks, pizza, and fatty meats like ribs, sausages, bacon, and hot dogs. Use these foods as occasional treats, not everyday foods.

9 compare sodium in foods
Use the Nutrition Facts label to choose lower sodium versions of foods like soup, bread, and frozen meals. Select canned foods labeled "low sodium," "reduced sodium," or "no salt added."

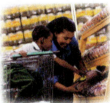

10 drink water instead of sugary drinks
Cut calories by drinking water or unsweetened beverages. Soda, energy drinks, and sports drinks are a major source of added sugar, and calories, in American diets.

Center for Nutrition
Policy and Promotion

Go to www.ChooseMyPlate.gov for more information.

DG TipSheet No. 1
June 2011
USDA is an equal opportunity provider and employer.

© Courtesy of the USDA.

Figure 17-8 Ten tips to creating an ideal MyPlate.

high blood pressure in many persons. Everyone, including children, is encouraged to consume less than 2,300 milligrams of sodium per day; that is the equivalent of approximately 1 teaspoon of salt. Persons older than 51 years of age, African Americans of any age, and persons with high blood pressure, diabetes, or chronic kidney disease are encouraged to reduce sodium intake to 1,500 milligrams per day.

Ways to consciously reduce sodium intake include the use of fresh rather than processed food and consuming smaller quantities of processed foods (cheesy foods, bacon, hot dogs, pizza, canned soups, and chili). Another strategy is to cook at home and gradually cut back on salt use. The choice of spices and herbs rather than salt to season foods helps to reduce dietary sodium intake. Reading food labels and selecting the product with the least amount of sodium is another way to reduce dietary sodium. Foods like pickles and olives, catsup, mustard, soy sauce, and salad dressings are high in sodium; use sparingly. Increasing intake of potassium-rich food, like potatoes (white and sweet), beans, bananas, oranges, and tomatoes, as well as yogurt and milk, can help to lower blood pressure.

Summary of DGAC Report

The 2015 DGAC report indicates that a healthy lifestyle is achievable if these guidelines are followed. The guidelines allow for flexibility in food choices to meet nutritional requirements. A program of regular physical activity in combination with the dietary plan can help with weight maintenance by balancing caloric intake and energy expenditure. Additional information may be found at the following sites: www.DietaryGuidelines.gov and www.ChooseMyPlate.gov.

NUTRITIONAL STATUS

Eating to meet nutritional needs is one of the major activities of daily living. Eating also meets important social and emotional needs when dining is carried out in the proper environment and with the proper support. Older people who live independently may prepare foods that satisfy their appetites, yet do not meet basic nutritional needs.

Easy-to-chew, high-calorie foods may provide energy in excess of body needs; the extra energy is stored as fat. Although the person's appetite is satisfied by these foods, they do not necessarily provide the nutrients needed. Essential vitamins, minerals, and proteins may be lacking.

Older people are at risk for becoming malnourished. An important part of the job of a nursing assistant is to monitor and report the food and fluid intake of the residents. Malnutrition can result in unintended weight loss and pressure ulcers. A guide called "Nutrition Care Alerts" has been developed by experts in nutrition and long-term care. The guide is to be used not only by nursing assistants but also by other members of the interdisciplinary health care team. Nutrition Care Alerts list the warning signs for unintended weight loss and dehydration and provides a list of actions that caregivers should take to avoid resident malnutrition.

- Warning signs for unintended weight loss:
- Needs help to eat or drink
- Eats less than half of the meals/snacks that are served
- Has mouth pain or dentures that do not fit
- Has a hard time using eating utensils
- Has a hard time chewing or swallowing
- Has sadness or crying spells, or withdraws from others
- Is confused, wanders, or paces
- Has diabetes, chronic obstructive lung disease, cancer, HIV, or other chronic diseases

? EXERCISE 17-5

COMPLETE THE FOLLOWING
Based on "MyPlate" in Figure 17-7, indicate the food groups.

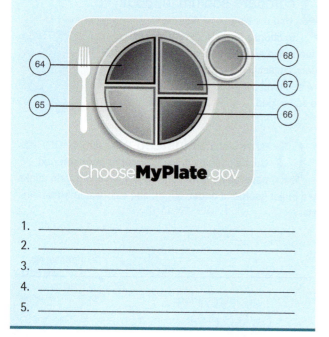

1. _____
2. _____
3. _____
4. _____
5. _____

If any of these signs are present, the nursing assistant should follow these steps:

- Report observations and warning signs to nurse and dietitian
- Reduce distractions from noise: turn off TV and phones
- Encourage resident to eat
- Honor food preferences
- Offer many kinds of foods and beverages
- Help residents who have trouble feeding themselves
- Allow adequate time to finish eating
- Notify nurse if resident has trouble using utensils
- Record meal/snack intake
- Provide oral hygiene before meals
- Position resident correctly for feeding

Facilities should have a protocol for standards of care for residents who experience weight loss of 5% or more in 30 days or 10% or more in the last 6 months. All residents should be weighed at least monthly and those at risk more often. It is important always to use the same scale, at about the same time of the day, and to take into account the weight of wheelchairs, leg rests, and clothing.

Residents who suffer dementia may be prone to weight loss and dehydration because they do not have sufficient food and fluid intake. These persons may forget to eat or they may not be able to visually identify the food and fluids to be consumed.

Research studies that were conducted at Boston University demonstrated that Alzheimer's disease affects areas of the brain that are responsible for vision that resulted in various visual defects. It was found that residents with advanced dementia consumed 25% more food and 84% more fluid if the substances were served from high-contrast dinnerware. Bright red plates, cups, and flatware were especially effective. It is important, however, to pair the food with the colored plate. For example, pizza slices would be more visually apparent on a white plate whereas mashed potatoes and chicken strips are more contrasting on a red plate. It may be helpful to use a contrasting placemat to make the plate more visible. Avoid using any patterned dinnerware or linens.

The serving of finger foods often encourages the resident with dementia to consume more food. Do not rush the resident; allow plenty of time for meals. Limit distractions. Remove clutter from the table and turn off any background noise such as the TV. If the resident doesn't eat an entire meal, offer various foods every few hours. For example, offer eggs and bacon, then in several hours offer toast strips, and then later offer a small fruit smoothie containing yogurt. In this way it may be possible to increase the amount of protein and calories the resident consumes.

DEHYDRATION

Water in adequate amounts is essential to normal body functioning. Most older adults need to consume about 2,000 to 3,000 mL or 2 to 3 quarts of liquid each day. If the body is functioning properly, the amount of fluids taken in will be balanced by the amount lost.

Dehydration (inadequate fluid level in the body) develops when fluid intake is not adequate. In addition, some drugs cause excessive amounts of fluids to be lost from the body. It is important to recognize the signs of dehydration. All signs of dehydration must be reported immediately so corrective actions can be taken.

The resident may not recognize thirst (Figure 17-9). Offer a variety of fluids frequently throughout the day. Encourage the resident to sip fluids while eating a meal. Offer some fruits with high water content, such as melon, pineapple, and citrus. Sometimes popsicles and root beer floats are welcomed treats that also add fluids to residents. Constantly monitor the resident for signs of dehydration and malnutrition: dry lips, cracked lips, white or parched tongue, scaly skin, and skin turgor (tenting).

The facility dietitian will calculate the daily fluid needs of residents who may be in danger of developing dehydration. The calculations are based on the weight of the person divided by 2.2 (weight in kilograms [kg]) times 25 to 35 mL of fluid. For example, a person who weighs 120 pounds would weigh

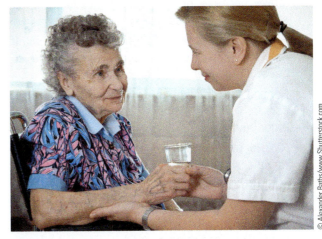

Figure 17-9 Residents may not recognize thirst so the nursing assistant should offer fluids frequently.

Schwab, J. 2010, Spring. *Out of sight, Out of mind: If you couldn't see your mashed potatoes you probably wouldn't eat them.* Retrieved July 16, 2011 from: http://www.bu.edu/cas/magazine/spring10/golomb/index.shtml

55 kg and would require 55 kg × 30 mL, or approximately 1,650 mL of fluid per day. If a resident has the tendency to retain fluids such as those persons with kidney failure or congestive heart failure, the dietitian will use 25 mL per kg to determine fluid needs. Fluid replacement for a person who may be losing fluids through fever or increased urination will need 35 mL per kg. Refer to the resident care plan to determine daily fluid needs for each resident.

Warning Signs of Dehydration

The Nutrition Care Alerts have identified the warning signs of dehydration:

- Drinks less than 6 cups of liquids daily
- Has one or more of the following:
  - Dry mouth
  - Cracked lips
  - Sunken eyes
  - Dark urine
- Needs help drinking from a cup or glass
- Has trouble swallowing liquids
- Has frequent vomiting, diarrhea, or fever
- Is easily confused or tired

Many residents do not take in enough fluids. This is especially true when they feel ill, have a fever, or have a decreased appetite. An essential task of nursing assistants is to remind and encourage residents to drink water or other fluids frequently.

- Always follow the care plan for each resident for fluid intake. Some residents may be on limited intake because of their medical conditions and should not be offered fluids.
- For other residents, be sure fresh water is within reach. Keep pitchers full. Some residents may request that ice be added to the water.
- Remind the resident to drink whenever you have contact with the resident. Offer flavored water or other beverages.
- A resident who has a fever requires careful monitoring of fluid intake.
- Increase attention to fluid intake during hot weather.
- If residents cannot drink unaided, offer fluids frequently and assist as needed.
- If a resident is to have intake monitored, record the amount of fluid consumed each time the resident drinks. If this is not possible, the amount of water left in a pitcher can be measured before the pitcher is refilled. The amount left is subtracted

from the total amount of water in the pitcher originally.

- Fluid intake over 24 hours is usually consumed during the day and evening shifts (0700–2300). It is important for nursing assistants on these shifts to encourage residents to drink adequate fluid.
- Provide alternatives for residents who do not like water. Check dietary card for beverage preferences. Check if resident prefers and is allowed ice in beverages.
- Serve water as well as other beverages at mealtime.

⊘ ON THE JOB

Residents may still become dehydrated even if they eat well-prepared, balanced meals.

The procedure for changing water is outlined in the facility procedure manual. Be sure you know the requirements for changing water, especially the steps to prevent the spread of infection. For example, if pitchers are taken to a central area to be refilled, be sure each resident receives his or her own pitcher and not one belonging to another resident. Pitchers must be covered before being taken back to the residents' rooms and should remain covered in the room. Facilities with ice machines/bins have specific infection control policies related to the use of the ice scoops. Follow agency protocol.

INTAKE AND OUTPUT (I&O)

The amount of fluid taken into the body and the amount of fluid lost should be just about equal. The intake and output (I&O) is frequently measured and recorded. Imbalances in intake and output can result in fluid imbalances such as edema (water retention) and dehydration.

Intake

Intake includes everything taken in that is liquid at room temperature. For example, included in the intake fluids are:

- Water or tea
- Gelatin, pudding, ice cream, popsicles
- Fluids given directly into a vein (IV)
- Fluids given by nasogastric tube or gastric tube

The output includes all fluids lost. This includes:

- Urine
- Perspiration
- Blood
- Diarrhea
- Vomiting
- Wound drainage
- Sputum

Calculating Fluid (Liquid) Intake (Output is covered in Lesson 18)

Calculating oral fluid intake is the responsibility of the nursing assistant. To do this correctly, you must know:

- The amount of fluid the container holds when full
- How to calculate the amount of fluid the resident drank from the container

The containers used include cups, glasses, soup bowls, water pitchers, milk cartons, ice cream cups, and gelatin and pudding cups. There are many types of containers and facilities do not all use the same kinds. Your facility will have a chart listing the sizes (amount of fluid the container can hold when full) of the containers used in the facility.

Fluids can be measured using either a standard household system (ounce, pint, quart) or the **metric system** (milliliter or cubic centimeter). A comparison of these measurements follows. Note that the abbreviation for milliliter is mL.

drop (gtt)		= .06 mL
teaspoon (tsp)		= 5 mL
tablespoon (tbsp)		= 15 mL
ounce (oz)		= 30 mL
pint (pt)	= 16 oz	= 480 mL
quart (qt)	= 32 oz	= 2 pt = 960 mL
gallon (gal)	= 128 oz	= 4 qt = 8 pt = 3,840 mL

You cannot actually measure what is gone from the container. Therefore, your calculation will be an estimate. It is important that the estimate be as accurate as possible. In facilities, fluid is recorded in **cubic centimeters (cc)** or **milliliters (mL)**. These measurements are the same amount. The preferred measurement is mL, but many facilities still use cc. All liquids and all foods that become liquid at room temperature (ice cream, sherbet, gelatin) are recorded

as fluid intake. All fluids taken with meals and between meals are recorded.

To simplify the calculation, some facilities consider a pint to be 500 mL, a quart 1,000 mL, and a gallon 4,000 mL. Some containers may be marked in ounces. The amount measured in ounces must be converted into mL. For example, a can of soda may be marked as 12 ounces. This equals 360 mL (12 × 30 mL where 30 mL is the same as 1 ounce).

- To calculate intake when the resident has finished drinking:
- Hold the container at eye level or place the container on a level surface and read contents at eye level.
- Determine whether $\frac{1}{4}, \frac{1}{3}, \frac{1}{2}, \frac{2}{3}$, or $\frac{3}{4}$ of the container of liquid has been consumed. Remember that containers are not filled to the top when full.
- Look at the facility's chart to see how much that type of container holds when it is full (Figure 17-10).
- Calculate the intake by multiplying the amount consumed times the amount the container holds when it is full.

Examples:

1. A juice glass holds 120 mL when full. The resident has consumed half of the juice. The intake is calculated: 1/2 × 120 (2 into 120) = 60 mL intake.
2. A water glass holds 180 mL when full. The resident has consumed 3/4 of the water. The intake is calculated: 3/4×180 (4 into 180 = 45) and multiply 45 times 3, which equals 135 mL intake.
3. An ice cream cup holds 150 mL when full. The resident has consumed all of the ice cream. Intake is recorded as 150 mL.

Water glass	= 6 oz	= 180 mL
Styrofoam cup	= 6 oz	= 180 mL
Juice glass (small)	= 4 oz	= 120 mL
Juice glass (large)	= 8 oz	= 240 mL
Full water pitcher (1 qt)	= 32 oz	= 960 mL
Coffee or tea pot	= 10 oz	= 300 mL
Coffee cup	= 5 oz	= 150 mL
Milk carton	= 8 oz	= 240 mL
Soup bowl (small)	= 6 oz	= 180 mL
Soup bowl (large)	= 10 oz	= 300 mL
Gelatin	= 4 oz	= 120 mL
Ice cream cup	= 5 oz	= 150 mL
Creamer	= 1 oz	= 30 mL

Figure 17-10 Average container amounts.

4. A soup bowl holds 180 mL when full. The resident has consumed 2/3 of the soup. The intake is calculated: 2/3 × 180 (3 into 180 × 60) and multiply 60 × 2. The intake is 120 mL.

When calculating fluids for a meal you may need to calculate the separate quantities, add them, and record the total intake for the meal. For example:

2/3 carton of milk	= 160 mL
1 small orange juice	= 120 mL
1/2 cup coffee	= 75 mL
1/3 glass water	= 60 mL

Total breakfast intake: 415 mL

A special form for recording I&O may be kept at the bedside to be used each day. Fluids taken in and lost are listed on the I&O sheet in the resident's health record (see Figure 17-11 in Procedure 17-37).

PROCEDURE 17-37
Measuring and Recording Fluid Intake

OBRA

1. Carry out each beginning procedure action.

2. Assemble the following:
   - Intake and output record at bedside
   - Pen for recording

3. Record intake on the I&O record at the bedside (Figure 17-11) by listing all fluids taken in. Total intake includes:
   - The amount of liquid the resident takes with meals
   - The amount of water and other liquids taken between meals
   - All other fluids given by mouth, intravenously, or by tube feeding. How these fluids are taken should also be recorded.

INTAKE AND OUTPUT

Room: 103 B   Name: Simon, Grace   Date:

Instructions: Record all I and O

2300-0700		0700-1500		1500-2300	
Intake	Output	Intake	Output	Intake	Output
Total		Total		Total	

Drinking Glass.........200 mL   Full Water Pitcher....950 mL   Milk Carton..............236 mL   Jello.........................90 mL
Styrofoam Cup........200 mL   Coffee or Teapot.....300 mL   Soup Bowl...............250 mL   Ice Cream Cup..........90 mL
Juice Glass (small)..100 mL   Coffee Cup.............150 mL   Soup Bowl (small)...100 mL   Creamer...................50 mL
Juice Glass (large)..250 mL

FOLEY CATHETER DRAINAGE: (Circle the following when applicable)

Color: Yellow   Amber   Brown   Red

Appearance: Cloudy   Clear   Sediment   Mucous   Bloody   24 hour INTAKE_____

Abdomen Distended   Catheter Irrigated   Catheter Changed   24 hour OUTPUT_____

Figure 17-11 An intake and output chart becomes part of the resident's record.

(continues)

PROCEDURE 17-37
Measuring and Recording Fluid Intake (Continued)

4. Copy information on the resident's chart from the bedside I&O record, according to facility policy. Report low intake to the nurse. Check the resident care plan to note individual needs.

5. Carry out each procedure completion action.

? EXERCISE 17-6

MEASURING AND RECORDING INTAKE

Measuring and recording intake are common nursing assistant assignments. It is important that you do it accurately.

Remember that when the whole of anything is divided into parts, each portion represents a fraction (part) of the entire amount. This fraction may be expressed as two numbers separated by a line. The bottom number represents all parts of the whole, and the top number represents the number of those parts that are still present.

For example:

$4/4$ means the whole is divided into four parts (the bottom number) and all four parts are present.

$1/2$ means the whole is divided into two parts and one part is present.

If a resident ate $1/2$ of a piece of toast, that means the whole toast has been cut into two parts, one of which was eaten. Therefore, if the resident is served a whole piece of toast and $1/2$ of the toast is left, you subtract what you found ($1/2$) from what you know is the total ($2/2$).

$$2/2 - 1/2 = 1/2 \text{ (subtract top number from the other)}$$

In each of the following, determine how much food or liquid has been taken.

Amount Left	Total to Start	Amount Taken
Example: $1/6$ glass of orange juice	$6/6$ glass	$6/6 - 1/6 = 5/6$ glass
1. $1/4$ glass of water	_____	_____
2. $1/2$ glass of cranberry juice	_____	_____
3. $2/3$ glass of milk	_____	_____
4. $3/4$ meat patty	_____	_____

Fluids are measured in milliliters (mL) so computations must be made using these measurements. For example:

A full pitcher of water holds 1,000 mL. You find the pitcher 1/2 full when you change the water. To determine how much water the resident has consumed:

1. Subtract the amount left from the whole:

$$2/2 - 1/2 = 1/2$$

2. Multiply $1/2 \times$ the total mL value of a whole carafe (1,000 mL)

$$1/2 \times 1,000 = 500 \text{ mL water taken}$$

Standard measurements are

Coffee/tea cup 240 mL
Foam cup 240 mL
Soup bowl 180 mL

Gelatin (1 serving) 120 mL
Water pitcher 1,000 mL

(*continues*)

? EXERCISE 17-6 (Continued)

5. Complete the equivalence chart by filling in the blank spaces.

U.S. Customary Units	Metric Units
a. 1 ounce	_____
b. _____	500 mL
c. 1 quart	_____
d. _____	15 mL
e. 1 gallon	_____
f. _____	30 mL

? EXERCISE 17-7

1. Complete the resident's intake record, using the information from the bedside records.

Peter Dismuke
Rm. N 117   Bedside Record
Dec 18

Time	Intake	Amount
1630	tea	120 mL
	ice cream	120 mL
	soup	120 mL
1820	water	100 mL
2100	ginger ale	100 mL
2200	water	90 mL

BAYSIDE SKILLED CARE FACILITY
FLUID INTAKE AND OUTPUT

Name _____   Room _____

Date	Time	Method of Adm.	Intake			Output		
			Solution	Amounts Rec'd	Time	Urine Amount	Others Kind	Amount
Total								

? EXERCISE 17-8

1. The bedside chart for Grace Borocho in Room 215D is shown below. Enter the information from the bedside chart in the intake record.

Bedside Chart

0700	juice	1 glass
	coffee	1 cup
0825	water	1 glass
1100	milk	1 carton
	soup	1 soup bowl
1300	water	1 glass
1430	gelatin	1 serving

INTAKE AND OUTPUT

Room: *215D*   Name: *BOROCHO, GRACE*   Date:

Instructions: *Record all I and O*

2300–0700		*0700–1500*		*1500–2300*	
Intake	Output	Intake	Output	Intake	Output
Total		Total		Total	

Drinking Glass........200 mL   Full Water Pitcher...950 mL   Milk Carton.............236 mL   Jello..........................90 mL
Styrofoam Cup........200 mL   Coffee or Teapot.....300 mL   Soup Bowl..............250 mL   Ice Cream Cup.........90 mL
Juice Glass (small)..100 mL   Coffee Cup.............150 mL   Soup Bowl (small)..100 mL   Creamer...................50 mL
Juice Glass (large)..250 mL

FOLEY CATHETER DRAINAGE: (Circle the following when applicable)

Color: Yellow   Amber   Brown   Red

Appearance: Cloudy   Clear   Sediment   Mucous   Bloody

Abdomen Distended   Catheter Irrigated   Catheter Changed

24 hour INTAKE_____

24 hour OUTPUT_____

DIETS

Some residents may need to have their diets modified because of health problems. Special diets are based on the food groups described previously, but consistency and method of preparation may be altered.

Standard Diets

Four standard diets are offered in long-term care facilities. These include:

1. Regular diet
2. Mechanical soft diet
3. Pureed diet
4. Liquid diet

Regular Diet

The regular diet is prepared for most residents. It includes varied selections from the food groups. It is rich in vitamins and minerals and provides adequate bulk and balanced calories (Figure 17-12).

Mechanical Soft Diet

The mechanical soft diet is based on the regular diet but includes liquids and semisolid foods that are more easily chewed and digested (Figure 17-13).

Pureed Diet

The pureed diet meets nutritional needs with foods that can be put into semiliquid or liquid form at room temperature (Figure 17-14). It may be given to residents with diseases of the intestinal tract or those who are unable to chew because of infection, stroke, or lack of teeth and difficulty swallowing.

Liquid Diets

Liquid diets are classified as clear liquid or full liquid. A *clear liquid diet* is a temporary diet because it is inadequate. It is used primarily to replace fluid that may be lost through vomiting or diarrhea. Clear liquids do not irritate, cause gas formation, or encourage bowel movements. This type of diet provides mainly fluid replacement and a few calories through the carbohydrate content. Feedings are usually given every 2, 3, or

4 hours as prescribed by the physician. Fluids that are allowed on a clear liquid diet (Figure 17-15) include:

- Tea and coffee with sugar, but no milk or cream
- Clear broths and bouillon
- Electrolyte replacement solutions (Gatorade or Pedialyte)
- Gelatin (occasionally)
- Popsicles
- Water or ice chips
- Ginger ale, 7 Up, colas
- Strained fruit or vegetable juices

Nutritionally adequate clear liquid diets (elemental diets), like Vivonex, can be ordered by the physician, if necessary.

A *full liquid diet* supplies nourishment and may be used for longer periods of time. Feedings of

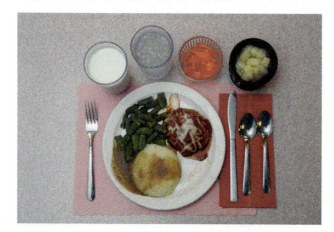

Figure 17-12 Well-balanced, smaller servings are more appealing to the elderly appetite.

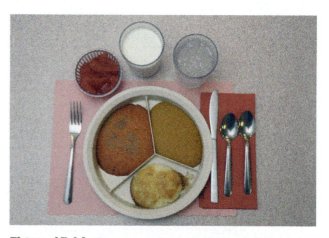

Figure 17-14 The pureed diet includes foods from each of the food groups. The foods were pureed in a blender.

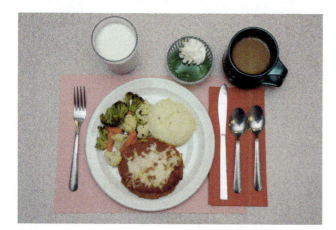

Figure 17-13 The mechanical soft diet is easy to chew and digest.

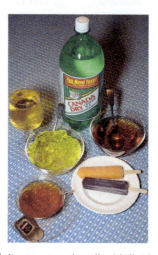

Figure 17-15 Items on a clear liquid diet include only liquids that you can see through.

6 to 8 ounces are given every 2 to 3 hours as pre-scribed. Full liquid diets are prescribed for persons who:

- Have difficulty chewing
- Have acute infections
- Have conditions involving the gastrointestinal system and are upgraded from clear liquids

A full liquid diet includes the following:

- Any type of milk product (unless lactose intolerant), plain ice cream, cream soups, plain yogurt, sherbets, puddings, malted milk
- Strained meat or poultry, eggs cooked in custards (raw eggs should not be used in milk shakes or eggnog because of the potential for bacterial contamination)
- Fruit and vegetable juices, strained fruits and vegetables
- Cereal gruel (strained cereals)
- Butter, margarine, or cream if not on a fat-free diet
- Any component or combination of clear liquids, sugars (honey, syrup, jelly, hard candy), salt or flavorings as tolerated, spices as tolerated

Building Cultural Awareness

- Remember that food may have an important relationship to cultural practices.
- Learn the cultural dietary preferences of the residents in your care. For example, Orthodox Jews do not eat pork or pork products; Seventh Day Adventists, Christian Scientists, and Mormons do not consume tea or coffee.
- Check with the nurse if food is brought in by the family to be sure it is permitted on the resident's diet. For example, American Indians (Native Americans) consume berries, corn, and dried meat after certain ceremonies and prayer. These foods may be brought to the resident from home.

Families of Chinese American residents may also bring in food that they believe will treat certain illnesses.

- Report to the nurse if the resident is not eating because of cultural preferences.

Therapeutic Diets

Therapeutic diets, also called special diets, are prepared for residents with specific needs (Figure 17-16). They include the:

- Diabetic diet
- Low-sodium diet
- Low-fat diet
- Calorie-restricted diet
- High-protein diet
- Low-residue diet
- Calorie-dense diet

The diabetic diet is usually a carefully balanced diet for residents who have diabetes mellitus and who must restrict concentrated sugar (e.g., candy or pastry) in their diet. They may eat only foods on their diet, but they must eat everything that is ordered for them. It is important that you report the exact amounts of foods eaten by the diabetic resident because their medication is calculated based on food intake. Some diabetic residents are able to control their sugar levels with a diet referred to a no concentrated sweet (NCS) diet.

The low-sodium diet is prescribed for the resident with a heart condition or one who retains fluids. The low-fat diet limits the amounts of fats in the diet and is served to residents who have gallbladder, cardiovascular, or liver disease. The calorie-restricted diet is given to residents in need of weight control (to avoid or correct obesity). The high-protein diet is provided for residents who are underweight and poorly nourished and when diseases such as cancer make unusual nutritional demands. Increased

Diabetic	Amounts of carbohydrates, fats, and proteins are balanced and prescribed. Concentrated sweets are restricted.
Low-sodium (sodium-restricted)	Amounts of sodium are specifically prescribed, such as 500 mg sodium. Sodium-rich foods, such as milk, bacon, and salted nuts, are excluded.
Low-fat	Foods with high fat content, such as whole milk and eggs, are restricted. Use of fats in preparation of food is eliminated.
Calorie-restricted	Number of calories is limited while ensuring an adequate intake of nutrients.
High-protein	Foods high in protein, iron, and vitamins are served in six small meals per day. Hot, spicy foods are excluded.
Low-residue	Roughage, fresh fruits and vegetables (except bananas and potatoes), nuts, and whole grains are limited.

Figure 17-16 Summary of therapeutic diets.

? EXERCISE 17-9

TRUE OR FALSE

Indicate whether the following statements are true (T) or false (F).

1. T F The primary source of body energy is provided by proteins.

2. T F Fruit is an excellent source of proteins.

3. T F Heat energy is measured in units called calories.

4. T F Fiber found in carbohydrate foods helps maintain bowel activity.

5. T F Vitamin D is a water-soluble vitamin and is found in whole-grain products.

6. T F Fats supply energy and heat to the body.

7. T F The charge nurse plans the residents' meals.

8. T F Easy-to-chew, high-calorie foods always provide sufficient nutrition.

9. T F Half your plate should be fruits and vegetables.

10. T F The elderly person may need to supplement the diet with vitamins and minerals.

11. T F Eating whole fruits is suggested instead of fruit juice because juices lack necessary fiber.

12. T F Nutrition care alerts list the warning signs for unintended weight loss and dehydration, and tells caregivers how to avoid resident malnutrition.

13. T F If a nursing assistant notices a sign of unintended weight loss in a resident, he or she should restrict the resident's options for food and beverage.

14. T F All residents should be weighed at least weekly.

? EXERCISE 17-10

MATCHING

Match the diet on the right to the resident need on the left.

Resident Need

1. _____ Mrs. Riley, 90 years of age, is poorly nourished, underweight, and has cancer.

2. _____ Mr. Rubenstein, a Jewish cantor, has emphysema.

3. _____ Mr. Smith is 84 years old with colitis. He needs to limit roughage intake.

4. _____ Mrs. Sanders has diabetes mellitus.

5. _____ Mrs. Robinson has gallbladder disease.

6. _____ Mr. Baum has heart disease.

7. _____ Mrs. Carr is 78 years of age and overweight.

8. _____ Mr. Brown is 86 years of age and refuses to wear his dentures.

9. _____ Mrs. McElvy is 81 years of age and is fed through a tube directly into her stomach.

10. _____ Mr. Haag is 94 years of age and, although still mobile, needs assistance with ADL.

Diet

a. diabetic

b. regular

c. mechanical soft

d. liquid commercial

e. low fat

f. calorie restricted

g. high protein

h. low sodium

i. kosher diet

j. low-residue diet

protein intake can also promote skin healing for persons with burns or pressure ulcers.

The low-residue diet is served to residents who need to limit roughage intake. It is given when residents have lower bowel problems such as colitis and diarrhea.

Residents who have unintentional weight loss, such as those undergoing chemotherapy for cancer or with dementia, may be prescribed a calorie-dense diet that helps them maintain their weight or even provide for weight gain. This diet allows for additional calorie intake without increased quantities of food.

Remember, special diets are *therapeutic*, which means they are used as *treatments*. Always check to be sure that the resident receives the right tray.

A progressive diet is ordered for many residents after digestive upset, as their conditions permit. The usual progression is:

- Ice chips/sips of water
- Clear liquids
- Full liquids
- Soft or light diet
- Regular diet

NURSING ASSISTANT RESPONSIBILITIES

Nursing assistants have a personal responsibility to provide good nutrition for themselves so they will stay healthy and have the energy to do their work. They also play an important role in helping residents to meet their nutritional needs.

It is important that each nursing assistant know and understand:

- The nutrients and amounts needed for health
- The importance of adequate water intake to prevent dehydration
- Ways diets can be modified to meet individual health needs

Mealtime is a busy time in the long-term care facility. The nursing assistant has a major responsibility to see that it goes smoothly and pleasantly. You will:

- Make sure the area is pleasant and odor-free.
- Assist residents to reach the dining room.
- Serve trays.
- Help residents who need assistance in eating.
- Use clothing protectors as needed.
- Always be sure the resident receives the proper diet (standard or therapeutic) by checking the tray card.

- Observe the amount of intake by the resident. Document as per agency protocol.
- Offer substitutes if the resident dislikes the food that is served.
- Be sure foods are served at the proper temperature; don't hesitate to warm foods if necessary.
- Make sure that used trays are not returned to the serving cart until all clean trays have been served.
- Keep food trays covered until served.
- Keep housekeeping carts and laundry hampers out of the corridor when food is served or keep them at least two room widths away from the food cart when they are placed in the corridor.
- Place the food cart against the wall when it is brought into the dining room.
- Keep doors to the food cart closed until the trays are served.

Eating may be one of the few generally enjoyable activities left to older persons. In addition to meeting nutritional needs, meals should also be sensually and socially satisfying. Large dining areas permit residents to eat together and promote a social atmosphere. The meals are prepared by the dietary staff in large kitchens and brought to the dining area on tray carts (Figure 17-17).

In many facilities, special evening meals are organized so that residents who are able will dress up and eat in a restaurant-like atmosphere. Dining tables are set up homestyle and dinner is not served on trays.

This activity meets both social and nutritional needs and is greatly appreciated by residents.

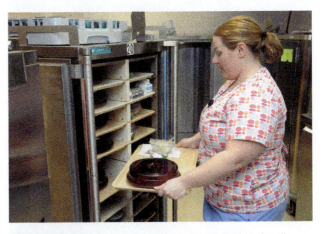

Figure 17-17 Residents' diets are prepared in the dietary department. The dietary aide takes the marked tray from the cart to serve to the resident. If a dietary aide is not available, the nursing assistant delivers the tray to the resident.

Assisting with Feeding

If residents can go to the dining room:

- Assist them to the toilet before mealtimes.
- Help them wash their hands.
- Help them into the dining room.

Wheelchairs can be rolled into the dining room if residents cannot walk. Some residents may remain in their wheelchairs. Other residents will transfer to dining room chairs. After washing your own hands, help serve the trays and assist as necessary (Figure 17-18).

- Cut meat into small, bite-size pieces. Allow resident time to chew thoroughly.
- Pour liquids. Do not fill containers too full. Cool hot drinks with milk or water to prevent burns.
- Butter bread using tongs or the bread wrapper, and cut into small pieces.
- Unfold and position napkin or apply clothing protector as needed.

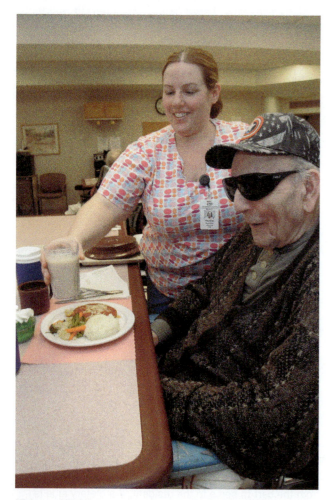

Figure 17-18 If residents need assistance, nursing assistants help them eat.

In some states nutritional assistants are hired at mealtimes to assist with feeding the residents. These persons are paid for their services and have special training to perform the needed tasks.

Feeding the Resident

Even when a resident is confined to bed or must be fed, you can make the experience more pleasant if you:

- Position the resident comfortably upright
- Provide clothing protector as needed
- Remove all unpleasant things from sight
- Never hurry the resident
- Allow the resident to help as much as possible
- Identify the food offered
- Always identify hot liquids
- Season food as the resident desires
- Use a different straw with each liquid
- Place food on unaffected side of the mouth if the resident is paralyzed
- Feed food from tip of spoon
- Provide a clothing protector
- Do not refer to these residents as "feeders"; use the term "assisted diners."
- Calculate amount of food that was consumed (Figure 17-19G).

Use of Food Thickeners

If the resident has difficulty swallowing, commercial food thickeners may be added to the diet. The type and amount of thickener is usually ordered by the speech therapist. The nursing staff, including nursing assistants, usually add the thickener at the time of feeding. When adding thickener, the nursing assistant must be sure that the:

- Correct thickener is added
- Correct amount of thickener is added
- Thickener is added according to the manufacturer's instructions
- The consistency of the thickened fluid is usually that of fruit nectar, honey, or pudding, or as prescribed.

When using food thickeners, follow the procedure for feeding the dependent resident. (See Procedure 17-39.) Be sure to allow enough time so the resident is not rushed. Direct the food and liquids toward the unaffected side of the mouth. Feed with the tip of a spoon that is not more than one-half full.

PROCEDURE 17-38
Assisting the Resident Who Can Feed Self

OBRA

1. Carry out each beginning procedure action.

2. Assemble equipment:
   - Bedpan/urinal
   - Wash water
   - Oral hygiene items
   - Tray of food

3. Offer bedpan/urinal. (If used, follow steps in Procedure 18-40 in Lesson 18.)

4. If permitted, elevate head of bed or assist resident out of bed.

5. Clear overbed table and position in front of resident (Figure 17-19A). Remove unpleasant equipment from sight. Remove sources of odors.

6. Provide water, soap, and towel to wash resident's hands and face (Figure 17-19B).

7. Assist with oral hygiene if desired.

8. Wash your hands. Obtain tray from dietary cart.

9. Check the diet with the dietary card and with the resident's identification band or photo according to agency protocol (Figure 17-19C).

10. Place tray on overbed table and arrange food in a convenient manner.

11. Describe the foods and where the foods are located on the plate (reference as to the face of a clock). See Figure 17-19D. Note this method is critical for the resident who has limited vision or is blind. It helps them to be independent as long as possible.

12. Assist in food preparation as needed (Figure 17-19E). Encourage resident to do as much as possible.

13. Remove tray as soon as resident is finished. Calculate food intake (Figure 17-19F).

14. Record fluids on intake record, if necessary.

15. Push overbed table out of the way.

(A)

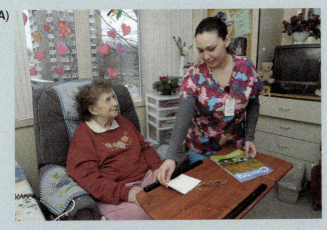

Figure 17-19A Clear off overbed table to make room for food tray.

(B)

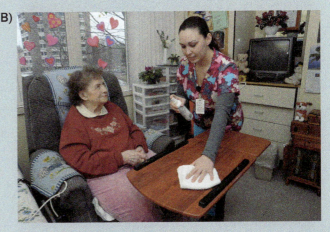

Figure 17-19B Cleanse overbed table.

(*continues*)

PROCEDURE 17-38
Assisting the Resident
Who Can Feed Self (Continued)

(C)

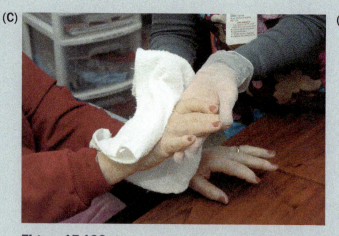

Figure 17-19C Give resident water to wash hands.

(D)

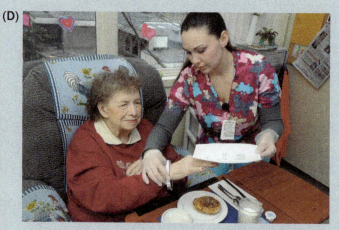

Figure 17-19D Check resident's arm band against the tray card to ensure that the resident is getting the right diet.

(E)

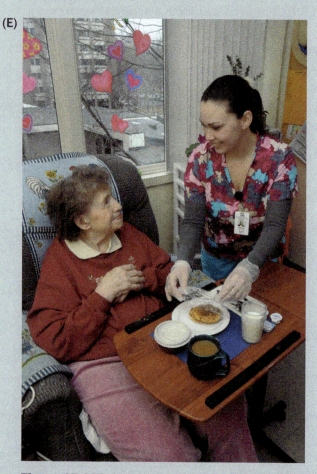

Figure 17-19E Assist resident in food preparation as needed.

(F)

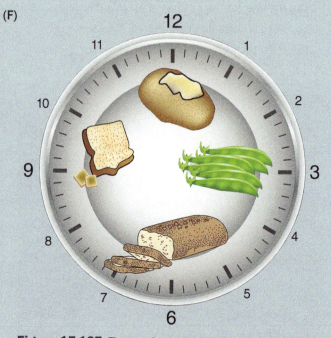

Figure 17-19F The numbers on a clock are used to help a visually impaired resident locate food.

(continues)

PROCEDURE 17-38
Assisting the Resident Who Can Feed Self (Continued)

16. Help perform oral hygiene to clean teeth or dentures and mouth.

17. Carry out each procedure completion action.

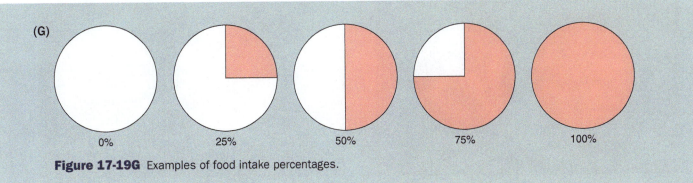

(G)

0%   25%   50%   75%   100%

Figure 17-19G Examples of food intake percentages.

NOTE: The nursing assistant in the photos for this procedure is wearing gloves while preparing the resident to eat. Some facilities require the wearing of gloves; others do not. Follow your facility policy.

PROCEDURE 17-39
Feeding the Dependent Resident

OBRA

1. Carry out each beginning procedure action.

2. Assemble equipment:
   - Bedpan/urinal
   - Wash water
   - Oral hygiene items
   - Tray of food

3. Offer bedpan or urinal. (If used, follow steps in Procedure 18-40 in Lesson 18.)

4. Provide oral hygiene if desired, and allow the resident to wash hands.

5. Remove unnecessary articles from the overbed table.

6. Elevate head of bed. Assist resident into a sitting or upright position with head slightly bent forward. If resident is out of bed, position resident in chair in an upright position with feet flat on the floor.

7. Place napkin, towel, or clothing protector under resident's chin (Figure 17-20A).

8. Obtain tray and check diet with the dietary card and the resident's identification band.

9. Place tray on overbed table (Figure 17-20B). Sit down facing resident so you are at eye level. The environment should be quiet and calm.

10. Butter bread and cut meat. Do not pour hot beverage until resident is ready for it. Be sure, however, that the beverage is cool enough to drink before offering it to the resident.

(continues)

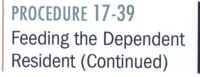

PROCEDURE 17-39
Feeding the Dependent Resident (Continued)

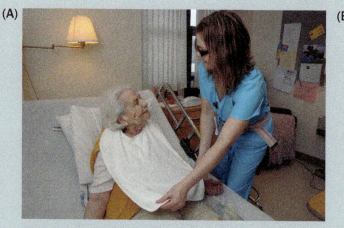

(A)

Figure 17-20A Place towel or clothing protector under the resident's chin.

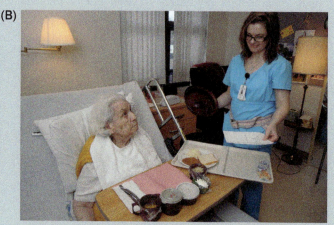

(B)

Figure 17-20B Uncover food and place it on the overbed table.

11. Use different drinking straws for each fluid or use a cup. Thick fluids are more easily controlled by using a straw. Do not use straws for residents with aspiration precautions. Use modified cups with spill-proof lids. Refer to resident care plan.

12. Holding spoon at a right angle:

    - Give solid foods from point of spoon (Figure 17-20C).
    - Alternate solids and liquids.
    - Rotate the offerings of food to give variety.
    - Describe or show resident what kind of food you are giving.
    - If resident has had a stroke, direct food to unaffected side of mouth and check for food stored in affected side (also known as "pocketing").
    - Test hot foods by dropping a small amount on the inside of your wrist before feeding them to the resident.
    - Never blow on the resident's food to cool it.
    - Never taste the resident's food.
    - Do not hurry the meal.

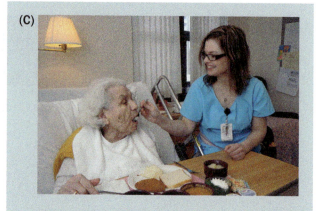

(C)

Figure 17-20C Give solid foods from the tip of the spoon.

13. Allow resident to hold bread or assist to the extent possible.

14. Use napkin to wipe resident's mouth as often as necessary.

15. Remove tray as soon as resident is finished. Calculate food intake (see Figure 17-19G). Report inadequate intake; a liquid nutritional supplement (Glucerna, Ensure, or Boost) may be substituted for the uneaten portion of the meal.

16. Provide oral hygiene.

17. Document fluid and solid food intake as per agency policy.

18. Carry out each procedure completion action.

❓ EXERCISE 17-11

TRUE OR FALSE

Indicate whether the following statements are true (T) or false (F).

1. T F Feeding procedures should be hurried because residents are very hungry.
2. T F You must make sure the resident is fed in the supine position.
3. T F Bedpans can be left covered on a chair while feeding a resident.
4. T F Never let the resident help feed himself or herself because that wastes time.
5. T F Be quiet and do not talk so that the resident can concentrate on eating.
6. T F Put food in the resident's mouth and let the resident try to guess what he or she is eating.
7. T F Give all fluids at the end of the meal to wash down the food.
8. T F Before tray time the resident should have the opportunity to visit the restroom or use a bedpan.
9. T F It is all right to place food carts near soiled linen barrels.
10. T F Used trays are returned after all clean trays have been served.
11. T F All foods should be served at a cool temperature so residents will not be burned.
12. T F Insertion of a nasogastric tube is an appropriate nursing assistant function.
13. T F Hyperalimentation provides high-density nutrients directly into the stomach through a gavage tube.
14. T F All facilities require that nursing assistants wear gloves when feeding residents.
15. T F You should keep seated residents upright after a meal for 30 minutes.

Choking

Choking is always a danger when feeding dependent or older residents because their swallowing ability is not always effective. Be sure to check the resident care plan for any precautions and suggestions before feeding. Watch carefully for signs of aspiration during intake. All health care providers working with the older persons should know how to do abdominal thrusts for choking victims (Heimlich maneuver). Be especially careful with dry, grainy foods such as bran or corn bread, because these are more difficult to swallow. Put such foods in milk or give in small amounts followed by liquid. Visually check the resident's mouth after eating for food that may have been pocketed in the cheeks. Provide mouth care. Keep seated residents upright for 30 minutes following a meal and residents who are fed in bed at a 45- to 60-degree angle. Care of the choking resident is covered in Lesson 8.

NOURISHMENTS AND SUPPLEMENTS

Nourishments are tasty refreshments, such as crackers, milk, juice, custards, and gelatins that residents enjoy between meals. Supplements are liquids or foods ordered by the physician to improve the nutritional status of the resident. Supplements are often given to increase weight. It is important that all ordered supplements are served in a timely manner and not be allowed to sit on the table for long periods of time.

Nursing assistants may be asked to serve nourishments or supplements, encourage residents to eat or drink them, and assist as necessary. If this is your assignment, be sure that you:

- Wash your hands before serving nourishments or supplements.
- Check the care plan and follow the dietary instructions carefully.
- Check that the right nourishment or supplement is given to the right resident.
- Allow a choice of nourishments if possible.
- Assist the resident if help is needed.
- Serve supplements at scheduled times. If they are served too close to meal time, the resident may feel too full to eat.
- Do not offer nourishments or supplements to residents who are not scheduled to receive them.
- If a resident asks for a supplement or a different supplement, check with your supervisor.
- Do not allow partially eaten nourishments or supplements to remain in the residents' rooms. Most nourishments or supplements are served in disposable containers.

• Record the nourishment or supplement served and the amount consumed according to facility policy. Record fluids on the intake form if required.

ALTERNATE METHODS OF FEEDING

There are several alternate ways to provide nutrition to a resident. These include:

• Enteral feedings
  • Nasogastric tube (NG tube) feedings (Figure 17-21A)
  • Gastrostomy tube (G tube) feedings (Figure 17-21B)
  • Jejunostomy tube (Figure 17-21C)
• Total parenteral nutrition (TPN)

Enteral Feeding

A nasogastric (NG) tube is a small tube introduced into the nose and through the pharynx and esophagus and into the stomach by the physician or nurse. A gastrostomy (G) tube is a small tube surgically or endoscopically (PEG) placed directly into the resident's stomach (Figure 17-21A and B). Feedings may be introduced through the gastrostomy or nasogastric tube using a syringe or feeding pump.

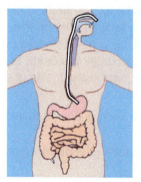
(A) Nasogastric Route

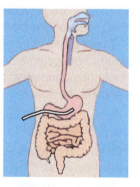
(B) Gastrostomy Route

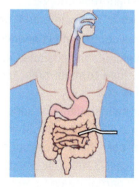
(C) Jejunostomy Route

Figure 17-21 Enteral feeding methods. (A) Nasogastric route. (B) Gastrostomy route. (C) Jejunostomy route.

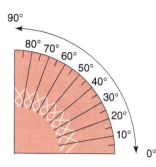

Figure 17-22 The head of the bed must be elevated 30 to 45 degrees or as specified on the plan of care whenever the tube feeding is running, and for at least 30 minutes after the feeding is completed. To prevent aspiration, never position the head of the bed lower than 30 degrees.

Tube feedings require special training and are performed by the nurse. Commercially prepared formula or liquid food is introduced directly into the tube (Figure 17-23C). The head of the bed must be elevated at 30 or 45 degrees, or according to facility policy, during the feeding and for 30 minutes after (see Figure 17-23). Great care must be taken to ensure that the tubes are properly positioned and are not pulled out or moved even slightly. You must inform the nurse if:

• You find the tube in the bed
• The resident complains of discomfort
• The resident is coughing or choking
• The resident feels nauseated, or vomits or retches
• The resident has diarrhea, constipation, a swollen stomach, or cramping
• There is redness, pain, heat, swelling, or oozing of fluid from the site where the tube is inserted into the body
• The resident has a cough or "wheezing" wet breathing sounds, or a feeling that something is caught in the throat

Other actions the nursing assistant can take include:

• Maintaining the head of the bed at least 30 degrees or more while the feeding is being given
• Maintaining the head of the bed at least 30 degrees for at least 30 minutes after a feeding
• Checking taping of the tube; if taping is loose, inform the nurse
• Reporting any retching (straining to but not vomiting), nausea, or vomiting immediately
• Ensuring that the end of the tube is closed between feedings
• Providing frequent mouth hygiene
• Not permitting tension on the tubes
• Being alert for kinks in the tubing
• Reporting signs of irritation near the tube entrance

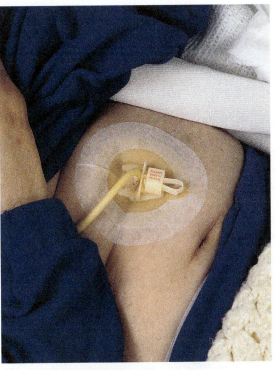

(B)

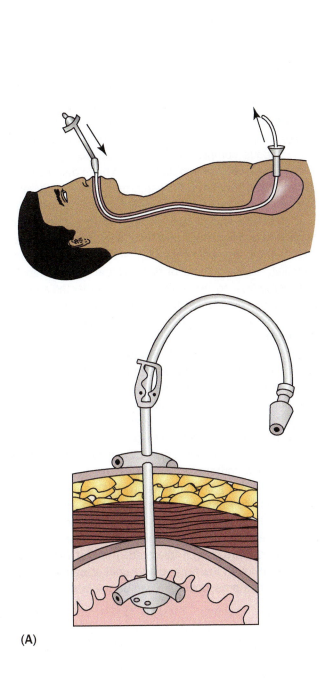

(A)

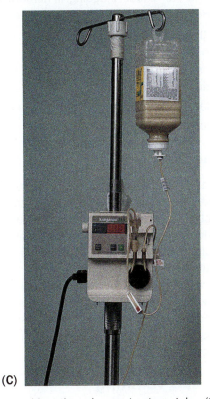

(C)

Figure 17-23 (A) Location of gastrostomy tube on abdomen. (B) Feeding a resident through a gastrostomy tube. (C) Using a feeding pump and prepared liquid nutrients.

- If food is given by pump, informing the nurse if:
  - The alarm goes off
  - The bag holding the solution is empty
  - The resident is coughing or choking

Total Parenteral Nutrition (TPN)

Total parenteral nutrition (TPN) or hyperalimentation is a technique in which **high-density** (concentrated) nutrients are introduced into a large vein such as the subclavian vein or the superior vena cava. The nurse manages TPN.

Notify the nurse if you notice that the system is leaking or if there is any redness around the area of the dressing.

DISORDERS OF THE DIGESTIVE SYSTEM

Constipation

Constipation is a common problem for older persons. Hard feces that are difficult to expel are a sign of constipation. This can be very uncomfortable for the resident and can cause bleeding if hemorrhoids are present. Regular bowel movements are aided by:

- Enough fluid intake to lubricate the colon and soften the feces
- Adequate fiber in the diet to act as bulk to promote intestinal activity
- Regular exercise to promote muscle tone
- Regular toileting opportunities

Dysphagia

Dysphagia (difficult swallowing) may be caused by decreased saliva production, paralysis due to a stroke, or obstructions such as malignancy of the esophagus. These residents are more prone to aspiration. The care plan should include a note to observe for aspiration and institute aspiration precautions.

The resident with dysphagia can more easily consume thick liquids and pureed foods than solid foods. If the difficulty is prolonged, it may be necessary to provide nourishment directly into the stomach or through hyperalimentation.

Nausea and Vomiting

Nausea and vomiting may be transient or persistent but should never be overlooked. These symptoms can be associated with a wide variety of disorders. Nausea is difficult to define because it is a subjective feeling; based on observation of the resident. It may be accompanied by the desire to vomit. Nausea can be precipitated by pain or unpleasant memories, an early sign of a disease process or infection, a side effect of a medication, a sign of food poisoning, or a physiologic change that occurs in the body such as during pregnancy or menstruation.

Vomiting is a complex series of events that results in the forceful expelling of the contents of the stomach through the mouth. It is important to determine the cause of the nausea and vomiting. Symptomatic relief may be provided through the use of antiemetic drugs and by temporarily avoiding oral intake of food and fluids.

Serious complications may result from prolonged vomiting: electrolyte imbalance, acid-base disturbance, dehydration, malnutrition, aspiration pneumonia, and tears in the mucous lining of the stomach and esophagus.

The CNA should observe and record the presence of nausea and vomiting and help to determine the cause, describe the amount, character, and frequency of the vomiting. Note the time of day and the relationship to food or medication intake. Determine whether the emesis contains any undigested food or has a coffee-ground appearance (may indicate the presence of bleeding). Do not discard the emesis until the nurse has observed it and determines whether there is a need for laboratory analysis of the specimen. Observe for signs of dehydration.

Food and fluids will usually be withheld for several hours or longer. Maintain NPO status as long as prescribed. Provide oral care every 2 hours. When oral intake resumes, the resident usually begins with clear liquids such as Gatorade, apple juice, ginger ale, broth, or gelatin. Allow carbonated beverages to sit and become "flat" to prevent gastric irritation or distention from the carbon dioxide in the beverages. Avoid the use of plain water because it contains no electrolytes or nutrients and can lead to electrolyte imbalance. Sometimes dry toast or crackers can be tolerated. The diet will usually progress through low-fat and soft until a regular diet or the resident's prescribed diet can be tolerated.

Hernias

A **hernia** occurs when a structure such as the intestine pushes out of its normal body position. Hernias are also known as **ruptures**. These may develop as the intestines push through a weakened area in the abdominal wall.

There are different kinds of hernias, depending on location. Types of hernias include femoral, umbilical, incisional, epigastric but the two types of hernias most common in older persons are:

- **Inguinal hernias**
- **Hiatal hernias**

Inguinal Hernia

This is a protrusion of the intestines through the wall in the groin area. It is felt as a small lump, especially when the resident strains.

Hiatal Hernia

In a hiatal hernia, the stomach pushes upward into the thoracic cavity, through the normal opening that allows the esophagus to pass through the diaphragm to the stomach. Signs and symptoms of hiatal hernia are:

- Dysphagia
- Pain and pressure in the chest as food and gastric fluid become trapped in the esophagus

The hydrochloric acid in the trapped gastric fluid can be very irritating, causing inflammation and ulceration of the esophagus.

Hiatal hernias tend to be a chronic problem. Residents feel better when they:

- Eat smaller meals
- Eat sitting up

They also feel more comfortable sleeping when the head of the bed is slightly raised. Antacids are sometimes ordered to overcome the acidity and reduce discomfort. Residents should avoid lying flat after meals.

Inflammation

Inflammation anywhere along the gastrointestinal tract can cause distress and the possibility of tissue breakdown and the formation of ulcers. Inflammation of the stomach (**gastritis**) can lead to **dyspepsia** (indigestion). A combination of overeating, foods that are too spicy, and natural aging changes can cause gastric distress. Also, ulcerations in the colon can cause blood in the stool and painful defecation.

Diverticulosis

Diverticuli are small, weakened areas in the wall of the colon (Figure 17-24). These areas form small pockets. Seeds and other hard food particles sometimes become trapped, causing inflammation (**diverticulitis**). When the diverticuli become inflamed, the resident complains of constipation and pain and is more susceptible to infection.

When diverticuli are multiple, the condition is called diverticulosis. Residents who have diverticulosis feel best when:

- A bland diet is eaten
- Weight is controlled
- Constipation is avoided
- Smaller, frequent meals are consumed

Sometimes part of the bowel must be removed to correct the problem.

Malignancy

Malignancies, or cancers, of the digestive system occur frequently in older people. Cancers may occur anywhere along the tract, but commonly occur in the lower colon. Because the lumen of the large intestine is fairly big, cancer can grow inside the colon for a relatively long time before it becomes large enough to cause an obstruction or change the character of the feces.

Hemorrhoids

Hemorrhoids are varicose veins of the rectum. Their presence can make defecation painful, and they sometimes bleed. Regularity and keeping feces soft to avoid straining are important in preventing complications.

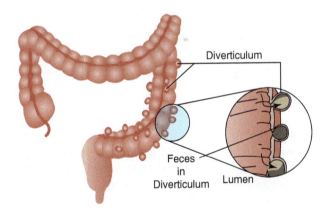

Figure 17-24 Diverticulosis.

? EXERCISE 17-12

CLINICAL SITUATIONS

Read the following situations and answer the questions.

1. Mrs. Young has a hiatal hernia. List ways you can assist her to feel more comfortable.

   _____

   _____

   _____

   _____

(continues)

? EXERCISE 17-12 (Continued)

2. Mrs. Montelongo has diverticulitis. What type of diet is best for her? _____ Two other situations that should be controlled to increase her comfort are _____ and avoiding _____.

3. Mr. Vincencio is receiving an intravenous solution of 1,000 mL 5% D/W with an infusion pump. List four actions you will take to provide the best nursing assistant care.

a.

_____

_____

b.

_____

_____

c.

_____

_____

d.

_____

_____

Mrs. Santos is a resident in the Upland nursing facility located in the southwestern part of America. She has had a bad cold and an elevated temperature. Her skin is dry, and her appetite is poor. It is late spring and the weather is unseasonably hot and dry.

4. What factors in Mrs. Santos' situation might lead to dehydration?

_____

5. How can the nursing assistants ensure adequate fluid intake?

_____

6. What signs would indicate that the resident is dehydrated?

_____

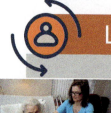

👤 LESSON SYNTHESIS: Putting It All Together

You have just completed this lesson. Now go back and review the Clinical Focus. Try to see how the Clinical Focus relates to the concepts presented in the lesson. Then answer the following questions.

1. Why is it especially important for Mrs. Hartley to receive proper nutrition and hydration at this time?

2. What kind of supplemental nourishments might be beneficial for her and when might you offer them?

3. From your observations, what might you suspect about Mrs. Hartley's level of hydration?

4. What beverage would you not serve to this resident?

17 REVIEW

A. Match each term with the proper definition

a. digestive system   f. flatulence

b. defecation   g. gastritis

c. digestion   h. nasogastric tube

d. dehydration   i. hyperalimentation

e. enzymes   j. obesity

1. _____ chemicals that help digest foods

2. _____ inflammation of the stomach

3. _____ bowel movement

4. _____ the condition of being overweight

5. _____ feeding tube

6. _____ total parenteral nutrition

7. _____ gastrointestinal tract

8. _____ gas

9. _____ excessive water loss

10. _____ mechanical and chemical process that breaks down food

B. Identify the parts of the digestive system by inserting the correct number of each part.

_____ appendix

_____ colon

_____ esophagus

_____ gallbladder

_____ liver

_____ mouth

_____ pharynx

_____ rectum

_____ small intestine

_____ stomach

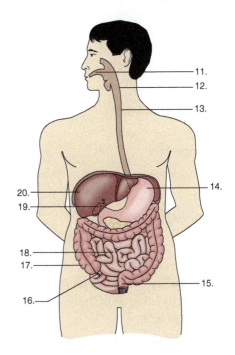

C. Indicate which of the following changes are associated with aging by circling yes (Y) or no (N).

21. Y N More sensitive taste

22. Y N Thinner saliva

23. Y N Reduced digestive enzymes

24. Y N More rapid absorption of nutrients

25. Y N Poorer tolerance to some foods

D. Select the one best answer for each of the following.

26. The primary source of energy for the body is

(A) fat

(B) minerals

(C) carbohydrates

(D) proteins

27. Which basic nutrient is essential for tissue building and repair?

(A) fats

(B) carbohydrates

(C) minerals

(D) proteins

28. Vitamins B and C are found in

(A) beef

(B) fruits and vegetables

(C) eggs

(D) vegetable oils

29. How much water should be taken in daily?

(A) 1 pint

(B) 3 glasses

(C) 2 cups

(D) 2 to 3 quarts

30. The 2015 Dietary Guidelines for Americans encourages people to follow all of the following recommendations except:

(A) Eat at least half of all grains as whole-grain foods.

(B) Half of MyPlate should be fruits and vegetables.

(C) Eat increased amounts of sugar, salt, and fats.

(D) Eat foods containing potassium.

31. Which of the four common diets prepared for long-term care residents includes liquids and semisolid foods that are more easily chewed and digested?

(A) pureed

(B) clear liquid

(C) regular

(D) mechanical soft

32. Which food is likely to be restricted on a low-fat diet?

(A) apples

(B) whole milk

(C) bananas

(D) white fish

33. Which food is excluded from a low-sodium diet?

(A) potato

(B) bacon

(C) whole-grain cereal

(D) carrot

34. Which food may be included on a low-residue diet?

(A) celery

(B) orange

(C) banana

(D) bran flakes

E.   Match the therapeutic diet (items a–e) with the specific requirements.

a. diabetic

b. low-sodium

c. low-fat

d. calorie-restricted

e. high-protein

35. _____ prescribed for resident with heart condition or one who retains fluid

36. _____ served to residents who are underweight or poorly nourished

37. _____ served to residents with cardiovascular, gallbladder, or liver disease

38. _____ carefully balanced, concentrated carbohydrates restricted

39. _____ given to residents who need weight control

F.   Determine the resident's intake using the chart on the I&O form at the end of this section. The resident has consumed:

40. ⅔ of a drinking glass of water   ___mL___

41. ¾ of a small glass of orange juice   _____

42. ⅔ of a small glass of apple juice   _____

43. ½ of a water pitcher   _____

44. ¾ of a water pitcher   _____

45. ⅓ of a cup of coffee   _____

46. ¼ of a carton of milk   _____

47. ¾ of a dish of gelatin   _____

      Total intake   _____

G. On the chart provided at the end of this section, make a record of the resident's intake and output for an 8-hour period.

48.

0730	Urine	300 mL
0800	Orange juice	90 mL
	Coffee	120 mL
0930	Water	60 mL
1130	Tea	120 mL
	Soup	120 mL
1300	Urine	400 mL
1315	Water	80 mL
1500	Cranberry juice	100 mL
1515	Vomitus	120 mL
1620	Tea	120 mL
	Sherbet	120 mL
1730	Urine	300 mL
1800	Water	150 mL
2100	Ginger ale	100 mL
2130	Urine	300 mL
2200	Water	90 mL

H. Match the metric amounts with their approximate equivalents.

a. 500 mL   d. 3,840 mL

b. 0.06 mL   e. 1,000 mL

c. 30 mL

49. _____ 1 minim

50. _____ 1 quart

51. _____ 1 gallon

52. _____ 1 pint

53. _____ 1 ounce

I. Show your understanding of fractions by completing the following problems.

54. ½ + ½ = _____

55. ⅔ + ⅓ = _____

56. ¼ + ¼ = _____

57. ¾ + ¼ = _____

58. Your resident drinks ⅔ of her juice. The glass held 120 mL. How much juice did she drink? Show how you determined your answer.

59. You picked up an empty coffee cup when your resident finished eating. How much did he drink if the cup held 150 mL and you filled it twice? Show how you determined your answer.

60. Your resident consumed a bowl of soup that contained 300 mL. How many ounces of soup did your resident consume? Show how you determined your answer.

J. Clinical Experiences

Read the clinical experiences and answer the questions about each long-term care resident.

Amelia Drage, age 92, spent her life as a homemaker. She contributed many hours to civic organizations. Her current frail condition means that she requires assistance in feeding. She is on a soft diet and receives nourishments.

61. The best combination of foods for her soft diet is

(A) coleslaw and milk

(B) toast and fresh fruit salad

(C) chicken and cottage cheese

(D) garden salad and eggs

62. When feeding her, remember

(A) do not remove equipment such as the emesis basin

(B) allow her to help herself as much as possible

(C) taste foods first to be sure they are not too hot

(D) offer the bedpan following the meal

63. When serving her nourishments,

(A) offer a full meal, since she is so frail

(B) leave the used dishes and glasses at the bedside because someone else can pick them up

(C) do not record the nourishments

(D) follow the dietary instructions carefully, using the nourishment list as a guide

Russell Barnes, age 82, has a large obstructing tumor of the esophagus. He is unable to take nourishment by mouth and transfer it to his stomach because of the tumor. A commercial nutritional formula is provided for him through a feeding tube. He has a gastrostomy tube in place.

64. The gastrostomy tube is in Mr. Barnes's

(A) esophagus

(B) pharynx

(C) stomach

(D) colon

INTAKE AND OUTPUT

Room: Name: Date:

Instructions:

Intake	Output	Intake	Output	Intake	Output
Total		Total		Total	

Drinking Glass.........200 mL   Full Water Pitcher....950 mL   Milk Carton...............236 mL   Jello...........................90 mL
Styrofoam Cup........200 mL   Coffee or Teapot.....300 mL   Soup Bowl...............250 mL   Ice Cream Cup..........90 mL
Juice Glass (small)..100 mL   Coffee Cup.............150 mL   Soup Bowl (small)...100 mL   Creamer....................50 mL
Juice Glass (large)..250 mL

FOLEY CATHETER DRAINAGE: (Circle the following when applicable)

Color: Yellow   Amber   Brown   Red

Appearance: Cloudy   Clear   Sediment   Mucous   Bloody   24 hour INTAKE_____

Abdomen Distended   Catheter Irrigated   Catheter Changed   24 hour OUTPUT_____

---

65. While taking care of Mr. Barnes, you note the tube is out of place and lying in the bed. You should

(A) throw the tube away as it probably is not needed

(B) notify the nurse immediately

(C) reinsert the tube so you will be ready for the next feeding

(D) leave the tube alone because the nurse can take care of it when she checks the resident

66. Your care of Mr. Barnes following a feeding includes

(A) elevating the head of the bed at 40 degrees for 30 minutes

(B) allowing him to lie on the tube

(C) keeping the bed flat for 30 minutes

(D) keeping the end of the tube open between feedings

Joe Spando is 78 years old and has chronic obstructive pulmonary disease, a hiatal hernia, and diverticulosis. He was a jockey as a young adult and smoking was a way of life. Even now he insists on his smoking time, which he enjoys under supervision.

67. Mr. Spando's hiatal hernia means that his

(A) intestines protrude through the wall in the groin area

(B) colon is inflamed

(C) rectum has varicose veins

(D) stomach protrudes up into the thoracic cavity

68. This resident probably suffers from

(A) painful defecation

(B) dysphagia

(C) blood in his stool

(D) pain in his rectum

69. He will probably be most comfortable if he

(A) eats while lying down

(B) eats three big meals a day

(C) sits up after meals

(D) sleeps with the head of the bed flat

Lisa Ling has been complaining of nausea. She has vomited four times. You have been instructed to keep her NPO for your shift.

70. Vomiting can predispose Ms. Ling to *all but one* of the following:

(A) Electrolyte imbalance

(B) Dehydration

(C) Aspiration pneumonia

(D) Edema

71. When caring for Ms. Ling, the CNA responsibilities include *all but one* of the following:

(A) Describe the amount and character of the emesis.

(B) Note the relationship to food intake.

(C) Send a specimen to the laboratory.

(D) Observe for signs of dehydration.

72. Food intake will resume gradually following an episode of vomiting. Choose the one diet that will be avoided for Ms. Ling.

(A) Clear liquid

(B) Soft

(C) High fat

(D) Regular

73. The 2010 Dietary Guidelines for Americans (DGAC) stresses the importance of balanced nutrition and exercise. It is designed for all of the following *except:*

(A) Persons age 2 and beyond.

(B) A plant-based diet

(C) Maintaining healthy weight.

(D) Adding sugars and solid fats to the diet.

74. The purple portion of MyPlate includes *all but one* of the following foods.

(A) Spinach

(B) Eggs

(C) Peanut butter

(D) Ground beef

75. Which of the following foods are considered to be a vegetable and a plant-based protein?

(A) Whole wheat

(B) Cornmeal

(C) Kidney beans

(D) Avocados

76. How many teaspoons of salt should the average American consume each day?

(A) 1

(B) 2

(C) 3

(D) 5

LESSON 18
MEETING THE RESIDENTS' ELIMINATION NEEDS

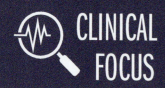

CLINICAL FOCUS

Think about how you may help a resident meet elimination needs as you study this lesson.

OBJECTIVES

After studying this lesson, you should be able to:

• Define vocabulary words and terms.

• Identify ways people eliminate wastes from the body.

• Identify the parts and functions of the digestive system.

• Identify the parts and function of the urinary tract.

• Review changes in the urinary system as they relate to the aging process.

• Explain the collection and care of urine and stool specimens.

• Explain the measurement and recording of fluid output.

• Describe common urinary system conditions affecting long-term residents.

• Demonstrate the following:
  Procedure 18-40 Giving and Receiving the Bedpan
  Procedure 18-41 Giving and Receiving the Urinal
  Procedure 18-42 Assisting with Use of the Bedside Commode
  Procedure 18-43 Assisting Resident to Use the Bathroom
  Procedure 18-44 Giving Routine Stoma Care (Colostomy)
  Procedure 18-45 Collecting a Stool Specimen

CASE STUDY

Jessica Beebe, age 79, has been assigned to your care. She seems listless, complaining of an upset stomach and cramps. She refused breakfast and you note some fecal soiling on the bedding. When you ask her about her last bowel movement, she cannot remember. You report the situation to the charge nurse, who examines Ms. Beebe for fecal impaction. It is decided that Ms. Beebe will benefit from a soapsuds enema.

VOCABULARY

anuria (ah-NEW-ree-ah)

bladder (BLAD-er)

Bowman's capsule (BOH-manz KAP-syoul)

catheter (KATH-eh-ter)

caustic (KAW-stik)

colon (KOHL-on)

colostomy (koh-LAHS-toh-mee)

condom (KON-dum)

constipation (kon-stih-PAY-shun)

continent (KON-tih-nent)

cystocele (SIS-toh-seel)

diarrhea (die-ah-REE-ah)

distended (dis-TEN-ded)

dysuria (dis-YOU-ree-ah)

emesis (EM-eh-sis)

enema (EN-eh-mah)

excreta (ecks-KREE-tah)

fecal impaction (FEE-kal im-PACK-shun)

glomerulus (gloh-MER-you-lus)

hematuria (hem-ah-TOO-ree-ah)

ileostomy (ill-ee-OS-toh-me)

incontinence (in-KON-tih-nens)

indwelling catheter (IN-dwell-ing KATH-eh-ter)

meatus (mee-AY-tus)

micturition (mick-too-RISH-un)

nephron (NEF-ron)

nocturia (nock-TUR-ee-ah)

occult (a-KULT)

oliguria (ol-ih-GYOU-ree-ah)

ostomy (OS-toh-mee)

prostate gland (PROS-tayt gland)

rectocele (REC-toh-seel)

renal calculi (REE-nal KAL-kyou-lee)

retention (ree-TEN-shun)

sepsis (SEP-sis)

septicemia (sept-tih-SEE-mee-ah)

specimen (SPES-ih-men)

sphincter (SFINK-ter)

stoma (STOH-mah)

stool (stool)

suppository (sup-POZ-ih-toh-ree)

suprapubic (soo-pra-PU-bik)

uremia (you-REE-mee-ah)

uremic frost (you-REE-mick frost)

ureter (yur-REE-ter)

urethra (you-REE-thrah)

urinalysis (yur-rih-NAL-ih-sis)

urination (yur-rih-NAY-shun)

voiding (VOYD-ing)

INTRODUCTION

The human body produces waste products continuously. Eliminating waste products regularly is one of the basic human needs.

Waste products (excreta) that must be eliminated (excreted) include:

- Solid wastes
  - Feces from the digestive tract
- Liquid wastes
  - Urine from the urinary system
  - Perspiration (water and salts) from the skin
  - Water in the feces
  - Water from the lungs
- Gaseous wastes
  - Carbon dioxide (CO_2) from the lungs

In Lesson 17 you learned how nutrients are processed from foods. The undigested portion of the food (roughage or bulk) continues to move through the colon to the anus, where it leaves the body as feces.

In this lesson you will learn ways to:

- Help residents maintain regular elimination
- Assist residents who need special help in eliminating wastes

- Care for residents as they eliminate solid wastes from the digestive system and liquid wastes from the urinary system

A resident who is **continent** is able to control the elimination of waste products. **Incontinence** is the inability to predict and control elimination. Therefore, an incontinent resident has no control over elimination. Incontinence leads to emotional and physical problems that hinder social interaction.

THE CONTINENT RESIDENT

Nursing assistant responsibilities in helping continent residents to meet their elimination needs (Figure 18-1) include:

- Being aware of the resident's need to reach the proper facilities in time.
- Being observant so that you can be available to help the resident reach the toilet or commode. Answer call lights promptly for residents who use a bedpan. Be ready to assist them when they are finished.
- Always noting and reporting the frequency and character of the excreta.

EQUIPMENT TO ASSIST ELIMINATION

Residents are encouraged to use regular bathroom facilities if their conditions permit. They may need help to reach the toilet in time and assistance with their clothing.

Several devices can make it easier and safer for residents to achieve more independence in elimination. An elevated toilet seat (Figure 18-2) means the resident does not have to bend as much as they would to use a regular toilet seat. Grab bars on the wall next to the toilet help stabilize the resident when sitting down and getting up. They also help stabilize the resident in the proper position for toileting. Proper positioning makes it easier for the resident to void.

When assisting with elimination procedures:

- Wear disposable gloves.
- Wash hands immediately before and after procedure.
- Provide privacy.
- Make resident comfortable in a seated position, if possible during elimination procedures.
- Ensure safety.
- Immediately answer call light, as resident may be finished.

Figure 18-1 Nursing assistant actions when assisting with elimination procedures.

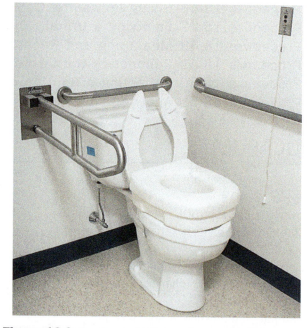

Figure 18-2 An elevated toilet seat promotes independent toileting.

The preferred position for women is to sit upright with the feet flat on the floor. Men may prefer to stand.

A commode or portable toilet (Figure 18-3) may be left in the room for convenience, but the container must be emptied and cleaned after each use and the cover closed. A commode with a rolling base and support arms may be placed over the toilet for security. The

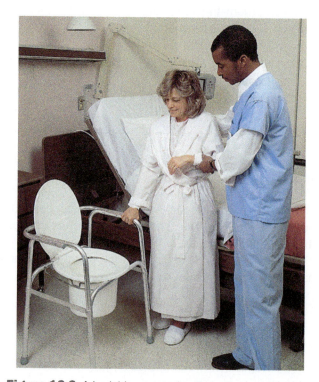

Figure 18-3 A bedside commode allows the resident to assume the best position for elimination.

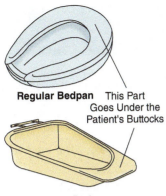

Figure 18-4 Regular bedpan (top); orthopedic (fracture) bedpan (bottom).

wheels of this type of commode must be locked once it is in place. Residents in bed who can be placed on a commode probably will be more comfortable and have a more natural elimination than when using a bedpan.

Bedpans are not comfortable in any position when left in place for any length of time (Figure 18-4). An orthopedic bedpan (fracture pan) is used when it is difficult for the resident to move. This type of bedpan is preferred for the resident who does not get out of bed.

As you provide care, remember to perform all beginning procedure and ending actions. Always follow the principles of medical asepsis.

- Apply principles of Standard Precautions when handling, emptying, and cleaning bedpans, urinals, and commodes.

- Perform hand hygiene before and after applying disposable gloves.
- Cover bedpans and urinals and close the covers of commodes after use until emptied.
- Avoid contamination of environmental surfaces with gloves.
- Encourage residents to perform perineal care after toileting, or assist as necessary.
- Restrict use of bedpan or urinal to specific resident; each resident has a personal bedpan or urinal that is stored in the bedside stand.

Safety Precautions

Following certain precautions can help prevent incidents during toileting.

- Be sure that resident knows how to use the emergency call signal in the bathroom and can reach it when using the toilet.
- Encourage resident to use grab bars for support.
- Lock wheels of commode after positioning it over toilet.
- Be sure resident is positioned comfortably on toilet before leaving. Do not leave a resident who is confused or disoriented.
- Do not restrain resident on the toilet or commode.
- Provide as much privacy as possible.
- Answer call lights promptly (resident may have completed toileting).

PROCEDURE 18-40
Giving and Receiving the Bedpan

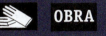

1. Carry out each beginning procedure action.
2. Assemble equipment:
   - Disposable gloves
   - Bedpan and cover
   - Bed protector
   - Basin
   - Washcloth
   - Toilet tissue
   - Soap
   - Towel
3. Lower the head of the bed if necessary.
4. Put on gloves.
5. Take the bedpan and tissue from the bedside stand.

(continues)

PROCEDURE 18-40
Giving and Receiving the Bedpan (Continued)

- Place the bedpan on the bedside chair. Never place it on the bedside stand or overbed table, or on the floor.

- Put the remainder of the equipment on the bedside table.

6. Place bedpan cover at the foot of the bed.

NOTE: Never carry or allow a used bedpan to sit uncovered. If a bedpan cover is not available, cover the bedpan with a towel, pillowcase, or paper towels.

7. Fold top bed covers back at a right angle. Raise the resident's gown. If the resident is thin or has a pressure sore, consult the nurse for the appropriate action. The nursing care plan may have specific instructions for such cases. For example, it may be necessary to pad the bedpan with a folded towel or take some other action.

8. Ask resident to flex knees and rest weight on heels, if able.

9. Help the resident to raise buttocks by:

- Place bed protector under buttocks if needed.

- Putting one hand under the small of the resident's back and lifting gently and slowly with one hand.

- With the other hand, place the bedpan under the resident's buttocks.

- The bedpan may also be placed by rolling the resident to one side, positioning the bedpan against the buttocks and rolling the resident back on it (Figure 18-5).

- Alternatively, if a trapeze is in place over the bed, place the bedpan under the resident as the resident lifts self using the trapeze.

- The resident's buttocks should rest on the rounded shelf of the regular bedpan. The narrow end should face the foot of the bed.

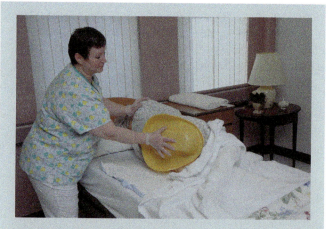

Figure 18-5 Roll resident away from you while supporting resident with one hand on the resident's hip. Place bedpan against resident's buttocks with other hand. Then roll resident back onto bedpan.

10. Remove gloves and dispose of properly. Perform hand hygiene. Replace top bedcovers. Raise the head of the bed to a comfortable height.

11. Make sure the toilet paper and call light are within easy reach of the resident. Leave the resident alone unless contraindicated in the nursing care plan.

NOTE: If a specimen is to be taken, instruct the resident that toilet tissue is not to be placed in the bedpan. In this case, the nursing assistant will clean the resident and provide perineal care.

12. Watch for resident's call light.

13. Answer resident's call light immediately. Perform hand hygiene and put on disposable gloves. Use a paper towel to turn on faucet and another one to turn off faucet.

14. Fill the basin with warm water (105–110°F) and place next to soap, washcloth, and towel on overbed table.

15. Remove bedpan from under resident.

- Ask the resident to flex knees and rest weight on heels. Place one hand under the small of the back and lift gently to help raise the buttocks off bedpan. Take the bedpan with the other hand. Cover it and place it on the chair.

- If the resident is unable to raise the buttocks, hold down the bedpan with one hand and roll the resident off the bedpan to the side and remove the bedpan. Hold the bedpan firmly with one hand and place it on the chair. Cover the bedpan.

(continues)

PROCEDURE 18-40
Giving and Receiving the Bedpan (Continued)

16. Assist the resident to a clean area of the bed, if necessary. Provide perineal care.
17. Change linen or protective pads as necessary. Replace bedclothes.
18. Assist the resident to wash hands after the procedure.
19. Take the bedpan to the bathroom or utility room and observe contents. Measure, if required.
20. Empty bedpan.
21. Rinse the bedpan with cold water and clean and store per facility policy.
22. Remove gloves and discard according to facility policy. Perform hand hygiene.
23. Carry out each procedure completion action.

PROCEDURE 18-41
Giving and Receiving the Urinal

OBRA

1. Carry out each beginning procedure action.
2. Assemble equipment:
   - Disposable gloves
   - Urinal and cover (Figure 18-6)
   - Toilet tissue
   - Basin
   - Soap
   - Washcloth
   - Towel

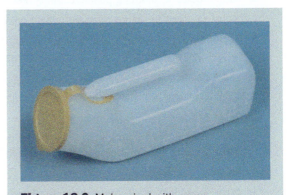

Figure 18-6 Male urinal with cover.

3. Put on gloves. Lift the top bedcovers and place the urinal under the covers so the resident may grasp the handle. Instruct resident to place his penis in the urinal opening. If he cannot do this, you must place the urinal in position and ensure that the penis is placed in the opening.
4. Remove gloves and dispose of them properly. Perform hand hygiene. Make sure the call light is within easy reach of the resident. Leave resident alone if possible. Watch for his call light.
5. Answer resident's call light immediately. Perform hand hygiene. Use a paper towel to turn on faucet. Fill a basin with warm water (105–110°F), and place next to the soap, washcloth, and towel, so resident can wash and dry hands.
6. Put on gloves. Ask resident to hand the urinal to you. Cover it. Provide perineal care if needed. Rearrange bedclothes if necessary.
7. Take the urinal to the bathroom or utility room and observe the contents. Measure, if required. Do not empty urinal if anything unusual (such as blood) is observed. Rather, save the contents of the urinal for your supervisor's inspection.
8. Empty the urinal. Use a paper towel to turn on the faucet and another paper towel to turn off the faucet. Rinse with cold water and clean with warm soapy water. Rinse, dry, and cover urinal. Remove gloves and dispose of them properly. Perform hand hygiene.
9. Place urinal inside resident's bedside table. Clean and replace other articles.
10. Carry out each procedure completion action.

PROCEDURE 18-42
Assisting with Use of the Bedside Commode

OBRA

1. Carry out each beginning procedure action.

2. Assemble equipment:

   - Disposable gloves
   - Portable commode
   - Toilet tissue
   - Basin
   - Washcloth
   - Soap
   - Towel

3. Position commode beside bed, facing head. Lock wheels and open lid. Be sure receptacle is in place under seat.

4. If bed and side rails are elevated, lower side rail nearest you and place bed in lowest horizontal position. Make sure bed wheels are locked.

5. Put on gloves.

6. Assist resident to sitting position. Swing resident's legs over edge of bed.

7. Assist resident to put on robe. Put shoes on resident. Assist resident to stand. If needed, use a transfer belt.

8. Support resident with hands on either side of the belt. Remember to use proper body mechanics. Pivot resident to the right and lower to commode. Do not restrain resident on the commode.

9. Leave call light and tissue within reach.

10. Remove gloves and discard according to facility policy. Perform hand hygiene.

11. When resident signals, return promptly. Perform hand hygiene and put on gloves. Use a paper towel to turn on the faucet and another paper towel to turn off the faucet. Fill the basin with warm water (105–110°F). Bring basin to bedside along with soap, towel, and washcloth.

12. Assist resident to stand. Wipe anal area or perineum, if required.

13. Allow resident to wash and dry hands. Remove gloves and dispose of according to facility policy. Perform hand hygiene.

14. Assist resident to return to bed. Adjust bedding and pillows for comfort.

15. Leave call light within easy reach.

16. Put on gloves. Remove receptacle from commode and cover. Close lid of commode.

17. Take receptacle to bathroom. Note contents and measure, if required.

18. Empty and clean receptacle per facility policy. Replace in commode. Remove and dispose of gloves properly.

19. Put commode in proper place. If it remains in the room, place it out of the way.

20. Carry out each procedure completion action.

PROCEDURE 18-43
Assisting Resident to Use the Bathroom

OBRA

1. Answer call light promptly.
2. Carry out each beginning procedure action.
3. Assist resident to toilet. Shut door for privacy.
4. Help resident position himself with the back of his legs against the toilet and facing you.
5. Assist as needed to:

   - Lift skirt or gown
   - Undo belt and lower trousers
   - Lower underwear

6. Assist resident to sit comfortably on toilet with feet flat on floor.
7. Place call light within reach of resident.
8. Adjust clothing to cover resident as much as possible or place towel over lap.
9. Leave toilet tissue close at hand. Indicate your willingness to return and assist resident to clean genital/anal area after toileting.
10. Leave resident alone if safe. Do not leave a resident who is confused, disoriented, or weak.
11. Return immediately when resident signals.
12. Perform hand hygiene. Put on disposable gloves. Assist resident to stand. (Gather up skirt with one hand to keep clean.)
13. Clean genital/anal area as needed.
14. Remove gloves and discard according to facility policy. Perform hand hygiene.
15. Help resident redress.
16. Note contents of toilet and flush.
17. Help resident wash and dry hands.
18. Perform hand hygiene.
19. Assist resident to a comfortable area with call light and water close at hand.
20. Carry out each procedure completion action.

? EXERCISE 18-1

TRUE OR FALSE
Indicate whether the following statements are true (T) or false (F).

1. T F Never allow a used bedpan to sit uncovered.
2. T F A plastic bedpan should always be warmed before placing under a resident.
3. T F The wheels of a commode should be locked before positioning a resident on it.
4. T F Always rinse bedpans and urinals with hot water before cleansing with soapy water.
5. T F When handling a bedpan or urinal, always wear gloves.

(continues)

? **EXERCISE 18-1 (Continued)**

COMPLETION
Complete the following statement.

6. Six steps that must be followed when assisting with elimination procedures include:

a. _____

b. _____

c. _____

d. _____

e. _____

f. _____

ELIMINATION FROM THE LOWER DIGESTIVE TRACT

Solid wastes are eliminated through the lower digestive tract or large intestine (colon) (Figure 18-7). The colon is divided into the:

- Ascending colon—located up the right side of the abdomen
- Transverse colon—wastes are moved through it to the opposite side
- Descending colon—located down the left side of the body
- Rectum in the pelvis and the anal opening to the outside of the body

Digested food leaves the stomach in liquid form and enters the small intestine. Here some of the water and the nutrients are absorbed. As the wastes move into the large intestine, they change to the more solid form known as feces. When the stool remains in the lower colon for a long period of time, for example, if the resident ignores the urge to have a bowel movement, more and more water is absorbed and the stool can become hard. Normal stool should be brown in color and formed but soft.

Bowel movements are recorded in the resident's record. Observe the bowel movement and report anything unusual about the feces (also known as stool).

- Infections and some medications, such as antibiotics, can cause loose, watery stools (diarrhea).
- Iron can make the stool black; in some residents iron can cause loose stools, whereas others experience constipation (difficult bowel movements).

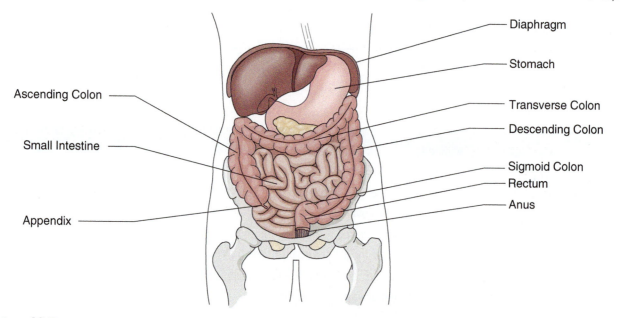

Figure 18-7 Elimination of solid wastes involves the organs of the lower digestive tract.

- Dark stool may also indicate the presence of blood from the intestines; bright red blood in the stool may be from distended and bleeding blood vessels in the rectum (hemorrhoids). Sometimes blood is present in stool, but it is not visible to the eye. This is referred to as occult blood.

Conditions resulting from lower digestive tract dysfunction include:

- Constipation
- Flatus (gas)
- Diarrhea
- Anal incontinence

AGE-RELATED CHANGES OF THE LOWER DIGESTIVE TRACT

Constipation (difficulty in emptying the bowels) is a problem for many residents in long-term care. This is due to food passing more slowly through the digestive tract. In addition, the residents do not:

- Take in adequate fluids
- Exercise sufficiently
- Take in enough bulk (fiber) to stimulate peristalsis

Other causes include depression, disease, and certain drugs.

The resident with constipation may not have an appetite and may complain of abdominal discomfort. The abdomen may be distended (stretched). If fecal impaction—the most serious form of constipation—is present, there may be frequent instances of diarrhea.

Nursing assistant actions to help residents who are constipated include:

- Encouraging as much activity as possible
- Encouraging a high fiber diet, as prescribed
- Offering fluids frequently
- Assisting the resident to the bathroom and allowing adequate time for defecation
- Administering bowel aids as ordered

Fecal impaction results when the stool mass stays lodged in the lower portion of the colon (sigmoid). The function of that portion of the colon is to reabsorb fluid from the feces back into the body. The longer the fecal mass remains in that portion of the colon, more and more fluid is absorbed and the stool mass becomes dry and hard and difficult to eliminate through the rectum. Mucus tends to dissolve the outer portion of the stool mass; this then oozes from the rectum, like diarrhea. Whenever you note the resident has frequent, small amounts of mucus-like diarrhea, immediately report this to the nurse who will check the resident for a fecal impaction.

Checking for Fecal Impaction

In some facilities, nursing assistants are permitted to check for fecal impaction. This is done by wearing gloves, applying a small amount of lubricant to the index finger, and with the resident lying on their left side and their right leg flexed, gently inserting the index finger inside the rectum to feel for the presence of stool, which could be hard like pebbles or soft like jelly. Findings should be immediately reported to the charge nurse. If it is determined that a resident has a

---

? EXERCISE 18-2

COMPLETION
Complete the following statement.

1. Five actions that can help the constipated resident include:

   a. _____
   _____

   b. _____
   _____

   c. _____
   _____

   d. _____
   _____

   e. _____
   _____

fecal impaction, an order is placed for a **suppository** or **enema** to provide relief. *Be sure your facility permits nursing assistants to perform this procedure.*

BOWEL AIDS

Nursing assistants may give oil-retention enemas and soapsuds enemas. In some facilities, they may be permitted to insert lubricating suppositories. Each of these procedures requires a specific order.

Enemas

An enema is the introduction of fluid into the rectum, through the anal sphincter, to remove feces (stool) or flatus (gas). The fluid is expelled a short time after introduction, along with the waste products. The need to empty the bowel is signaled by a feeling of urgency. Sometimes a small amount of warm oil is given to soften the stool (oil-retention enema). This is followed by a cleansing soapsuds enema.

Prepackaged commercial enema solutions may be used. A specific order is required for an enema before it is given. Some facilities do not permit nursing assistants to give enemas of any kind. You are responsible for knowing the regulations of your facility.

General Considerations
Some general considerations to keep in mind when giving an enema are:

- If the resident is to use the bathroom after the enema, make sure the bathroom is not in use before giving the enema.

- When possible, the enema should be given before breakfast or morning care.
- Do not give an enema within an hour after a meal.
- Remember that you must have a physician's order for any enema and that you can give an enema only *if it is a nursing assistant responsibility in your facility.*
  Enemas commonly ordered are:
- Commercial preparations
  - Phospho soda
  - Oil
- Saline
- Soapsuds enema (SSE)
- Tap water enema (TWE)

The procedure for administering an oil-retention enema and a commercially prepared enema is essentially the same. The only difference is in the solution that is administered.

The oil-retention enema is administered to soften the feces and is usually followed by a cleansing enema.

Rectal Suppositories

Rectal suppositories are used to stimulate bowel evacuation or administer medication. Medicinal suppositories must be inserted by the nurse. You may be asked to insert the type of suppository that lubricates stool and promotes elimination. Check your facility policy to be sure this is a nursing assistant function. The suppository must be placed beyond the rectal **sphincter** (circular muscle that controls the anal opening) and against the bowel wall so it can melt and lubricate the rectum.

? EXERCISE 18-3

TRUE OR FALSE
Indicate whether the following statements are true (T) or false (F).

1. T F Enemas may be given by a nursing assistant without a specific order.
2. T F Oil-retention enemas are usually followed by a cleansing enema.
3. T F An oil-retention enema is usually kept in the colon overnight.
4. T F Enemas are best given just before breakfast.
5. T F Suppositories need to be placed beyond the rectal sphincter.

COMPLETION
Complete the following statement.

6. Fluids often ordered as enemas are:

_____
_____
_____

OSTOMIES

The surgical removal of a section of diseased bowel requires the creation of an artificial opening (**ostomy**) in the abdominal wall for solid waste elimination. When the colon is brought through the abdominal wall, the opening is called a **colostomy**. If a portion of the small intestine (usually the ileum) is used to create an ostomy, this is referred to as an **ileostomy**. The mouth of the opening is called a **stoma** (Figure 18-8). The ostomy may be temporary or permanent. The location of the ostomy (Figure 18-9) determines if the feces are formed, soft and mushy, semiliquid, or liquid.

The resident with a colostomy does not have normal sphincter control. This means the resident cannot voluntarily control emptying of the bowel in the same manner as emptying through the anus. If the colostomy is located in the bowel where stool is formed, regularity of elimination may be established. As elimination is controlled, the stoma may be covered with a simple dressing between evacuations. Liquid to mushy fecal drainage from a stoma is collected in a disposable

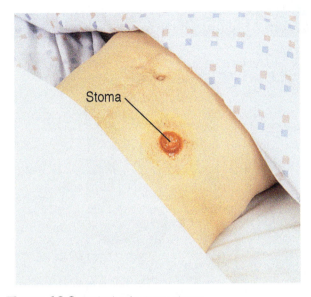

Figure 18-8 Typical colostomy stoma.

drainage pouch that is attached over the stoma. It is the responsibility of the CNA to empty the pouch during each shift or whenever the pouch is full.

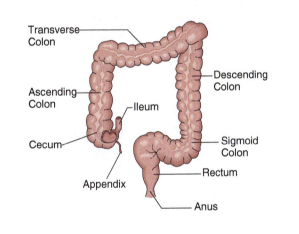

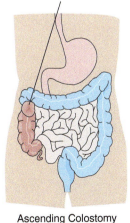 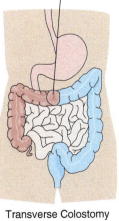 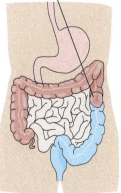 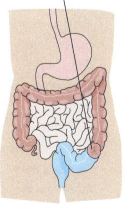

Figure 18-9 The site of the colostomy determines the character (color and consistency) of the feces.

? EXERCISE 18-4

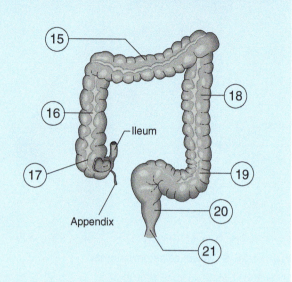

Write the names of the parts of the large intestine (colon), shown in the accompanying figure. Be sure you spell the names correctly.

1. _____   5. _____
2. _____   6. _____
3. _____   7. _____
4. _____

Stoma Care

Proper care is needed to keep the tissue around the stoma healthy. The waste eliminated from the stoma may be irritating to the tissue, especially the liquid or semiliquid feces because digestive enzymes are present. Other problems may include leakage and odor.

You can assist the resident with a colostomy by:

- Encouraging the resident to eat food helpful in controlling elimination. Restricting foods determined to cause flatus or loose feces (depending on location of ostomy) can make management of the ostomy easier.
- Performing routine stoma care
- Keeping the area around the opening clean and dry
- Protecting the skin around the stoma according to facility policy. Follow the care plan exactly.
- Adding deodorizer to ostomy bag, if instructed, to reduce odor
- Attaching the pouch securely over the stoma
- Reporting the nature of the colostomy output
- Reporting to the nurse if area around the stoma is red, irritated, or nonintact

If the colostomy pouch is reusable, it should be washed with soap and water and dried while a clean alternate is applied. If the pouch is not reusable, dispose of it according to facility policy. Always wear gloves when handling an ostomy pouch of any type.

PROCEDURE 18-44
Giving Routine Stoma Care (Colostomy)

   OBRA

1. Carry out each beginning procedure action.

2. Assemble equipment:

- Disposable gloves
- Washcloth and towel
- Basin of warm water (105–110°F)
- Bed protector
- Bath blanket
- Disposable colostomy bag and belt
- Bedpan
- Skin lotion as directed
- Prescribed solvent/dropper
- Cleansing agent
- Adhesive wafer
- 4 × 4 inch gauze square
- Toilet tissue

(continues)

PROCEDURE 18-44
Giving Routine Stoma Care (Colostomy) (Continued)

3. Place bath blanket over resident. Fanfold top bedding to foot of bed.

4. Perform hand hygiene and put on disposable gloves.

5. Place bed protector under the resident's buttocks.

6. Place bedpan and cover on bed protector on chair.

7. Remove the soiled disposable stoma bag (pouch) and place in bedpan—note amount and type of drainage.

8. Gently clean area around stoma with toilet tissue to remove feces and drainage (Figure 18-10A). Dispose of tissue in bedpan.

9. Wash area around stoma with soap and water. Rinse thoroughly and dry.

10. If ordered, apply barrier cream lightly around the stoma—too much lotion may interfere with proper seal of fresh ostomy bag.

11. It may be necessary to remove the adhesive wafer. To select the proper size of wafer, a commercial guide can be used to size the stoma (Figure 18-10B).

12. Replace adhesive wafer (Figure 18-10C). Place clean ostomy bag over stoma and secure belt.

13. Remove bed protector. Check to be sure bottom bedding is not wet. Change if necessary.

14. Remove gloves and discard according to facility policy. Perform hand hygiene.

15. Replace bath blanket with top bedding, making resident comfortable.

16. Using a paper towel to protect hands, gather and cover soiled materials and bedpan. Take to utility room. Dispose of materials according to facility policy.

17. Empty, wash, and dry bedpan. Store according to facility policy.

18. Carry out each procedure completion action.

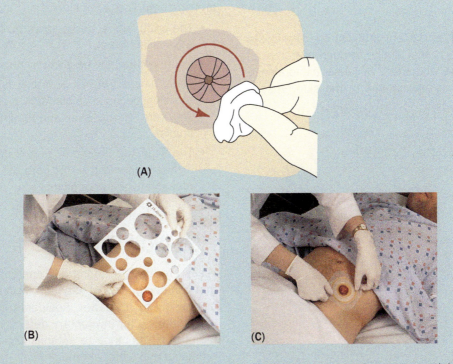

(A)

(B)

(C)

Figure 18-10 (A) The area around the stoma is cleaned thoroughly but gently and dried before a new pouch is applied. (B) Check the size of the stoma to be sure the proper size of barrier is used. (C) A new barrier adhesive wafer is applied around the stoma.

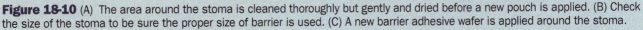

? EXERCISE 18-5

COMPLETION
Complete the following statements.

1. Three problems associated with a colostomy are:

    a. _____
        _____

    b. _____
        _____

    c. _____
        _____

2. Nursing assistants assist in colostomy care by:

    _____
    _____
    _____

3. A reusable colostomy pouch should be cared for by:

    _____
    _____
    _____

Care of the Resident with an Ileostomy

An ileostomy is a permanent artificial opening in the ileum (Figure 18-11) that drains through a stoma on the surface of the abdomen. Because the drainage from ileum is liquid and caustic to the skin, special considerations are needed to care for the resident with an ileostomy. These considerations include:

- The professional nurse cares for the resident with a fresh ileostomy.
- Routine care may be given by nursing assistants.
- The drainage from an ileostomy is very irritating to the skin because it contains digestive enzymes. The care of the skin surrounding the stoma is crucial.
- The fit of the ileostomy ring is critical to prevent leakage. This is true for both the disposable and reusable types of appliances.

FECAL INCONTINENCE

Feces are highly irritating and contain many microbes that can be sources of infection. Fecal incontinence is distressing to residents. Residents must be cleaned immediately after involuntary defecation and every attempt must be made to establish continence through retraining and dietary management.

When there are frequent liquid stools, a drainable fecal incontinence collector may be needed (Figure 18-12).

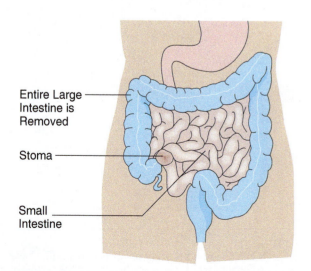

Entire Large Intestine is Removed

Stoma

Small Intestine

Figure 18-11 An ileostomy brings a section of the ileum through the abdominal wall.

? EXERCISE 18-6

COMPLETION
Select the correct terms from the following list. Some words may be used more than once.

anus	ileostomy	prelubricated
bedpan	infection	stoma
bleeding	irritating	strong
closed	left side-lying	suds
colon	lubricated	taken into
diarrhea	medication	105
fecal impaction	opening	2–4
freely	pale to deep yellow	12
gently		

1. Normal urine is _____ and clear and should not have a(an) _____ odor.

2. Unusual feces may be the result of _____, _____, _____, or iron.

3. The amount of urine varies with the amount of water _____ the body.

4. The best position for a resident receiving an enema is _____ position.

5. The temperature of a soapsuds enema should be approximately _____°F.

6. The soap solution should be added to the water and mixed _____ so that no _____ will form.

7. The tip of an enema tube must be well _____ before insertion.

8. The enema tubing tip should be inserted into the _____ approximately _____ inches.

9. The container of enema solution should be raised _____ inches above the level of the anus.

10. The tip of a commercially prepared enema is _____ and is already premeasured and ready to use.

11. A colostomy is an artificial _____ made in the _____.

12. The opening of the colostomy is called the _____.

13. If a portion of the small intestine is used to create an ostomy, it is called a _____.

14. The most serious form of constipation is _____.

15. When fecal impaction is present there may be frequent instances of _____.

16. The drainage from a colostomy can be very _____ to the skin so care of the skin around the _____ is crucial.

COLLECTING A STOOL SPECIMEN

A stool specimen is usually required when infection, bleeding, or parasites in the colon are suspected. You may be asked to collect a stool specimen. When carrying out this task:

- Wear gloves.
- Collect the specimen in a bedpan, commode receptacle, toilet insert, or from a fecal collection bag or bed linens.
- Do not place toilet paper in the collection container.
- Do not allow the specimen to touch the outside of the collection container.
- Use tongue depressors to handle the specimen.
- Make sure that the specimen is properly labeled and promptly transported.

URINARY SYSTEM

Most liquid wastes are eliminated from the body through the urinary system in the form of urine.

The urinary system consists of the kidneys (filter blood and form urine) and the ureters and urethra

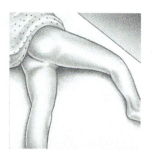
1. Position patient on side.

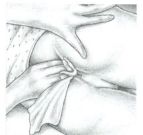
2. Clean and dry skin.

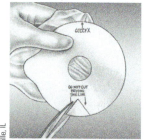
3. Trim barrier, if needed.

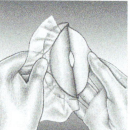
4. Remove release paper.

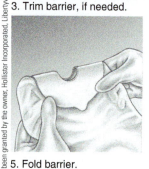
5. Fold barrier.

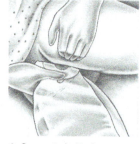
6. Separate buttocks.

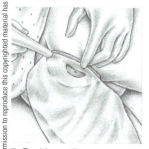
7. Position collector.

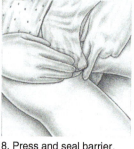
8. Press and seal barrier.

Figure 18-12 Fecal incontinence collection system.

Permission to reproduce this copyrighted material has been granted by the owner, Hollister Incorporated, Libertyville, IL

DRAINABLE FECAL INCONTINENCE COLLECTOR WITH FLEXTEND SKIN BARRIER

Preparation and Application

1. Turn resident on one side, bending the upper knee up toward the chest.
2. Clean and dry the perineal area thoroughly.
3. If necessary, trim the skin barrier to fit perineal area.
   - For females with a narrow perineal bridge, the skin barrier should be cut to fit.
   - Follow the cutting guide, leaving as much of the skin barrier as possible. The barrier should not cover the labia or the vaginal opening.
4. Remove the release paper.
5. Fold the skin barrier in half.
6. Separate the buttocks.
7. Position the pre-cut hole over the anus. Do not enlarge pre-cut hole.
8. Apply and press firmly.
   - Apply barrier to perineal area first, pressing firmly after positioning correctly. Using your other hand, press the barrier firmly, holding for 30 seconds to allow it to adhere properly.
9. To empty, open drain cap and direct the stool into an appropriate receptacle. For best results, connect to a bedside drainage collector.
10. To remove, gently ease the barrier from the resident's skin, using fabric tab.

Preparation and Application

- Remove oily substances or powders from the skin that interfere with skin barrier adhesion.
- Skin gel wipes on skin may decrease wear time.
- DO NOT cut the barrier opening.
- Trim excess hair with scissors. DO NOT use a razor.

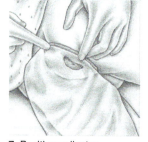
7. Position collector.

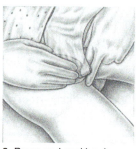
8. Press and seal barrier.

PROCEDURE 18-45
Collecting a Stool Specimen

OBRA

1. Carry out each beginning procedure action.
2. Assemble equipment:
   - Disposable gloves
   - Bedpan and cover or collection container
   - Bed protector
   - Specimen container and cover
   - Biohazard specimen transport bag

(continues)

PROCEDURE 18-45
Collecting a Stool Specimen (Continued)

- Label including:
  - Resident's full name
  - Room number
  - Date and time of collection
  - Physician's name
  - Examination to be performed
  - Other information required
- Toilet tissue
- Tongue depressors
- Basin

3. Perform hand hygiene and put on disposable gloves.

4. Uncover container used to collect bowel movement (bedpan or commode receptacle). (If toilet insert is used, specimen will be collected from insert.) If resident is incontinent of feces, use tongue depressors to obtain specimen from bed linens, brief, or protective padding. A specimen may also be obtained from a fecal incontinence collection bag when it is changed.

5. Following defecation, resident is to wash hands. Fill basin with water at 105–110°F. Assist resident if needed. If resident is incontinent, carefully clean and dry area around anus. Change bed linens as needed.

6. Take container with bowel movement to the bathroom. Use tongue blades to remove specimen and place in specimen container (Figure 18-13). Do not contaminate the outside of the specimen container or the cover. If possible, take a sample (about 1 teaspoon) from each part of the specimen.

7. Empty collection container into toilet. Clean or dispose of collection container according to facility policy. If resident was incontinent, dispose of soiled brief or padding as biohazardous waste. Place soiled linen in proper hamper.

8. Remove and dispose of gloves according to facility policy.

9. Perform hand hygiene.

10. Cover container and attach completed label. Make sure cover is on container tightly. Place container in biohazard transport bag.

11. Take or send specimen to laboratory promptly. (Stool specimens are never refrigerated.)

12. Carry out each procedure completion action.

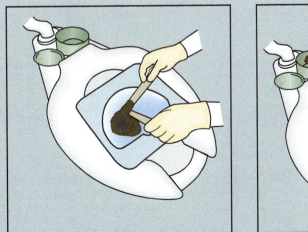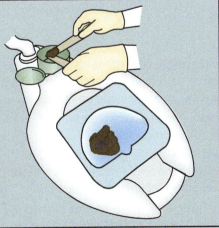

Figure 18-13 Use tongue blades to transfer the stool specimen from the collection container (left) to the specimen container (right).

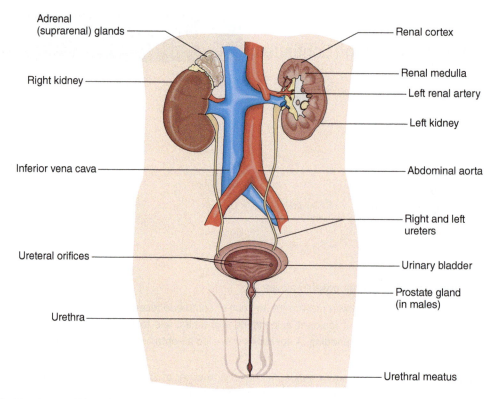

Figure 18-14 Structures of the urinary system.

(tubes that carry the urine to the outside of the body) (Figure 18-14). The urinary system:

- Forms urine
- Stores urine
- Excretes urine
- Regulates electrolyte balance (sodium, potassium, calcium)
- Manages fluid balance and maintains blood pressure
- Removes waste products from the body—mainly urea and uric acid

Kidneys

The kidneys are two bean-shaped organs about 6 inches long. They are located on either side of the spinal column in the lumbar area. They are made up of the:

- Cortex—the dark reddish-brown outer part that contains the urine-producing unit called the **nephron** (Figure 18-15).
- Medulla—the lighter colored middle part contains collecting tubules that receive the formed urine.
- Renal pelvis—the central basin-like area into which the urine passes. The renal pelvis directs the urine out of each kidney and into the ureters.

The kidneys are selective filters that remove wastes to be excreted in the urine but also return

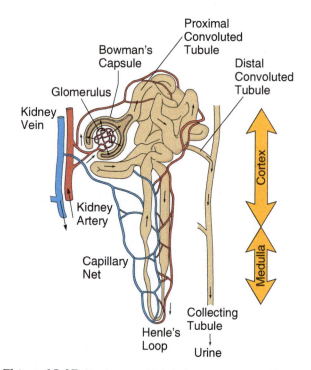

Figure 18-15 Nephron and related structures. Small arrows indicate the flow of blood through the nephron. Urine produced by the nephron flows through the collecting tubule.

needed substances to the body, such as sugar, sodium, potassium, and amino acids. Blood cells and other protein cells do not filter through the system and, when present, can be a sign of injury to the kidney.

Ureters

The ureters are tubes about 12 inches long that lead from each kidney to the urinary bladder. Peristalsis (wave-like motions) in the ureter moves the urine from the kidney to the bladder.

Urinary Bladder

The bladder, a hollow muscular organ in the pelvis, has the following functions:

- Receives the urine from the ureters
- Stores urine until it can be eliminated from the body (holds about 500–600 mL, or when overly distended, 1,000 or more mL)

The exit from the bladder is guarded by a small, circular (sphincter) muscle that prevents urine from escaping involuntarily.

Urethra

The urethra is a small tube that carries the urine from the bladder out of the body. The opening to the outside is called the meatus. The male and female urethra differ as follows:

The female urethra:

- Is about 1½ inches long
- Transports urine only

The male urethra:

- Is 8 to 10 inches long
- Is surrounded by a gland called the prostate gland, which is part of the reproductive system
- Transports urine
- Transports semen

Enlargement of the prostate gland can press on the urethra, making the passage of urine difficult. This often happens in men as they reach later middle age.

Urine Formation

The nephron is a filtering system of tubules and blood vessels that produces urine. It is estimated that each kidney contains 1 million nephrons.

Blood arriving at the kidneys carries waste products such as acids and salts. These waste products must be eliminated from the body. Urine is a liquid waste solution containing water and dissolved substances. Urine is produced as follows:

- Waste products, helpful products, and large quantities of water are passed (filtered) through the capillary walls of the glomerulus (capillary bed) into

Bowman's capsule, forming a liquid called filtrate. (See Figure 18-15.)

- The filtrate moves slowly along the convoluted tubules where some water and helpful substances like sugar and important electrolytes are reabsorbed into the blood.
- The liquid remaining in the convoluted tubules is urine and contains wastes.
- The urine passes into the collecting tubules of the medulla, then out of the kidney to the ureter and into the urinary bladder.
- *Normal* urine is acid in pH and pale to deep yellow in color.
- *Dilute* urine has more water and fewer dissolved substances, so it is colorless to pale yellow.
- *Concentrated* urine has less water and more dissolved substances, so it is darker in color and has a stronger odor.
- The amount of urine produced depends on the amount of intake and various physical conditions. Inadequate water intake leading to dehydration results in a small amount of concentrated urine. Normal urine output is usually considered to be 1,000 to 1,500 mL per day.

The substances in the urine provide good information about the chemistry of the body and how well it is functioning. Tests are frequently performed on the urine (urinalysis).

During your care of the resident, note the amount, color, and odor of the urine, and the presence of any sediment, including blood.

URINE ELIMINATION

The act of eliminating urine from the bladder is known by various terms:

- Micturition
- Urination
- Voiding

Voiding or *urinating* are the terms most frequently used to describe emptying the bladder.

When 150 to 300 mL of urine is present in the bladder, the urge to urinate can be sensed. Voiding can occur voluntarily or involuntarily when the bladder fills. Urine is released as the sphincter muscle relaxes and the bladder walls contract. With training, the signal that the bladder is filling is brought to the level of conscious thought so that voiding can be voluntarily controlled.

? EXERCISE 18-7

IMAGE LABELING
Write the names of the organs of the urinary tract. Be sure the names are spelled correctly.

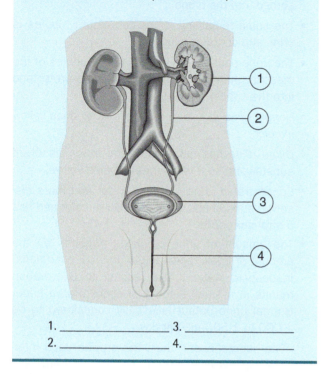

1. _____ 3. _____
2. _____ 4. _____

- Kidneys decrease in size.
- Scar tissue replaces some renal cells.
- Reduced blood flow through the kidneys means lower urine production.
- Reduced renal concentration leads to nocturia.
- Less efficient bladder emptying.
- Reduced filtration ability.

Figure 18-16 Changes in the urinary system as the result of aging.

When 150 to 300 mL of urine is present in the bladder, the urge to urinate can be sensed. Voiding can occur voluntarily or involuntarily when the bladder fills.

URINARY RETENTION AND INCONTINENCE

Older residents face two major problems related to the urinary system: retention and incontinence.

Urinary retention is due to poor bladder tone or incomplete emptying because of an obstruction. Poor tone may be related to the aging process or prolonged catheter drainage. Obstruction may be due to tumor growth. In men, obstruction is often due to the enlargement of the prostate gland. Urinary retention due to a tumor may require surgery to relieve the obstruction.

Urinary retention is due to one or more factors including:

- Inability to reach toileting facilities in time
- Emotional withdrawal
- Lack of awareness of need
- Physical changes
- Infection of the urinary tract
- Fecal impaction
- Neurologic damage such as in a stroke
- Inability to communicate the need to use the toilet
- Mental confusion
- Ineffective muscle control

Urinary incontinence may be temporary or established. If attention is given to the underlying causes, the temporary use of incontinence pads may be all that is needed. When the incontinence is prolonged, tests to determine the cause may be ordered. If needed, a urinary retraining program will be started. This program generally means the resident is encouraged or assisted to the bathroom before and after meals and once through the night until bladder control is restored.

CHANGES IN THE URINARY SYSTEM CAUSED BY AGING

As a person ages, the kidneys decrease somewhat in size and some renal cells are lost and replaced by scar tissue. This means the kidneys are less efficient filters. The blood vessels carrying the blood to the kidneys for filtration undergo changes that reduce the amount of blood delivered. The lower blood flow decreases urine production.

Loss of pelvic muscle tone and strength makes bladder emptying less efficient. Urine may be retained in the bladder (retention). Urine production influences the acid-base and fluid balances of the body.

Urine is produced continuously. In younger persons, it is more concentrated during the night. An older person loses some concentrating ability and experiences more need to empty the bladder at night. This problem is called nocturia. Make sure the call light is available, there is no clutter in the pathway, and that lighting is adequate for safe ambulation at night. Figure 18-16 summarizes the urinary system changes caused by aging.

Nursing Assistant Actions

Urinary incontinence is uncomfortable and embarrassing to the resident. In addition, prolonged exposure of the skin to urine is a major cause of skin breakdown. The warm, moist conditions also encourage bacterial growth. Pathogens on the skin grow quickly and move upward through the urinary tract to cause serious urinary infections. These can lead to life-threatening **septicemia** (**sepsis**). Wet linen that is not changed promptly has an offensive, repugnant odor. Residents who are incontinent fear having "accidents" and tend to limit social interactions with others.

Every effort must be made to help the resident become continent. Little reference should be made to the temporary incontinence. Nursing assistants can do much to give emotional support and reassurance to residents who are incontinent. Nursing assistant responsibilities include:

- Assisting residents to toilet regularly
- Anticipating toileting needs and answering call lights promptly
- Always being courteous and patient when assisting residents with toileting
- Maintaining a positive attitude when changing soiled garments and bed linen and never being critical
- Performing good perineal care and being sure resident is clean and dry
- Checking the skin for signs of irritation whenever you toilet or bathe resident or perform perineal care
- Giving special attention to residents who are confused or forgetful because they may be unable to clearly state their need for assistance

INTERNAL URINARY CATHETER DRAINAGE

At times, it may be necessary to assist urinary elimination by the use of an **indwelling catheter**. The **catheter** is a slender rubber or plastic tube that is inserted into the bladder using sterile technique. The urine drains out of the bladder through the catheter. A balloon around the neck of the catheter is inflated once the catheter is in place. The inflated balloon

---

? EXERCISE 18-8

COMPLETION

Select the correct terms from the following list to complete each statement.

bladder	difficult	less	soft
blood	dissolved	lighter	urine
brown	empty	more	water
carbon dioxide	feces	night	1½
decrease	filters	salts	8–10"

1. The female urethra is _____ long.

2. The male urethra is _____ long.

3. The waste product eliminated through the kidneys is called _____.

4. Enlargement of the male prostate gland can make passage of urine _____.

5. The solid wastes eliminated through the colon are called _____.

6. Other organs that excrete wastes from the body are the lungs that excrete _____ and the skin that excretes _____ and _____.

7. Normal feces would be _____ in color, _____ in consistency, and formed.

8. Concentrated urine has _____ water and more _____ substances.

9. Dilute urine has _____ water and is _____ in color.

10. As people age:

   a. The kidneys _____ in size and are less efficient _____.

   b. There is less _____ flow to the kidneys.

   c. Pelvic muscle tone and strength decrease making it more difficult to empty the _____.

   d. The ability to concentrate urine during the _____ is less.

   e. They experience the need to _____ their bladder more often at night.

keeps the catheter in place so that it will not easily fall out. The other end of the catheter is connected to a drainage tube and collection bag (Figure 18-17A). This is a closed system and is sterile as long as it is not opened. Opening the system greatly increases the risk of infection. The insertion of a sterile catheter is

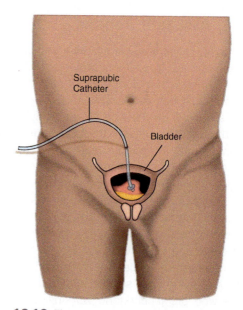

Figure 18-18 The suprapubic catheter is surgically inserted through the abdominal wall. The urethra may be nonfunctional.

the responsibility of the nurse. Sometimes it is necessary for the physician to insert a catheter into the bladder through a surgical incision in the abdomen. This is referred to as a **suprapubic** catheter (Figure 18-18). Some residents with neurological disorders may have orders for periodic, intermittent catheterization with a straight catheter.

Catheter Care

The nursing assistant provides daily care of the catheter when the resident has an indwelling catheter for urinary drainage. This care consists of the following actions:

- Applying the principles of standard precautions, using PPE appropriately
- Keeping the urinary meatus clean
- Washing the area around the meatus twice daily with a solution approved by your facility
- Checking regularly for signs of irritation or urinary discomfort and reporting to the nurse
- Securing the tubing in such a way that there is no strain on the catheter or tubing. A catheter strap should be applied if ordered or appropriate for the resident's condition. It may be contraindicated if the resident has cardiac or vascular problems.
- Maintaining the drainage bag below the level of the bladder
- Clamping and unclamping the catheter tubing at specific times. The clamping allows the bladder to fill, stimulating muscle tone.

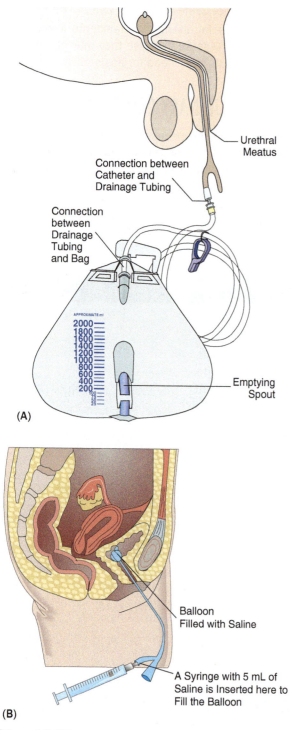

Figure 18-17 (A) Indwelling catheter connected to a urine drainage bag in a male resident. (B) Indwelling catheter in a female resident.

- Not opening the closed system unless emptying the urinary drainage bag
- Making sure the tubing is not kinked or obstructed
- Ensuring that the collection bag does not touch the floor
- Measuring the amount of drainage in the collection bag at the end of each shift, noting the character of the urine, and reporting and recording the information
- Checking the entire drainage setup each time care is given and at the beginning and end of your shift
- Reporting changes in the character or quantity of urine
- All observations that apply to care of an indwelling catheter apply to a suprapubic catheter, except that the nurse will care for and change the abdominal dressing. Follow your facility policies regarding bathing a resident who has a suprapubic catheter. Usual nursing assistant actions include daily washing of the abdomen with soap and water around the suprapubic catheter site.

Ambulating with a Catheter

When residents are ambulatory or using a walker or wheelchair, you must be careful about placement of the urinary drainage bag. Remember that the drainage bag must always be lower than the bladder so the urine cannot flow back into the bladder. The bag may be secured to the resident's leg or clothing when the resident ambulates or the resident may carry the bag.

When the resident is seated in a wheelchair, the tubing should run below and under the wheelchair so the drainage bag can be secured to the wheelchair back. The drainage bag or tubing must never touch the floor and should always be in an enclosed bag.

Infection Risk

You must carefully follow the procedure for disconnecting the catheter. The resident who has an indwelling catheter is at risk for infection. There are several sites where infection can enter the drainage system:

- Urinary meatus, where the catheter is inserted
- Connection between the catheter and drainage tube
- Connection between the drainage bag and drainage tubing
- Opening used to empty the drainage bag

Disconnecting the Catheter

It is preferable never to disconnect the drainage setup, but at times, it is necessary. If sterile caps and plugs are available, they should be used.

PROCEDURE 18-46
Giving Indwelling Catheter Care

OBRA

1. Carry out each beginning procedure action.
2. Assemble equipment:
   - Disposable gloves
   - Bed protector
   - Bath blanket
   - Plastic bag for disposables
   - Washcloth, towel, basin, and soap if kit is unavailable
   - Tape
   - Catheter bag cover
3. Elevate bed to comfortable working height. Be sure opposite side rail is up and secure. Position resident on back, with legs separated and knees bent, if permitted.
4. Cover resident with bath blanket and fanfold bedding to foot of bed.
5. Ask resident to raise hips. Place bed protector underneath resident.
6. Position bath blanket so that only genitals will be exposed.
7. Perform hand hygiene and put on gloves and draw bath blanket back.

(continues)

PROCEDURE 18-46
Giving Indwelling Catheter Care (Continued)

8. For the male resident:

   - Gently grasp penis and draw foreskin back, if not circumcised (Figure 18-19).

   - Cleanse around meatus and glans. Wash with soap and water and rinse using a circular motion. Cleanse the catheter for 4 inches from the meatus outward, pat dry in the same manner. Make sure to return the foreskin (if not circumcised) to its normal position.

   For the female resident:

   - Separate the labia.

   - Cleanse downward from front to back, use one stroke only.

   - Repeat cleansing, using a new section of the washcloth each time, as needed. You may need to use several washcloths.

   - Using a clean section of the washcloth, cleanse 4 inches down the catheter tubing.

   - Rinse and pat dry in same manner.

9. Remove gloves. Perform hand hygiene.

10. Check catheter to be sure it is secured properly to the leg (Figure 18-20). Readjust leg strap for slack, if needed. If a Velcro strap is not used, use tape (Figure 18-21).

11. Check to be sure tubing is coiled on bed (see Figure 18-20) and hangs straight down into drainage container. Empty bag and measure if necessary. Do not raise bag above level of resident's bladder. Place catheter bag in protective cover.

12. Replace bedding and remove bath blanket.

13. Fold bath blanket and put in linen hamper.

14. Lower bed. Adjust side rails for positioning, if used.

15. Carry out each procedure completion action.

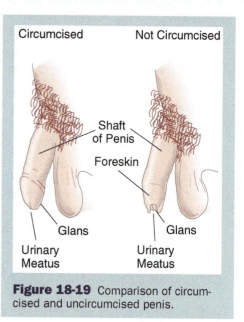

Figure 18-19 Comparison of circumcised and uncircumcised penis.

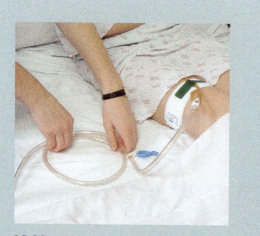

Figure 18-20 Check the catheter tubing to be sure it is secured but not obstructed by the Velcro® leg band and that its coiled on the bed.

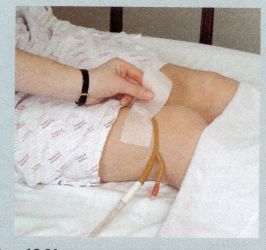

Figure 18-21 The catheter tubing can also be taped to the thigh using hypoallergenic tape (preferably).

INTAKE AND OUTPUT (I&O)

Intake

Intake includes everything taken in that is liquid at room temperature, such as:

- Water or tea
- Gelatin, junket, or pudding
- Fluids given directly into a vein (IV)

Output

Normal fluid output includes all fluids that leave the body, including:

- Urine
- Perspiration
- Moisture from the lungs
- Moisture from the bowels

Excessive fluid loss results in dehydration (inadequate water content in body tissue). This loss can occur through:

- Diarrhea
- Vomiting
- Excessive urine output (diuresis)
- Excessive perspiration (diaphoresis)

Retention of fluids results in edema (swelling of body tissues). This may be caused by:

- Kidney dysfunction
- Cardiovascular disease
- Liver disease

Recording Output

An accurate recording of intake and output is basic to the care of many residents. Intake and output totals are usually kept on the same form. Records are kept when ordered by the physician and when residents:

- Are dehydrated
- Receive intravenous infusions
- Have a urinary catheter
- Are perspiring profusely or vomiting
- Have specific diagnoses such as congestive heart failure or renal disease that require accurate monitoring of I&O

If the resident is incontinent, indicate the number of times on the output record. Do not forget to check the resident often and to change the bed linen each time it is wet. After each incident, clean resident and give perineal care. Change soiled clothing.

PROCEDURE 18-47
Emptying a Urinary Drainage Bag

OBRA

1. Carry out each beginning procedure action.

2. Assemble equipment:

   - Disposable gloves
   - Graduated container
   - Sterile cap or sterile 4 × 4 (needed if container has no bottom drain tube)
   - Antiseptic wipes
   - Clamps

3. Perform hand hygiene and put on gloves.

4. Place paper towel on the floor under the drainage bag. Place a graduated container (graduate) on paper towel under drain of collection bag.

5. Remove drain from holder (Figure 18-22) and open. Using aseptic technique, allow the urine to drain into the graduate. Do not allow the tip of the tubing to touch the sides of the graduate.

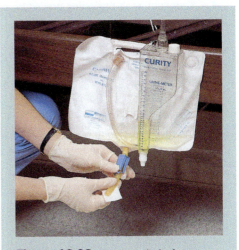

Figure 18-22 Remove drain from holder and cleanse with an antiseptic wipe.

(continues)

PROCEDURE 18-47
Emptying a Urinary Drainage Bag (Continued)

6. Close the drain and replace it in the holder (Figure 18-23). If accidental contamination occurs, wipe the drain tip with an antiseptic wipe in one circular motion before returning it to the holder. Dispose of antiseptic wipe in plastic bag.

7. Pick up paper towel, touching top surface only, and discard.

8. Check position of drainage tube.

9. Take graduate to bathroom and empty it.

10. Wash and dry graduate and store it according to facility policy.

11. Carry out each procedure completion action.

12. Copy information on resident's record from intake and output sheet according to facility policy.

NOTE: Reverse the procedure to reconnect the catheter. If you find an unprotected, disconnected tube in the bed or on the floor, do not reconnect it. Report it at once.

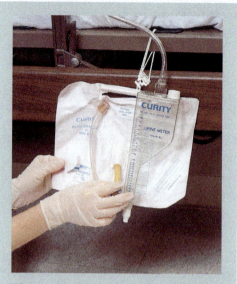

Figure 18-23 Cleanse the drain with an antiseptic wipe and return the drain to the holder.

PROCEDURE 18-48
Measuring and Recording Fluid Output

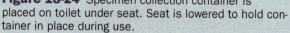

1. Carry out each beginning procedure action.

2. Assemble equipment:
   - Disposable gloves
   - Graduate pitcher
   - Pen for recording

3. Perform hand hygiene and put on disposable gloves.

4. Instruct a resident who is able to ambulate to the bathroom to use the hat-shaped specimen collection container (Figure 18-24).

5. Pour urine from bedpan, urinal, or collection container into graduate pitcher and measure (Figures 18-25 and 18-26).

6. Empty urine.
   - If urine is accidentally spilled, estimate amount and make notation that it is an estimate.

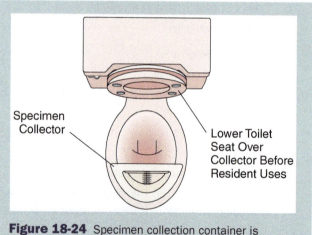

Figure 18-24 Specimen collection container is placed on toilet under seat. Seat is lowered to hold container in place during use.

(continues)

PROCEDURE 18-48
Measuring and Recording Fluid Output (Continued)

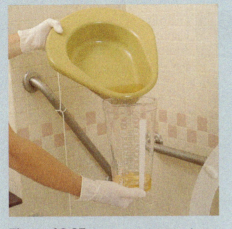

Figure 18-25 Pour urine into graduate pitcher. Make sure there is no toilet paper in the bedpan.

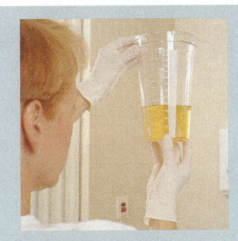

Figure 18-26 Read the amount of urine in the graduate pitcher at eye level (hold level). The measuring scale is marked in cc or mL.

NOTE: Some health care facilities have guidelines for estimating the amount of urine or blood on pads or linen by the diameter of the wet area.

7. Rinse graduate pitcher with cold water. Clean according to facility policy.
8. Clean bedpan or urinal or specimen container and store properly, according to facility policy.
9. Remove and dispose of gloves according to facility policy. Perform hand hygiene.
10. Record amounts immediately under output column on bedside intake and output record (Figure 18-27). All liquid output should be recorded. Output includes:

   - Urine
   - Vomitus—also called **emesis**
   - Drainage from a wound or the stomach
   - Liquid stool—record an estimated amount
   - Blood loss—record an estimated amount if on sheets or dressings, otherwise measure with a graduate
   - Perspiration—record an estimated amount

NOTE: Fluids used to irrigate the bladder or for an enema are not included in calculating the output.

11. Carry out each procedure completion action.
12. Copy information on resident's record from intake and output sheet according to facility policy.

   - Perspiration and blood loss may be described as little, moderate, or excessive.
   - Also record the number of times linens or dressings have been changed or reinforced because of such fluid losses.

13. Blood loss is determined by the size of the wet area on dressings and by measuring amounts in vacuum containers.

PROCEDURE 18-48
Measuring and Recording Fluid Output (Continued)

Date	Time	Method of Adm.	Solution	Intake Amounts Rec'd	Time	Output Urine Amount	Kind	Amount
7/16	0700	PO	water	120 mL		500 mL		
	0830	PO	coffee	240 mL				
			or. ju.	120 mL				
	1030	PO	cran. ju.	120 mL				
	1100					300 mL		
	1230	PO	tea	240 mL				
	1400	PO	water	150 mL				
Shift	1500			990 mL		800 mL		
Totals	1530	PO	gelatin	120 mL				
	1700	PO	tea	120 mL				
			soup	180 mL				
	2000					512 mL		
	2045						vomitus	500 mL
	2205						vomitus	90 mL
Shift	2300			420 mL		512 mL		590 mL
Totals	2345						vomitus	80 mL
	0130	IV	D/W	500 mL				
	0315					400 mL		
Shift	0700			500 mL		400 mL		80 mL
Total								
25 Hour				1910 mL		1712 mL	vomitus	670 mL
Totals								

Figure 18-27 Bedside intake and output sheet. In this example, the output amounts are highlighted.

? EXERCISE 18-9

COMPLETION

1. Augusta Pratt has an indwelling urinary drainage system and has an order for I&O.

   a. Explain how you will give daily care to her perineum and what precautions you will take.

   _____

   _____

   _____

(continues)

? EXERCISE 18-9 (Continued)

Intake	Output
0700 100 mL water PO	1500 urinary drainage 600 mL
0830 240 mL tea PO	1700 vomitus 150 mL
1030 120 mL cranberry PO	2300 urinary drainage 750 mL
1230 240 mL broth PO	2345 vomitus 80 mL
1400 150 mL water PO	0700 urinary drainage 700 mL
1530 120 mL sherbert PO	
1700 120 mL tea PO	
2000 100 mL H$_2$O PO	
2200 150 mL H$_2$O PO	
2345 500 mL D/W IV	
0600 30 mL H$_2$O PO	

LEG BAG DRAINAGE

Some residents find it easier to ambulate when urine drainage is collected in a leg bag instead of the larger urinary drainage bag. Wearing a leg bag enhances dignity and independence, since the bag is not noticeable by others. The leg bag is held to the resident's leg by adjustable straps around either the thigh or the lower leg (Figure 18-28). Points to keep in mind when residents use a leg bag are:

- The leg bag is smaller and must be emptied more often.
- The bag must be placed so there is a straight drop down from the catheter.

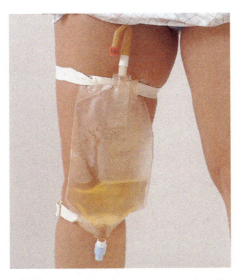

Figure 18-28 The leg bag is held in place by adjustable straps. Because it is smaller than the standard drainage bag, it must be emptied more often.

- Tension on the catheter tubing must be minimal.
- Care must be taken not to introduce germs when connecting and disconnecting the bag and catheter.
- Be alert for skin irritation and/or breakdown under the straps or the leg bag. Immediately report any unusual findings to the nurse.

EXTERNAL URINARY DRAINAGE (MALE)

External urinary drainage is preferred for male residents who require drainage for long periods of time. In this form of drainage, an internal catheter is not inserted in the urethra. Thus, there is less danger of infection.

A condom (sheath) or some other type of appliance is placed on the penis. The condom is attached to drainage tubing and a collection bag. The condom is removed every 24 hours and the penis is cleansed.

COMMON CONDITIONS

Rectocele and Cystocele

The urinary bladder, ureters, and the urethra are found in the pelvic cavity. Some of the female reproductive organs are also in the pelvis. Each group of organs can be affected by disease or stress in the other group.

Frequent pregnancies and general loss of muscle tone due to the aging process may cause the bladder to protrude into the vagina (cystocele) and the rectum into the vagina (rectocele).

The weakness of the bladder wall can cause urinary incontinence, especially with extra stress such as laughing or coughing. The weakened rectal wall can lead to constipation and hemorrhoids. Surgery can be helpful in repairing the cystocele and rectocele.

Renal Calculi

Renal calculi, or kidney stones, form as various salts and compounds settle out of the forming urine. Starting as tiny grains of sediment, they become larger and larger until they block part of the drainage system,

---

? EXERCISE 18-10

TRUE OR FALSE

Indicate whether the following statements are true (T) or false (F).

1. T F A resident with a colostomy does not have normal sphincter control.
2. T F The nursing assistant usually cares for a fresh ileostomy stoma.
3. T F Insertion of a sterile urinary catheter is an appropriate nursing assistant duty.
4. T F When emptying a urinary drainage bag, it is permissible to place the tip of the tubing in the bottom of a graduate while the bag drains.
5. T F The single-use leg bag should be discarded in a biohazardous waste container.
6. T F It is not necessary to wash the resident's genital area before collecting a clean catch specimen.
7. T F It is all right to send bits of toilet paper with a routine urine specimen.
8. T F When collecting a clean-catch urine specimen, take the sample from the beginning of the urine flow.

PROCEDURE 18-49
Connecting the Catheter to Leg Bag and Emptying the Leg Bag

 OBRA

NOTE: Always check with the nurse before using a leg bag.

1. Carry out each beginning procedure action.
2. Assemble equipment:
    - Disposable gloves
    - Antiseptic wipes
    - Leg bag and tubing
    - Emesis basin
    - Bed protector
    - Graduate pitcher
    - Paper towels
    - Sterile cap/plug
    - Clamp
3. Perform hand hygiene and put on gloves.
4. Place bed protector under the connection between catheter and drainage tube.
5. Clamp the catheter.

(continues)

PROCEDURE 18-49

Connecting the Catheter to Leg Bag and Emptying the Leg Bag (Continued)

6. Disconnect the catheter and drainage tubing. Do not put them down or allow them to touch anything.

7. Insert a sterile plug in the end of the catheter. Place a sterile cap over the exposed end of the drainage tube.

NOTE: If accidental contamination occurs, wipe the area with antiseptic wipes before inserting the sterile plug or replacing the sterile cap over the exposed end of the drainage tubing. Dispose of antiseptic wipes in plastic bag.

8. Remember that the drainage tube must not touch the floor.

9. Remove catheter plug.

10. Insert the end of the leg bag tubing into the catheter (Figure 18-29).

11. Release the catheter clamp.

12. Secure the leg bag with the adjustable straps to the resident's leg so there is no tension on the tubing. Be sure there is a straight drop down of tubing from the catheter to the bag for urine flow. Check for leakage.

13. Remove bed protector and discard.

14. Remove gloves and discard according to facility policy. Perform hand hygiene.

15. Assist resident to get out of bed. The single-use leg bag should be discarded in a biohazardous waste container.

16. Carry out each procedure completion action.

NOTE: To reconnect the regular drainage bag, reverse the procedure.

To Empty the Leg Bag:

17. Position resident safely.

18. Perform hand hygiene and put on gloves.

19. Release the adjustable straps holding leg bag so it can be moved away from leg.

20. Place paper towel on floor under drainage outlet of leg bag.

21. Place graduate on paper towel under drainage outlet.

22. Remove cap, being careful not to touch tip. Drain urine into the graduate. Do not put cap down and do not touch inside of cap. If accidental contamination occurs, wipe the area with antiseptic wipes before replacing cap. Dispose of antiseptic wipes in a plastic bag.

23. Wipe drainage outlet with an antiseptic wipe and replace cap.

24. Refasten the adjustable straps to secure drainage bag to leg.

25. Make sure resident is comfortable and safe.

26. Discard paper towel.

27. Measure urine and note amount if required.

28. Discard urine. Clean graduate, cover, and store.

29. Remove gloves and discard according to facility policy.

30. Carry out each procedure completion action.

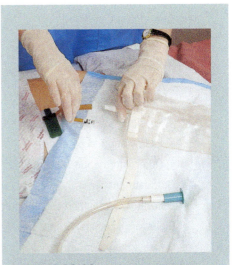

Figure 18-29 Connecting leg bag to catheter tubing. Do not let the catheter tubing touch anything that could contaminate it. Note that the tubing to the drainage bag is covered with a sterile cap to protect it until it is reconnected to the catheter.

PROCEDURE 18-50
Collecting a Routine or Clean-Catch Urine Specimen

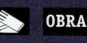 **OBRA**

1. Carry out each beginning procedure action.

2. Assemble equipment:

   - Disposable gloves
   - Bedpan/urinal
   - Sterile **specimen** container and cover
   - Label including:
     - Resident's full name
     - Room number
     - Facility identification
     - Date and time of collection
     - Physician's name
     - Examination to be done
     - Other information requested
   - Graduate pitcher
   - Laboratory requisition slip, properly filled out
   - Biohazard specimen transport bag
   - Gauze squares or cotton
   - Antiseptic wipes

3. Completely fill out the label of the specimen container.

To Collect a Routine Urine Specimen:

4. Perform hand hygiene and put on disposable gloves.

5. Offer bedpan or urinal.

6. Instruct resident not to discard toilet tissue in the pan with the urine. Provide a small plastic bag in which to place the soiled tissue.

7. After resident has voided, cover pan and place on bed protector on chair. Offer wash water to resident.

8. If resident can ambulate to bathroom, place specimen collector in toilet.

9. Assist resident to bathroom. Ask resident to void into specimen collector. Instruct resident to discard soiled toilet tissue in plastic bag provided. Tissue must not be placed in collector.

10. Provide privacy.

11. Put on gloves. Remove specimen collector from toilet. If resident is on I&O, note amount of urine (Figure 18-30). If resident used bedpan, pour urine into graduate to measure. Note amount. Remove

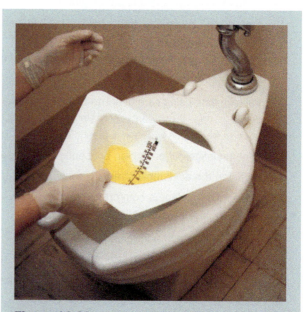

Figure 18-30 Remove specimen collector from toilet. Note amount of urine if resident is on I&O.

(continues)

PROCEDURE 18-50
Collecting a Routine or Clean-Catch Urine Specimen (Continued)

gloves and discard according to facility policy. Perform hand hygiene.

12. Remove cap from specimen container. Place cap (inside up) on shelf or other flat surface in bathroom or utility room. Do not touch inside of cap or container.

13. Put on gloves. Carefully pour about 120 mL urine into specimen container from collector (Figure 18-31). Make sure the amount of urine taken for the laboratory specimen is included in the output total for the shift.

14. Remove and discard gloves according to facility policy.

15. Perform hand hygiene.

16. Place cap on specimen container. Do not contaminate outside of container. Attach completed label to container (Figure 18-32). Place specimen container in biohazard specimen transport bag and attach laboratory requisition slip (Figure 18-33).

17. Carry out each procedure completion action.

18. Follow facility policy for transporting specimen to laboratory.

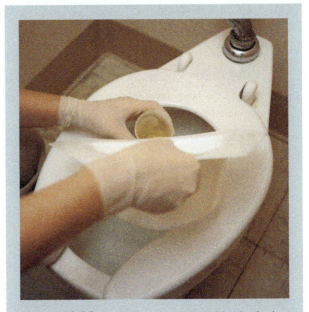

Figure 18-31 Carefully pour about 120 mL of urine from specimen collector into specimen container.

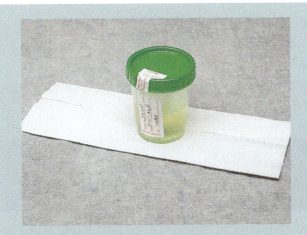

Figure 18-32 After specimen is placed in container and cap is put on, place label on container.

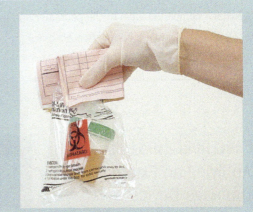

Figure 18-33 Properly labeled specimen container is placed in a biohazard specimen transport bag and laboratory requisition is attached.

To Collect a Clean-Catch Specimen:

Complete steps 1 and 2 noted at the beginning of this procedure, then:

19. Perform hand hygiene and put on disposable gloves.

20. Wash resident's genital area properly or instruct resident to do so. If soiled due to incontinence, perform perineal care.

(continues)

PROCEDURE 18-50
Collecting a Routine or Clean-Catch Urine Specimen (Continued)

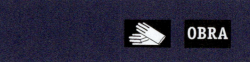

21. For female residents:

    - Spread the labia.
    - Cleanse downward from front to back over urinary meatus, left side and right side.
    - Use a clean wipe for each stroke. Discard in appropriate manner.
    - Keep the labia separated so the folds do not recover the meatus, collect the urine specimen.

22. For male residents:

    - Using the antiseptic wipes, cleanse the tip of the penis from the urinary meatus down, using a circular motion.
    - Discard in plastic bag.

23. Instruct resident to void, allowing the first part of the urine to escape. Then:

    - Catch the urine stream that follows in the sterile specimen container.
    - Allow the last portion of the urine stream to escape.

NOTE: If resident's I&O is being monitored, or if the amount of urine passed must be measured, catch the first and last part of the urine in a bedpan, urinal, or specimen collection container.

24. Place the sterile cap on the urine container immediately to prevent contamination of the urine specimen.

25. Allow resident to wash hands. Assist as necessary.

26. With the cap securely tightened, wipe the outside of the specimen container with a clean paper towel.

27. Remove and dispose of gloves according to facility policy.

28. Perform hand hygiene.

29. Attach completed label to the container and place specimen in the biohazard transport bag.

30. Carry out procedure completion actions.

31. Follow facility policy for transporting specimen to laboratory.

PROCEDURE 18-51
Applying an External Urinary Drainage Device

1. Carry out each beginning procedure action.

2. Assemble equipment:

    - Disposable gloves
    - Basin of warm water
    - Condom with drainage tip or external drainage device
    - Bed protector
    - Bath blanket
    - Towel

(continues)

PROCEDURE 18-51
Applying an External Urinary Drainage Device (Continued)

3. Arrange equipment on overbed table.

4. Raise bed to comfortable working height.

5. Be sure opposite side rail is up and secure for safety.

6. Cover resident with bath blanket and fanfold bedding to foot of bed.

7. Perform hand hygiene and put on gloves.

8. Place bed protector under resident's buttocks.

9. Adjust bath blanket to expose genitals only.

10. Carefully wash and dry penis. Observe for signs of irritation. Check to be sure condom (external device) has "ready stick" surface.

11. Apply external device and drainage tip to penis by placing condom at top of penis and rolling toward base of penis. Leave space between drainage tip and glans of penis to prevent irritation (Figure 18-34). If resident is not circumcised, be sure that foreskin is in normal position.

12. Apply tape provided with condom to secure it to the penis (Figure 18-35).

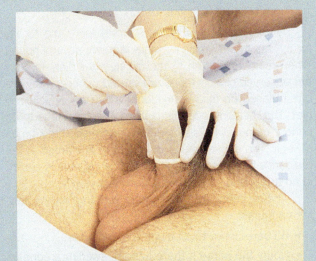

Figure 18-34 When condom is placed on penis, leave room between the drainage tip and the glans of the penis to prevent irritation. Roll condom to base of penis.

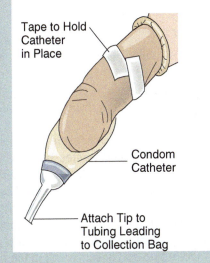

Tape to Hold Catheter in Place

Condom Catheter

Attach Tip to Tubing Leading to Collection Bag

Figure 18-35 Correctly applied and secured condom ready to be attached to tubing leading to drainage bag.

13. Condom (external device) is now ready to be connected to drainage tubing leading to collection bag.

14. Remove gloves and discard according to facility policy.

15. Perform hand hygiene.

16. Adjust bedding and remove bath blanket and place in laundry hamper.

17. Lower bed. Adjust side rails if used for positioning.

18. Carry out procedure completion actions.

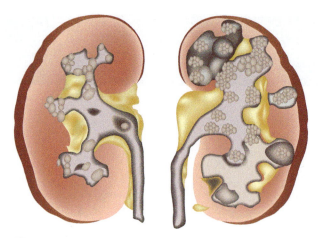

Figure 18-36 Renal calculi.

often a ureter (Figure 18-36). When blockage occurs the resident experiences extreme pain. Pain associated with urine elimination is known as dysuria. Most kidney stones are passed when fluids are forced, but surgery may be required to relieve the obstruction.

The urine may be strained through gauze or filter paper before being measured and discarded to determine when the stone is passed. Blood may cause the urine to become pink to deep red in color. Blood in the urine is called hematuria.

Renal Failure

Renal failure (uremia) may occur suddenly but it is usually a chronic situation that develops gradually over a period of years. Causes include changes in the blood vessels that serve the kidneys, hypertension, and the aging process.

The resident in chronic renal failure does not eliminate effectively, so water and wastes build up in the body. Urine output is reduced (oliguria). In the terminal stage of renal failure, urine output ceases altogether (anuria). Blood pressure increases and edema and chemical imbalance develop throughout the body. The resident may complain of headache, nausea, and a bad taste in the mouth. Uric acid is eliminated in the perspiration. The uric acid accumulates as white crystals on the skin and is called uremic frost. The perspiration has an unpleasant odor. Careful attention is needed to keep the skin clean and free from breakdown.

Figure 18-37 Dialysis filters wastes from the resident's blood. Blood leaves the body from an artery, is filtered by the machine, and is returned to the body through a vein.

Renal failure is treated by:

- Surgery to implant a healthy kidney
- Dialysis (hemodialysis or peritoneal) is a procedure that uses a machine to filter wastes and impurities from the blood (Figure 18-37).

Residents receiving dialysis may leave the facility for the treatment, which normally requires several hours. When residents return to the facility after dialysis, they are observed closely for dizziness and fainting. They are often placed on fluid restriction, I&O, and a specialized diet. The resident receiving dialysis may have little to no urinary output. Dialysis is often performed three times a week. Two connectors (cannulas) are implanted in the resident's body, usually in an arm. One cannula is placed in an artery and the other is placed in a vein.

When caring for the resident with implanted dialysis cannulas:

- Be careful not to dislodge the cannulas.
- Notify the nurse if there is pain, swelling, redness, or drainage in the arm.
- Do not use the arm for blood pressure measurements.
- Do not apply tight clothing to the arm.
- Encourage resident to follow any special exercises that may have been ordered.

? EXERCISE 18-11

MATCHING
Match the condition on the right with the definition on the left.

Definition
1. _____ painful urination
2. _____ protrusion of bladder wall into vagina

Condition
a. retention
b. rectocele

(continues)

? EXERCISE 18-11 (Continued)

3. _____ blood in the urine   c. cystocele
4. _____ renal failure   d. renal calculi
5. _____ diminished urine output   e. uremia
6. _____ protrusion of rectal wall into vagina f. dysuria
7. _____ involuntary elimination   g. incontinence
8. _____ inability to empty the bladder completely h. nocturia
9. _____ kidney stones   i. hematuria
10. _____ getting up to urinate at night   j. oliguria

LESSON SYNTHESIS: Putting It All Together

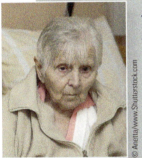

© Anetta/www.Shutterstock.com

You have just completed this lesson. Now go back and review the Clinical Focus. Try to see how the Clinical Focus relates to the concepts presented in the lesson. Then answer the following questions.

1. What do you think Ms. Beebe's problem is?

2. What made the nursing assistant think to ask Ms. Beebe when she had her last bowel movement?

3. What actions could the nursing staff take that might help the resident avoid a similar situation in the future?

4. Why is the attitude of the staff an important factor in the success or failure of managing elimination problems?

18 REVIEW

A. Match each term (items a–e) with the proper definition.

- constipation
- diarrhea
- feces
- micturition
- retention

1. _____   loose, liquid stools

2. _____   inability to urinate

3. _____   hard stool that is difficult to evacuate

4. _____   solid waste

5. _____   another term for urination

B. Complete the sentence by providing the proper term.

6. Elimination of feces is called _____.

7. Blood in the urine is called _____.

8. Painful urination is _____.

9. Inability to control elimination is _____.

10. An artificial opening in the wall of the abdomen for the elimination of feces is called a(an) _____.

C. Fill in the blanks by selecting the correct word or phrase from the list.

liquid	sit upright
left side	I&O sheet
floor	incontinent
coiled	dehydration
oil-retention enema	tongue depressors
voiding	stoma

11. The best position for the resident receiving an enema is on the _____ with the knees flexed.

12. One type of enema that should be retained for 20 minutes is the _____.

13. When collecting a stool specimen, use _____ to transfer the sample from the bedpan to the specimen container.

14. The best position to encourage voiding in a female resident is to have her _____.

15. A person who is unable to control urine output voluntarily is said to be _____.

16. Intake includes everything taken in that is _____ at room temperature.

17. Intake and output are recorded on the _____.

18. When a resident has a colostomy, the opening is called the _____.

19. During a routine urinary drainage check, the tubing should be _____ on the bed.

20. A urine collection bag must never touch the _____.

21. A common term for eliminating urine from the bladder is _____.

22. Excessive fluid loss from the body results in _____.

D. Select the one best answer for each of the following.

23. Feces that is not expelled and remains in the rectum is referred to as:

(A) Diarrhea

(B) Fecal impaction

(C) Fecal incontinence

(D) Constipation

24. Average adult urinary output is approximately:

(A) 500 mL per day

(B) 1,000 mL per day

(C) 1,500 mL per day

(D) 4,000 mL per day

25. Gloves should be worn in each instance except when

(A) applying an external urinary device

(B) giving perineal care

(C) applying a leg drainage bag

(D) filling out the label for a specimen container

26. A resident with a colostomy eliminates feces through an opening into the

(A) anus

(B) ileum

(C) jejunum

(D) colon

27. Normal urine color is

(E) red

(F) yellow

(G) colorless

(H) brown

E. Clinical Experience

Mrs. Duff has an indwelling catheter and is in a wheelchair. You are assigned to her care. Answer the following questions.

28. May the collection bag touch the floor at any time?

29. Should the collection bag or tubing be higher or lower than the resident's bladder?

30. Is perineal care necessary?

31. How often should the drainage be emptied?

32. When Mrs. Duff is in her wheelchair, how should the urinary drainage tubing be positioned?

6

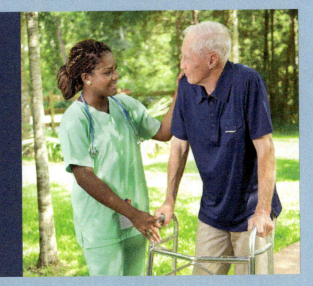

Special Nursing Assistant Activities

MEASURING AND RECORDING RESIDENTS' DATA

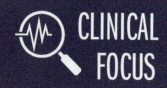

CLINICAL FOCUS

Think about situations in which the measuring and recording of data are an important part of your duties as you study this lesson.

OBJECTIVES

After studying this lesson, you should be able to:

- Define vocabulary words and terms.

- Explain how to properly select and use equipment to measure vital signs.

- Identify the range of normal values.

- State the reasons for measuring weight and height.

- Demonstrate the following:

  Procedure 19-52 Measuring an Oral Temperature (Electronic Thermometer)
  Procedure 19-53 Measuring a Rectal Temperature (Electronic Thermometer)
  Procedure 19-54 Measuring an Axillary Temperature (Electronic Thermometer)
  Procedure 19-55 Measuring a Tympanic Temperature
  Procedure 19-56 Counting the Radial Pulse Rate
  Procedure 19-57 Counting the Apical-Radial Pulse
  Procedure 19-58 Counting Respirations
  Procedure 19-59 Taking Blood Pressure
  Procedure 19-60 Weighing and Measuring the Resident Using an Upright Scale
  Procedure 19-61 Measuring Weight with an Electronic Wheelchair Scale
  Procedure 19-62 Weighing the Resident in a Chair Scale
  Procedure 19-63 Measuring and Weighing the Resident in Bed

CASE STUDY

Geraldine Hoden, 72 years old, is a resident in your facility. Mrs. Hoden has heart problems that cause her to retain fluid (edema). She becomes short of breath with any physical exertion. Mrs. Hoden is taking medication to strengthen and regulate her heart activity. She also has a history of hypertension. Mrs. Hoden is alert and cooperative.

VOCABULARY

accelerated (ack-SELL-er-ay-ted)
antihypertensive (an-ti-high-per-TEN-siv)
apex (AY-pecks)
apical/radial pulse (AP-ih-kal/RAY-dee-al puls)
bradycardia (brad-ee-KAR-dee-ah)
Celsius (SELL-see-us)
centimeter (SEN-tih-mee-ter)
cyanotic (sigh-ah-NOT-ick)
depressant (dee-PRESS-ant)
diastolic (die-ah-STOL-ick)
expiration (ecks-pih-RAY-shun)
Fahrenheit (FAIR-en-hight)
fasting (FAST-ing)
hypertension (high-per-TEN-shun)
hypotension (high-poh-TEN-shun)
inspiration (in-spih-RAY-shun)
kilogram (KILL-oh-gram)
mercury (MER-kyou-ree)

oral (OR-al)
pulse (puls)
pulse deficit (pulsDEF-ih-sit)
pulse rate (puls rayt)
radial artery (RAY-dee-alARE-ter-ee)
rales (rahls)
respiration (res-pih-RAY-shun)
rhythm (RITH-um)
sheath (sheeth)
sphygmomanometer (sfig-moh-mah-NOM-eh-ter)
stethoscope (STETH-oh-skohp)
systolic (sis-TOL-ick)
tachycardia (tack-ee-KAR-dee-ah)
temporal artery (TEM-per-al AR-ter-ee)
thermometer (ther-MOM-eh-ter)
tympanic (tim-PAN-ick)
vital signs (VIGH-tal signs)
volume (VOL-youm)

MEASURING VITAL SIGNS

Each resident must have **vital signs** (*vital* means living) measured and recorded on admission. Vital signs are also frequently measured throughout the resident's stay. The vital signs are:

- Temperature
- Pulse rate
- Respiratory rate
- Blood pressure
- Pain (considered the fifth vital sign since 2001 when Joint Commission rolled out its Pain Management Standards)

The vital signs give information about the general health of the individual and changes in the health status. It is essential that these measurements be accurate and that you record them properly.

To do this accurately you must know how to:

- Read a clinical thermometer using the **Celsius** and **Fahrenheit** scales
- Read a **sphygmomanometer** (blood pressure cuff)

In addition to vital signs, you will also measure residents' weight and height on a regular basis. To do this accurately you must know how to:

- Read a scale for weight in pounds and **kilograms**.
- Read a scale for height in feet and inches and in **centimeters**.

Procedures for measuring weight and height are described later in this lesson.

CLINICAL FOCUS

Think about Geraldine Hoden and her diagnosis. Why is it important to monitor her weight? Make a correlation between her weight (loss/gain) and her medical condition.

Celsius, kilograms, and centimeters are metric measurements. Facilities that use the metric system for these temperature, weight, and height measurements will have thermometers and scales with the metric values. You do not have to convert measurements from one system to the other.

Equipment Needed

Clinical **thermometers** are used to determine temperature. A watch with a second hand is needed to count the pulse and respiratory rate. A **stethoscope** and sphygmomanometer are needed to measure the blood pressure. Each vital sign is discussed separately, although actual measurements are usually done as a combined activity.

TEMPERATURE

Temperature is the measurement of body heat. One of two temperature scales may be used: Fahrenheit or Celsius. Normal body temperature is about 98.6° Fahrenheit (37° Celsius).

Temperatures are usually measured orally. The temperature can also be taken with a thermometer placed and held in the rectum (rectal temperature) or, the thermometer can be placed in the armpit (axillary temperature) if the resident:

- Is unable to keep the mouth closed
- Has respiratory difficulty
- Is receiving oxygen
- Is receiving oral tube feeding

The rectal temperature registers 1° higher and the axillary temperature registers 1° lower than an **oral** temperature in the same person (Figure 19-1).

The temperature of the blood in the vessels of the eardrum may also be measured. This is known as **tympanic** temperature. The temperature taken in the axilla is the least accurate reading. Rectal and tympanic temperatures give a measurement of core body temperature; the temperature is not as affected by other factors in the environment like inhaling cold air or drinking cold or hot fluids.

Temporal artery temperature also gives an accurate measure of body temperature. The temperature is measured in a noninvasive manner over the temporal artery on the forehead; it measures the temperature of blood in the artery.

It is interesting to note that normal body temperatures do not vary greatly between older persons and other adults. Temperature regulation, however, is more difficult for older persons because of changes in the heart rate, decreased elasticity in the blood vessels, and possible loss of subcutaneous fat layers. Residents may wear extra layers of clothing to keep warm, but at the same time they may find it difficult to sense when they are overheated.

Body temperature can be increased by:

- Infection
- Dehydration
- Physical exercise
- Hot water
- Hot weather
- Brain damage
- Some medications (such as chemotherapy)

  Body temperature can be decreased by:
- Shock
- Cold weather
- Sponge bath
- Medications
- Approaching death

The condition of the resident will determine the safest route that is used to measure body temperature. Contraindications to the use of the oral and rectal routes are listed below.

Contradictions—Oral Temperatures: An oral temperature is not taken if the resident is

- Confused, disoriented
- Restless
- Unconscious
- Chilled
- Coughing
- Unable to breathe through the mouth
- Very weak
- On seizure precautions
- On oxygen via nasal cannula

Contradictions—Rectal Temperatures: A rectal temperature is not taken if the resident has

- Diarrhea
- Fecal impaction
- Combative behavior
- Rectal bleeding
- Hemorrhoids
- Recent rectal surgery
- Colostomy

Clinical Thermometers

The types of thermometers currently used in long-term care facilities may be electronic, digital, or disposable

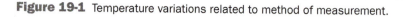

	Oral	Axillary	Rectal	Tympanic membrane	Temporal artery
Average temperature	98.6°F	97.6°F	99.6°F	98.6°F	99.6°F
Acceptable range	97.6–99.6°F	96.6–98.6°F	98.6–100.6°F	98.6°F	99.6°F
	(36.5–37.1°C)	(36–37°C)	(37–38.1°C)	(37°C)	(37.5°C)

Figure 19-1 Temperature variations related to method of measurement.

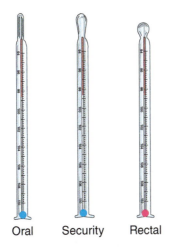

Figure 19-2 Clinical thermometers: From left to right— oral, security, rectal.

(paper or plastic). The nursing assistant must be familiar with the use of all types of thermometers.

Improvements in technology and safety issues have made the use of the glass thermometer a thing of the past. You may recall seeing the glass thermometers shown in Figure 19-2. Formerly the central core of the thermometer was filled with a heat sensitive fluid like **mercury**. Because of the toxic hazards associated with the use of mercury, glass thermometers are now filled with an alcohol-based or gallium tin solution; neither of which is harmful if the thermometer should break. Glass thermometers posed other hazards as well. Because glass breaks easily, a resident might bite the glass tube and swallow glass fragments or cut the mouth. In addition, thermometers have broken while taking rectal temperatures, especially if the resident rolled from the side-lying position even though your hand may have been holding the thermometer in place. Glass thermometers also took longer to register an accurate temperature: at least 3 minutes orally, 2 minutes rectally, and up to 10 minutes for an axillary temperature.

General Thermometer Safety

- Check equipment before beginning procedure to make sure it is in functioning order.
- Do not leave the resident alone with a thermometer in place.
- Hold rectal and axillary thermometers in place.
- When measuring a rectal temperature, lubricate the probe cover before inserting in rectum.
- Discard probe cover per facility policy

The Electronic Thermometer

The electronic thermometer is battery operated. The temperature is registered in large numbers on the

screen. The *probe* is the portion that is placed directly upon the resident. The probes or probe stems are colored blue for oral or axillary use and red for rectal use. The probe is covered with a disposable **sheath** that stays on during use and is then discarded (Figure 19-3).

The tympanic (ear) thermometer (Figure 19-4) measures the temperature from blood vessels in the tympanic membrane in the ear. This provides a reading close to the core body temperature. The instrument

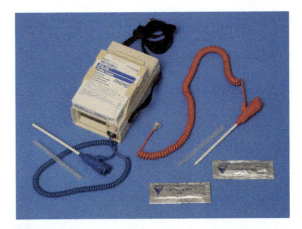

Figure 19-3 An electronic thermometer. The temperature is registered in large, easy-to-read numerals. The disposable plastic sheath is placed over the probe tip. (The blue probe is for oral temperatures and the red probe is for rectal temperatures.) The blue probe is then inserted into the resident's mouth in the usual manner.

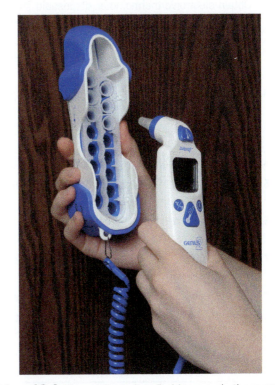

Figure 19-4 The cordless, handheld tympanic thermometer. The lens on the handset indicates the digital temperature reading.

has a built-in converter that provides the equivalent temperature in rectal or oral values (in both Fahrenheit and Celsius systems). The type of thermometer reading (mode) is selected by the user.

Many facilities use tympanic (aural) thermometers. The temperature is taken by measuring the heat given off by the tympanic membrane (in the ear). This method has several advantages:

- Tympanic thermometers are accurate and easy to use.
- The temperature registers in a few seconds. Because of this, taking the temperature of an agitated resident is safer and faster.
- Temperatures that cannot be taken orally can be taken by the tympanic method, eliminating the need to take rectal or axillary temperatures.

- Some tympanic thermometers allow you to select a core, oral, or rectal mode. This means the reading will correlate with the mode selected. Choose the mode according to your facility's policy.
- Wait for 15 minutes to take the temperature if the resident has been outdoors or if the resident has been lying on the ear you will use.
- Remove hearing aids if taking a tympanic temperature.
- If the resident is ill with a fever, the axillary or temporal artery routes will be more accurate.
- *Note:* Do not use the tympanic route if the resident has a lot of earwax build-up. An accurate recording will not be possible.

PROCEDURE 19-52
Measuring an Oral Temperature (Electronic Thermometer)

OBRA

1. Carry out each beginning procedure action.
2. Obtain electronic thermometer, disposable sheaths, and gloves (if this is your facility policy). (Gloves are not necessary with an oral temperature using this type of thermometer. Know and follow your facility policy.)
3. Ask resident if he or she has had hot or cold liquids to drink or has smoked within the last 15 minutes. If the answer is "yes," wait 15 minutes before taking oral temperature.
4. Cover probe (blue) with protective sheath.
5. Insert covered probe under resident's tongue into a heat pocket (Figure 19-5).
6. Hold probe in position. Instruct the resident to keep the mouth closed around the probe.
7. A beep signals that temperature has been determined, take reading and record on pad.

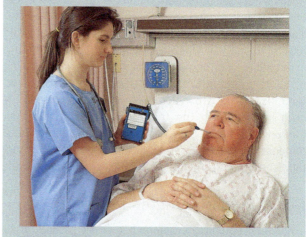

Figure 19-5 Inserting the blue probe of the electronic thermometer in the resident's mouth.

8. Discard sheath in wastebasket. Do not touch sheath. Remove gloves and discard according to facility policy.
9. Return probe to proper position and entire unit to charging.
10. Carry out each procedure completion action.
11. Record the reading.

PROCEDURE 19-53
Measuring a Rectal Temperature (Electronic Thermometer)

1. Carry out each beginning procedure action.
2. Assemble equipment:
   - Disposable gloves
   - Electronic thermometer with red probe
   - Sheaths
   - Lubricant
3. Lower head of the bed flat or as tolerated. Ask resident to turn on side. Assist resident, if necessary. Have resident bend upper leg as far as possible.
4. Put on disposable gloves.
5. Place a small amount of lubricant on the tip of the sheath (Figure 19-6).
6. Fold the top bedclothes back to expose anal area.
7. Separate buttocks with one hand. Insert sheath-covered probe about 1 to 1½ inches into rectum or as recommended by manufacturer. Hold in place. Replace bedclothes as soon as thermometer is inserted.
8. Read temperature when registered on digital display and beep sounds. Note reading on pad.
9. Remove probe and discard sheath. Wipe lubricant from resident. Discard tissue.
10. Remove gloves and discard according to facility policy.
11. Record the reading followed by letter "(R)" (in parentheses) indicating rectal route.
12. Carry out each procedure completion action.

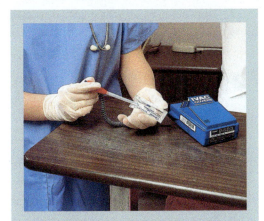

Figure 19-6 Lubricating the tip of the sheath-covered probe.

PROCEDURE 19-54
Measuring an Axillary Temperature (Electronic Thermometer)

OBRA

1. Carry out each beginning procedure action. *Note:* Use disposable gloves if there may be contact with open lesions, wet linens, or body fluids.
2. Equipment needed: same as for oral temperature measurement using an electronic thermometer (see Procedure 19-52).
3. Wipe axillary area dry and place covered probe in place. Keep resident's arm close to the body. Hold probe in place until temperature records on digital display and beep sounds.
4. Remove thermometer probe. Dispose of sheath.
5. Record the reading followed by letter "(A)" (in parentheses) indicating axillary route.
6. Carry out each procedure completion action.

PROCEDURE 19-55
Measuring a Tympanic Temperature

OBRA

1. Carry out each beginning procedure action.

2. Assemble equipment:

   ▪ Disposable gloves if there may be contact with blood or body fluids, open lesions, or wet linens

   ▪ Tympanic thermometer

   ▪ Probe covers

3. Place a clean probe cover on the probe.

4. Select the appropriate mode on the thermometer, if possible.

5. Check the lens to make sure it is clean and intact (Figure 19-7).

6. Put on disposable gloves if you may have contact with blood or body fluids, open lesions, or wet linens.

7. Position the resident so you have access to the ear you will be using.

8. Gently pull the ear pinna back and up (Figure 19-8). This straightens the ear canal so the thermometer can be placed for an accurate reading.

9. Place the probe in the resident's ear, aiming it directly toward the tympanic membrane. Insert the probe until it seals the ear canal (Figure 19-9). Do not apply pressure.

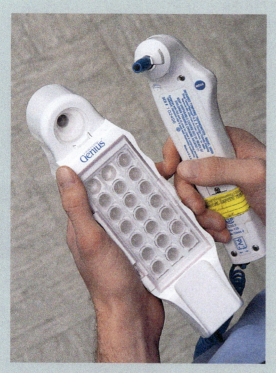

Figure 19-7 Check the lens of the tympanic thermometer to make sure it is clean and intact.

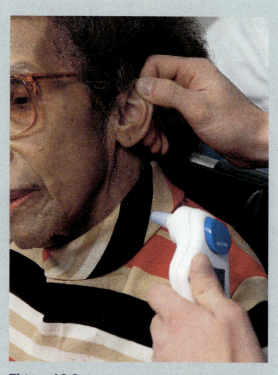

Figure 19-8 Gently pull the ear pinna back and up.

10. Press the activation button (Figure 19-10). Leave the thermometer in the ear for the time recommended by the manufacturer.

11. When you have a reading, remove the probe from the resident's ear and dispose of the cover.

(continues)

PROCEDURE 19-55
Measuring a Tympanic Temperature (Continued)

12. Record the reading followed by letter "(T)" (in parentheses) indicating tympanic route.

13. Carry out each procedure completion action.

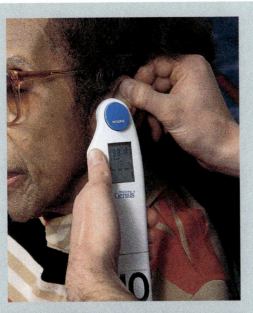

Figure 19-9 Place the probe in the resident's ear, aiming it toward the tympanic membrane. Insert probe until it seals the ear canal.

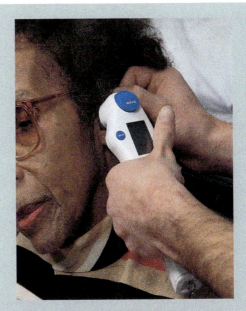

Figure 19-10 Press the activation button and leave the thermometer in the ear for the time recommended by the manufacturer.

Other Types of Thermometers

The temporal artery scan thermometer (Figure 19-11A) is a noninvasive method of taking the resident's temperature. The infrared scanner is stroked across the forehead and reads the temperature of the blood in the temporal artery, which is close to the skin surface in the brow. This arterial temperature is similar to the temperature of the blood in the heart (Figure 19-11B). The digital reading on the scanner is available within a few seconds.

As with any procedure, specific actions must be followed. Before taking the temperature, follow the beginning procedure actions:

- Attach disposable scanner cover.
- Use the exposed side of the head, not the side that has been on a pillow or under a hat or scarf.
- Gently slide the scanner across the center of the forehead, midway between the eyebrows and the hairline. Maintain direct contact with the skin.
- If the brow is moist with perspiration, use the area behind the earlobe on the exposed side of the head. (The perspiration will give a cooling effect on the body and give a lower, inaccurate temperature reading.)
- Read the display and record the temperature.
- Remove and discard the disposable scanner cover.
- Follow agency protocol for cleaning scanner if necessary.
- Follow procedure completion actions.

Disposable thermometers (plastic or paper) are used in some facilities for residents in isolation. These thermometers are chemically treated; the dots on the thermometer are read to obtain the resident's temperature (Figure 19-12). Because the unit is disposable, no sheath is needed to protect the thermometer. *Remove the thermometer carefully from the mouth.* The thermometers are made from hard plastic and can cause injury to the lips and inner surfaces of the mouth if removed quickly.

Another form of electronic thermometer is the small, handheld, battery-operated type (Figure 19-13).

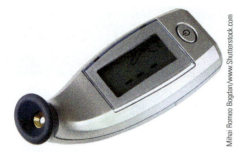

Figure 19-11A Temporal artery thermometer.

Figure 19-12 The chemical-dot thermometer is used only for oral temperatures. It is used once, then discarded.

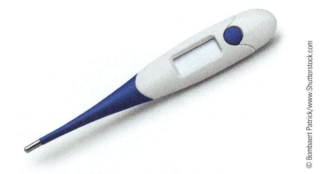

Figure 19-13 The battery-operated digital thermometer is commonly used in long-term care facilities. Always cover the thermometer with a disposable probe cover before use.

This type of digital thermometer is covered with a plastic sheath when taking a temperature. The procedure for using this thermometer is the same as for that of the electronic thermometer. Comply with facility policies for disinfecting the thermometer between uses.

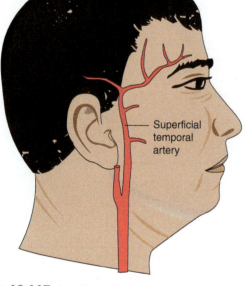

Superficial
temporal
artery

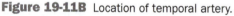

Figure 19-11B Location of temporal artery.

CLINICAL FOCUS

If Mrs. Hoden was confused and disoriented, what method would you use to take her temperature? Explain your choice.

? EXERCISE 19-1

BRIEF ANSWERS

Answer the following statements about nursing assistants' actions with A for appropriate or I for inappropriate. If the action is inappropriate, write the appropriate action in the space provided.

1. _____ The nursing assistant prepares to measure a resident's oral temperature while he or she is receiving a nasogastric tube feeding. _____

2. _____ The nursing assistant notices excessive ear wax in a resident's ear so decides a tympanic temperature is not appropriate.
   _____

3. _____ The nursing assistant is told to obtain a temporal temperature and knows this means the temperature will be taken over the resident's cheek. _____

4. _____ A resident has diarrhea so the nursing assistant measures the temperature using a rectal thermometer.
   _____

(*continues*)

? EXERCISE 19-1 (Continued)

5. _____ An oral thermometer, which reads 98°F, is wiped and placed immediately under a resident's tongue. _____

6. _____ The nursing assistant uses an electronic thermometer probe that is colored blue to measure a rectal temperature. _____

7. _____ The nursing assistant lubricates the tip of the sheath prior to obtaining a rectal temperature. _____

8. _____ A nursing assistant holds the thermometer at waist level when reading the temperature. _____

9. _____ A nursing assistant inserted a rectal thermometer and left the room to fill the water pitcher while the temperature was registering. _____

10. _____ A nursing assistant put on disposable gloves before beginning to measure a temperature of the resident rectally. _____

11. _____ A resident has one broken arm in a splint and an IV running into the wrist of the opposite arm so a nursing assistant measures the pulse rate by placing his or her fingers on the temporal region. _____

12. _____ The pulse is irregular so the nursing assistant is careful to count the rate for one-half minute and multiply by two. _____

13. _____ A nursing assistant uses a tympanic thermometer without a probe cover. _____

14. _____ A nursing assistant finds a resident's respiratory rate is 11 respirations per minute but does not feel this value is low enough to report. _____

15. _____ A nursing assistant finds the blood pressure just taken is higher than the previous reading and reports this to the nurse. _____

? EXERCISE 19-2

COMPLETION

1. Which thermometer would you choose to determine the resident's temperature in each of the following situations. Check under the appropriate type.

Thermometer
The Resident

	Rectal	Oral	Tympanic
a. has diarrhea			
b. is unconscious			
c. is coughing			
d. has a fecal impaction			
e. is combative			
f. has hemorrhoids			
g. is unable to breathe through nose			
h. is very weak			
i. is disoriented			
j. has a colostomy			

PULSE AND RESPIRATION

The **pulse** and **respiration** of the resident are usually counted during the same procedure.

Pulse is the pressure of the blood felt against the wall of an artery as the heart beats (contracts) and rests (relaxes). The pulse is more easily felt in arteries that are fairly close to the skin surface and can be gently pressed against a bone by the fingers. The pulse rate and its character provide a good indication of how the cardiovascular system is able to meet the body's needs.

Radial Pulse

The pulse is usually measured over the **radial artery** (at the base of the wrist on the thumb side) (Figure 19-14). The age, gender, size, and condition of the resident affect the character of the pulse. Pulse character means:

- Rate (speed)
- **Volume** (fullness; bounding or thready)
- **Rhythm** (regularity)

Pulse character should always be noted when counting the pulse.

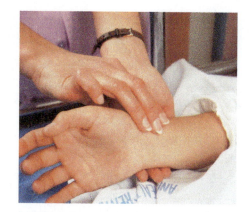

Figure 19-14 Locate the pulse on the thumb side of the wrist with tips of your fingers.

 CLINICAL FOCUS

If you take Mrs. Hoden's pulse and respirations right after she has been up to the bathroom, what results would you expect and why?

PROCEDURE 19-56
Counting the Radial Pulse Rate

OBRA

1. Carry out each beginning procedure action. *Note:* Use disposable gloves if there may be contact with open lesions, wet linens, or body fluids.

2. Place resident in a comfortable position. The palm of the hand should be down and the arm should rest across the resident's chest.

3. Locate the pulse on the thumb side of the wrist with the tips of your first three fingers. Do not use your thumb because it contains a pulse that may be confused with the resident's pulse. Refer to Figure 19-15 for the location of other sites on the body where the pulse rate can be counted.

4. When the pulse is felt, exert slight pressure. Use second hand of watch and count for 1 minute. It is the practice in some facilities to count for 30 seconds, multiply the value by two, and then record the rate for 1 minute. For accuracy, a 1-minute count is preferred and must be done if the pulse is irregular. Figure 19-16 lists average pulse rates.

5. Carry out each procedure completion action.

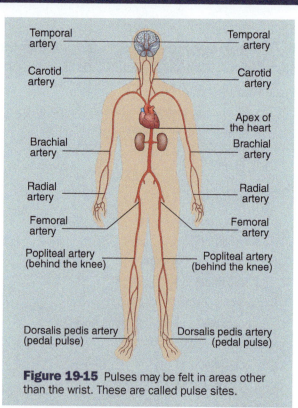

Figure 19-15 Pulses may be felt in areas other than the wrist. These are called pulse sites.

(continues)

PROCEDURE 19-56
Counting the Radial
Pulse Rate (Continued)

Adult men	60–70 beats per minute
Adult women	65–80 beats per minute
Children older than 7 years	75–100 beats per minute
Preschoolers	80–110 beats per minute
Infants	120–160 beats per minute

Figure 19-16 Average pulse rates.

Apical Pulse

The apical pulse is taken when measuring fast, weak, or irregular heartbeats. This pulse is measured by placing the stethoscope on the chest at the apex or point of the heart and counting the beats for one full minute. The apex of the heart is the lowest point of the heart. It can easily be located on the left side in the 5th intracostal space, approximately 2 to 3 inches from the sternum (breastbone). On a woman it may be located under the left breast (Figure 19-17A).

The heart rate is usually the same as the pulse rate. At times, however, some of the heartbeats are not strong enough to be transmitted and felt along the radial artery. This results in a difference between the heart rate and the pulse rate. This difference is called a pulse deficit. Pulse deficits are found in some forms of heart disease. If a pulse deficit is suspected, it may be necessary to count the heart rate and the pulse rate at the same time. One person (usually the nurse) determines the heart rate by placing a stethoscope on the chest over the apex of the heart. The second person (possibly the nursing assistant) counts the radial pulse at the same time and the rates are compared. This is called taking an apical/radial pulse. Pulse rates under 60 or over 100 should be reported.

- Tachycardia—unusually fast pulse rate (over 100 bpm)
- Bradycardia—unusually slow pulse rate (under 60 bpm)

Any irregularities in the rate, rhythm, or volume of the resident's pulse should be reported immediately.

Respiration

Respiration supplies the cells in the body with oxygen and rids the body of excess carbon dioxide. When respirations are inefficient, carbon dioxide gas builds up in the bloodstream, making the skin dusky, bluish, or cyanotic.

There are two parts to each respiration:

- Inspiration (inhalation)
- Expiration (exhalation)

The character (rhythm and volume) and the rate of respirations must be noted. Respirations are described as:

- Normal
- Shallow
- Deep
- Labored
- Difficult

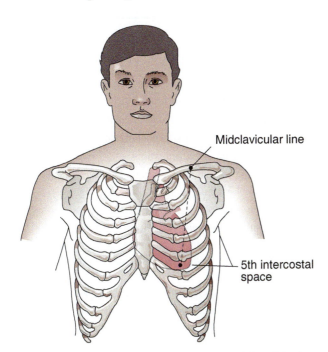

Midclavicular line

5th intercostal space

Figure 19-17A The apical pulse is located 2 to 3 inches to the left of the sternum (breastbone) in the 5th intracostal space.

PROCEDURE 19-57
Counting the Apical-Radial Pulse

1. Carry out each beginning procedure action.

2. Clean stethoscope earpieces and diaphragm with disinfectant.

3. Two people measure the heart rate and the radial pulse at the same time. The nurse places the stethoscope earpieces in the ears and the stethoscope diaphragm over the apex of the resident's heart. (The diaphragm may be warmed in the hands before placing it on the resident's chest.) The heartbeats are counted for 1 minute.

4. At the same time, the nursing assistant counts the radial pulse for 1 minute (Figure 19-17B).

5. Compare the results and note them on the pad.

6. Clean earpieces and diaphragm of stethoscope with disinfectant.

7. Carry out each procedure completion action. Record date, time, pulse values as in example, and character, such as weak and irregular.

Example:

Apical pulse	A 108
Radial pulse	R 82

Pulse deficit is 26

(108 − 82 = 26)

NOTE: Use disposable gloves if there may be contact with open lesions, wet linens, or body fluids.

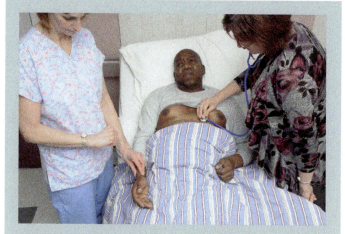

Figure 19-17B The nurse takes the apical pulse while the nursing assistant takes the radial pulse.

The normal respiration rate for adults is 12 to 20 per minute. If the rate is more than 25 per minute, it is **accelerated** and is reported. If the rate is less than 12 per minute, it is too low and is reported. Special terms are used to describe different types of breathing (Figure 19-18).

The rate is determined by counting the rise and fall of the chest for 1 minute while using a watch equipped with a second hand.

Breathing is partially under voluntary control; that is, a person is able to stop breathing for a short period of time. This frequently happens when a resident realizes that breathing is being watched and counted. The breathing pattern is altered unintentionally. To avoid this, the respirations are counted immediately following the pulse count. The resident's hand is kept in the same position on the chest and your fingers remain on the pulse.

- Tachypnea—rapid, shallow breathing.
- Dyspnea—difficult or labored breathing.
- Shallow—breaths that partially fill the lungs.
- Apnea—a period of no respirations.
- Cheyne-Stokes respirations—a period of dyspnea followed by periods of apnea.
- Stertorous—snoring-like respirations.
- **Rales** (gurgles)—moist respirations. At times, fluid (mucus) will collect in the air passages. This causes a bubbling type of respiration. Rales are common in the dying resident.
- Wheezing—difficult breathing accompanied by a whistling or sighing sound due to narrowing of bronchioles (as in asthma) or an increase of mucus in bronchi.

Figure 19-18 Special terms describe different breathing patterns.

PROCEDURE 19-58
Counting Respirations

OBRA

1. After counting the pulse rate, leave your fingers on the radial pulse.
2. Start counting the number of times the chest rises and falls during a period of 1 minute.
3. Note depth and regularity of respirations.
4. Record the time, rate, depth, and regularity of respirations.

? EXERCISE 19-3

COMPUTATIONS

1. What reading will you record for each pulse rate when you have counted the pulse for only 30 seconds?

Counted Pulse	Computation	Recorded Pulse
a. 30	_____	_____
b. 45	_____	_____
c. 46	_____	_____
d. 34	_____	_____
e. 38	_____	_____

2. What is the pulse deficit in each of the following situations? Show how you computed your answers.

Apical Pulse	Radial Pulse	Computation Pulse Deficit
a. 108 82	_____	_____
b. 112 88	_____	_____
c. 102 66	_____	_____
d. 118 72	_____	_____
e. 106 84	_____	_____

- Illness
- Emotions
- Elevated temperature
- Age
- Exercise
- Position
- Drugs

Figure 19-19 Factors affecting respiratory rates.

Factors affecting respiratory rates are listed in Figure 19-19.

BLOOD PRESSURE

The American Heart Association blood pressure classification for normal blood pressure is: systolic pressure of less than 120 mmHg and a diastolic pressure of less than 80 mmHg. Prehypertension readings are considered to be: systolic pressure of 120 to 139 mmHg and a diastolic pressure of 80 to 90 mmHg.

The factors that influence blood pressure are listed in Figure 19-20.

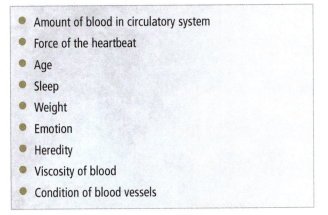

- Amount of blood in circulatory system
- Force of the heartbeat
- Age
- Sleep
- Weight
- Emotion
- Heredity
- Viscosity of blood
- Condition of blood vessels

Figure 19-20 Factors influencing blood pressure readings.

There is greater resistance to blood flow in arteries that have lost their elasticity or ability to stretch due to disease. This causes higher blood pressure. Blood pressure is also increased by:

- Exercise
- Eating
- Stimulants
- Emotional anxiety
- Some drugs

Blood pressure is decreased by:

- **Fasting** (not eating)
- Rest
- **Depressants** (drugs that slow down body functions)
- Excessive loss of blood
- **Antihypertensives** (drugs that lower blood pressure in persons who have hypertension)

If the resident is resting, any reading between 60 and 90 diastolic (lower reading) is considered normal. Blood pressure rises slightly with age.

Hypertension is high blood pressure (greater than 120/90). Uncontrolled hypertension can lead to stroke, kidney disease, or heart damage. **Hypotension** is low blood pressure (below 100/70). Excessive hypotension can lead to shock. In either case, unusual or changed findings must be recorded and reported.

Blood Pressure Equipment

Blood pressure equipment includes the sphygmomanometer (Figure 19-21) and the stethoscope (Figure 19-22). The commonly used sphygmomanometer consists of a cuff with a rubber bladder inside with two tubes—one connected to the pressure control bulb and the other to the pressure gauge

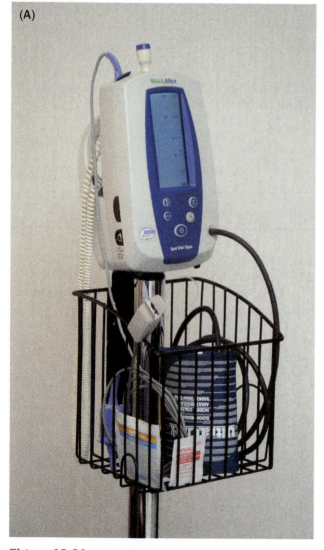

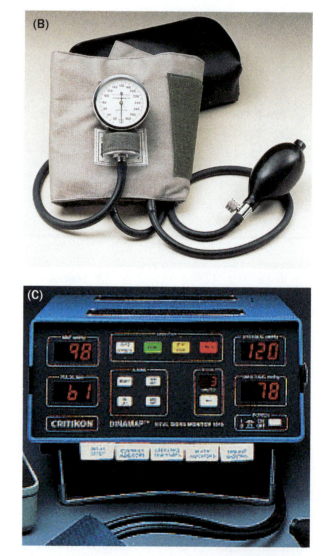

Figure 19-21 Types of sphygmomanometers: (A) Mercury-gravity sphygmomanometer; (B) dial (aneroid) sphygmomanometer; (C) electronic sphygmomanometer.

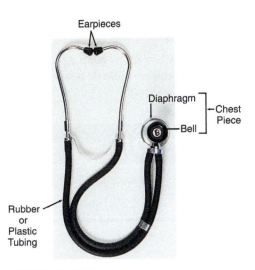

Figure 19-22 Stethoscope.

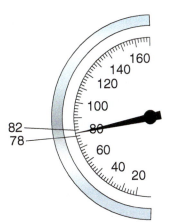

Figure 19-23 The gauge is marked with a series of large lines at 10-mm (millimeter) intervals.

(see Figure 19-21). The gauge may be a round dial or a column of mercury. Both are marked in numbers. Be sure to use a cuff of the proper size. Cuffs that are too wide or too narrow for the arm will give inaccurate readings. The length of the bladder portion of the cuff should be about 80% of the circumference of the resident's arm.

How to Read the Gauge

The gauges are marked with a series of large lines at 10-mm (millimeter) intervals (Figure 19-23). In between the large lines are shorter lines, each of which indicates 2 mm. For example, the small line above 80 mm is 82 mm, and the small line below 80 mm is 78 mm. For accuracy, the gauge should be at eye level when reading. The mercury column gauge must not be tilted. The level of the top of the column of mercury or the pointer of the dial is taken for the reading. Two readings are recorded:

- **Systolic**—first sound heard. It represents the highest pressure in the arteries.

- **Diastolic**—the level at which sound stops. The smaller number indicates when this change in sound is heard. This number represents the artery at rest.

The blood pressure is recorded as a fraction with the larger number on top. For example, 112/68 means:

- 112 is the systolic pressure
- 68 is the diastolic pressure

Precautions

Determine the best site to take the blood pressure. Make sure that a tight shirtsleeve will not constrict the arm and alter the blood pressure. If necessary, remove the resident's arm from the sleeve of the shirt or blouse, and ensure the resident has adequate privacy. To prevent further damage to an extremity, avoid taking a blood pressure on the extremity if any of the following are present:

- An intravenous infusion or port for medications
- Impaired circulation
- Paralysis
- A/V shunt (for dialysis access)
- Edema
- Fracture or other trauma
- Bulky dressings
- Burns
- Recent mastectomy (removal of breast) on that side
- Pulse oximeter on a finger on that side

These precautions should be listed on the resident's plan of care. Check with the nurse before taking a blood pressure if you are unsure of the proper extremity to use.

Potential Causes of Inaccurate Blood Pressure Readings

- Use of wrong size cuff
- Improperly wrapped cuff
- Incorrect arm position
- Incorrect position of body (sitting or lying down; always be consistent)
- Using different arms (consistently use right or left arm)
- Not having the gauge at eye level
- Deflating the cuff too slowly or too rapidly
- Taking the blood pressure several times in a row
- Distractions in the room such as loud talking, or increased volume on radio or television

⊘N THE JOB

Make sure you have the right size blood pressure cuff for the resident.

⚠ GUIDELINES FOR. . . PREPARING TO MEASURE BLOOD PRESSURE

BEFORE USING THE STETHOSCOPE:

1. Clean the earpieces with an alcohol wipe and clean the diaphragm with a different alcohol wipe.
2. Point the earpieces forward when inserting them in your ears.
3. Use the diaphragm portion of the stethoscope (Figure 19-24).
4. Be sure the diaphragm portion is open so you will hear the beats.

BEFORE USING A SPHYGMOMANOMETER:

1. If using a mercury manometer—if the mercury moves up the column very slowly, it may have oxidized. Report this to the nurse and use another sphygmomanometer.

2. If using an aneroid manometer—make sure the needle is on zero before inflating the cuff (Figure 19-25). If it is not, report this to the nurse and use another sphygmomanometer.
3. Be aware of any precautions to be observed before taking the resident's blood pressure, as well as potential causes of inaccurate blood pressure readings.

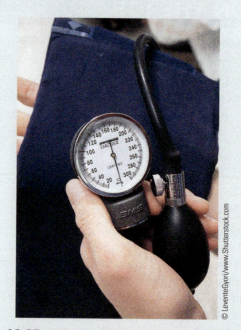

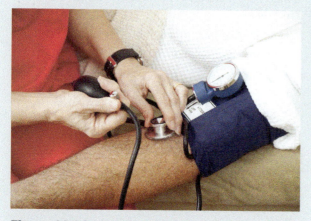

Figure 19-24 Use the diaphragm portion of the stethoscope when taking a blood pressure.

Figure 19-25 Make sure the needle is in the small box or oval to assure the device is accurately calibrated before inflating the cuff of the aneroid manometer.

© LeventeGyori/www.sShutterstock.com

Pain

Pain is considered the fifth vital sign as the absence or presence of pain can impact the readings of the measureable vital signs. It is important to evaluate:

- How chronic the pain is (when did it start, how long does it last)

- How severe the pain is (rated on a scale of 1–10)

- Activity that causes or decreases pain

- Measures that alleviate pain (medication, positioning, environmental)

? EXERCISE 19-4

MATCHING
Match the vital sign term on the right with the meaning on the left.

MEANING TERM

1. _____ elevated body temperature
2. _____ moist respirations
3. _____ difficult, labored breathing
4. _____ rapid pulse
5. _____ no respiration
6. _____ periods of dyspnea followed by apnea
7. _____ slow pulse
8. _____ snoring-like respirations
9. _____ elevated blood pressure
10. _____ rapid, shallow breathing

a. tachypnea
b. bradycardia
c. dyspnea
d. fever
e. apnea
f. rales (gurgles)
g. tachycardia
h. stertorous
i. Cheyne-Stokes
j. hypertension

? EXERCISE 19-5

COMPLETION
Select the correct terms from the following list to complete each statement.

at	earpieces	not be measured
brachial artery	elevated	raises
change	improper fraction	size
cuff	inaccurate	systolic
diaphragm	last	sound

1. The highest point of blood pressure measurement is the _____ reading.

2. Hereditary factors can cause a(an) _____ blood pressure.

3. Deflating the cuff too slowly can result in a(an) _____ reading.

4. All blood pressure readings should be made with the gauge _____ eye level.

5. The diastolic pressure is measured at the _____ or _____ that is heard.

6. The blood pressure is most often taken over the _____.

(continues)

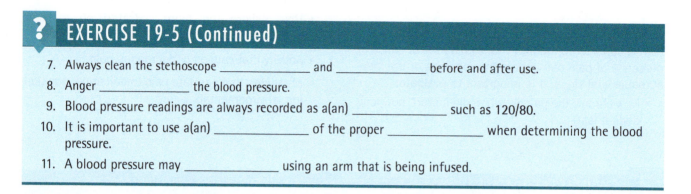

? EXERCISE 19-5 (Continued)

7. Always clean the stethoscope _____ and _____ before and after use.

8. Anger _____ the blood pressure.

9. Blood pressure readings are always recorded as a(an) _____ such as 120/80.

10. It is important to use a(an) _____ of the proper _____ when determining the blood pressure.

11. A blood pressure may _____ using an arm that is being infused.

WEIGHING AND MEASURING THE RESIDENT

Maintaining a record of the height and weight of all residents is important for several reasons:

- Medication dosages may be calculated based on height and weight.

- Weight is monitored to determine if the resident is retaining fluid (edema).

- Weight indicates if the resident's nutritional intake is adequate.

Baseline (original) measurements are obtained on admission. Residents are weighed at least monthly thereafter. Some residents may need to be weighed more often.

PROCEDURE 19-59
Taking Blood Pressure   OBRA

1. Carry out each beginning procedure action.

2. Assemble equipment:

   - Sphygmomanometer with appropriate size cuff
   - Stethoscope
   - Alcohol wipes

3. Remove resident's arm from sleeve or roll sleeve 5 inches above elbow; it should not be tight or binding.

4. Locate the brachial artery with your fingers. The brachial artery is located in the inner aspect of the elbow; follow the "little" finger up to the antecubital space and feel for the pulsations (Figure 19-26A and B).

5. Place resident's arm palm upward, supported on bed or table. Resident should be comfortable.

6. Wrap the cuff smoothly and snugly around resident's arm. Center the bladder over the brachial artery. The bottom of the cuff should be 1 inch above the antecubital space (inner elbow) (Figure 19-27) and should cover about two-thirds of the upper arm.

7. Place the bulb in your dominant hand. In your other hand, place the diaphragm portion of the stethoscope over the brachial artery where you previously located the pulse with your fingers (Figure 19-28).

   - Inflate the cuff quickly to about 30 mmHg above the level where pulse sounds disappear.
   - Release the air slowly—about 2 to 3 mmHg per second.
   - Listen closely while keeping your eyes on the gauge. The first sound you hear is the systolic pressure.
   - Continue to listen until the sound stops. Note the closest number on the gauge; this is the diastolic pressure. Continue to listen for 10 mmHg below this sound.

8. Quickly deflate the cuff. If it is necessary to recheck the blood pressure, wait at least 15 to 30 seconds before reinflating the cuff.

(continues)

PROCEDURE 19-59
Taking Blood Pressure (Continued)

(A)

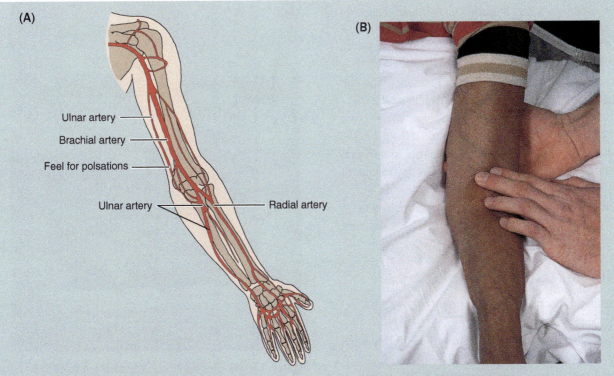

Ulnar artery
Brachial artery
Feel for polsations
Ulnar artery
Radial artery

(B)

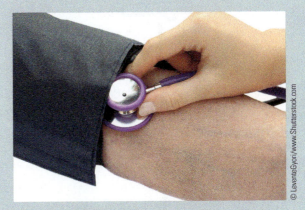

Figure 19-26 (A) Note location of the brachial artery. (B) Locate the brachial artery with your fingers.

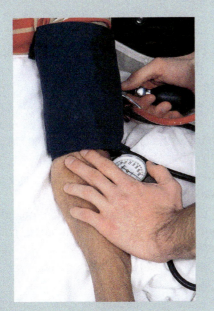

Figure 19-27 The bottom of the cuff should be 1 inch above the antecubital space (inner elbow).

Figure 19-28 Position the diaphragm of the stethoscope over the brachial artery.

© LeventeGyori/www.Shutterstock.com

9. Clean the earpieces and diaphragm of the stethoscope with alcohol wipes. Return equipment to appropriate area.

10. Carry out each procedure completion action.

Methods of Measurement

Height and weight may be measured using the metric system: centimeters for height and kilograms for weight. If your facility uses this method, the scales will be calibrated for the metric system. There is no need to convert from the inch and pound system to the metric system. There are several types of scales:

- An upright scale is used only for residents who can stand unattended on the platform (Figure 19-29).
- Chair scales are used for residents in wheelchairs who cannot stand on an upright scale (Figure 19-30).
- A bed scale is used to weigh residents in bed who cannot stand on an upright scale and who cannot sit in a wheelchair (Figure 19-31).

Height is measured with the ruler attached to an upright scale or with a tape measure when the resident is in bed.

Obtaining Accurate Weights

To obtain an accurate measurement of weight, you must:

- Weigh the resident at the same time of day each time.
- Have the resident wear the same type of clothing each time.

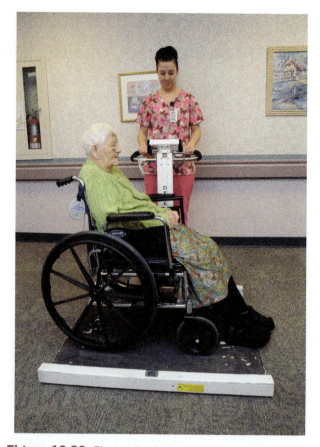

Figure 19-30 Electronic chair scales are used for residents in wheelchairs who cannot stand on an upright scale.

- Use the same method and the same scale each time, if possible.
- Scale should be routinely calibrated to ensure accuracy.

You must learn to read the scale correctly. There are two bars on the upright scale shown in Figure 19-31. The balance bar should hang free to start.

- The lower bar indicates weights in large 50-pound increments.
- The upper bar indicates smaller pound weights (Figure 19-32). The even-numbered pounds are marked with numbers.
- The long line between each number indicates the odd-numbered pounds.
- Each small line indicates one-fourth of a pound, or 4 ounces.

The two figures are added and recorded as the person's total weight. The sum is recorded according to facility policy in either pounds or kilograms.

Large weight =   100 pounds
Small weight = + 22 pounds
          Total =   122 pounds

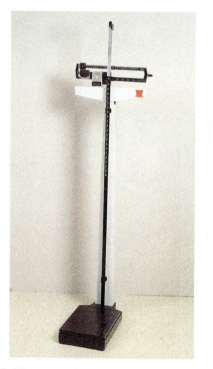

Figure 19-29 An upright scale is used only for residents who can stand unattended on the platform.

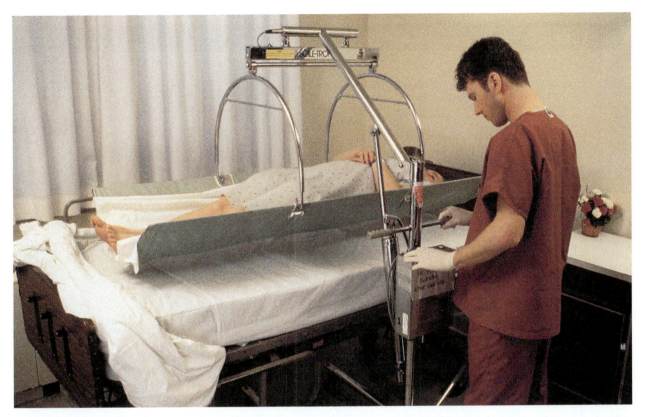

Figure 19-31 A mechanical lift with scale is used to weigh residents in bed who cannot stand on the upright scale and cannot sit up in a wheelchair.

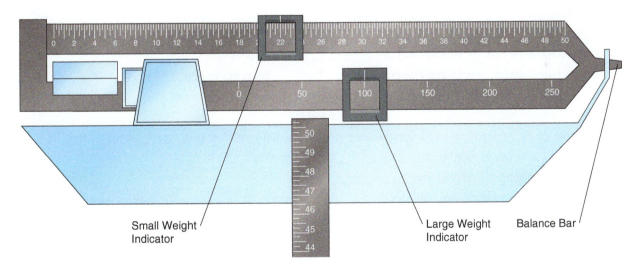

Small Weight Indicator   Large Weight Indicator   Balance Bar

Figure 19-32 The upper bar indicates smaller pound weights. The weight shown on the lower bar is added to the weight shown on the upper bar.

Measuring the resident may be done during the weighing procedure with an upright scale. The information is recorded in feet and inches or in centimeters, according to facility policy.

Example:

A height measurement of 62 inches may be recorded as 62 inches or 5 feet 2 inches or 155 cm.

RECORDING VITAL SIGNS

Temperature, pulse, and respiration (TPR) and height and weight values are recorded in a notebook and then transferred to the resident's chart (Figure 19-35) by a secretary or a nurse.

? EXERCISE 19-6

BRIEF ANSWERS

Select the correct terms from the following list. Some words may be used more than once.

blood	infection	temperature
brain damage	kilograms	thermometer
Celsius	living	volume
dehydration	pound	wrist
emotions	pounds	65–80
exercise	rate	¼
Fahrenheit	rhythm	4
free	scale	60–70
functions	stethoscope	50
heart		

1. Vital signs mean _____.

2. Vital signs provide information about essential body _____.

3. The vital signs include measurement of body _____, heart _____, breathing _____, and _____ pressure.

4. Two scales used on clinical thermometers are _____ and _____.

5. Weights are measured in pounds or _____.

6. Temperature is measured using a _____.

7. Blood pressure is measured with a cuff and _____.

8. Weight is measured with a _____.

9. The most common place to measure the pulse is at the _____.

10. The character of the pulse refers to the speed or _____, the fullness or _____, and the regularity of _____.

11. The average pulse rate for an adult man is _____ beats per minute.

12. The average pulse rate for an adult woman is _____ beats per minute.

13. An apical pulse is counted with the bell of the stethoscope placed over the apex of the _____.

14. Weight is measured in _____ and ounces and in _____.

15. When weighing a resident using an upright scale, the balance bar should hang _____.

16. The lower bar indicates weights in _____-lb increments.

17. The upper bar indicates weights in _____ increments.

18. The small line on the upper bar indicates _____ ounces or _____-lb increments.

19. Four factors that increase body temperature include:

    a. _____

    b. _____

    c. _____

    d. _____

PROCEDURE 19-60
Weighing and Measuring the Resident Using an Upright Scale

OBRA

1. Carry out each beginning procedure action. *Note:* Use disposable gloves if there may be contact with open lesions, wet linens, or body fluids.

2. Check previous weight as documented. Then escort the resident to the scales.

3. Place a paper towel on the platform of the scale.

4. Be sure the weights are to the extreme left and the balance bar (bar with weight markings) hangs free.

   - The lower bar (large indicator) is calibrated (marked) in increments (amounts) of 50 pounds.
   - The upper bar (small indicator) is calibrated in increments of single pounds.
   - The even-numbered pounds are marked with numbers.
   - The long line between even numbers indicates the odd-numbered pounds.
   - Each small line indicates one-fourth of a pound.

   a. Prior to weighing the resident, allow the resident the opportunity to use the bathroom or bedpan.

   b. Assist the resident to remove shoes and step up onto the scale platform, facing the balance bar. The balance bar will rise to the top of the bar guide. The resident should not hold the bar or other parts of the scale.

5. Move the large weight to the right to the closest estimated resident weight.

6. Move the small weight to the right until the balance bar hangs freely halfway between the upper and lower bar guides.

7. Add the two figures and record the total as the resident's weight in pounds or kilograms, according to the type of scale used.

8. Assist the resident to turn on the platform until facing away from the balance bar. Raise the height bar until it is level with the top of the resident's head.

9. The reading is made at the movable point of the ruler (Figure 19-33).

10. Note the number of inches indicated. Record this information in inches ("), feet (') and inches ("), or centimeters (cm) according to the type of scale. The height shown in Figure 19-33 is 62 inches. This may be recorded as 62 inches or 5 feet 2 inches (62 ÷ 12 = 5 feet 2 inches). Record value on your note pad.

11. Assist the resident off the platform. Help resident to put on shoes, if necessary, and return to the room.

12. Carry out each procedure completion action.

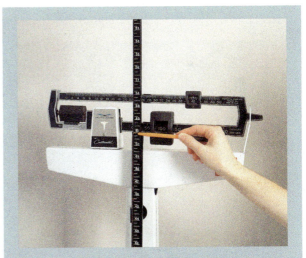

Figure 19-33 The resident's height is read at the movable point of the ruler.

PROCEDURE 19-61
Measuring Weight with an
Electronic Wheelchair Scale

1. Carry out each beginning procedure action.

2. Assemble equipment:

   - Wheelchair scale (Figure 19-34A)

3. Determine empty weight of wheelchair by weighing it on the scale. Know whether the wheelchair weight is to be with or without foot pedals and cushions to ensure accuracy of recording.

4. Take wheelchair to resident's room. Help the resident into the wheelchair and take the resident to the electronic wheelchair scale.

5. Open metal ramp sides on scale to rest on floor. This allows wheelchair access to scale.

6. Press "on" button.

7. Make sure scale reads zero before you weigh the resident (Figure 19-34B).

8. Roll wheelchair with resident onto platform of scale. Lock wheels of wheelchair.

9. Digital readout will show weight.

10. Record weight of resident and wheelchair. Subtract wheelchair weight to obtain resident weight.

11. Unlock wheels of wheelchair. Roll wheelchair with resident off scale.

12. Fold scale ramps back in place.

13. Carry out each procedure completion action.

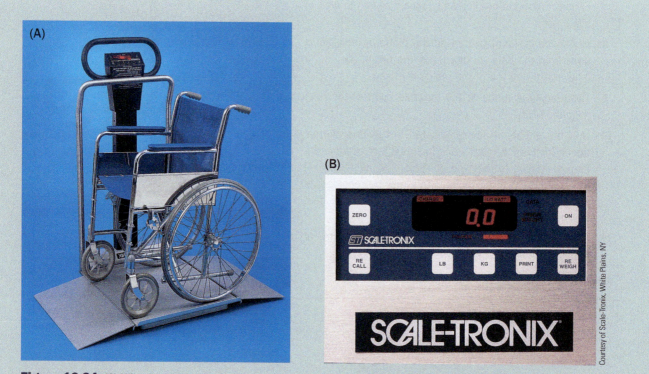

Courtesy of Scale-Tronix, White Plains, NY

Figure 19-34 (A) Wheelchair scale. (B) Press "on" button to zero scale automatically.

PROCEDURE 19-62
Weighing the Resident in a Chair Scale

OBRA

1. Carry out each beginning procedure action.
2. Assemble equipment:
   - Chair scale
3. Take resident in wheelchair to chair scale.
4. Apply transfer belt to resident and assist in a pivot transfer to chair on scale. Instruct resident to sit down when the chair is felt against the back of the legs. Be sure resident's feet are on footrest of scale.
5. Walk behind the scale to obtain the reading. Record weight.
6. Transfer resident back to wheelchair.
7. Carry out each procedure completion action.

PROCEDURE 19-63
Measuring and Weighing the Resident in Bed

OBRA

1. Carry out each beginning procedure action.
2. Obtain assistance from coworker.
3. Assemble equipment:
   - Overbed scale
   - Tape measure
   - Pencil
4. Check scale sling and straps for frayed areas or poorly closing straps.
5. Lower side rail on your side, if necessary. Make sure side rail is up on other side.

To measure the resident:

6. Fanfold top linen to foot of bed.
7. Position resident flat on back with arms and legs straight and body in good alignment.
8. Make a small pencil mark at the top of the resident's head on the sheet.
9. Make a second pencil mark even with the feet.
10. Using the tape measure, measure the distance between the two pencil marks.
11. Note this on a pad with resident's height in feet and inches.

To weigh the resident:

12. Place plastic cover on sling, if available, to prevent contamination.
13. Turn resident on one side and place sling on the bed. Roll or fanfold in half.
14. Roll the remaining portion of the sling under the resident; make sure the resident is centered on the sling.
15. Bring the scale over the bed, make sure the legs of the scale are under the bed. Open and lock the wheels.
16. Turn on the scale and calibrate to zero.

(continues)

PROCEDURE 19-63
Measuring and Weighing
the Resident in Bed (Continued)

17. Lower the arms of the scale and attach hooks through the holes in the sling.

18. Pump the scale until the sling is completely off the surface of the bed.

19. Remind the resident to remain still. Read the weight on the digital display after the numbers have stopped fluctuating. Record the weight.

20. Lower the resident back in the bed and remove the arms of the scale.

21. Unlock scale wheels and remove the scale from under the bed.

22. Turn the resident to the side, roll the sling midway, roll the resident to the other side and remove the sling.

23. Remove the sling and disposable cover, if used. If not, clean and disinfect sling according to facility protocol.

24. Replace the pillows and bed linens and make the resident comfortable.

25. Lower the bed to the lowest horizontal height.

26. Carry out procedure completion action.

Bay Shore Convalescent Home
4782 Bay Shore Drive
Watertown, Mich.

Vital signs are to be checked on all residents once each day unless ordered otherwise.

Date 4/10/XX

Resident	Room	Temp.	Pulse	Resp	B/P	Comments
Estrada, Luisa	101A					
Hartong, Mary	101B					
Diette, Marie	102A					
Aquino, Lucy	102B					
Ihli, Fred	103A					
Dyment, Frank	103B					
Lightfoot, Wm.	104A					
Lee, Sayo	104B					
Salcido, Rose	105A					
Tham, Peou	105B					
Wilde, Rose Marie	106A					
Hubbard, Marta	106B					
Lam, Lotruc	107A					
Uy, Aime	107B					
Valasco, Mary	108A					
Lobliner, Esther	108B					
	109A					
Moak, Loreta	109B					
Ocha, Vario	110A					
	110B					

Figure 19-35 Vital signs may be taken and recorded on the unit sheet and later transferred to the resident's record.

LESSON SYNTHESIS: Putting It All Together

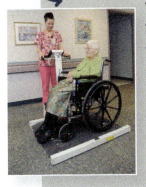

You have just completed this lesson. Now go back and review the Clinical Focus. Try to see how the Clinical Focus relates to the concepts presented in the lesson. Then answer the following questions.

1. The physician has ordered that Mrs. Hoden be weighed daily. Why do you think this is important?

2. Which method would be the most appropriate for weighing Mrs. Hoden?

3. An apical/radial pulse is taken on Mrs. Hoden because she has a pulse deficit. What does this mean?

4. What type of respirations would you expect to note on Mrs. Hoden?

19 REVIEW

A. Select the one best answer for each of the following.

1. The term vital signs includes

(A) height and weight

(B) temperature, pulse, respirations, blood pressure, pain

(C) temperature, pulse, and respirations

(D) blood pressure

2. Temperature can be increased by

(A) medications

(B) shock

(C) dehydration

(D) cold weather

3. Oral temperatures should be taken on residents who are

(A) confused and disoriented

(B) on seizure precautions

(C) unconscious

(D) conscious

4. A temperature taken in the ear is called

(A) oral

(B) axillary

(C) rectal

(D) tympanic

5. When taking a rectal temperature, insert the lubricated rectal probe (electronic thermometer) into the anus approximately:

(A) ¼ inch

(B) ½ inch

(C) 1 inch

(D) 2 inches

6. On an adult, the pulse is usually taken at which artery?

(A) brachial

(B) radial

(C) femoral

(D) carotid

7. The average pulse rate per minute for adult women is

(A) 80 to 110

(B) 60 to 70

(C) 65 to 80

(D) 75 to 100

8. Blood pressure can be decreased by

(A) exercise

(B) eating

(C) emotional anxiety

(D) resting

9. Medications prescribed to lower blood pressure are called

(A) antihypertensives

(B) stimulants

(C) depressants

(D) antibiotics

10. The first sound heard when taking blood pressure is called

(A) diastolic

(B) systolic

(C) pulse pressure

(D) apical

11. When taking a resident's temperature, one of the following is *not* considered to be an invasive route:

(A) oral

(B) rectal

(C) tympanic

(D) temporal artery

12. When taking the blood pressure, you recognize diastolic pressure as:

(A) the last sound heard

(B) the first sound heard

(C) 20 mmHg below the first sound heard

(D) the highest pressure in the arteries

13. Which of the following would be considered a normal respiratory rate for your resident?

(A) 8

(B) 10

(C) 18

(D) 26

14. Prehypertension is referred to as blood pressure over:

(A) 100/72 mmHg

(B) 120/90 mmHg

(C) 110/68 mmHg

(D) 120/70 mmHg

15. Blood pressure will not be taken on the resident's right arm in *all but one* of the following situations:

(A) Resident says her arm "itches."

(B) There is an intravenous infusion in the right hand.

(C) If the resident has an A/V shunt for renal dialysis.

(D) The resident had a right radical mastectomy.

16. To obtain an accurate weight for the resident, *all but one* of the following is essential:

(A) Weigh at the same time of day.

(B) Use any scale that is available.

(C) Resident wears the same type and amount of clothing.

(D) Use the same wheelchair with leg supports.

B. Match each term (items a–j) with the proper definition.

a. sphygmomanometer

b. tachycardia

c. thermometer

d. volume

e. fasting

f. hypotension meter

g. bradycardia

h. hypertension

i. pulse deficit

j. rales

17. _____ low blood pressure

18. _____ bounding

19. _____ moist respirations

20. _____ not eating

21. _____ rapid heart rate

22. _____ slow heart rate

23. _____ used to determine blood pressure

24. _____ used to determine temperature

25. _____ high blood pressure

26. _____ difference between radial and apical pulse rates

C. Fill in the blanks by selecting the correct word or phrase from the list.

apnea	rales
axillary	rate
bradycardia	rectal
centimeters	rhythm
cyanotic	sphygmomanometer
dyspnea	stethoscope
expiration	tachycardia
inspiration	vital signs
kilograms	volume

27. Temperature, pulse, respiration, blood pressure, and pain are: _____.

28. The instrument used to listen to the heart is a(an): _____.

29. The instrument used to measure blood pressure is a(an): _____.

30. A(An) _____ temperature is usually 1° higher than an oral temperature.

31. A(An) _____ temperature is usually 1° lower than an oral temperature.

32. In the metric system, height is measured in _____.

33. In the metric system, weight is measured in _____.

34. When taking a pulse, you should note _____, _____, _____.

35. A rapid pulse rate is called _____.

36. A slow pulse rate is called _____.

37. The two parts to each respiration are called _____ and _____.

38. The term _____ means a dusky, bluish color to the skin.

39. A period of no respirations is called _____.

40. Labored breathing is called _____.

ADMISSION, TRANSFER, AND DISCHARGE

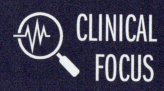

CLINICAL FOCUS

Think about situations that require admission to, or transfer and discharge from, the long-term care facility as you study this lesson.

OBJECTIVES

After studying this lesson, you should be able to:

• Define vocabulary words and terms.

• List reasons why residents are admitted to long-term care facilities.

• Describe the emotional reactions of the resident and the family to admission.

• Identify reasons why admission to a long-term care facility may be more difficult for a teenager or young adult.

• Identify the responsibilities of the nursing assistant related to admission procedures.

• List reasons why residents may be transferred out of the facility.

• Identify the responsibilities of the nursing assistant related to transfer procedures.

• List reasons why residents are discharged from long-term care facilities.

• Describe the actions involved in the discharge of a resident.

• Identify the responsibilities of the nursing assistant related to discharge procedures.

• Demonstrate the following:
  Procedure 20–64   Admitting the Resident
  Procedure 20–65   Transferring the Resident
  Procedure 20–66   Discharging the Resident

CASE STUDY

Jack Tyler, 28 years old, has multiple sclerosis. He is no longer able to care for himself and has made the decision to enter a long-term care facility.

VOCABULARY

community services (kom-MYOUN-ih-tee SIR-vih-sez)
diagnosis-related group (DRG) (die-ag-NOS-is ree-LAY-ted groop)
discharge planner (DIS-charj PLAN-er)

discharge planning (DIS-charj PLAN-ing)
kidney dialysis (KID-nee die-AL-ih-sis)
personal inventory (PER-SON-AL IN-VEN-TOR-EE)

ADMITTING THE RESIDENT

Reasons for Admission

A resident may be admitted to a long-term care facility because the individual:

- Requires 24-hour-a-day supervision and nursing care
- Requires specialized treatments
- Requires rehabilitation services before returning home
- Has a progressive, chronic disease that requires more care
- Has Alzheimer's disease or another dementia and can no longer be cared for at home
- The resident may be admitted from
  - An acute care hospital
  - Home
  - Another extended care facility

There may be varying circumstances surrounding the admission. Some residents are admitted to the hospital for emergencies requiring immediate care. An example of this would be a person who fell and broke a hip or the person who had a stroke. The individual can stay in the hospital for a limited number of days according to the **diagnosis-related group (DRG)** that covers the person's diagnosis. At the end of this time most people are not yet ready to care for themselves. The **discharge planner** (the person who arranges care after discharge from the hospital) may arrange for home care or for the person to be admitted to a long-term care facility until the person is more independent. In these situations the family and resident may need to make a quick decision about placement (Figure 20-1).

Some residents are admitted because they have Alzheimer's disease or another dementia. These diseases are progressive and eventually require 24-hour-a-day supervision. Most families do not have the energy or resources to cope with the situation at home. Other chronic diseases such as Parkinson's disease or multiple sclerosis may progress to the point that the individual is unable to perform the activities of daily living (ADLs) without maximal assistance.

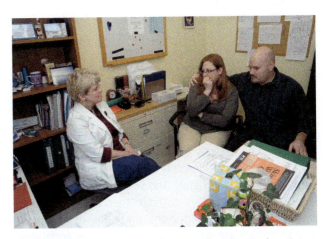

Figure 20-1 In some cases, a decision about a long-term care facility may have to be made in a hurry.

In some situations, residents require specialized care because they need:

- Artificial ventilation to breathe
- **Kidney dialysis** (treatment when kidneys fail)
- Complicated wound care
- Rehabilitation services
- Continuous intravenous therapy
- Continuous wound vacuum for wounds

Anxiety about Admission

Some admissions are considered permanent, which means the resident will live in the facility for the rest of his or her life. Other admissions are temporary and the resident will eventually be discharged.

The new resident who is considered a permanent admission probably has experienced many losses. Admission means a further loss of independence. He or she may have lost a spouse and now, along with failing strength and health, the comfort and security of familiar surroundings are about to be lost. Families often feel guilty because the family member cannot be provided for at home. They may also be physically and emotionally exhausted from giving care for several years before this admission. Burdens also may be intensified by the financial costs of admission. Residents who need to apply for Medicaid may feel embarrassed because they cannot pay their own way.

Both the family and the resident will feel uncertain and somewhat fearful of the new environment. They will need support and encouragement. Their anxiety may make it difficult for them to remember things that you explain to them and they may feel overwhelmed. Be prepared to repeat statements. Reassure them that their feelings are natural and help them express these feelings. Make their first impression of you and the facility a positive one.

The admission of a teenager or younger adult to the long-term care facility is difficult, especially if it considered a permanent admission. This type of admission may be the result of a motor vehicle accident, head trauma associated with a variety of situations such as swimming/diving accidents, war-related injuries, or neurological conditions such as multiple sclerosis or amyotrophic lateral sclerosis (ALS); these neurologic conditions are discussed in Lesson 29.

The illness or disability of a family member affects every person in the family. The young person as well as the parents may be devastated to learn that the child will not be able to experience the privileges of adulthood. The individual will not be a part of the peer community that is so vital to teenage development. As you complete your admission responsibilities, remember how difficult this process is for both the resident and the family.

Preadmission Activities

Arranging for admission to a long-term care facility involves many activities that occur before the resident arrives. The family is often responsible for participating in these procedures, especially if the resident is in the hospital. The family will need to:

- Choose (with the resident's input if possible) a facility
- Meet with someone from the Social Services or Admissions department to arrange for the admission
- Apply for Medicaid, if necessary, to pay for the cost of services
- Verify whether insurance benefits and coverage are applicable

If the resident is coming from a hospital, the discharge planner at the hospital will need to:

- Confirm admission with the Social Services or Admissions department of the facility to be sure a bed is available and that the facility can provide the care and treatment the person needs
- Complete transfer forms to ensure continuity of care
- Arrange for the resident's transfer (usually by ambulance) from the hospital to the facility

The Social Services or Admissions department staff of the receiving facility will need to:

- Meet with the discharge planner to determine what services are needed. The social worker or admissions director may visit the resident to make an initial assessment.
- Meet with the nursing staff of the receiving facility to determine if special equipment, such as traction, will be needed
- Meet with the family (and resident if possible) to explain the facility's services and the responsibilities of the family and resident
- Explain and provide a copy of the Residents' Rights to family and resident
- Determine the method of payment for services
- Inform appropriate departments of the resident's pending admission and the services that will be needed
- Inform any residents who may be sharing the room of the new resident's arrival

Inservice meetings or training for the staff may be needed if the resident has an unusual diagnosis, requires special treatment, or needs special equipment.

Day of Admission

On the day of admission, you and/or maintenance will be expected to check the room to be sure it is ready for the new resident's arrival.

- Check the room lights to be sure they are working.
- Check the call light to be sure it is working. Attach it to the bed.
- Check bed controls and attach them to the bed.
- Check the bed for clean sheets, a pillow, and a spread. Lock the wheels of the bed. Place the bed in lowest position.
- Move the overbed table, if necessary, so it is not in the way.
- Place a pitcher and glass on the bedside table if the resident is allowed to drink thin liquids. Wait to fill the pitcher with fresh water until the resident arrives.
- Place personal care items in the bedside table. The arrangement of items may be different for each facility. Remember that "dirty" items such as bedpans and urinals will be wrapped in plastic and should not be stored with clean items like the wash basin and toothbrush.
- Check the resident's bathroom for:
  - Cleanliness
  - Soap in soap dispenser
  - Paper towels in dispenser

- Towels and washcloths for the resident
- Toilet tissue
- Check dresser drawers for cleanliness.
- Check the closet for hangers.

The bed may be opened (top covers folded to end of bed) or left closed depending on the condition of the resident. The nurse or the unit secretary will set up a chart, care plan, and other forms to be used on admission.

Admission Assessments

The members of the interdisciplinary health care team will each make an assessment of the new resident (Figure 20-2). This includes the Minimum Data Set (MDS) 3.0 form required by OBRA and other assessments required by the facility. This information will be used to start the plan of care.

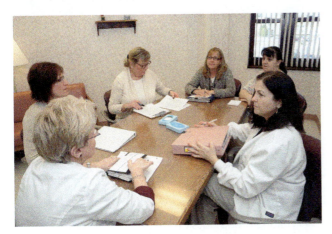

Figure 20-2 Each member of the interdisciplinary team participates in the admission of a new resident.

BUILDING CULTURAL AWARENESS

Remember that persons from different cultural groups may respond differently to admission and health care procedures. Consider issues of personal space, touching, and eye contact. Members of some cultures may have beliefs about nature and the cause of illness and types of health care practices that differ from yours.

Meeting the New Resident

First impressions are important. Remember that this is a new and strange experience for the resident and family. Someone from the facility is designated to meet the resident and family at the entrance to the facility, if possible, and accompany them to the assigned room. The social worker, admissions director, or nurse may be responsible for this procedure.

The resident's first impression is a lasting one. Your appearance and your attitude will set the tone for the resident's opinion of the facility.

Responsibilities of the Nursing Assistant

The nurse and social worker need to complete a number of procedures once the resident is in the room. At the appropriate time you will need to complete the nursing assistant's part of the admission procedure.

PROCEDURE 20-64
Admitting the Resident

1. Wash hands and assemble equipment:

   - Equipment for taking temperature
   - Worksheet for recording information
   - Stethoscope
   - Sphygmomanometer
   - Watch with second hand
   - Appropriate scale

2. Prepare unit as described earlier in this chapter, if that has not yet been done.

3. Identify the resident both by asking the name and checking the identification bracelet.

(continues)

PROCEDURE 20-64
Admitting the Resident (Continued)

4. Introduce yourself.

5. Introduce resident to roommates, if appropriate.

6. Help resident to undress if instructed by the nurse to do so. If resident will remain dressed, have resident sit in a comfortable chair.

7. Orient resident to the room and show how to use the call light, the telephone, the television, and so on.

8. Assist resident with unpacking and setting up personal items, such as photographs, cell phone and charger, religious or reading articles, and electronic device, i.e., IPad, laptop

9. Label resident's belongings according to facility policy and complete the Inventory List.

10. Fill the water pitcher with fresh water and ice (if appropriate).

11. Take and record resident's vital signs.

12. Obtain and record the resident's height and weight.

13. Make arrangements to tour the facility with the resident (Figure 20-3).

14. Carry out each procedure completion action.

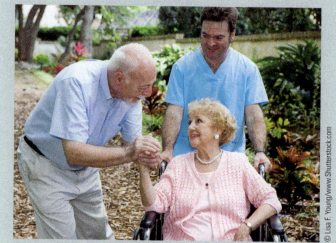

Figure 20-3 The nursing assistant can take the new resident on a tour of the facility.

In most facilities the social worker or nurse will inform the resident and family about:

- Facility rules such as limitations on smoking
- Visiting periods
- Availability of services and activities

The resident (if possible) and the family will be taken on a tour of the building so they know the location of:

- Stairs and elevators
- Dining room
- Activity areas
- Visiting areas outside the resident's room
- Offices of administrative staff
- Public telephones
- Public restrooms
- Rehabilitation services areas

You should be familiar with this information so you can accurately answer any questions the resident may have later.

? EXERCISE 20-1

COMPLETION
Complete the chart on admission activities. Indicate which activities are the responsibility of the nursing assistant.

ACTIVITY	NURSING ASSISTANT	
1. Check room to be sure it is ready for admission.	Yes	No
2. Determine the method of payment for services.	Yes	No

(continues)

? EXERCISE 20-1 (Continued)

3. Inform residents who may be sharing the room with a new arrival.	Yes	No
4. Check room lights to be sure they are working.	Yes	No
5. Check bed controls and attach to bed.	Yes	No
6. Check bed for clean sheets, a pillow, and spread.	Yes	No
7. Explain and provide copy of the resident's rights to family and resident.	Yes	No
8. Place personal items in bedside table.	Yes	No
9. Check closet for hangers.	Yes	No
10. Make an assessment of the new resident.	Yes	No

Completing a Personal Inventory

A personal inventory is completed for every resident who is admitted. This is a special form that lists and describes all items the resident brings to the facility (Figure 20-4). All items must be labeled with the resident's name. Follow the facility policy for this procedure. This task may be completed by the nurse, the unit secretary, the nursing assistant, or house-keeping staff.

The personal inventory includes:

- All items of clothing
- Jewelry, including wedding rings and watches
- Personal equipment such as razors, combs, brushes
- Religious items such as bibles, rosaries
- Books, magazines, plants, photographs, afghan, quilt
- Furniture such as a chair, dresser, television
- Assistive devices: glasses, dentures, hearing aids, cane, walker

The items listed are also described. Be careful in your descriptions. For example, do not describe a ring as a "diamond in a gold setting." The correct description is "clear stone in a yellow metal setting." This is done because the staff is not qualified to determine whether the stone is a diamond or whether it is glass. After the inventory is completed, sign the form. The resident or a family member also signs the form. Residents are discouraged from keeping large sums of money or valuable items in their rooms. Facilities are required to provide accounts for residents so they can deposit and withdraw money as it is needed. Other valuable items can be placed in the facility safe.

Helping the Resident Adapt to the Facility

Remember that living in the long-term care facility is a very different experience for the resident. It will take the resident time to adapt to the environment, the routine, and the caregivers. Some residents may have a temporary period of confusion and disorientation until they become familiar with the facility. Residents may feel overwhelmed by the amount of information they are expected to remember. Be patient in repeating and reinforcing the information. Offer to write down times of activities, meals, and therapy sessions so they have something to refer to once you leave the room.

Introduce the resident to other residents and caregivers. Take time to talk with new residents so they feel safe and secure in their new home. Fire drills and other routine procedures may be frightening. Explain what is happening and guide the resident through the process. If the new admission is a teenager or young adult, be sure to introduce him or her to other residents in the same age group.

Welcome the family and consider them members of the care team. Follow your facility policies regarding such issues as:

- Family members taking residents outside the facility
- Family members feeding residents or providing other types of care
- Smoking on the premises, if allowed

Form 883/2   BRIGGS, Des Moines, Iowa 50306
PRINTED IN U.S.A.

INVENTORY LIST

QTY.	ARTICLES	QTY.	APPLIANCES	QTY.	PROSTHETIC DEVICES		ACQUIRED AFTER ADMISSION	
							Date	Item
	Belts		T.V. - Ser. #:		Dentures: ☐ Upper			
	Blouses		Radio - Ser. #:		☐ Lower ☐ Partial	Date		
	Coats		Hair Dryer		Eye Wear			
	Dresses		Electric Razor		Cane			
	Gloves				Walker - Ser. #:			
	Hats				W/chair - Ser. #:			
	Housecoats - Robes		JEWELRY		Brace			
	Jackets		Ring (Describe)					
	Nightgowns - Pajamas							
	Purses		Watch (Describe)		OTHER			
	Shaving Kit							
	Shoes		Other					
	Shorts							
	Slacks							
	Slippers							
	Slips		FURNITURE					
	Socks/Hose							
	Suitcases							
	Suits				VALUABLES RELEASED FROM SAFE			
	Sweaters							
	Ties							
	Undershirts							
	Underwear							

I received on discharge in satisfactory condition the above articles and a copy of this list.
Disposition of belongings: _____

▶ _____   _____   ▶ _____   _____
Signature of Patient/Resp. Party   Date   Signature of Facility Representative   Date

NOTE ▶ Patient/Responsible Party is responsible for assuring that all personal belongings are properly marked. All items brought in after admission are added to this inventory at the request of Patient/Responsible Party.

QTY.	ARTICLES	QTY.	APPLIANCES	QTY.	PROSTHETIC DEVICES		ACQUIRED AFTER ADMISSION	
							Date	Item
1	Belts (black)		T.V. - Ser. #:		Dentures: ☐ Upper			
2	~~Blouses~~ Shirts (polo)		Radio - Ser. #:		☐ Lower ☐ Partial	Date		
	Coats		Hair Dryer		Eye Wear			
	Dresses	1	Electric Razor		Cane			
	Gloves				Walker - Ser. #:			
	Hats				W/chair - Ser. #:			
1	~~Housecoats~~ - Robes (red)		JEWELRY		Brace			
	Jackets	1	Ring (Describe)					
	Nightgowns - Pajamas		Yellow metal wedding band					
1	Purses		Watch (Describe)		OTHER			
	Shaving Kit		Timex silver metal	1	Bible			
1 pr	Shoes (black laced)		Other	8	handkerchiefs, white			
	Shorts							
2	Slacks (knit, black, grey)							
1 pr	Slippers (brown felt)							
	Slips		FURNITURE					
6 pr	Socks/~~Hose~~ (black)							
	Suitcases							
	Suits				VALUABLES LOCKED IN SAFE			
	Sweaters							
	Ties							
6	Undershirts (white T)							
6	Underwear (white jockey)							

I certify that this is a correct list of my clothes and belongings which I wish to retain in my possession and for which I take ENTIRE RESPONSIBILITY. I have received a copy of this list.

▶ *Joseph Cervanti*   1/25/2XXX   ▶ *Della Sheeling*   1/25/2XXX
Signature of Patient/Resp. Party   Date   Signature of Facility Representative   Date

If the patient is unable to sign, state reason: _____
▶ Signature of Witness: _____

PATIENT NAME—LAST	FIRST	MIDDLE	HOSP. NO.	ROOM NO.
Cervanti	Joseph	—		203 B

INVENTORY LIST

Form 883/2   BRIGGS, Des Moines, Iowa 50306
PRINTED IN U.S.A.

Figure 20-4 The personal inventory lists and describes all items that the resident brings into the facility.

? EXERCISE 20-2

BRIEF ANSWERS
Select the correct terms from the following list to complete each statement.

combs	incorrect	religious
dentures	introduce	required
discouraged	personal inventory	resident
glasses	property	resident or family member
hearing aids		

1. The personal inventory includes all items of the _____.

2. Personal equipment such as razors, _____, and brushes should be listed.

3. Assistive devices to be included in the personal inventory include _____, _____, _____, canes, and walkers.

4. Residents are _____ from keeping large sums of money or valuable items in their rooms.

5. It would be _____ to describe a white stone in a ring as a diamond.

6. Books, magazines, and plants should be listed in the _____.

7. Rosaries are considered _____ items and should be listed.

8. A chair or dresser is listed as personal _____.

9. The nursing assistant and _____ both sign the completed personal inventory form.

10. Facilities are _____ to provide accounts for residents so they can deposit or withdraw money as it is needed.

11. If the new admission is a teenager or young adult, be sure to _____ him to other residents in the same age group.

? EXERCISE 20-3

CLINICAL SITUATION
Read the following situations and answer the questions.

Mrs. Goldstein has just been admitted to your facility. She lost her husband approximately 2 years ago after 54 years of marriage. He had been ill for several years before his death. Her one daughter accompanied her to the facility. Mrs. Goldstein seems very fragile and tired. You know her costs are covered by Medicare. She confides to you that she feels "so badly" that she needs to accept help in this way.

1. What losses do you think Mrs. Goldstein has suffered and how do you think this has affected her?
   _____
   _____

2. Do you feel she is comfortable about her current financial situation?
   _____

3. Do you think anxiety might make her admission more difficult?
   _____
   _____

4. What can you do to make this life transition easier for her and her daughter?
   _____
   _____

(continues)

? EXERCISE 20-3 (Continued)

5. Mrs. Wheeler is a new resident that you are admitting. She is agitated, looking about, and clinging to her daughter. She is in a wheelchair and will be living with Mrs. Crawley in Room 12. Her daughter also appears anxious. Although you have explained the call system, she asks again if you are sure her mother can be heard if she needs help. List ways you can make the transition to a long-term care facility easier for this resident and her family.

_____

_____

_____

_____

TRANSFERRING THE RESIDENT

There are two types of resident transfers:

- Within the facility, transferring the resident from one room or nursing unit to another
- Outside the facility to another health care agency
- There are several reasons why a resident may be transferred within the facility:
  - The resident's condition changes, requiring a different level of care
  - Residents in the same room do not get along
  - Resident requests a different room
- One is diagnosed with some illness requiring isolation

When a transfer within the facility occurs, all items go with the resident to the new room or unit (Figure 20-5).

- Clothing and all personal items belonging to the resident
- Items in the bedside stand

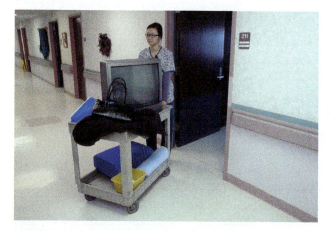

Figure 20-5 All items go with the resident when she is transferred to another room in the same facility.

- Chart, care plan, other medical records, and medications if resident is moving to another unit
- Medications

A resident may be transferred out of the facility to another health care agency because the resident needs:

- The services of an acute care hospital
- Evaluation and treatment for psychiatric problems

If the resident is transferred outside the facility, personal possessions, medical records, and personal care items remain in the facility. The only item that goes with the resident is a transfer record. The transfer record contains information for the receiving facility (Figure 20-6).

DISCHARGING THE RESIDENT

Discharging of residents from the long-term care facility has become a common occurrence. Residents are discharged because they:

- Have improved enough to go home
- Do not need the high-level services of the facility but can function in a less restrictive environment such as an assisted living facility
- Require care that can be provided by another long-term care facility

The discharge procedure is usually simple if the resident is going to another facility. The social worker and nurse relay information to the receiving facility. The resident's belongings are sent to the new facility with the resident or family member.

Discharge to the resident's home is more complicated and requires a number of actions called **discharge planning**. Discharge planning is a cooperative procedure that involves all members of the interdisciplinary health care team. The social worker is the coordinator for discharge planning and is

SUGGESTIONS FOR COMPLETING FORM
1. The purpose of this form is to insure continuity of care in transfer from a skilled care facility to an acute care facility or another skilled care facility.
2. The form is not intended to supply information of long-term nature.
3. Original should accompany resident with transfer. Carbon copy should be retained in resident's record.

INSTRUCTIONS:
This form has two sides. After completing front side, pull out carbon; turn form over; reinsert carbon face down. When writing, press firmly.

RESIDENT TRANSFER FORM
(INTER-AGENCY REFERRAL)
(Reference tags: F203 - F205)

RESIDENT'S LAST NAME	FIRST NAME	MI	SEX ☐M ☐F	SOCIAL SECURITY NUMBER

RESIDENT'S ADDRESS (Street, City, State, Zip)	DATE OF BIRTH	RELIGION

DATE OF THIS TRANSFER

FACILITY NAME AND ADDRESS TRANSFERRING TO

PHYSICIAN IN CHARGE AT TIME OF TRANSFER

Will this physician care for resident after admission to new facility? ☐YES ☐NO

DATES OF STAY AT FACILITY TRANSFERRING FROM
ADMISSION   DISCHARGE

PAYMENT SOURCE FOR CHARGES TO RESIDENT
A. ☐ SELF OR FAMILY
B. ☐ PRIVATE INSURANCE
C. ☐ BLUE CROSS BLUE SHIELD
D. ☐ EMPLOYER OR UNION
E. ☐ PUBLIC AGENCY (Give name)
F. ☐ OTHER (Explain)

NAME AND ADDRESS OF FACILITY TRANSFERRING FROM

NAME AND ADDRESSES OF ALL HOSPITALS AND EXTENDED CARE FACILITIES FROM WHICH RESIDENT WAS DISCHARGED IN PAST 60 DAYS.

CLINIC APPOINTMENT SCHEDULED   DATE   TIME   ☐CLINIC APPOINTMENT CARD ATTACHED

DATE OF LAST PHYSICAL EXAMINATION   DATE OF LAST BOWEL MOVEMENT

RELATIVE OR GUARDIAN (Name, Address, Phone Number, Relationship to Resident)

WAS THIS PERSON NOTIFIED REGARDING THIS TRANSFER? ☐ YES ☐ NO

WAS THIS PERSON (OR WAS THE RESIDENT) GIVEN INFORMATION ON HOW TO CONTACT THE STATE OMBUDSMAN? ☐ YES ☐ NO

EMPLOYMENT RELATED: ☐YES ☐NO

DIAGNOSES AT TIME OF TRANSFER
(a) PRIMARY

(b) SECONDARY

VITALS AT TIME OF TRANSFER: Ht. _____   Wt. _____
T _____ P _____ R _____ B/P _____

REASON FOR TRANSFER

CHECK ALL THAT APPLY

DISABILITIES
☐Amputation
☐Paralysis
☐Contracture(s)
☐Pressure Ulcer

IMPAIRMENTS
☐Mental
☐Speech
☐Hearing
☐Vision
☐Sensation

INCONTINENCE
☐Bladder
☐Bowel
☐Saliva

ACTIVITY TOLERANCE LIMITATIONS
☐None ☐Moderate ☐Severe

RESIDENT KNOWS DIAGNOSIS?
☐Yes ☐No

POTENTIAL FOR REHABILITATION
☐Good ☐Fair ☐Poor

DIET, DRUGS, AND OTHER THERAPY
at Time of Discharge

Diet Order:
Therapy:

Current Medications	Strength & Frequency	Time Last Dose	Amt. Sent

☐May **NOT** use generic substitutes
*(Physician or nurse must sign below - See verification of meds.)

IMPORTANT MEDICAL INFORMATION
(State allergies if any)

ADVANCE DIRECTIVES
☐Yes ☐Attached ☐None

BED HOLD POLICY
Given to resident ☐ Yes ☐ No
Attached ☐ Yes ☐ No, reason: _____

TB Test	Date _____	Type _____	Result _____
Chest X-Ray	Date _____	Result _____	
C.B.C.	Date _____	Result _____	
Biochem	Date _____	Result _____	
Urinalysis	Date _____	Result _____	

SUGGESTIONS FOR ACTIVE CARE

BED
Position in good body alignment and change position every _____ hrs.
Avoid _____ position.
Prone position _____ times/day as tolerated.

SITTING
_____ hr(s). _____ times/day.

WEIGHT BEARING
☐Full ☐Partial ☐None
on _____ leg.

EXERCISES
Range of motion _____ times/day
to _____ by
☐resident ☐nurse ☐family.
Stand _____ minutes _____ times/day.

LOCOMOTION
Walk _____ (distance) _____ (no.) times/day.

SOCIAL ACTIVITIES
Encourage: (☐group ☐individual) activities
(☐within ☐outside) home.

Transportation: ☐Ambulance ☐Car
☐Car for handicapped ☐Bus

VERIFICATION OF MEDS X _____
*Signature of Physician or Nurse
Date ___/___/___

CFS 2-4/2P © 1992 Briggs Corporation, Des Moines, IA 50306 (800) 247-2343
R195   Printed in U.S.A.

RESIDENT TRANSFER FORM
☐Continued on Reverse

Figure 20-6 The transfer record goes with the resident from one facility to the next.

RESIDENT TRANSFER FORM (continued)

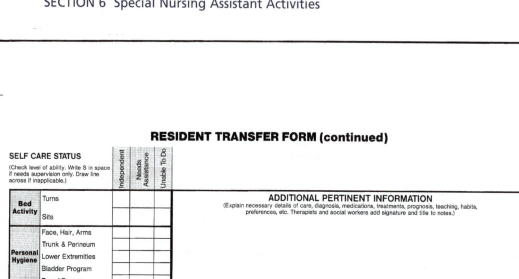

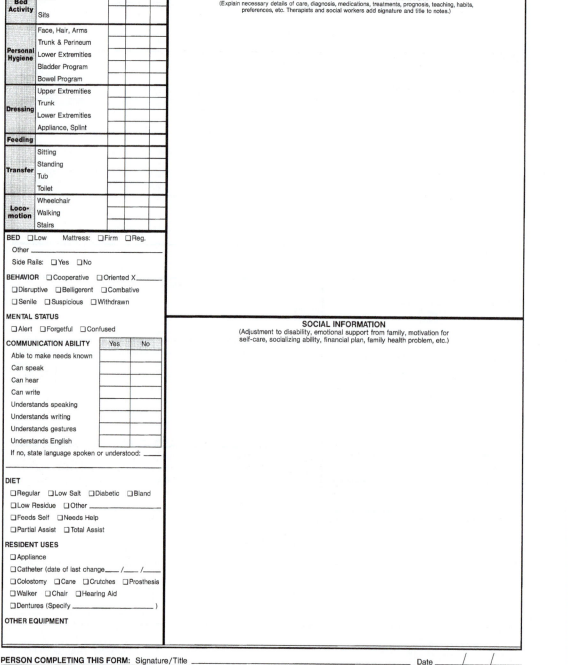

SELF CARE STATUS (Check level of ability. Write S in space if needs supervision only. Draw line across if inapplicable.)		Independent	Needs Assistance	Unable To Do
Bed Activity	Turns			
	Sits			
Personal Hygiene	Face, Hair, Arms			
	Trunk & Perineum			
	Lower Extremities			
	Bladder Program			
	Bowel Program			
Dressing	Upper Extremities			
	Trunk			
	Lower Extremities			
	Appliance, Splint			
Feeding				
Transfer	Sitting			
	Standing			
	Tub			
	Toilet			
Loco-motion	Wheelchair			
	Walking			
	Stairs			

BED ☐Low   Mattress: ☐Firm ☐Reg.

Other _____

Side Rails: ☐Yes ☐No

BEHAVIOR ☐Cooperative ☐Oriented X_____

☐Disruptive ☐Belligerent ☐Combative

☐Senile ☐Suspicious ☐Withdrawn

MENTAL STATUS

☐Alert ☐Forgetful ☐Confused

COMMUNICATION ABILITY	Yes	No
Able to make needs known		
Can speak		
Can hear		
Can write		
Understands speaking		
Understands writing		
Understands gestures		
Understands English		

If no, state language spoken or understood: _____

_____

DIET

☐Regular ☐Low Salt ☐Diabetic ☐Bland

☐Low Residue ☐Other _____

☐Feeds Self ☐Needs Help

☐Partial Assist ☐Total Assist

RESIDENT USES

☐Appliance

☐Catheter (date of last change____ /____ /____

☐Colostomy ☐Cane ☐Crutches ☐Prosthesis

☐Walker ☐Chair ☐Hearing Aid

☐Dentures (Specify _____)

OTHER EQUIPMENT

ADDITIONAL PERTINENT INFORMATION
(Explain necessary details of care, diagnosis, medications, treatments, prognosis, teaching, habits, preferences, etc. Therapists and social workers add signature and title to notes.)

SOCIAL INFORMATION
(Adjustment to disability, emotional support from family, motivation for self-care, socializing ability, financial plan, family health problem, etc.)

PERSON COMPLETING THIS FORM: Signature/Title _____ Date ____/____/____

RESIDENT TRANSFER FORM

Reprinted with permission of Briggs Corporation, Des Moines, IA 50306; 800-247-2343

Figure 20-6 (Continued) The transfer record goes with the resident from one facility to the next.

? EXERCISE 20-4

TRUE OR FALSE

Indicate whether the following statements are true (T) or false (F).

1. T F Residents may be transferred when they require a different level of care.

2. T F When a resident is transferred to another room within the facility, all personal items accompany the resident.

3. T F When a resident is transferred out of the facility, personal care items remain in the facility.

4. T F Nursing assistants need to know the method of transport before assisting with a transfer to another facility.

5. T F Nursing assistants should transport medical records, care plan, and medications with the resident during a transfer within the facility.

6. T F Supplies and equipment used for the resident's care remain in the original room when a resident is transferred within the facility.

7. T F Nursing assistants should introduce the transferred resident to the new staff.

8. T F Nursing assistants must make sure that residents are dressed appropriately when transferred out of the facility.

9. T F The nursing assistant is responsible for relaying information to the new facility when a resident is transferred out of the facility.

10. T F Discharge planning is a cooperative procedure that involves all members of the interdisciplinary health care team.

responsible for arranging for **community services**. Community services may include intermittent services including:

1. A registered nurse for ongoing assessment, monitoring, supervision of other caregivers, planning of care, teaching, and implementation of treatments

2. A home health aide for personal care including bathing, positioning, passive range-of-motion exercises, taking vital signs, and doing simple treatments

3. Rehabilitation staff for physical therapy, occupational therapy, and speech therapy

4. A homemaker for completing routine household chores such as light cleaning, laundry, cooking, and grocery shopping

5. Home-delivered meals. These are delivered for the noon meal and meet the nutritional requirements of the resident. Meals for persons on diabetic, low-salt, low-fat, and low-cholesterol diets can usually be arranged.

PROCEDURE 20-65
Transferring the Resident

1. Find out if the resident is to be transferred within the facility or out of the facility.

2. If within the facility, find out if the resident will be moved by wheelchair or in the bed.

3. If out of the facility, find out if the resident will be taken to the exit by wheelchair to a car or if the resident will be transferred by ambulance.

4. Carry out each beginning procedure action.

5. For transfer within the facility, the following items will be moved with the resident:

   - Resident's belongings
   - Personal care items from bedside table
   - Supplies or equipment used for resident's care
   - Medical records, care plan, and medications (if moving to another unit)

(continues)

PROCEDURE 20-65
Transferring the Resident (Continued)

6. Help resident dress if necessary.

7. Move resident to new unit as indicated.

8. Help resident get settled in new room.

9. Introduce resident to staff and other residents.

10. Tell the resident good-bye and wish him well.

11. Carry out each procedure completion action.

If resident is being transferred out of facility:

1. If resident is going by car, make sure the resident is well groomed and dressed appropriately for the weather (Figure 20-7), then assist into wheelchair and take to exit. Assist in transferring into car.

2. If resident is going by ambulance, follow nurse's instructions.

3. The nurse will give appropriate records and transfer form to family or ambulance drivers.

4. Tell the resident good-bye.

5. Carry out each procedure completion action.

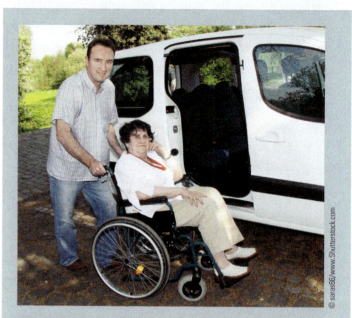

Figure 20-7 Make sure the resident is well groomed and dressed appropriately when transferred from the facility.

Factors to Consider Before Discharge

Before discharge planning proceeds, the interdisciplinary team must consider several factors:

1. Does the resident have the potential to regain enough independence to go home?

2. Is there a person (spouse, family member, or friend) willing to serve as a liaison (go-between) for the resident when he or she goes home? The person living alone will usually need someone to call or check on him or her, run errands, help with money management, and oversee the household management.

3. Are adequate community services available? If the resident needs continuing physical therapy, for example, there must be an agency that provides this service. In some areas of the country there are not enough therapists to meet the demand.

4. Does the resident need 24-hour-a-day supervision or care? Medicare and private insurance will not pay for this type of care. Most people could not afford to pay for it themselves. (Continuous care may cost several hundreds of dollars per day.)

5. Will the structure of the resident's home allow the resident to function adequately and safely? For example, is there a bedroom and bathroom on the same floor?

These factors are especially critical if the resident will be living alone. If the resident, the family, and the care team determine that discharge is a reasonable expectation, then planning proceeds.

1. The interdisciplinary team will prepare a discharge plan of care. This plan provides information to the resident and caregivers (family, friends, or community service providers) on how to help the resident maintain health (Figure 20-8).

2. The social worker arranges for the community services.

3. The physical therapist or a restorative nurse may take the resident home for a short visit to evaluate the resident's ability to function in the home

POST-DISCHARGE PLAN OF CARE

(Reference tags: F203, F204; Cross reference tags: F157, F284)

The following discharge information is to help you maintain your health and independence.

You are being discharged : ☐ home   ☐ to a residential care facility (see facility name and address below).

Facility _____   Phone _____

Address _____   City/State/Zip _____

THE FOLLOWING COMMUNITY RESOURCES ARE AVAILABLE TO MEET YOUR INDIVIDUAL NEEDS ▶

State Ombudsman _____   Phone _____

Address _____   City/State/Zip _____

Visiting Nurse _____   Phone _____

Address _____   City/State/Zip _____

Other Agency _____   Phone _____

Address _____   City/State/Zip _____

COMMUNITY RESOURCES AND SERVICES PLANNING ▶

Nursing needs: _____
_____

Personal care: _____
_____

Transportation: _____

Meals: _____

Housekeeping: _____

Social support/Family system/Special requests: _____
_____

Financial status/needs: _____

Financial access/Payment for services: _____

Therapy services: _____
_____

Other: _____

Person completing this section: _____   ___/___/___
             Signature and title   *Date*

SCHEDULED APPOINTMENTS ▶

Appointment With	Date	Purpose	Telephone

NAME—Last	First	Middle	Attending Physician	Chart No.

CFS 2-2/2P © 1992 Briggs Corporation, Des Moines, IA 50306 (800) 247-2343
Printed in U.S.A.

POST-DISCHARGE PLAN OF CARE
☐ Continued on Reverse

Reprinted with permission of Briggs Corporation, Des Moines, IA 50306, 800-247-2343

Figure 20-8 Care plan for the resident who is to be discharged home.

POST-DISCHARGE PLAN OF CARE (continued)

DIETARY AND NUTRITIONAL NEEDS ▶

Suggested food/fluids: _____

Special instructions: _____

Avoid: _____

❑ Copy of diet given   ❑ Diet explained to resident/caregiver   ❑ Restrictions explained (if applicable)

Person completing this section _____   ___/___/___
                                  Signature and title   *Date*

ACTIVITIES AND LEISURE PURSUITS ▶

Suggested activities: ❑ T.V./Movies   ❑ Radio   ❑ Reading   ❑ Senior Center   ❑ Talking books

❑ Volunteer Work   ❑ Other_____

Special instructions: _____

Activities to avoid: _____

Person completing this section _____   ___/___/___
                                  Signature and title   *Date*

MEDICATIONS ▶

Medication	Dose and Frequency	Purpose and Special Instructions	Amount Sent With Resident	Prescription Sent With Resident	Prescription Called To Pharmacy

Person completing this section _____   ___/___/___
                                  Signature and title   *Date*

WOUND CARE, TREATMENTS, THERAPY ▶ Procedures you should do

Procedure	Purpose	Frequency

Person completing this section _____   ___/___/___
                                  Signature and title   *Date*

IMPORTANT NAMES AND PHONE NUMBERS ▶

Physician _____   Phone _____
          Name and address

Pharmacy _____   Phone _____
          Name and address

These discharge instructions have been reviewed with me in a language I understand. All questions have been answered to my satisfaction. I have received the medications or written prescriptions as indicated above.

Signature **X**_____   ___/___/___
          Resident / Caregiver   *Date*

Please contact us if you have further questions.

Facility_____   Telephone _____

NAME–Last	First	Middle	Attending Physician	Chart No.

POST-DISCHARGE PLAN OF CARE

Reprinted with permission of Briggs Corporation, Des Moines, IA 50306; 800-247-2343

Figure 20-8 (Continued)

PROCEDURE 20-66
Discharging the Resident

1. Check with the nurse to be sure the resident has an order to be discharged.

2. Carry out each beginning procedure action.

3. Collect equipment:

   - Wheelchair
   - Cart to transport items to exit

4. Help the resident to dress if necessary.

5. Collect the resident's personal belongings and verify all items are present

   - Check them against the admission inventory list.
   - Help resident pack.
   - Check bathroom, closets, dressers, and bedside table for overlooked items.

6. Check with nurse to see if there are other items such as records, unused supplies, or medications that will go home with the resident.

7. Help resident into wheelchair and take resident to exit.

   - Help resident transfer into car.
   - Be sure all items go with resident.
   - Be gracious as you say good-bye.

8. Return wheelchair

9. Return to resident's room

   - Strip bed. Dispose of soiled linens.
   - Discard disposable items.

10. Notify housekeeping so room can be cleaned

11. Record discharge according to facility policy

    - Time
    - Method of transport
    - Person(s) accompanying resident
    - Resident's reaction
    - Signature

12. Report completion of procedure to nurse

---

setting. The therapist will make recommendations, if necessary, that may include:

- Rearranging rooms (e.g., turning the living room into the bedroom)
- Building a ramp from the outside entrance
- Installing a telephone that is accessible to the resident
- Renting equipment such as a seat for the shower or tub

- Suggesting safety measures, such as the removal of throw rugs and electrical cords on the floor

4. The interdisciplinary health care team will determine what the resident and family need to learn before discharge and who will be responsible for teaching. Some examples follow. Not all residents need all of these, and some residents will need teaching not included here.

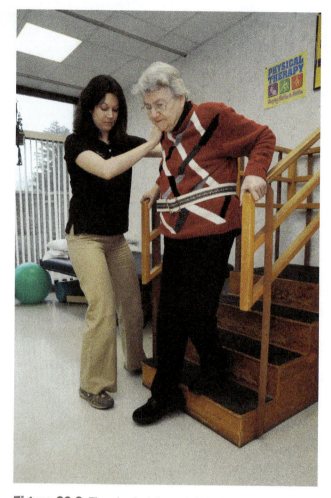

Figure 20-9 The physical therapist teaches the resident how to go up and down stairs in preparation for going home.

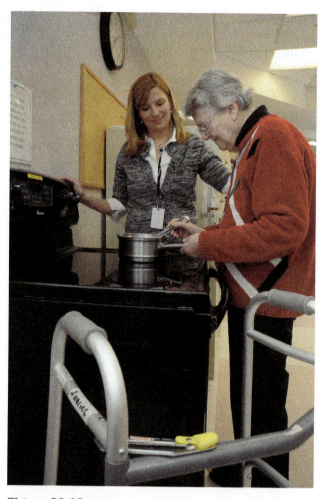

Figure 20-10 The occupational therapist teaches the resident how to manage ADL before she goes home.

- The physical therapist will teach the resident how to transfer in and out of bed, how to ambulate with an artificial leg (prosthesis), how to walk up and down stairs (Figure 20-9).

- The occupational therapist will teach the resident how to dress and undress, how to use the telephone, or how to cook (Figure 20-10).

5. The dietitian will teach the resident and family the basics of planning and preparing diabetic meals.

6. The nursing staff will teach the resident how to give his own insulin (Figure 20-11), how to check his blood sugar, how to recognize signs and symptoms of complications, or how to change a colostomy or wound dressings.

A discharge date will be arranged and all members of the team, including the resident and family, will strive to meet the goals that will enable the resident to return home.

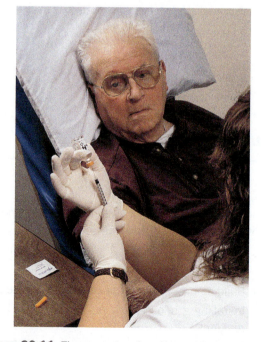

Figure 20-11 The nurse teaches the resident how to inject insulin.

? EXERCISE 20-5

COMPLETION

Complete the form to demonstrate your understanding of the activities of the interdisciplinary health care team. Select the correct team member from the list provided.

ACTION TEAM MEMBER

1. _____ makes recommendations about making telephones more accessible

2. _____ teaches resident and family the basics of planning and preparing special diets

3. _____ arranges for community services

4. _____ teaches resident how to give her/his own medicine

5. _____ teaches resident how to ambulate with an artificial leg

6. _____ teaches residents how to recognize complications of their conditions

7. _____ makes recommendations about building ramps

8. _____ teaches resident how to care for her or his own colostomy

9. _____ teaches resident how to use the telephone

10. _____ teaches resident how to dress and undress

11. _____ suggests safety measures such as removal of throw rugs

12. _____ teaches resident how to care for a wound dressing

a. social worker
b. physical therapist
c. occupational therapist
d. dietitian
e. nursing staff

? EXERCISE 20-6

CLINICAL SITUATION

1. Mr. Smith is being discharged to his son's home. List your actions to make this transition easier.

_____

_____

_____

_____

(8) LESSON SYNTHESIS: Putting It All Together

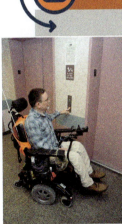

You have just completed this lesson. Now go back and review the Clinical Focus. Try to see how the Clinical Focus relates to the concepts presented in the lesson. Then answer the following questions.

1. Would you expect Mr. Tyler to feel anxiety on admission to the long-term care facility? What is a likely reason for this anxiety? How may the interdisciplinary team help Mr. Tyler to overcome this anxiety?

2. How can you make him feel more comfortable and secure in his new environment?

3. What information would you want to learn about Mr. Tyler's present condition? How will you do this?

4. How will the nursing staff use the information that you obtain in formulating a care plan that is appropriate for this resident?

20 REVIEW

A. Select the one best answer for each of the following.

1. Most residents are admitted to long-term care facilities because

(A) their families no longer want to deal with them

(B) the resident no longer wants the responsibility of keeping up a home

(C) the resident is tired and needs rest

(D) the resident requires health care services

2. When the resident is admitted, the nursing assistant is responsible for gathering the following information upon admission to the facility:

(A) food likes and dislikes

(B) disease diagnoses

(C) family contacts

(D) vital signs, weight, and height

3. The length of hospital stays for acute illness is limited because

(A) of staff shortages

(B) of the inconvenience to the family

(C) of diagnosis-related groups

(D) the resident wants to go home

4. Before admission, the family will need to

(A) choose a facility if the resident is unable to do so

(B) draw the resident's money out of the bank

(C) sell the resident's home

(D) try to care for the resident at home

5. The members of the interdisciplinary health care team will obtain assessments of new residents for the purpose of

(A) starting the plan of care

(B) keeping the resident busy

(C) making the family think the staff is attentive

(D) determining the cost of the resident's stay

6. When a new resident is admitted, the nursing assistant will do all but

(A) take the resident's vital signs

(B) weigh and measure the resident

(C) help the resident put away personal possessions

(D) charge the resident for the care

7. When a resident is transferred from one nursing unit to another within the facility, the nursing assistant will

(A) move the resident's belongings to the new room

(B) give the resident any medication that is due before moving

(C) call the resident's family for permission before moving the resident

(D) move all the furniture in the room to the new room

8. Residents may be discharged because they

(A) have improved enough to go home

(B) have complained to the administrator

(C) want special items for breakfast every day

(D) are difficult to care for

9. Community services include all but

(A) services of a registered nurse

(B) home-delivered meals

(C) services of a home health aide

(D) taking the resident to the movies

10. Community services are usually coordinated and arranged for by the

(A) administrator

(B) family

(C) director of nursing

(D) social worker

B. Answer each statement true (T) or false (F)

11. T F First impressions of the family and resident are extremely important.

12. T F The hospital discharge planner selects the long-term care facility for patients who need that service.

13. T F The family may need to apply for Medicaid if the resident has exhausted his funds.

14. T F Copies of the Residents' Rights are only given to residents who are able to read and understand them.

15. T F The physician makes out the personal inventory after the resident is admitted.

16. T F Residents are advised not to bring any personal possessions with them to the long-term care facility.

17. T F A resident may be transferred to another room because of friction between roommates.

18. T F Some admissions to long-term care facilities are considered permanent.

19. T F Families are discouraged from visiting residents.

20. T F Most families have concerns about admitting a family member to a long-term care facility.

WARM AND COLD APPLICATIONS

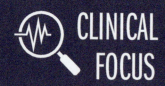 **CLINICAL FOCUS**

Think about the reasons for warm and cold applications and the safety precautions to observe when they are carried out as you study this lesson.

OBJECTIVES

After studying this lesson, you should be able to:

• Define vocabulary words and terms.

• State the effects of warm and cold applications.

• Give reasons why warm and cold applications may be ordered.

• Describe precautions in carrying out warm and cold application procedures.

• Demonstrate the following:
 Procedure 21-67   Applying a Disposable or Reusable Cold Pack
 Procedure 21-68   Applying an Ice Bag

VOCABULARY

asepto syringe (ay-SEP-toh sih-RINJ)
diathermy (DIE-ah-ther-mee)
hypothermia (high-poh-THER-mee-ah)
ice bag (ise bag)

vasoconstriction (vas-oh-kon-STRICK-shun)
vasodilation (vas-oh-die-LAY-shun)
warm soak (war m sohk)
wet compress (wet KOM-press)

CASE STUDY

Mr. Lipskin is assigned to your care. He tires easily and is returned to his bed for rest in the afternoon. As he was getting into bed, he slipped and hit his forearm against the side of the bed. To counteract pain and swelling from the injury, a disposable cold pack is ordered and applied to his arm.

Warm and cold applications require a physician's order. Some facilities permit only licensed care providers to perform warm and cold applications. In other facilities, nursing assistants are permitted to carry out these procedures under the supervision of the nurse. All warm and cold applications must be performed carefully to prevent injury to the resident. *Be sure you know and follow the policy of your facility and are adequately prepared and supervised.*

Older people have less sensitivity to changes in temperature. They may not realize when an application is too hot or cold. If the temperature is too high, burns may result. Other types of tissue damage may occur if the temperature is too cold. Warm and cold applications that are left on too long can also cause damage.

SAFETY

The older resident has a more complex response to pain than a younger person because pain can come from a variety of causes and conditions. However, older persons are at greater risk for injury from heat or cold therapies. *Note: Heat is especially dangerous.* When using warm or cold applications on older residents, it is very important that you:

- Check the area to be treated against the same area on the other limb. Observe the appearance of the skin before, during, and after the treatment. Report your observations to the nurse.
- Frequently check the area that is being treated, every 3 to 5 minutes.
- Report unusual changes. You should check for excessive redness, blanching (whitening), or other discoloration. Report any complaints of discomfort, numbness, or pain.
- Do not rely on the resident's ability to inform you of any problems; check carefully yourself. The resident may not be aware that a problem exists.
- Follow facility policy for discontinuing the treatment.

Applications of warm and cold may be either moist or dry (Figure 21-1). Moisture makes both heat and cold deeper and more penetrating. Therefore, moist heat or moist cold is more likely to cause injury. Extra care must be taken to protect the resident when moist treatments are used. Be sure you know:

- Exact method to be used
- Correct temperature and placement
- Proper length of time the warm or cold application is to be performed

Dry Warm Applications
Disposable warm pack

Moist Warm Applications
Warm soaks

Compresses

Tub bath

Sitz bath

Dry Cold Applications
Ice cap

Ice bag

Disposable cold pack

Moist Cold Applications
Compresses

Soaks

Figure 21-1 Types of warm and cold applications.

- How often to check the area being treated
- Never put packs in direct contact with the skin

COMMERCIAL PREPARATIONS

Easy-to-use commercial warm and cold packs are available for dry applications. Read the directions, for one type of pack, a single blow to the pack before application activates the heat or cold, while some other packs are twisted. The pack is discarded after one use.

Reusable packs are also available, but infection control issues make them less desirable.

USE OF WARM APPLICATIONS

Warm applications are ordered to:
- Relieve muscle spasms
- Reduce pain
- Decrease joint stiffness
- Promote healing
- Combat local infection
- Decrease tissue swelling
- Improve mobility before exercise periods
- Soothe the resident

The value of heat treatments (diathermy) lies in the fact that heat dilates or increases the size of blood vessels (vasodilation). This brings more blood to the area to promote healing. Warmth is very soothing when there is pain.

There must be a specific order for a warm application. Some groups of people require extra care when they receive warm applications (Figure 21-2).

> **Caution: Consider the age and condition of the resident when using warm or cold treatments.**
>
> **Proceed with caution with:**
> - Elderly residents
> - Uncooperative residents
> - Unconscious residents
> - Paralyzed residents
> - Residents with tissue damage
> - Residents with very thin skin
> - Residents with poor circulation

Figure 21-2 Use caution when applying warm and cold treatments.

Cautions

Follow these cautions when working with residents.

- Constant warmth must be carefully monitored.
- Moisture intensifies the effect of warmth. Use extra caution.
- Never allow a resident to lie on a constant heat unit, because heat may be trapped and build up to dangerous levels.
- Temperature of a constant heat unit should be between 95° and 100°F.
- Always use a bath thermometer to check solution temperatures.
- Always remove the body part being soaked before adding warm solution.

- Always stay with the resident during the treatment.
- Protect areas not being treated from excessive exposure.
- Warmth is not applied to the head because it could cause blood vessels in the area to dilate, resulting in headaches.
- Rubber or plastic should never touch the resident's skin. Be sure all appliances are covered with cloth.

Moist Warm Applications

Any warm application will be applied by a therapist or therapy assistant. Moisture intensifies heat and requires extra care. For each of the warm treatments, the therapist will follow the facility policy for:

- Method of applying the treatment
- Length of time treatment is to be applied
- How often resident is to be checked for condition of skin in the treatment area and general response to the treatment
- Signs that treatment should be discontinued

Moist warm treatments that a CNA may assist with include:

- **Warm soaks**—The resident, or the part of the resident's body that is being treated, is immersed in a tub filled with water at a specific temperature, usually 105°F.
- **Wet compresses**—Wet compresses are moistened with a solution and placed on the affected area.
  - An **asepto syringe** may be used to add water to the compresses to keep them moist.

? EXERCISE 21-1

COMPLETION

Complete the following statements by writing in the correct words.

1. Three facts the nursing assistant must know before administering any heat treatment are:

   a. _____

   b. _____

   c. _____

2. Four reasons that heat applications are ordered include:

   a. _____

   b. _____

   c. _____

   d. _____

(continues)

3. Six situations that require extra watchfulness when giving heat and cold treatments include giving treatments to residents who are:

   a. _____

   b. _____

   c. _____

   d. _____

   e. _____

   f. _____

4. Two ways to apply moist heat include:

   a. _____

   b. _____

USE OF COLD APPLICATIONS

Applications of cold are given only with a physician's order. The application of cold:

- Constricts or decreases the size of blood vessels (**vasoconstriction**) and reduces swelling
- Decreases sensitivity to pain
- Reduces temperature
- Slows inflammation
- Reduces itching

Cautions

Moisture intensifies the effect of cold just as it does heat. Caution must be used in the application of moist cold.

- Excessive cold can damage body tissues.
- Report color changes such as blanching (turning white) or cyanosis (becoming bluish).
- Report feelings of numbness or discomfort experienced by resident.
- Stop the cold treatment if shivering develops. Cover resident with blanket and report immediately to the nurse. Cold applications may be dry or moist.

Dry Cold Applications

Several methods exist for applying therapeutic cold. For the elderly, careful attention to the application is required to prevent injury.

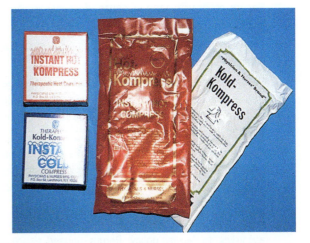

Figure 21-3 Examples of heat and cold disposable packs before activating the chemicals.

- **Disposable cold pack**—This single-use commercial pack can be stored until needed (Figure 21-3). Reusable commercial packs are also available (for both warm and cold applications). The pack remains effective for approximately 15 to 30 minutes. If the cold pack must be activated, follow the manufacturer's instructions exactly. When activating the pack, do not hold it in front of your face. If a leak occurs, the chemicals inside the pack may splash. Check the area being treated every 10 minutes.
- **Ice bag**—The reusable waterproof canvas container can be filled with ice to provide temporary local cold. An ice bag is never placed directly on the affected area because the weight of the bag will cause the resident discomfort.

PROCEDURE 21-67
Applying a Disposable or Reusable Cold Pack

1. Carry out each beginning procedure action.

2. Assemble equipment:

   - Disposable, commercial cold pack

   - Cloth covering (towel, warm water bag cover, or other cover specified by the facility)

   - Tape or rolls of gauze

3. Expose area to be treated. Note condition of area.

4. Place cold pack in cloth covering.

5. If disposable, strike or squeeze cold pack to activate chemicals. (Follow manufacturer's instructions). If using a gel pack procure from the freezer.

6. Place covered cold pack on proper area and cover with a towel (Figure 21-4). Note time of application.

7. Secure cover with tape or gauze, if necessary, to hold in place.

8. Leave resident in comfortable position with call light within easy reach.

9. Return to bedside every 10 minutes. Check area being treated for discoloration or numbness. If these signs and symptoms occur, discontinue treatment and report them to your supervisor.

10. If no adverse symptoms occur, remove pack in 20 minutes, or after amount of time given in your instructions. Note condition of area. Continuous treatment requires application of a fresh pack.

11. Remove pack from cover and if disposable type discard according to facility policy. Return unused gauze and tape. Reusable gel packs should be cleansed according to facility policy and returned to the freezer storage area.

12. Put cover in laundry hamper.

13. Carry out each procedure completion action.

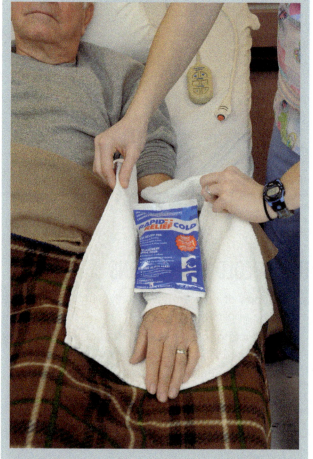

Figure 21-4 Once the cold pack is in place, cover the entire application with a towel.

PROCEDURE 21-68
Applying an Ice Bag

1. Carry out each beginning procedure action.

2. Assemble equipment:

   - Ice bag

   - Cover (usually cotton, such as a towel, or cover specified by your facility)

   - Paper towels

(continues)

PROCEDURE 21-68
Applying an Ice Bag (Continued)

- Spoon or similar utensil
- Ice cubes or crushed ice

3. Prepare ice bag as follows:

    a. Fill ice bag with cold water and check for leaks.

    b. Empty the bag.

    c. If ice cubes are used, rinse them in water to remove sharp edges. The use of crushed ice gives more flexibility to the bag and is more comfortable for the resident.

    d. Fill ice bag one-half to two-thirds full, using ice scooper, paper cup, or large spoon (Figure 21-5). Avoid making ice bags too heavy. Do not allow scoop to touch ice bag.

    e. To remove air from ice bag:

        - Rest ice bag flat on a paper towel on a flat surface.

        - Put top in place, but do not screw on.

        - Press bag until air is removed.

    f. Fasten top securely.

    g. Test for leakage.

    h. Wipe dry with paper towels. Place in cloth cover.

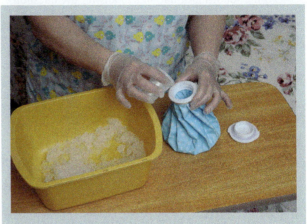

Figure 21-5 Fill ice bag half full.

NOTE: As an alternative, a gel pack stored in the freezer can be used for cold applications. These packs can be refrozen and reused if this is the facility policy.

4. Apply ice bag to the affected part. Make sure that the skin is protected by a towel before applying the cold pack.

5. Refill ice bag before all ice is melted.

6. Check skin area under the ice bag every 10 minutes. Report to supervising nurse immediately if skin is discolored or white or if resident reports skin is numb.

7. Continue the cold application for the amount of time specified by your supervisor, usually 20 minutes. If the resident feels cold, cover with a blanket, but do not cover the area being treated.

8. Carry out each procedure completion action.

9. When the treatment is complete, wash the bag with soap and water, rinse, dry completely, and then screw top on. Wipe with a disinfectant if this is your facility policy. Leave air in ice bag to prevent sides from sticking together.

10. If a reusable cold pack is used, wash it thoroughly with soap and water or wipe with a disinfectant, according to facility policy. Return pack to the refrigerator. Discard a disposable pack.

? EXERCISE 21-2

CLINICAL SITUATION
Read the following situation and answer the questions.

Mrs. Rose fell and hurt her wrist. The nurse asked you to place an ice pack on it for her. Complete the statements regarding her care.

1. The ice used should be _____ or _____.
2. When filling the ice cap, always handle the ice with _____.
3. The ice cap should be filled _____ full.
4. Make sure to always expel _____ from the ice bag before closing.
5. Always test the ice bag for _____.
6. The ice cap must be covered with _____.
7. Make sure the metal cap is _____ on the affected part.
8. Report to the nurse if you notice the skin is _____ or _____, or if the resident reports the skin is _____.
9. After use, the ice bag should be washed with _____ and allowed to dry.
10. Air is left in the clean ice bag to _____.

Moist Cold Application

Wet compresses—the same cautions apply to cold as to warm compresses. They may be kept wet with an asepto syringe and cold by placing a covered ice bag against the area that is affected.

Follow facility policy for:

- Method of applying the treatment
- Length of time treatment is to be applied
- How often resident is to be checked for condition of skin in the treatment area and general response to the treatment
- Signs that treatment should be discontinued

? EXERCISE 21-3

COMPLETION
Complete the following statements by writing in the correct words.

1. Before capping, ice bags should not be filled more than _____.
2. In some facilities, only _____ nursing assistants are permitted to carry out heat and cold procedures.
3. Heat applications are especially _____.
4. Never rely on the resident's ability to inform you of _____ related to heat and cold.
5. The area being treated needs to be checked _____.
6. The temperature of heat treatment solutions should always be checked with a _____.
7. Rubber or plastic should _____ touch the resident's _____.
8. Moist treatments present the _____ danger because moisture _____ either heat or cold.
9. A good way to keep wet compresses moist is to add water with an _____.
10. When giving a warm arm soak, the temperature of the water should be checked _____.
11. When adding water to a warm soak treatment, always _____ the part being soaked before _____ water.

(continues)

? EXERCISE 21-3 (Continued)

12. To activate a disposable cold pack, the nursing assistant should _____ the cold pack.

13. A disposable cold pack should be removed within _____ minutes.

14. An acceptable way to secure a disposable cold pack in place is to use _____ and _____.

15. Before beginning any procedure, you must always wash your _____.

16. If there is potential for contact with body secretions or discharges, the nursing assistant must always wear _____.

17. Disposable cold packs are effective for approximately _____ minutes.

18. Packs should never be in _____ contact with skin.

19. When activating a disposable pack do not hold it in front of your _____.

20. _____ refers to the skin turning white.

21. Cyanosis refers to the skin turning _____.

LESSON SYNTHESIS: Putting It All Together

You have just completed this lesson. Now go back and review the Clinical Focus. Try to see how the Clinical Focus relates to the concepts presented in the lesson. Then answer the following questions.

1. How was the disposable cold pack activated?
2. How might it have been secured in place?
3. Is the pack placed directly on the area of the body to be treated?
4. How often should you check the area in contact with the pack?
5. What signs or symptoms should be reported to the nurse during the treatment?

21 REVIEW

A. Write the definition for each of the following terms.

1. diathermy _____
2. warm soak _____
3. vasoconstriction _____
4. vasodilation _____
5. ice bag _____

B. Answer each statement true (T) or false (F).

6. T F Warm and cold treatments are part of the job description for all nursing assistants.

7. T F Older persons are usually more sensitive to warm and cold treatments.

8. T F A physician's order is required for all warm and cold applications.

9. T F Moisture increases the effect of both warm and cold treatments.

10. T F Heat may be applied to the head because it causes vasoconstriction and relieves headache.

11. T F All heat or cold appliances must be covered with cloth so that rubber or plastic never touches the skin.

12. T F Residents should not be left alone when receiving a heat treatment.

13. T F Always place a filled ice bag on top of the area being treated.

C. Select the one best answer for each of the following.

14. Which resident is at greatest risk for injury during a heat treatment?

a. resident who is conscious

b. resident who is cooperative

c. resident who is paralyzed

d. resident who has warm pink skin

15. Ice bags are

a. filled to the top

b. partially filled with air before adding ice

c. filled with the largest ice cubes

d. tested for leaks before filling

D. Clinical Situations

16. Mrs. Maupin has an order for a diathermy to be applied for back pain. Shauna, the nursing assistant, notes that her lower back has become discolored and is more painful. What action should Shauna take?

17. Shauna's supervisor tells her to apply cold to Mrs. Bronson's injured ankle. Shauna replies that she needs more information to give proper care to Mrs. Bronson. What information does Shauna need?

Introduction to Restorative Care

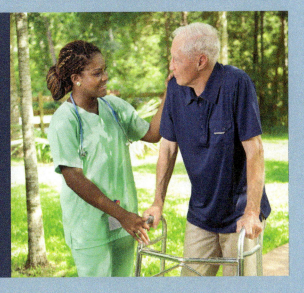

RESTORATIVE AND REHABILITATIVE CARE OF THE RESIDENT

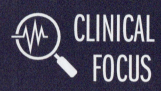

CLINICAL FOCUS

Think about the care you would give to residents with disorders for which restorative care is appropriate as you study this lesson.

OBJECTIVES

After studying this lesson, you should be able to:

- Define vocabulary words and terms.

- List the complications associated with inactivity.

- Describe the reasons why some residents have self-care deficits.

- Describe the principles of restorative care.

- Explain the benefits of restorative care.

- Describe the responsibilities of the nursing assistant for implementing restorative care.

- State the guidelines for doing passive range-of-motion exercises.

- State the guidelines for positioning residents in bed and chair.

- Describe the purpose of an orthosis.

- List the reasons for implementing bowel and bladder programs.

- Describe the responsibilities of the nursing assistant for implementing bowel and bladder programs.

- Explain correct body mechanics for carrying out all procedures in this lesson.

- Demonstrate the following:
  Procedure 22-69   Passive Range-of-Motion Exercises
  Procedure 22-70   Moving the Resident in Bed

CASE STUDY

Mrs. Murphy was admitted to the facility while on your day off. She is 5 feet, 9 inches tall, with a heavy frame. She is 78 years old and had a stroke 2 months ago. She is unable to use her left arm or leg. Mrs. Murphy is relearning mobility skills and how to perform the activities of daily living. You are assigned to care for her and must assist her in these tasks.

VOCABULARY

active assistive range of motion (ACK-tiv ah-SIS-tiv rainj of MOH-shun)

active range of motion (ACK-tiv rainj of MOH-shun)

activities of daily living (ADLs) (ack-TIV-ih-tees of DAY-lee LIV-ing)

adaptive devices (ah-DAP-tiv dih-VICE-es)

amputation (am-pyou-TAY-shun)

arthritis (are-THRIGH-tis)

atrophy (AT-roh-fee)

body alignment (BAH-dee ah-LINE-ment)

chronic disease (KRON-ick dih-ZEEZ)

contracture (kon-TRACK-shur)

deconditioned (dee-kon-DISH-und)

disability (dis-ah-BILL-ih-tee)

dislocation (dis-loh-KAY-shun)

disorientation (dis-oh-ree-en-TAY-shun)

embolus (EM-boh-lus)

flaccid (FLASS-id)

footboard (FOOT-bord)

functional ability (FUNK-shun-al ah-BILL-ih tee)

functional incontinence (FUNK-shun-al in-KON-tin-ens)

goniometer (gah-nee-AH-meh-ter)

hemiplegia (hem-ee-PLEE-jee-ah)

incontinence (in-KON-tin-ens)

instrumental activities of daily living (IADLs) (in-strew-MEN-tal ack-TIV-ih-tees of DAY-lee LIV-ing)

interdisciplinary health care team (in-ter-DISS-ih-plin-air-ee helth kair teem)

lateral (LAT-er-al)

mixed incontinence (mixed in-KON-tin-ens)

mobility skills (moh-BILL-ih-tee skills)

orthosis (or-THOH-sis)

orthostatic hypotension (or-tho-STAT-ik high-po-TEN-shun)

osteoporosis (oss-tee-oh-poh-ROH-sis)

overflow incontinence (o-ver-flo in-KON-tin-ens)

paralysis (pah-RAL-ih-sis)

paraplegia (pair-ah-PLEE-jee-ah)

passive range of motion (PASS-iv rainj of MOH-shun)

perceptual deficit (per-SEP-tyou-al DEF-ih-sit)

pneumonia (new-MOH-nee-ah)

postural hypotension (POS-tur-al HIGH-po-ten-shun)

postural support (POS-chur-al sup-PORT)

pressure ulcer (PRESH-ur UL-sir)

progressive mobilization (proh-GRESS-iv moh-bill-ih-ZAY-shun)

prone (prohn)

protraction (proh-TRACK-shun)

quadriplegia (kwahd-rih-PLEE-jee-ah)

rehabilitation (ree-hah-bill-ih-TAY-shun)

residual limb (rih-ZID-you-al lim)

restorative care (ree-STOR-ah-tiv kair)

retraction (ree-TRACK-shun)

self range of motion (self rainj of MOH-shun)

sensory deprivation (SEN-soh-ree deh-prih-VAY-shun)

sensory stimulation (SEN-soh-ree stim-you-LAY-shun)

shearing (SHEER-ing)

sling (sling)

spasticity (spas-TIS-ih-tee)

splint (splint)

strengths (strenths)

stress incontinence (stres in-KON-tin-ens)

subluxation (sub-luck-SAY-shun)

supine (SOO-pine)

task segmentation (task seg-men-TAY-shun)

thrombus (THROM-bus)

turning sheet (TURN-ing sheet)

urge incontinence (urg in-KON-tin-ens)

RESTORATIVE CARE AND THE INTERDISCIPLINARY HEALTH CARE TEAM

Restorative care is a process in which the interdisciplinary health care team assists the resident to reach an optimal level of ability.

Several sections of OBRA refer to restorative care. The Residents' Rights state that the residents' independence must be promoted. The section on nursing assistant training requires that all nursing assistant courses include basic restorative skills. These include:

- Training of the resident in self-care according to the resident's abilities
- Assisting residents in transferring, ambulating, eating, and dressing
- Maintenance of range of motion
- Proper turning and positioning in bed and chair
- Bowel and bladder training
- Care and use of prostheses and orthoses

The Minimum Data Set (MDS) 3.0 includes a section on physical functioning and structural problems. The nurse is responsible for collecting these data, but the nursing assistants can provide valuable information about the resident's abilities.

Restorative care and rehabilitation are similar and in many cases identical. Some of the differences are that:

- **Rehabilitation** involves the skills of therapists including any or all of these individuals: physical therapist, occupational therapist, speech/language pathologist.
- Rehabilitation is more intense and is time-limited, such as physical, occupational, and speech. That means the resident is working harder to meet a goal with a definite time limit. Medicare covers the cost of the therapists' services for a specified period of time or as long as progress is made.
- Rehabilitation nurses coordinate the care and services of the residents in rehabilitation programs. They work with the therapists to see that the programs are carried out consistently 24 hours a day.
- Rehabilitation is a specialized health care service. Many skilled care facilities now employ full-time therapists and other rehabilitation (restorative) staff to meet the needs of residents. As a nursing assistant, you may be given additional training

to work with the professionals in the rehabilitation department.

- Restorative care is a nursing responsibility with assistance from other members of the interdisciplinary health care team. Nurses assess the residents and plan restorative programs. The nursing assistants implement the programs.

Restorative care is successful when members of the team:

- Have a positive attitude about the residents and their capabilities
- Have confidence in their own abilities as care providers
- Are willing to learn from other care providers, residents, and their families
- Learn to think creatively to increase residents' quality of life
- Cooperate with other staff as team members
- Realize that "ideal" working situations seldom exist, but attempt to bring "ideal" and "real" closer together through problem-solving techniques
- Continually learn and acquire new skills by participating in educational programs

PURPOSES OF RESTORATIVE AND REHABILITATIVE CARE

All nursing care should be considered restorative care. The interdisciplinary health care team is concerned with:

- Increasing the resident's physical abilities. This may include mobility skills (the ability to move from one place to another) and the ability to care for oneself (Figure 22-1).
- Preventing complications that result from mental and physical inactivity
- Maintaining the resident's current abilities
- Helping the resident adapt to limitations imposed by a disability (the inability to perform certain activities because of a physical or mental impairment)
- Increasing the resident's quality of life

Many of the residents receiving rehabilitation will be discharged from the facility. Some of the residents receiving restorative care will also be able to go home.

Some of the residents living in long-term care facilities will never be able to return to their homes.

Federal regulations mandate that the resident is to attain or maintain the highest level of function possible. Surveys are based on identification of risks and preventable decline. If decline occurs, it must be evident that everything possible was done to prevent it.

People need hope and quality in their lives, even when they are living with a **chronic disease** (a disease or condition that is permanent). If residents are forced to be dependent and are not allowed to make decisions, then there is little reason for living.

Restorative care provides hope and quality by empowering the resident, that is, encouraging and allowing the resident to be as independent as possible. There may be reasons why some residents really cannot do things for themselves. In these cases, the team must do for residents what they are unable to do for themselves. However, the residents should still be allowed to make decisions regarding their care. If residents are no longer mentally competent to make decisions, the team will be responsible for all aspects of their care.

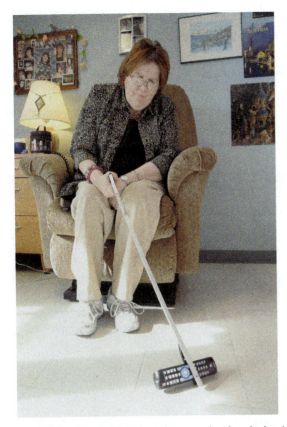

Figure 22-1 This resident is using an adaptive device to increase her independence.

For this reason, the staff may feel it is pointless to try to improve their abilities.

When residents are admitted to long-term care facilities, "good care" does not mean that the health care providers will do everything for the residents. It is to promote independent actions as much as possible. In a short period of time, this approach will result in residents becoming helpless. In other words:

- Residents are stripped of all motivation for independence. They have no reason to act independently.

- Muscles weaken and atrophy, circulation slows down, and all body systems gradually lose the ability to function. Both mind and body deteriorate.

- When residents are placed in positions of dependency, they also lose their self-esteem. They no longer see themselves as people of value.

- Residents become disinterested in what is happening around them. Life has little meaning; they may become depressed.

- Residents' needs should be continually assessed. The level of response is ongoing. Measures that are not effective now may be successful in 3 to 6 months.

Principles for Restorative and Rehabilitative Care

The following principles provide the foundation for restorative care:

1. **Begin treatment as soon as possible.** This means that plans for maintaining or increasing the resident's level of independence are made as soon as the resident is admitted to the facility.

2. **Stress the resident's ability, not disability.** The resident's **strengths** are used to help the resident adapt to any limitations. This means that care providers think in terms of what the resident can do, not what the resident cannot do.

3. **Activity strengthens and inactivity weakens.** Complications result from physical and mental inactivity. These can cause further disability or even be life-threatening.

4. **Treat the whole person.** It is important to attend to the residents' emotional and mental health needs as well as their physical well-being. The interdisciplinary team also works with the residents' families. Families directly influence the emotional and mental health of the residents.

PREVENTING COMPLICATIONS FROM INACTIVITY

Restorative and rehabilitative care attempts to prevent the complications that result from inactivity. These complications can affect older persons more quickly than younger persons because of the changes that are taking place in their bodies. Refer to Table 22-1 for a summary of possible complications and preventive nursing assistant actions.

ACTIVITIES OF DAILY LIVING

One purpose of restorative care is to increase the resident's physical abilities. This includes mobility skills and the ability to carry out activities of daily living (ADLs).

Complications by Body System	Prevention
Musculoskeletal System	
• Muscles become weak and atrophy. This means that muscles that are not used shrink and become useless (Figure 22-2). • Contractures can develop, making movement impossible. The joints become stiff when they are not moved. In a short time the tissue around the joints also stiffens. Soon the joint cannot be moved at all (Figure 22-2) **Figure 22-2** Contractures are a complication of immobility.	• Carry out exercise programs planned for the residents' capabilities. • Do range-of-motion exercises. • Use correct positioning techniques when in bed or sitting up. • Use splints and other devices to maintain the proper joint position.
Musculoskeletal System	
• Osteoporosis may develop with nonuse during exercise. When the legs do not bear weight, calcium begins to leave the bones and enter the bloodstream. This causes brittle bones; fractures may occur without reason. Both men and women can develop osteoporosis.	• Offer the resident opportunities to stand and bear weight on the legs, for example, during transfer procedures.
Integumentary System	
• Pressure ulcers may develop over a joint, where two bones meet such as the hip, elbow, or shoulder or areas where the bone is in close proximity to the skin (tail bone at the base of the spine). If a resident sits or lies on one spot, blood cannot circulate to that area. The cells in the skin and tissue begin to die, causing an ulcer to develop (Figure 22-3). **Figure 22-3** Pressure ulcers are also a complication of immobility.	• Reposition the resident every 1 or 2 hours. • Do range-of-motion exercises twice a day. • Provide adequate nutrition and fluids. • Observe skin frequently to note any signs of pressure. • Use pressure-relieving devices. (See Lesson 16.)

Table 22-1 Complications Resulting from Inactivity

(continues)

Complications by Body System	Prevention
Cardiovascular System	
• The heart becomes deconditioned. The heart is a muscle and weakens when the body is inactive. In its weakened state, the heart takes longer to return to a normal pace after activity. If this happens, the resident must rest between physical activities. • Blood does not circulate as efficiently. This can lead to embolus and thrombus. A thrombus is a blood clot that forms in a blood vessel. If the thrombus breaks loose and moves through the circulatory system, it is called an embolus. • Because of changes in the cardiovascular and nervous systems, residents who assume a sitting or standing position too rapidly may experience dizziness due to drop in blood pressure. Blood pools in the lower portion of the body below the heart and does not reach the brain quickly enough. This is referred to as orthostatic hypotension or postural hypotension. Certain medications that are used to treat high blood pressure also may precipitate this condition. When a person has been in bed for long periods of time or is taking medications to lower the blood pressure, get the resident up slowly. First, allow the resident to sit on the side of the bed; ask if they are experiencing any dizziness. If not, proceed to slowly get them out of bed.	• Follow all instructions for assisting the resident with ambulation (walking) and exercise programs. • Follow all instructions for ambulation and exercise.
Respiratory System	
• The lungs do not expand as efficiently when a resident is immobile. Secretions collect in the lungs and bacteria grow in the secretions, causing pneumonia, an infection of the lungs.	• Provide the resident with fluids to drink. • Position the resident so the lungs can expand. • Encourage the resident to take deep breaths.
Gastrointestinal System	
• Without exercise or activity, the appetite decreases, causing weight loss. • Risk of pressure ulcers increases with weight loss and lack of nutrition. • Peristalsis slows down, causing indigestion and constipation (the inability to move the bowels).	• Tell the nurse if the resident likes or dislikes certain foods. • Encourage resident to drink adequate fluids. • Assist the resident with ambulation and exercise. • Assist the resident to develop a bowel elimination schedule. Provide privacy for toileting.
Urinary System	
• The bladder does not always empty completely if a person is not able to sit properly on the toilet or commode. This increases the risk of bladder infection. • Incontinence can result from inability to get to the bathroom. • Urinary stones may develop from the calcium in the bloodstream resulting from osteoporosis.	• Encourage adequate fluid intake. • Assist the resident to the toilet regularly and provide privacy.
Psychosocial Reactions	
• Depression can occur from physical and mental inactivity. Depression is an emotional condition that causes the resident to be slow to respond to questions, retreats to his or her room, does not join in activities, and is sad and lonely. • Inactivity and sensory deprivation can lead to disorientation. Sensory deprivation occurs when there is a lack of stimulation to the senses—vision, hearing, smelling, tasting, and touching. A person who is disoriented is confused about time, place, and who he or she is.	• Cooperate with activities department to provide sensory stimulation programs. These are activities that increase the resident's awareness of the surroundings.

Table 22-1 (Continued)

These are the tasks that adults do throughout a day to meet their basic needs. The ADLs are:

- Bathing
- Grooming—hair care, nail care, oral care, shaving, and applying makeup
- Dressing and undressing
- Eating
- Toileting
- Mobility (the ability to move about)

ADLs are taught to people when they are children. Healthy adults do these tasks automatically. If the resident cannot complete any or all of the ADLs, a self-care deficit exists. A self-care deficit may be due to:

- Diseases such as multiple sclerosis, arthritis, Parkinson's disease, Alzheimer's disease, or cerebral palsy
- A stroke or injuries that have damaged the brain or spinal cord
- Vision impairment
- Emotional illness
- Fractured extremity

Problems can result from these conditions that limit the resident's ability to do self-care. Examples of these problems are:

- Decreased strength
- Lack of endurance
- Limited range of motion
- **Paralysis**
- **Perceptual deficits**
- Depression
- Disorientation

Paralysis occurs because of damage to the brain or spinal cord. It means the resident cannot move one or more of the extremities. Brain damage from a stroke frequently causes **hemiplegia**, which means paralysis on one side of the body. Spinal cord injuries can cause **quadriplegia** (paralysis from the neck down) or **paraplegia** (paralysis from the waist down).

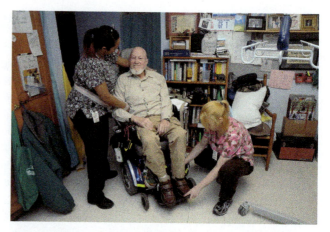

Figure 22-4 Brain damage from a stroke may cause paralysis.

Perceptual deficits usually occur because of damage to the brain from disease or injury (Figure 22-4). Examples of perceptual deficits include the inability to:

- Organize a task. ADLs cannot be completed unless the resident is able to prepare for the task, get the necessary items together, and then complete the task.
- Sequence a task. A resident with this inability may put on a dress before the slip or shoes before the socks.
- Exercise judgment. This deficit may be noted if a resident puts on a wool coat in hot weather, when appropriate clothing is available.
- Identify common objects such as eating utensils and grooming items. When this occurs, the resident may look at a fork, but not know what it is.
- Use common items. The resident may be able to identify an item such as a comb or toothbrush, but be unable to pick it up and use it, even though there is no physical reason for the problem.
- Initiate or start a task without assistance.

? EXERCISE 22-1

COMPLETION

Select the correct term(s) from the following list to complete each statement.

optimum   self-care deficit
brain   spinal cord
strengths
tasks
judgments

(continues)

? EXERCISE 22-1 (Continued)

1. Restorative care is a process in which the resident is assisted to reach a(an) _____ level of ability.

2. When a person cannot carry out any of the activities of daily living, he or she is said to have a(an)

   _____.

3. It is important to stress a resident's _____ rather than his or her disabilities.

4. Paralysis occurs because of damage to the _____ or _____.

5. The resident with perceptual deficit may be unable to organize _____ or exercise _____.

INSTRUMENTAL ACTIVITIES OF DAILY LIVING

Higher-level tasks are called **instrumental activities of daily living** or **IADLs**. These include skills that adults need to function independently. Examples of IADLs include:

- Managing money
- Managing a household
- Driving a car

In some situations the adult may not be able to physically complete these tasks but is able to competently direct others to do so.

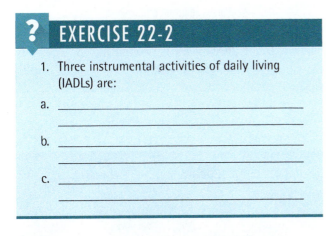

? EXERCISE 22-2

1. Three instrumental activities of daily living (IADLs) are:

   a. _____
      _____

   b. _____
      _____

   c. _____
      _____

SETTING UP RESTORATIVE PROGRAMS

Residents with self-care deficits are evaluated by therapists and nurses. The results of the evaluation will determine whether a resident's **functional ability** (ability to do ADLs) can be increased. In other words, can the interdisciplinary team help this resident to relearn ADLs?

- This is discussed with the resident and the family. If the resident, family, and staff agree that the resident's physical abilities can be increased, then a restorative program is planned by the interdisciplinary team.

- The members of the interdisciplinary team meet together at the care plan conference. Methods for solving the resident's problems and concerns are discussed with the resident and family.

When the resident is unable to do any ADLs independently, it is generally best to concentrate on relearning just one ADL at a time. The first step is to find out what the resident wants to work on first. The interdisciplinary team then works with the resident and family to plan the process. They will:

- Establish goals.
- Each ADL consists of several steps. This is called **task segmentation** (Table 22-2).
- The resident will not be able to do all steps right away. Some residents may never be able to do all of the steps.
- Goals, therefore, are very small. For example, if the resident is in a restorative program for eating, the first goal for the resident may be to hold a glass, bring it to her mouth, and drink from it.
- All goals are functional (purposeful). For example, instead of saying the resident will walk 30 feet, the goal will state: Resident will walk to the dining room for breakfast.
- Plan approaches.
- Approaches include the techniques and procedures carried out by care providers to assist resident to relearn the ADL.

The resident may participate in other physical or occupational rehabilitation programs. These programs are planned to help the resident acquire skills needed to complete a task. For example, exercises may be done that will increase range of motion, strength, or endurance.

ADL	Steps of Activity	ADL	Steps of Activity
Grooming	• Washes, brushes, combs hair		• Buckles belt
	• Brushes teeth		• Puts on/takes off shoes/socks
	• Gets equipment ready	Eating	• Gets to table
	• Places paste on brush		• Uses spoon, fork, knife appropriately
	• Brushes teeth		• Opens/pours
	• Rinses mouth		• Brings food to mouth
	• Cleans/puts equipment away		• Chews, swallows
	• Shaves		• Uses napkin
	• Gets equipment ready	Toileting	• Gets to commode/toilet
	• Shaves face		• Manipulates clothing
	• Cleans/puts equipment away		• Sits on toilet
	• Nail care		• Eliminates in toilet
	• Gets equipment ready		• Cleans self
	• Cleans nails		• Flushes toilet
	• Trims nails		• Gets clothing in place
	• Cleans/puts equipment away		• Hands
Bathing	• Gathers supplies	Mobility	• Gets self to side of bed
	• Gets to tub/sink/shower		• Maintains upright position
	• Undresses		• Comes to standing position
	• Regulates water		• Places self in position to sit in chair
	• Washes/rinses upper body		• Locks wheelchair brakes
	• Washes/rinses lower body		• Turns body to sit
	• Dries body		• Lowers self into chair
	• Puts away supplies		• Propels wheelchair
Dressing/ Undressing	• Obtains/selects clothing		• Repositions self in chair
	• Puts on/takes off slipover top		• Raises self from chair
	• Puts on/takes off cardigan-style top		• Places self in position to sit on edge of bed
	• Manages buttons, snaps, ties, zippers		• Walks alone/with assistance
	• Puts on/takes off skirt/pants		• Uses assistive device

Table 22-2 Task Segmentation

Approaches Used in Restorative Programs

- Setup
  - Residents with self-care deficits cannot set up or prepare for ADLs. You may need to provide the setup (Figure 22-5). *Example:* The setup for mealtime includes bringing the tray to the resident and assisting with uncovering food, opening containers, removing eating utensils from package, and preparing food, if necessary.
- Verbal cues
  - Verbal cues are short, simple phrases to prompt the resident to do something. *Example:* Give the

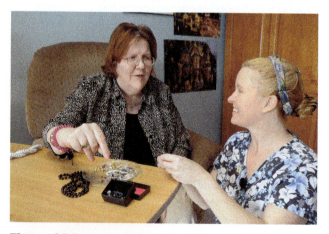

Figure 22-5 Many residents can complete ADLs if you set up the articles they need.

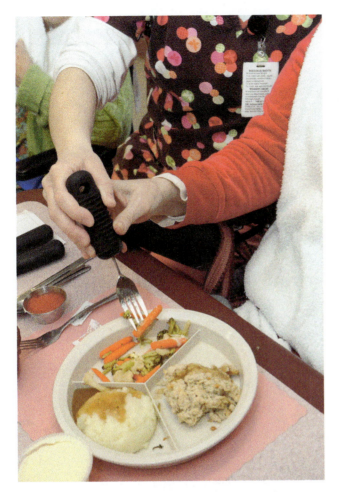

Figure 22-6 The nursing assistant is using hand-over-hand technique to help the resident regain eating skills.

resident a prepared washcloth and then say, "Please wash your face."

- Hand-over-hand technique
  - For this technique, your hand is placed over the resident's hand to guide it (Figure 22-6). *Example:* For eating program, place a spoon with food in the resident's hand. Place your hand over the resident's hand. Guide the spoon to the resident's mouth. Eventually, the resident will be able to do this without assistance.
- Demonstration
  - Act out what you want the resident to do. *Example:* Before giving the resident a toothbrush, make the motions of brushing your teeth with the toothbrush.

The care plan will indicate the approach to be used. The decision is made by the physical therapist, occupational therapist, or restorative nurse.

Adaptive devices are sometimes used to simplify ADLs (Figure 22-7A–C). An adaptive device is an ordinary item that is changed in some way so that it can be used by individuals with specific disabilities. These devices allow people to do things they may not otherwise be able to do. If adaptive devices are ordered, be sure they are used each time the ADL is carried out.

Guidelines for mobility programs and toileting are presented later in this lesson.

Not all residents have potential for restorative programs. For those who do not, the goals are concerned with preventing complications and maintaining current abilities as long as possible. Restorative programs may remain in place after the resident reaches the highest goal possible. This is done to be sure that the resident does not lose the skill. Some residents with progressive diseases such as Alzheimer's reach the point where even maintenance is difficult. Preventing complications such as pressure ulcers and contractures is then the major goal.

THE RESTORATIVE ENVIRONMENT

A restorative environment is not only for residents in restorative programs. The staff can provide an environment and act in such a manner that all residents will benefit. The interdisciplinary team can help promote this environment:

- Give residents a sense of control and the opportunity to make decisions.
- Remember that mental and physical activities are essential to the resident's well-being. Opportunities for physical exercise and various types of activities must be offered to residents.
- Encourage and assist residents to be well dressed and well groomed at all times (Figure 22-8).
- Use touch freely in appropriate ways with residents and only with their permission (Figure 22-9).
- Provide cues for orientation throughout the building such as large clocks, calendars, pictures, and color codes.
- Respect the resident's identity, individuality, and privacy at all times.
- Respect and understand the resident's sexuality and need for intimacy.
- Give residents opportunities to help others. All people need to feel useful.
- Encourage and assist residents to remain a part of the community and encourage the community to be a part of the facility.
- The environment should be safe, serene, and colorful.

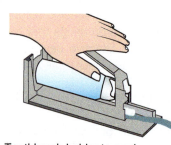

A. Toothbrush holder to apply toothpaste with one hand

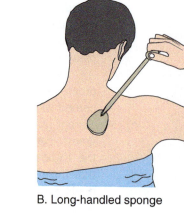

B. Long-handled sponge

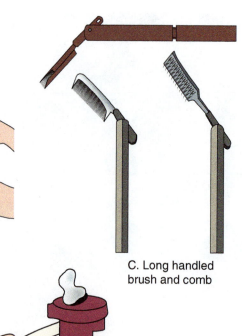

C. Long handled brush and comb

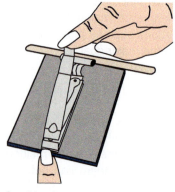

D. Combination nail clipper and file for one-handed use

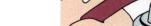

E. Aerosol can adapter with trigger to push button

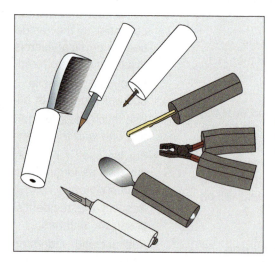

F. Grooming aids with built-up handles for easier gripping

Figure 22-7A   Adaptive devices used for grooming and bathing.

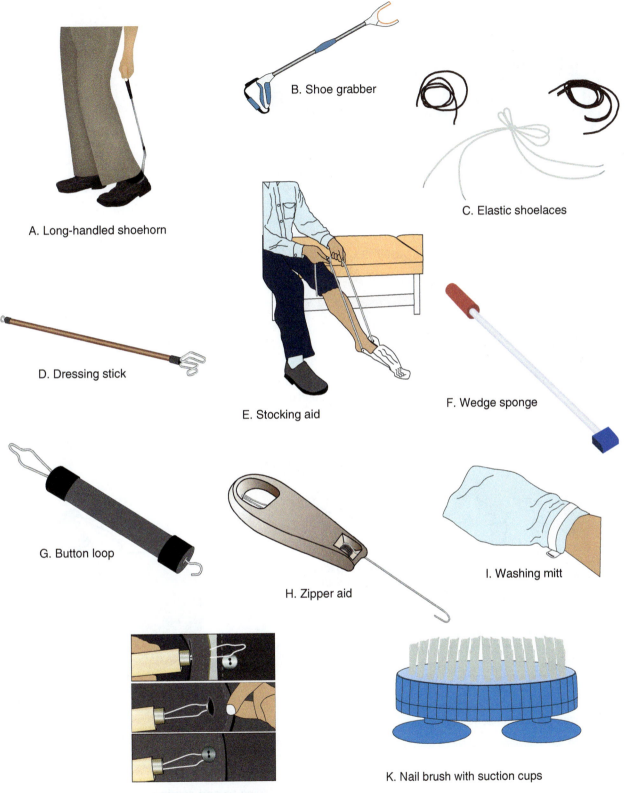

A. Long-handled shoehorn

B. Shoe grabber

C. Elastic shoelaces

D. Dressing stick

E. Stocking aid

F. Wedge sponge

G. Button loop

H. Zipper aid

I. Washing mitt

J. Button loop in use

K. Nail brush with suction cups

Figure 22-7B Dressing aids.

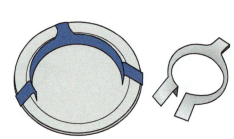

A. Food bumper snaps on to keep food on plate

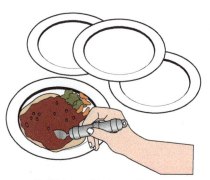

B. Plates with inner lip to keep food in place

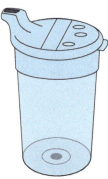

D. Feeding cups

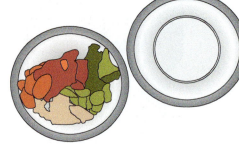

C. Plate with high curved edge to help push food onto utensil

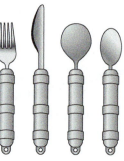

E. Cutlery with built-up handles for easier gripping

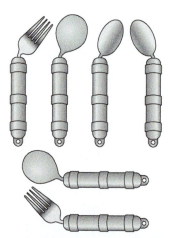

F. Angled cutlery for people with limited arm and wrist movement

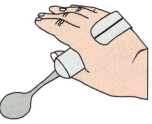

G. Hand clip for people who can't grip handles

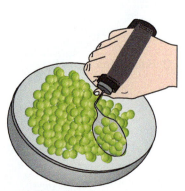

H. Gripper for people who cannot grip standard or built up handles

Figure 22-7C Adaptive devices used for eating.

PROGRESSIVE MOBILIZATION

Progressive mobilization is a process used to increase a resident's mobility skills. Mobility includes:

- Moving in bed
- Changing position in bed
- Moving to and coming to a sitting position on the edge of the bed
- Coming to a standing position
- Transferring into a bathtub, shower, and car or out of bed and into a chair
- Ambulating or moving about in a wheelchair

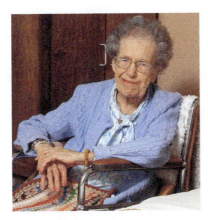

Figure 22-8 All residents should be assisted to look attractive and well groomed.

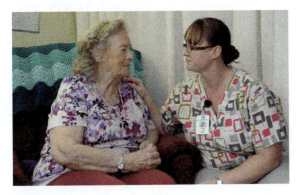

Figure 22-9 Touching residents is important for restorative care.

Not all residents are able to complete every step of progressive mobilization. All residents should be given the opportunity to reach their own potential. Progressive mobilization, like all restorative programs, must begin at the simplest level. A resident may not be able to do any of these skills independently but may be able to do each skill with assistance.

RANGE OF MOTION

Exercise is a basic physical need. Residents who are unable to do active exercises are exercised through passive range-of-motion exercises by the care provider. The physical or occupational therapist may order additional exercises to increase specific abilities or to strengthen certain muscles.

Range-of-motion exercises are one technique used to prevent the formation of contractures (see Figure 22-2). It is the responsibility of each person on the health care team to recognize risks for contracture formation and to implement preventive therapy. The therapists and professional nurses are trained to use a special instrument called a goniometer to assess the resident for the presence of contractures, to determine how a potential contracture affects the resident's functional capacity, and to set rehabilitation goals and interventions.

? EXERCISE 22-3

FILL IN THE BLANKS

1. Members of the interdisciplinary team meet to plan for restorative care during a(an) _____ conference.

2. Placing a hand over a resident's hand to help train the resident to perform a task is called _____.

3. A shoehorn with an extra-long handle used by a resident to make it easier to put on his or her shoes is an example of a(an) _____.

BRIEF ANSWERS
Briefly answer the following.

4. What is meant by progressive mobilization? _____

_____

5. Six mobility skills that are followed in progressive mobilization are:

a. _____

b. _____

c. _____

d. _____

e. _____

f. _____

There are four stages of contracture development:

- Stage I has an onset of 0 to 4 days and within 2 weeks has a 0- to 15-degree loss in range of motion
- Stage II advances in 1 to 2 more weeks through 15 to 45 degrees of loss in range of motion
- Stage III has a 45- to 90-degree loss
- Stage IV has a 90+ degree loss of range of motion

A *fixed contracture* is one that allows the resident no range of motion. It is caused by fibrosis with a muscle. The only treatment is surgery, which is expensive, not appropriate for all residents, and offers no guarantee of success.

Contractures are painful, much like a continuous, severe cramp in the muscle. In the presence of contractures, blood flow is impeded and pressure ulcers can form. It is imperative that the appropriate range-of-motion exercises be completed when ordered:

- **Passive range of motion**
  The care provider moves the joints for the resident.
- **Active assistive range of motion**
  The care provider supports the joints and assists in the movement while the resident attempts to do independent movement.
- **Active range of motion**
  The resident is able to move the joints without assistance.
- **Self range of motion**
  The resident uses the strong extremity to move the affected extremity. *Example:* A resident with a stroke may use the strong arm to passively move the paralyzed arm.

⚠ GUIDELINES FOR... NURSING ASSISTANT RESPONSIBILITIES IN GENERAL RESTORATIVE PROGRAM

GENERAL

1. Know the cause of the resident's self-care deficit.
2. Know the resident's goals as stated on the care plan.
3. Be consistent. Read the care plan and follow the specific approaches each time you work with the resident.
4. Keep your directions simple but not childish when you are helping the resident relearn an activity.
5. Avoid distractions. Do ADLs in a private, quiet area. Restorative programs are incorporated into the resident's daily care. For example, if the resident is in a grooming program to relearn how to comb her hair, then the program is carried out when the hair would usually be combed.
6. Use adaptive devices consistently and correctly.
7. Do not show impatience. Be encouraging and give praise.
8. Treat the resident with dignity at all times.
9. Realize that the resident's progress may be uneven and inconsistent. A resident may do better one day than another.

GROOMING

1. A grooming program may be for combing/brushing hair, applying makeup, doing nail care, shaving, or oral care.
2. The resident should sit in a comfortable chair that supports the resident's body.
3. Place the necessary items on the overbed table. Place the table in front of the resident and adjust it to the appropriate height so the resident can reach every item.
4. Avoid putting too many items on the table at once. Do not put the items close together or the resident may have trouble picking the correct item.

BATHING

1. Residents in bathing programs should also be allowed to:
   - Wash their hands after toileting
   - Wash their face and hands after eating
   - Follow the program for morning and evening care as well as for bathing
2. A setup is usually needed:
   - Prepare the water (basin, tub, or shower).
   - Obtain all the necessary items (towels, washcloths, soap).
   - Help the resident choose clothing to put on after the bath.

EATING

1. Assist the resident to go to the bathroom.
2. Provide opportunity for handwashing.

(continues)

⚠ GUIDELINES FOR... NURSING ASSISTANT RESPONSIBILITIES IN GENERAL RESTORATIVE PROGRAM (Continued)

3. Be sure the resident has dentures in if needed and that the mouth is clean.

4. Seat the resident in a regular dining chair at a dining table.

5. Avoid distractions. Turn off televisions and radios.

6. Prepare the tray: open cartons, butter the bread, cut the meat, add seasonings as the resident wishes, and pour liquids. Avoid touching any food with your bare hands. The resident may eventually be able to do these things independently.

DRESSING/UNDRESSING

The following adaptations will make the program more likely to succeed:

1. Use loose-fitting styles or clothing one size larger.

2. Encourage the family to bring clothing that fastens in front rather than in back. Velcro closings are usually easier to manipulate than zippers, buttons, or snaps.

3. Suggest garments with large buttons rather than small ones. It is easier to match buttons with the right buttonholes if the resident starts to button from the bottom of a shirt or blouse rather than the top.

4. Suggest that elastic thread be used for cuff buttons so they do not need to be undone each time.

5. Encourage the resident to wear slip-on shoes or shoes with Velcro closings.

⚠ GUIDELINES FOR... PASSIVE RANGE-OF-MOTION EXERCISES

1. Always tell the resident what you are doing and why. Encourage the resident to help you when possible.

2. Passive exercises of the neck are not generally done on older people. Arthritis is a common problem and passive exercises can injure the neck. Instead, encourage the resident to move the head independently.

3. Move each joint to its fullest range for that resident. Remember that the maximum range in an older person may be small.

4. Never force movement or cause pain. If the resident cannot speak, watch the face for signs of pain, such as a grimace or a grunt.

5. Use gentle, physical contact. Always support the extremities at the joints. Use the palms of your hands to cup the joints.

6. Do each motion at least three to five times (as directed). The exercises should be done at least twice a day. Do each joint unless you have been instructed to omit specific joints or a specific movement for a joint.

7. Do each motion slowly, smoothly, gently, and rhythmically. A resident's stiff joints may gradually loosen as you continue the exercises.

8. Come to a complete stop in an anatomically neutral position at the end of each movement before starting the next movement.

Nursing assistants in long-term care facilities may complete passive range-of-motion exercises with residents several times a day.

Definitions of Joint Movements

Specific terms describe joint movements. Not all joints are capable of the same movements.

1. Flexion—bending a joint; decreasing the angle of the joint (Figure 22-10)
   - Palmar flexion—bending the hand down toward the wrist

   - Dorsiflexion—bending the hand back or bending the foot back
   - Plantar flexion—bending the foot forward toward the sole

2. Extension—the opposite of flexion—to straighten the joint out, increasing the angle of the joint (Figure 22-11)

3. Abduction—moving an extremity away from the body (Figure 22-12)
   - Horizontal abduction—bringing the arm out so the elbow is parallel to shoulder

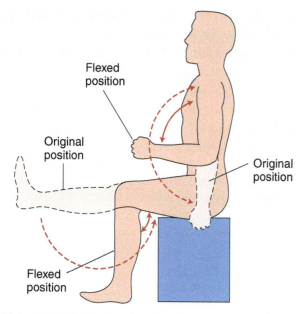

Figure 22-10 Flexion—bending a joint.

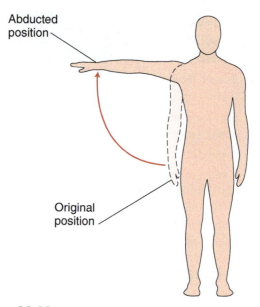

Figure 22-12 Abduction—moving an extremity away from the body.

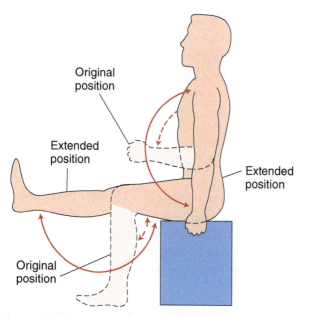

Figure 22-11 Extension—straightening a joint.

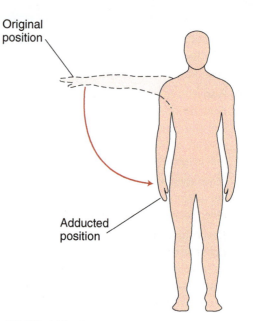

Figure 22-13 Adduction—moving an extremity back to the body.

4. Adduction—the opposite of abduction—moving the extremity back to the body (Figure 22-13)
   - Horizontal adduction—bringing the arm up and crossing it over the chest
5. Rotation—turning around an axis (Figure 22-14)
   - Internal rotation—turning toward the median line

- External rotation—turning outward from the median line
6. Pronation—turning the forearm so the palm is facing downward
7. Supination—the opposite of pronation—turning the forearm so the palm is facing upward

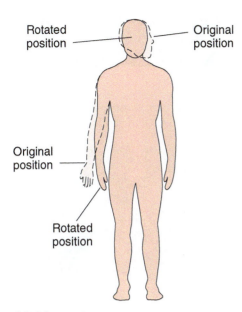

Figure 22-14 Rotation.

8. Radial deviation—lateral movement of wrist toward thumb side of hand
9. Ulnar deviation—lateral movement of wrist toward little finger side of hand
10. Inversion—turning inward
11. Eversion—the opposite of inversion—turning outward
12. Opposition—bringing palmar surface of thumb to the finger joint

It is important that you review the section on body mechanics in Lesson 9. You will need to use your muscles correctly as you help residents with their mobility. This will help prevent painful and costly injuries to both you and the residents.

PROCEDURE 22-69
Passive Range-of-Motion Exercises

1. Carry out each beginning procedure action.
2. Position the resident in good **body alignment**. This means the resident's spine is straight and the resident's extremities are straight in relation to the body. The body is straight in the bed. Bring the resident close to your side of the bed.
3. Place a bath blanket over the covers. Then bring the covers to the foot of the bed. Expose only the extremity that you are working on.
4. Remember to use correct body mechanics to avoid straining your back. While working on one side of the bed, perform the exercises on the arm and leg on that side. Go to the other side of the bed and complete the exercises on the arm and leg on that side.
5. When all four extremities have been exercised, carry out procedure completion actions.
6. Report any unusual resident reactions or problems to the nurse.

Shoulder

Support the elbow and wrist during all shoulder exercises.

1. Flexion and extension
   - With shoulder in adduction, flex the resident's elbow and raise entire arm over the head (flexion) (Figure 22-15). *Note:* This movement is flexing the resident's elbow as well as the shoulder.
   - Bring arm back down parallel to body (extension) (Figure 22-16). *Note:* This movement is extending the resident's elbow as well as the shoulder.

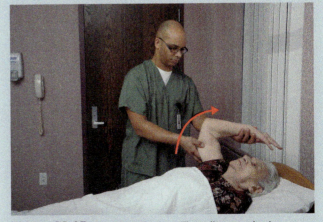

Figure 22-15 Shoulder flexion: Flex elbow and raise entire arm over head.

(continues)

PROCEDURE 22-69
Passive Range-of-Motion Exercises (Continued)

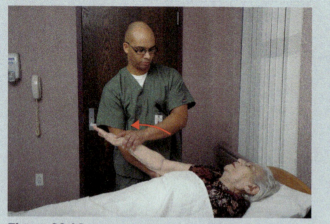

Figure 22-16 Supporting the upper arm and wrist, straighten the elbow.

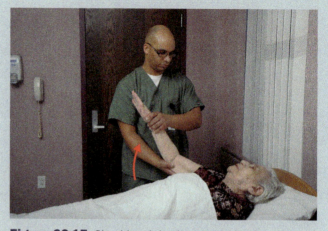

Figure 22-17 Shoulder abduction and adduction: Supporting elbow and wrist, bring the entire arm out at right angle from the body.

Repeat flexion and extension three to five times.

2. Abduction and adduction

   ▪ Bring entire arm out at right angle to body (abduction) (Figure 22-17).

   ▪ Return arm to position parallel with body and across the chest as far as possible (adduction) (Figure 22-18).

   Repeat abduction and adduction five to seven times.

3. Horizontal adduction and horizontal abduction

   ▪ With arm parallel to body, bring arm up and cross it over chest (horizontal adduction) (Figure 22-19).

   ▪ Bring arm back so elbow is parallel to shoulder (horizontal abduction) (Figure 22-20).

   Repeat horizontal adduction and horizontal abduction three to five times. Each is a single motion, not one continuous action.

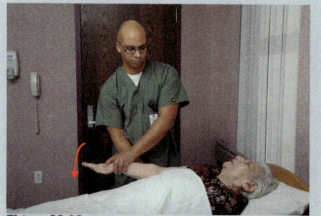

Figure 22-18 Return arm to position parallel to body.

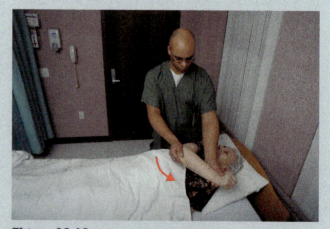

Figure 22-19 Horizontal adduction of shoulder.

(continues)

PROCEDURE 22-69
Passive Range-of-Motion Exercises (Continued)

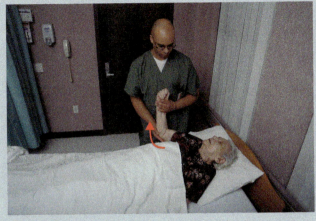

Figure 22-20 Horizontal abduction of shoulder.

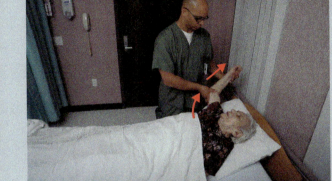

Figure 22-21 External rotation of shoulder.

4. External rotation and internal rotation

    ▪ With elbow parallel to shoulder, place forearm in up position with palm of hand up (external rotation) (Figure 22-21).

    ▪ Bring forearm down with elbow and shoulder remaining stationary (internal rotation) (Figure 22-22).

    Repeat external rotation and internal rotation five to seven times.

Elbow

Support the resident's wrist during the elbow exercises.

1. Flexion and extension

    ▪ With arm parallel to body and palm up, bend elbow (flexion) (Figure 22-23).

    ▪ Return arm to position parallel with body and palm up (extension) (Figure 22-24).

    Repeat flexion and extension of elbow five to seven times.

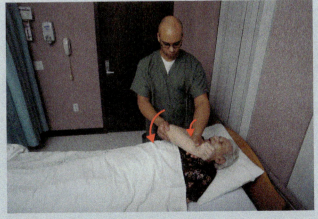

Figure 22-22 Internal rotation of the shoulder.

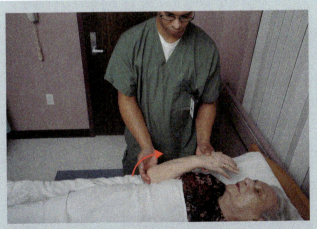

Figure 22-23 Flexion of the elbow: Bring lower arm toward upper arm.

(continues)

PROCEDURE 22-69
Passive Range-of-Motion Exercises (Continued)

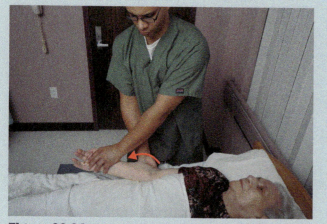

Figure 22-24 Extension of the shoulder and elbow.

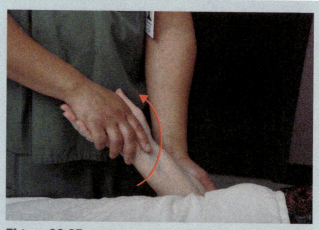

Figure 22-25 Supination: Grasp resident's hand as if to shake hands; turn hand so resident's hand is palm up.

2. Supination and pronation

    ▪ Place your hand in resident's hand as if to shake hands. Turn resident's hand with yours so the palm is down (pronation).

    ▪ Without moving your hand, turn resident's hand with yours so resident's palm is up (supination) (Figure 22-25).

    Repeat supination and pronation five to seven times.

Wrist

Support the forearm during wrist exercises. The elbow and shoulder will rest on the bed.

1. Flexion (palmar flexion), extension (dorsiflexion)

    ▪ Bend wrist forward (flexion, palmar flexion) (Figure 22-26).

    ▪ Straighten wrist so hand is even with forearm (extension) (Figure 22-27).

    Repeat flexion and extension five to seven times.

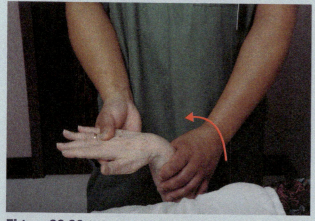

Figure 22-26 Wrist flexion and extension: Place hand over resident's hand while supporting wrist and bend wrist.

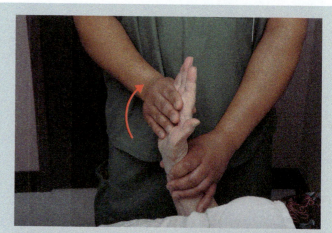

Figure 22-27 Supporting arm above wrist and hand, straighten wrist.

(continues)

PROCEDURE 22-69
Passive Range-of-Motion Exercises (Continued)

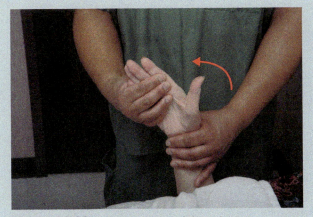

Figure 22-28 Ulnar deviation of the wrist.

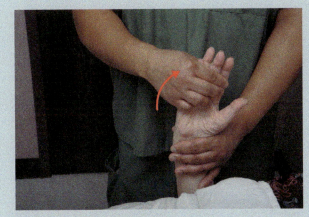

Figure 22-29 Radial deviation of the wrist.

2. Ulnar and radial deviation

 - Move the wrist away from the thumb toward little finger side (ulnar deviation) (Figure 22-28).
 - Move the wrist laterally toward thumb side (radial deviation) (Figure 22-29).

 Repeat ulnar and radial deviation five to seven times.

Fingers

Support the wrist and forearm during the finger and thumb exercises.

1. Flexion and extension

 - Curl the fingers together to make a fist (flexion) (Figure 22-30).
 - Straighten the fingers out (extension) (Figure 22-31).

 Repeat flexion and extension of the fingers five to seven times.

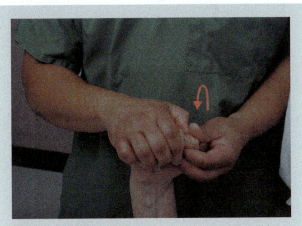

Figure 22-30 Finger flexion: Supporting wrist with one hand, cover resident's fingers and curl them to make a fist.

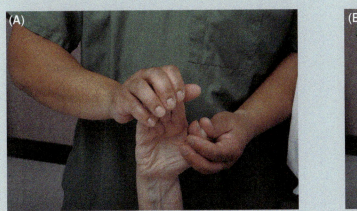

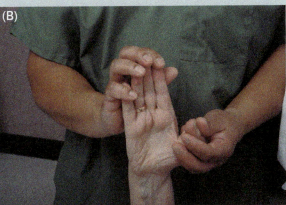

Figure 22-31 Finger extension: Slip fingers over resident's flexed fingers (A) and straighten the fingers (B).

(continues)

PROCEDURE 22-69
Passive Range-of-Motion Exercises (Continued)

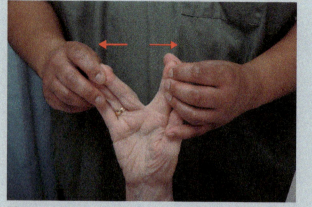

Figure 22-32 Abduction of the fingers.

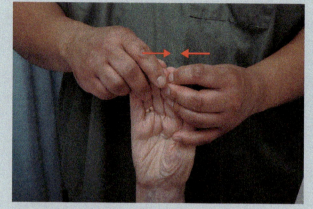

Figure 22-33 Adduction of the fingers.

2. Abduction and adduction

- Spread each finger apart from the one next to it (abduction) (Figure 22-32).

- Bring each finger back (adduction) (Figure 22-33).

Repeat abduction and adduction five to seven times.

Thumb

1. Flexion and extension

- Bend the thumb forward (flexion).

- Straighten the thumb out (extension).

Repeat flexion and extension of the thumb five to seven times.

2. Abduction and adduction

- Move the thumb away from the other fingers (abduction) (Figure 22-34).

- Move the thumb back toward the other fingers (adduction).

Repeat abduction and adduction five to seven times.

3. Opposition

- Move the thumb to the base of each finger and then back (Figure 22-35).

Repeat opposition five to seven times.

NOTE: Opposition is an exercise for the thumb, not the fingers. It is important that the thumb receive the movement.

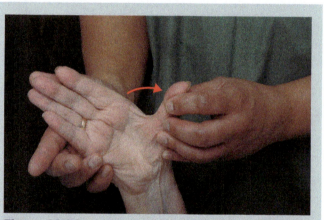

Figure 22-34 Abduction and adduction of thumb: Supporting hand, draw thumb toward and away from extended fingers.

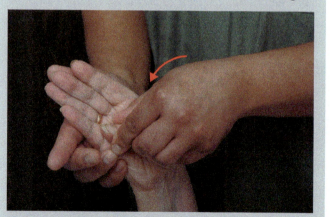

Figure 22-35 Thumb opposition: Supporting the hand, touch each finger with the thumb.

(continues)

PROCEDURE 22-69
Passive Range-of-Motion Exercises (Continued)

Hips

Support the knee and ankle during hip exercises.

1. Abduction and adduction

   - Place the palm of your hand under the resident's knee and the other hand under the heel.
   - Move the entire leg away from the body (abduction) (Figure 22-36).
   - Move the entire leg back toward the body (adduction) (Figure 22-37).

   Repeat abduction and adduction of the hip five to seven times.

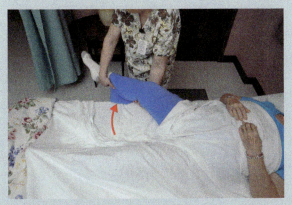

Figure 22-36 Abduction of the hip: Supporting resident's knee and ankle, move entire leg away from body.

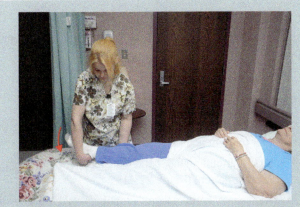

Figure 22-37 Adduction of hip: Supporting leg, return to center of body.

2. Flexion and extension

   - Place one hand under the resident's upper calf. Place your other hand under the heel with the resident's foot resting against your forearm.
   - Bend the resident's knee and hip toward the resident's trunk (flexion) (Figure 22-38).

   NOTE: You are flexing the knee at the same time as the hip.

   - Straighten the knee and hip (extension). Be sure to support the knee so it does not "flop" down (Figure 22-39).

   NOTE: You are extending the knee at the same time as the hip. Repeat flexion and extension of the hip and knee five to seven times.

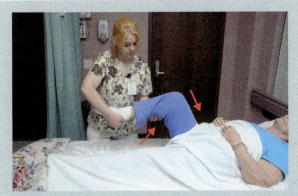

Figure 22-38 Hip and knee flexion: Supporting resident's upper calf and heel, flex knee and hip.

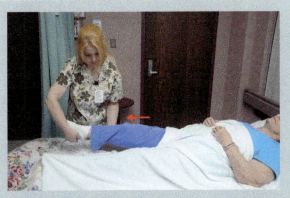

Figure 22-39 Knee extension: Supporting calf and heel, straighten knee.

(continues)

PROCEDURE 22-69
Passive Range-of-Motion Exercises (Continued)

3.   Internal rotation and external rotation

   ▪ Place one hand on the resident's leg just above the knee. Place the other hand on the resident's lower leg just above the ankle.

   ▪ With the resident's leg extended, roll the leg back and forth. Rolling the leg inward is internal rotation. Rolling the leg outward is external rotation (Figure 22-40).

   Repeat internal rotation and external rotation of the hip five to seven times.

Knee

Flexion and extension are the only knee movements. These were done with the hip.

Ankle

1.   Plantar flexion and dorsiflexion

   ▪ Bend resident's knee slightly and support lower leg with your forearm and hand.

   ▪ With your other hand, bend resident's foot downward (plantar flexion) (Figure 22-41).

   ▪ Then gently bend resident's foot backward (dorsiflexion, hyperextension).

   Repeat plantar flexion and dorsiflexion five to seven times.

2.   Inversion and eversion

   ▪ Support the resident's lower leg with one hand. Grasp the resident's foot with the other hand and gently turn it inward (inversion) (Figure 22-42).

   ▪ With your hands in the same positions, move the resident's foot outward (eversion) (Figure 22-43).

   Repeat inversion and eversion five to seven times.

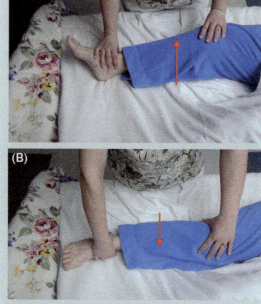

Figure 22-40 External (A) and internal (B) rotation of hip.

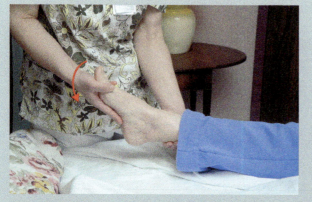

Figure 22-41 Plantar flex the ankle by drawing the foot in a downward position.

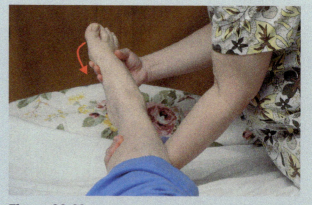

Figure 22-42 Ankle inversion: Grasp resident's foot and gently turn it inward.

(continues)

PROCEDURE 22-69
Passive Range-of-Motion Exercises (Continued)

Toes

1. Flexion and extension

   ▪ Bend (flexion) and straighten (extension) each toe.

   Repeat flexion and extension of the toes five to seven times.

2. Abduction and adduction

   ▪ Move each toe away from the next toe, one at a time (abduction) (Figure 22-44).

   ▪ Move each toe toward the next toe, one at a time (adduction) (Figure 22-45).

   Repeat abduction and adduction five to seven times.

   Additional exercises can be done with the resident in the prone (lying on the abdomen) position. However, many residents cannot lie in this position. Your facility may not include these exercises. Check with your supervisor and be sure you receive instruction before doing the additional exercises.

   Carry out procedure completion actions. Report to the nurse any pain or change in range of motion of the resident's joints. Position resident comfortably.

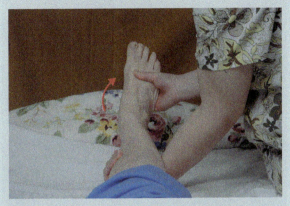

Figure 22-43 Foot eversion: Grasp resident's foot and gently turn it outward.

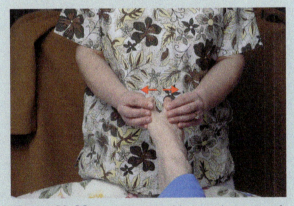

Figure 22-44 Toe abduction: Move each toe away from the next toe, one at a time.

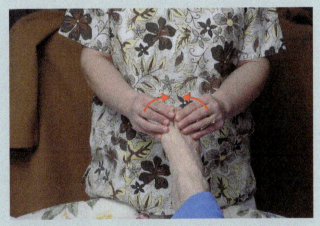

Figure 22-45 Toe adduction: Move each toe toward the next toe.

SELF RANGE-OF-MOTION EXERCISES

Self range-of-motion exercises are done by the resident. The resident can use a strong extremity to move a paralyzed or weak extremity (Figure 22-46). The physical therapist or restorative nurse will give you instructions if you are to assist a resident with self range-of-motion exercises.

ACTIVE RANGE-OF-MOTION EXERCISES

Residents can do many exercises independently that involve movement of the joints. Many long-term care facilities have health and fitness trails within the facility that have several stations and instructions for the resident. Active range-of-motion exercises can also be done by residents in wheelchairs.

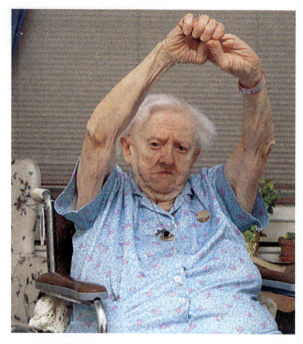

Figure 22-46 The resident is using her stronger arm to raise her weak arm.

POSITIONING THE RESIDENT

Residents who cannot move themselves about in bed need to be repositioned frequently. As a nursing assistant, you will carry out these procedures several times a day. Three basic positions are **supine** (lying on the back), **prone** (lying on the abdomen), and **lateral** (lying on either side). Each of these positions has variations.

Positioning procedures have several steps:

- Moving the resident's body so it is in correct body alignment
  - You may need to move the resident toward the head of the bed, the foot of the bed, or either side of the bed.
- Turning the resident to the desired position
  - To either the right or left side from the side, the back, or the abdomen
  - To the back from either side or the abdomen
  - To the abdomen from the back or other side
- Placing pillows or other supportive devices to maintain the position

⚠ GUIDELINES FOR... POSITIONING

1. A firm mattress helps to maintain correct body alignment.

2. Lock the wheels of the bed before beginning the positioning procedure.

3. Raise the bed to a comfortable working height. Remember to lower the bed when the procedure is finished.

4. Raise the quarter side rail on the other side of the bed unless there is another person helping you.

5. Handle the resident's body gently during mobility activities. Use the palms of your hands rather than your fingertips to support the extremities.

6. Incorporate range-of-motion exercises into positioning procedures. These exercises are in addition to those carried out routinely.

7. Encourage the resident's independence. Provide the assistance that is needed but avoid "over-helping."

8. Turn the resident at least every 2 hours. Inspect the skin for signs of breakdown each time. Gently massage around reddened areas with lotion. Rubbing over the reddened area may cause further skin damage.

9. Use a turning sheet to move a dependent resident in bed. This avoids friction and **shearing** the skin. Shearing occurs when the resident's body slides across the sheets; the skin moves in one direction

as deeper tissues move in the opposite direction causing skin irritation.

10. Support paralyzed extremities in extension. Prevent prolonged overstretching of weakened muscles. **Flaccid** paralysis means the extremity is limp and incapable of independent movement. **Spasticity** occurs in some paralyzed limbs. Spasticity can cause involuntary movements. It may cause the joints to assume positions of flexion. Contractures can happen easily in spastic limbs.

11. Avoid dependent positions of extremities. The wrists and feet should never hang. This will cause edema (swelling).

    Be supported by pillows, if necessary.

12. Check incontinent residents each time you move them. If they have soiled the bed, cleanse them thoroughly, following incontinence care steps. Change the sheets. Change clothing if soiled.

13. Straighten the sheets frequently. Wrinkles cause pressure areas on the resident's skin.

14. Items used for positioning are used only for a specific resident. Send sheets, pillows, and other washable items to the laundry as necessary. Do not let these items touch the floor.

15. Remember the privacy of the resident when completing all positioning procedures.

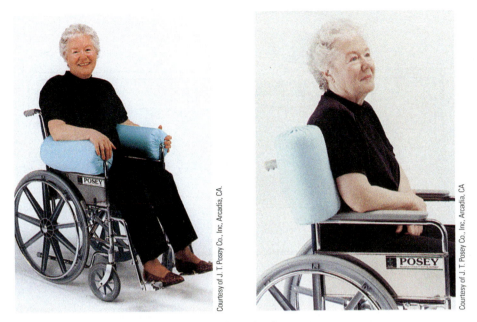

Courtesy of J. T. Posey Co., Inc, Arcadia, CA.

Courtesy of J. T. Posey Co., Inc, Arcadia, CA

Figure 22-47 Supports help position residents and maintain body alignment.

Purposes of Positioning

Positioning is done to:

- Improve circulation and respiratory function
- Maintain the resident's body alignment and good posture
- Prevent contractures, skin breakdown, pain, discomfort, thromboses, pneumonia, and edema
- Increase sensory stimulation. The sense of touch is stimulated when the assistant moves the resident. The sense of vision is stimulated when the resident is turned and sees a different part of the environment.

Supportive Equipment

Supportive equipment may be needed to position the resident. The procedure must be adapted for residents with catheters or other tubes. You may need further instructions from the nurse for positioning residents with contractures.

Postural supports are devices to help maintain the resident in good posture and body alignment. Examples of postural supports include:

- Trochanter rolls
- Bath blankets
- Pillows of various sizes and shapes
- Bath towels
- Footboards
- Splints or slings, if ordered
- Turning sheet

Other postural supports are prescribed for specific residents for specific purposes (Figure 22-47). Be sure you know how to apply these devices correctly.

A trochanter roll is used to prevent external rotation of the hip (Figure 22-48). It is put in place when the resident is in supine (on the back) position. If the hip contracts in this position, the resident will be unable to move the leg. You can make a trochanter roll with a bath blanket:

- Fold the blanket in thirds, lengthwise. The roll should be 12 to 14 inches wide.
- The blanket is placed lengthwise under the resident's hips. Roll the end that is on the affected side *under* until it is firmly against the resident's body. It should extend from above the hip to just above the knee.

Footboards are sometimes ordered to prevent plantar flexion of the feet. This causes contracture of the ankle.

- The footboard should be well-padded, smooth, and firm.
- The footboard must extend 2 inches above the toes. This will prevent skin breakdown on the toes.
- The bottoms of the feet rest against the footboard to maintain position.

Commercial footboards are available or sometimes a folded pillow can be placed between the soles of the feet and the foot of the bed to take the place of a footboard. Special shoes worn in bed are sometimes used to maintain feet in correct alignment. However, in most cases, ankle contractures can be

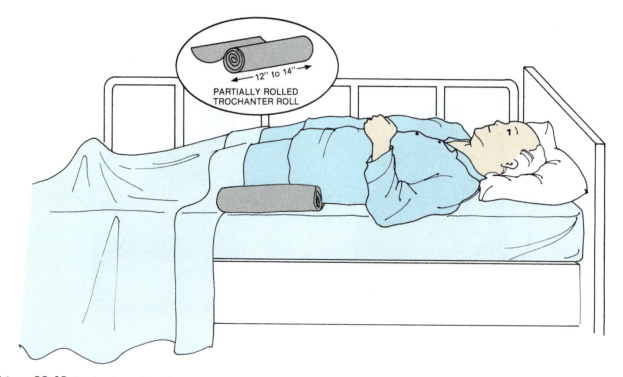

Figure 22-48 Trochanter roll in place to prevent external rotation of hip. Footboards are used to prevent foot drop, a severe contracture of the feet.

avoided by consistently doing passive range-of-motion exercises.

No matter what type of device is used to prevent footdrop, constantly monitor the resident's feet to relieve pressure and to ensure that skin breakdown does not occur. If you note any signs of irritation, immediately notify the nurse to prevent serious decubitus ulcers from forming.

• A bed cradle (Figure 22-49) is placed on the bed over the resident's legs. The bed covers are placed over the bed cradle. This keeps the weight of the covers off the resident's legs and feet. It prevents

the covers from forcing the feet into plantar flexion, which could cause a contracture.

A device called an **orthosis** can also be used to maintain position of an extremity. The correct use of these devices prevents contracture formation. Orthoses are also called **splints**.

• The splint must be applied correctly. Follow the manufacturer's directions for each splint.

• Keep the splint clean. If it becomes soiled, check with the nurse to see how it should be cleaned.

• Make sure the splint is not too tight, because it may impair circulation.

The physician may also order splints or orthoses for the lower extremities. A common type is called the ankle brace. The brace provides support for an unstable ankle and is applied to the lower leg before the shoe is put on.

When using splints:

• The splint may be ordered to be on and off the extremity at various times throughout the day. Be sure you know the correct procedure and schedule.

• Check the splint to be sure there are no pressure areas against the resident's skin.

• Folded washcloths should *never* be placed in the resident's hand. The rough surface of the cloth increases spasticity and the risk of contractures.

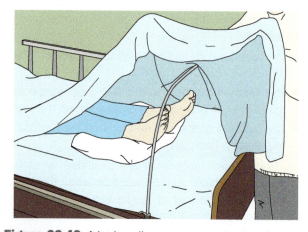

Figure 22-49 A bed cradle prevents pressure on the foot from the top covers.

Slings are sometimes used to prevent a paralyzed arm from hanging. The force of gravity pulls on the weight of the arm, causing subluxation. This occurs when the shoulder joint separates (a dislocation). It is a permanent and painful condition. A sling is not usually worn constantly because it forces the upper arm into a position of adduction and the elbow into flexion. If you apply a sling, remember:

- Read the manufacturer's instructions for application.
- Position the hands and fingers at about heart level.
- Support the hand and fingers with the sling. Avoid palmar flexion of the wrist.
- Check the sling for foreign bodies that may produce pressure spots.
- Position the sling to provide adequate support at the elbow so the shoulder is in good position.

- Hand should be 4 to 6 inches above the elbow.
- Apply the sling properly to prevent it from pulling on the resident's neck (Figure 22-50).

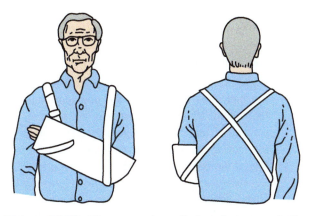

Figure 22-50 When properly applied, a sling supports the wrist and does not pull on the resident's neck.

PROCEDURE 22-70
Moving the Resident in Bed

OBRA

NOTE: A turning sheet should always be used to move dependent residents in bed. This avoids injury to the resident and the caregivers. Always use the principles of good body mechanics to avoid injury to your back.

1. Carry out each beginning procedure action.

    Use disposable gloves if there may be contact with open lesions, wet linens, or body fluids.

2. Be sure the turning sheet is in place on the bed.

3. Two people are needed, standing on opposite sides of the bed. Three or four people may be needed if the resident is very heavy or has many restrictions (e.g., tubing, traction devices).

4. Before beginning this procedure:

    - The bed must be flat.
    - Raise it to a comfortable working height.
    - Fanfold the top covers to the foot of the bed. Do not expose the resident's bare body.
    - Remove all supportive devices from the bed.
    - Put the resident in supine position.
    - Cross the resident's arms over the chest or abdomen.
    - If the resident lacks head control, position the turning sheet to extend up under the head.
    - Remove the pillow under the resident's head and prop it against the headboard.
    - Keep your feet separated, your back straight, and your knees and hips flexed as you complete these procedures to avoid back injuries.

These directions apply to all assistants who are helping with this procedure. There are one or two assistants on each side of the bed, depending on the size of the resident.

5. Grasp the turning sheet at the level of the resident's shoulders and thighs.

    - Using an overhand grasp, roll or gather the sheet until your hands touch the resident's body. Pull the sheet taut.

(continues)

PROCEDURE 22-70
Moving the Resident in Bed (Continued)

6. If the resident lacks head control, grasp the sheet at a level that allows you to maintain stability of the resident's head.

7. If you are moving the resident to the head of the bed, face the head of the bed with your feet about 12 inches apart and the toes of your outer foot forward (Figure 22-51). If you are moving the resident down in bed, face the foot of the bed with the toes of your feet about 12 inches apart and your outer foot forward. These positions allow you to flex your elbows and move the resident toward you, following the principles of body mechanics.

8. Before moving, place your weight on the forward foot.

   ▪ As you move, shift your weight to the other foot. (Avoid twisting. Move smoothly.)

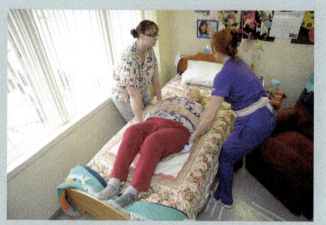

Figure 22-51 Moving a resident up in bed with a turning sheet.

9. If moving the resident to the side of the bed, the persons on the side of the bed to which the resident will be moved should:

   ▪ Place one foot forward (maintaining a broad base of support). Body weight is on this foot.

   ▪ As the resident is moved, body weight is shifted to the other foot.

10. The assistant(s) on the other side of the bed grasp the turning sheet to avoid dragging the resident's body. The person on this side does very little actual lifting.

11. One person gives the signal by counting to three

   ▪ All persons move on the count of three, flexing their elbows and moving the sheet toward the head of the bed.

12. Position the resident according to directions, lower the bed, and carry out procedure completion actions.

PROCEDURE 22-71
Turning the Resident to the Side

OBRA

NOTE: Directions are given for turning the resident onto the right side. Reverse directions for positioning a resident on the left side.

1. Carry out each beginning procedure action.

2. Follow procedure for moving the resident to the head of the bed if necessary (Procedure 22-70). Remember: Keep your feet about 12 inches apart. Bend your knees and keep your back straight. Get as close to the bed and resident as possible.

3. Now move the resident to the left side of the bed. Assistants on both sides face the bed.

4. Move the resident's right arm away from the body.

   ▪ Place the resident's left arm across the abdomen.

5. Cross the resident's left leg over the right leg.

(continues)

PROCEDURE 22-71
Turning the Resident to the Side (Continued)

6. To turn the resident without the turning sheet (turning the resident away from you):

   - The assistant on the resident's left side places the right hand so it cups the resident's left shoulder.

   - The other hand is placed so the palm is against the resident's hip (Figure 22-52).

NOTE: To turn the resident toward you, stand on the right side of the bed and place your hands as indicated (Figure 22-53).

7. If the resident is large, the assistant on the other side can place both hands beside the hands of the other assistant. On the count of three, turn the resident onto the right side.

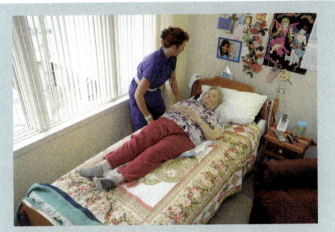

Figure 22-52 Turning the resident away from you.

8. To turn the resident with the turning sheet:

   - The assistant on the resident's left side grasps the turning sheet at the shoulders and hips.

   - The other assistant reaches across the resident and grasps the turning sheet at the knees and waist.

9. The assistant on the right side bends elbows to pull the sheet so the resident is turned. The other assistant grasps the sheet to assist in the turn (Figure 22-54).

10. Complete positioning procedure (see Procedure 22-72).

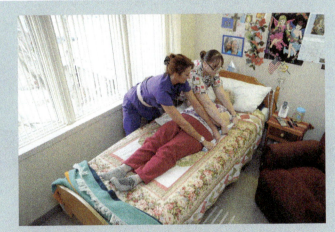

Figure 22-53 Turning the resident toward you.

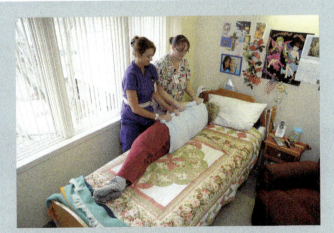

Figure 22-54 Turning the resident onto the side using a turning pad. For safety, make sure the resident is not too close to the edge of the bed.

PROCEDURE 22-72
Logrolling the Resident onto the Side

OBRA

NOTE: This procedure is used when the resident's spinal column must be kept straight. This technique may be used after spinal surgery or spinal injury. Directions are given for turning the resident onto the left side.

1. Carry out each beginning procedure action.

   Remember to use disposable gloves if there may be contact with open lesions, wet linens, or body fluids.

2. This procedure takes two or more people, depending on the size of the resident.

   - If the resident is small, two people can stand on the side to which the resident will be turning.
   - If the resident is large, another person can stand on the other side of the bed.

3. The bed is always kept flat for residents who need logrolling.

   - Elevate the bed to a comfortable working height.
   - Lower the side rails if used for positioning.

4. Make sure the turning sheet is in place under the resident. If the resident has poor head and neck control, the sheet should be wide enough to come up under the back of the head.

5. Place a pillow lengthwise between the resident's legs.

   - Fold the resident's arms over the chest.
   - The resident's head, neck, back and legs must be straight throughout the procedure.

6. The assistants on the left side reach across the resident and grasp the turning sheet, one assistant at the level of the head and shoulders, the other assistant at the level of the buttocks and legs. The sheet should be folded or rolled until the assistant's hands are close to the resident's body.

   - The assistants hold the folded sheet and turn the resident until he/she is lying on the left side.
   - If the resident is large, a third assistant can stand on the other side of the bed in the area of the legs. This assistant helps by supporting the top leg and pillow during the move. The resident should move as a unit (log).
   - The nurse closest to the resident's head gives the signal to turn: "1-2-3 turn."

7. Support the resident's body with pillows as needed. Be sure to maintain good body alignment.

8. Carry out procedure completion actions.

PROCEDURE 22-73
Supine Position

OBRA

NOTE: This procedure should be used to position a resident who is paralyzed on one side of the body (hemiplegia). The instructions would apply to the paralyzed side. The resident should be encouraged to move the strong side. These directions are also appropriate for anyone in the supine position.

1. Carry out each beginning procedure action.

2. Refer to previous procedures for turning the resident onto the back and moving to the head of the bed. Head of bed may be slightly elevated.

3. Center a flat pillow under the resident's head. It should come down to the resident's shoulders. This will prevent too much neck flexion.

4. If the resident's leg(s) tend to fall into external rotation, place a trochanter roll under the affected hip or both hips, as directed under the section on supportive equipment.

(continues)

PROCEDURE 22-73
Supine Position (Continued)

5. Place a folded towel or small, flat pillow under each shoulder. Place the shoulders in slight abduction.

6. Place the shoulders and elbows in extension. (The arms will be straight.)

   - The forearm is pronated. (The palm of the hand is against the bed.)

7. Place a pillow under each arm that extends from the elbow to the ends of the fingers.

   - The wrist and the fingers should be extended with the fingers in slight abduction (separated).

   - The hand, wrist, elbow, and shoulder on each side should be about the same distance from the bed.

8. Place a small pillow under the thighs and another pillow under each leg, extending from the knee to the ankle. This prevents pressure on the heel.

9. Place a folded pillow between the end of the bed and the soles of the resident's feet (Figure 22-55).

10. Make sure the top covers are not pressing on the tops of the resident's feet.

11. Carry out each procedure completion action.

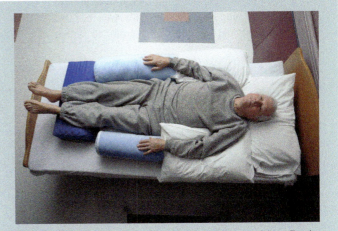

Figure 22-55 Supine or dorsal recumbent position. Resident is flat on back. Bed is flat or head is slightly raised. Pillows are placed under resident's head, shoulders, arm/hands, thighs, lower legs, and ankles. Foot alignment is maintained. Trochanter rolls or rolled pillows placed along hips/thighs prevent external rotation.

PROCEDURE 22-74
Semisupine or Tilt Position

OBRA

NOTE: Directions are given for the resident lying on the left side. This position prevents pressure on the sacrum, coccyx, and hip.

1. Carry out beginning procedure actions.

2. Gather equipment:

   - Pillows

3. Start with the resident in supine position. Roll the resident's trunk and shoulder away from you so that there is a 45-degree angle between the resident's back and the bed.

4. Place a pillow behind the resident's back for support.

5. Bring the resident's left shoulder forward. Flex the elbow of the left arm and place the lower left arm palm up on a pillow.

6. Flex the elbow of the right arm and bring the forearm across the chest with palm down.

(continues)

PROCEDURE 22-74
Semisupine or Tilt Position (Continued)

7. Extend both legs. Place right leg a little behind left leg. Support right leg with two pillows. Pillows should extend from groin to ankle (Figure 22-56).

8. Carry out procedure completion actions.

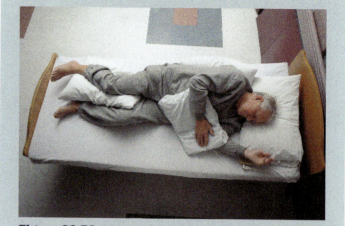

Figure 22-56 Semisupine or tilt position. In this position, the resident is supported on the side with weight distributed across the shoulders. This position takes pressure off the sacrum, coccyx, and hip.

PROCEDURE 22-75
Lateral (Side-Lying) Position

OBRA

NOTE: Directions are given for positioning a resident on the right side. Use the same guidelines for positioning on the left side. It is especially important that this procedure be followed when a resident with hemiplegia is positioned on the unaffected side.

1. Carry out each beginning procedure action.

2. Follow previous procedures for moving the resident in bed (Procedure 22-70) and turning the resident to the side (Procedure 22-71).

3. Place a flat pillow under the resident's head. It should extend 3 to 4 inches beyond the resident's face.

4. When the resident is on his side, the bottom shoulder and hip should be in **protraction** (brought forward). This means you should not pull the shoulder and hip back. To do so will place the shoulder in **retraction** and eventually will cause contracture of those joints.

5. The right shoulder should be slightly abducted and can be in a position of internal or partial external rotation, or extension. For partial external rotation, it will have to be supported on pillows.

   ▪ Use the position that is most comfortable for the resident.

   ▪ Be sure the wrist and fingers are extended and fingers slightly abducted.

6. Slightly flex the right knee.

7. Support the left arm on pillows so that the resident's elbow and wrist are supported.

   ▪ The left shoulder is protracted.

   ▪ The elbow is very slightly flexed.

   ▪ The hand is pronated (palm down).

   ▪ The wrist and fingers are extended with fingers slightly abducted.

(continues)

PROCEDURE 22-75
Lateral (Side-Lying) Position (Continued)

- The shoulder, elbow, and wrist should be about the same height from the bed.

8. Support the left leg on pillows that extend from the knee to the foot.

   - Place the hip and knee in slight flexion. The hip is protracted.
   - The ankle, knee, and hip should all be about the same distance from the bed.

9. If the resident tends to fall back, place a pillow against the resident's back for support (Figure 22-57).

10. Place the top covers loosely over the resident.

11. Carry out each procedure completion action.

NOTE: The right (top) foot and hand should not dangle over the ends of the pillows.

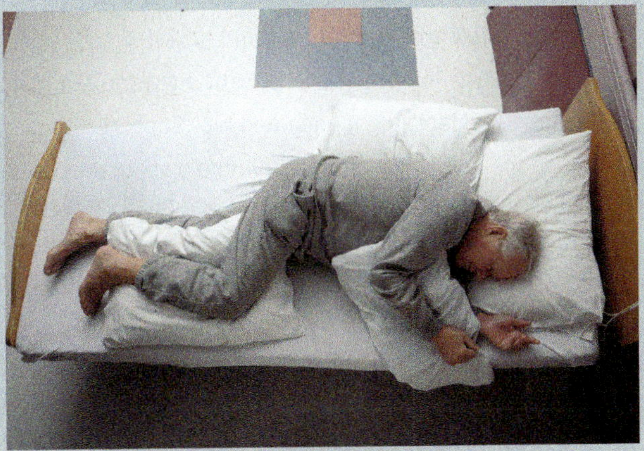

Figure 22-57 Lateral (side-lying) position. In this position, the resident's shoulders and pelvis are maintained in proper alignment.

PROCEDURE 22-76
Lateral Position on the Affected Side

OBRA

1. Follow Steps 1 through 4 in Procedure 22-75.
2. The affected (bottom) shoulder is protracted with elbow extended and forearm pronated.
3. The affected hip is protracted with hip and knee slightly flexed.
4. The unaffected side can be positioned as described in Procedure 22-75, *or*
5. If resident will be in this position only a few minutes, omit the pillows and encourage the resident to actively move these strong extremities.
6. Carry out each procedure completion action.

PROCEDURE 22-77
Semiprone Position

OBRA

This position relieves pressure on the iliac crest and the greater trochanter. Directions are given for the resident lying on the left side.

1. Carry out beginning procedure actions.
2. Gather equipment:

   - Sheepskin
   - Pillows
   - Two foam blocks, each 3 × 6 × 18 inches

(continues)

PROCEDURE 22-77
Semiprone Position (Continued)

3. Place the sheepskin under the resident so it reaches from the shoulders to the knees.
4. Place the left arm in extension and tuck it slightly beneath the resident's body.
5. Place a pillow in front of and at right angles to the resident's chest.
6. Flex the resident's right knee and hip. Support with pillows that are parallel to the leg.
7. Grasp the resident's left arm from the back of the resident. Turn the resident onto the chest facing away from you. Gently pull the left arm toward you and push on resident's hip.
8. Extend the right arm upward and toward the head of the bed. Place it on the head pillow with the fingers and palm against the bed.
9. Flex the upper arm on a pillow.
10. Lift up the sheepskin and place a foam block under the sheepskin above the iliac crest.
11. Place the other foam block under the sheepskin just below the iliac crest (Figure 22-58). You should be able to slide your hand between the hip and the bed.
12. Carry out procedure completion actions.

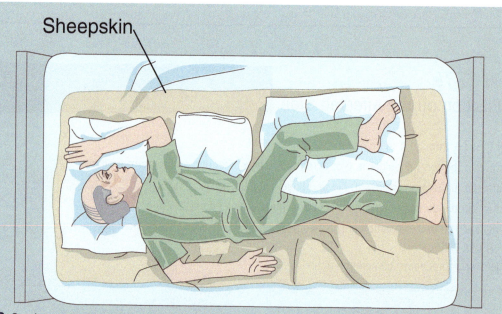

Sheepskin

Figure 22-58 Semiprone position. The resident is lying on a full sheepskin for pressure relief. The resident is almost lying on his stomach. Foam blocks under the sheepskin help to relieve pressure on the iliac crest and greater trochanter.

PROCEDURE 22-78
Fowler's Position

OBRA

Fowler's position is a variation of supine position. In the semi-Fowler's position, the backrest of the bed is raised 30 degrees from the horizontal position. For the Fowler's position, the backrest is raised 45 to 60 degrees from the horizontal position. In the high Fowler's position, the backrest is at 90 degrees from the horizontal position. This position is used most often for residents who have trouble breathing.

PROCEDURE 22-78
Fowler's Position (Continued)

NOTE: A resident at risk for skin breakdown along the lower spine and buttocks should not have the backrest elevated more than 30 degrees (unless there is a nasogastric or gastrostomy tube in place or for 30 minutes after eating). A higher position causes shearing of the skin over the lower spine and buttocks.

1. Carry out each beginning procedure action.
2. Use the turning sheet to move the resident's body into good alignment.
3. Raise the backrest to the desired level.
4. Place one, two, or three pillows behind the resident's head and shoulders.
5. The knees may be slightly flexed and supported with small pillows. This will prevent the resident from sliding down in bed.
6. A pillow can be placed between the resident's feet and the end of the bed.
7. Pillows may be placed under each arm. These should extend from the elbows to fingertips to support the shoulders (Figure 22-59).
8. Place top covers loosely over resident.
9. Carry out each procedure completion action.

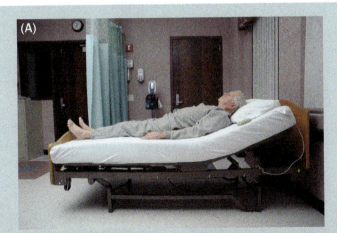

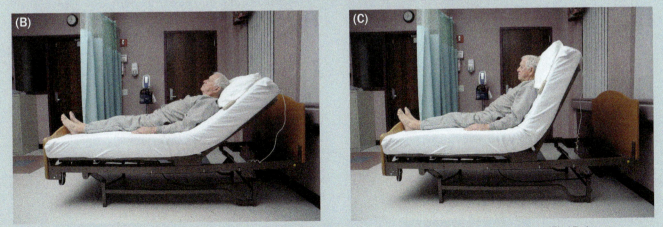

Figure 22-59 Fowler's position. The head of the bed is elevated at a low angle of (A) 30 degrees (low), (B) 45 degrees (Fowler's), or (C) 90 degrees (high).

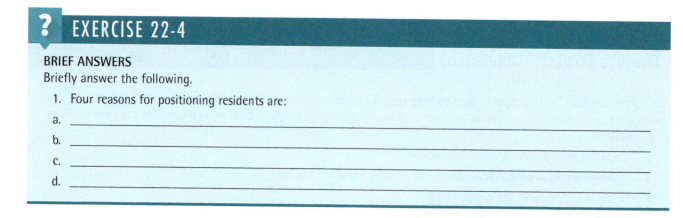

? EXERCISE 22-4

BRIEF ANSWERS
Briefly answer the following.

1. Four reasons for positioning residents are:

   a. _____

   b. _____

   c. _____

   d. _____

TURNING THE DEPENDENT RESIDENT WITH A TURNING SHEET

A **turning sheet** is used to move a dependent resident in bed. Using a regular flat bed sheet:

- Fold the sheet in half, end to end.
- Place this on the resident's bed when the bed is made. Change it as needed.
- Place the folded side toward the head of the bed. Let the ends hang freely over the sides of the bed.
- Place it on the bed so that it extends from the resident's shoulders to knees.

POSITIONING THE DEPENDENT RESIDENT

Special Points for the Resident with Arthritis

Residents with **arthritis** (disease of the joints) are at risk for developing contractures. Be sure you avoid positions of flexion as much as possible.

1. Use a small, flat pillow under the head extending down to the shoulders.
2. Do not place pillows under the knees in supine position.
3. Prone position helps prevent flexion contractures of the hips and knees and should be considered for residents with arthritis.

Special Points for the Resident with Lower Extremity Amputation

Hip flexion contractures can develop easily after a resident has a leg **amputation** (removal of a limb). Knee flexion contractures may develop in residents with below-the-knee amputations. To prevent these:

1. Avoid placing pillows under the **residual limb** (stump).

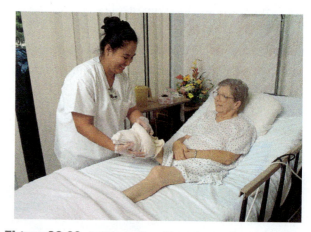

Figure 22-60 Avoid placing pillows under the resident's residual limb. The nursing assistant will place the residual limb flat on the bed.

2. Keep the residual limb flat on the bed with knees extended (Figure 22-60).
3. Keep hips flat on surface of bed.
4. Keep legs adducted.
5. Some residents will be encouraged to lay prone for a prescribed period of time; consult the plan of care for each resident who has had an amputation.
6. Some residents may complain of "phantom pain," a tingling, burning, or cramping sensation in the portion of the leg that has been amputated. Sometimes the phantom pain can be severe. These phantom sensations are thought to be caused by changes in the nervous system. The person with the amputation senses that the missing limb is still present.

Special Points for the Resident with Paralysis

1. If the affected extremities tend to go into flexion, use extension as much as possible when positioning.

2. If the affected extremities tend to go into extension, use flexion when positioning.

3. When paralysis is present in any resident (e.g., stroke, spinal cord injury, multiple sclerosis), use smooth, slow movements avoid causing spasms.

Bridging

Bridging is a technique that prevents pressure on a specific area by the placement of pillows or cushions.

- Trochanter area: Place pillows under trunk and lower extremities when resident is on side, leaving trochanter area free from pressure.
- Ankle: Support foot and lower leg, leaving ankle area suspended.
- Heels: Support entire lower legs with pillows. Maintain good alignment of feet.
- Sacrum: Support both sides of trunk and pelvis, leaving sacral area free from pressure.

Positioning the Resident in a Chair or Wheelchair

Correct positioning for dependent residents sitting in chairs is just as important as it is when they are in bed. The resident's hips and knees should be at 90-degree angles. The feet should be flat on the floor

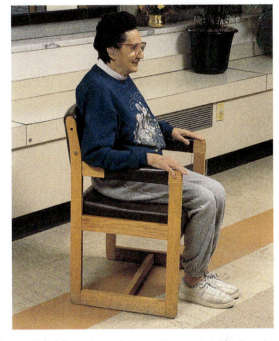

Figure 22-61 Correct chair position maintains the elbows, hips, knees, and ankles at 90 degrees.

(Figure 22-61). Pressure ulcers and contractures can occur just as readily in the chair. Wheelchairs are for transportation and are not designed to be used for long periods of sitting. If this is unavoidable, be sure that the resident is allowed to stand and move about at intervals.

PROCEDURE 22-79
Chair Positioning

OBRA

1. Carry out each beginning procedure action.

2. Head and spine should be erect and in alignment.

3. The resident's arms should rest on the arms of the chair or in the resident's lap. If the shoulders appear to be pushed upward:

   - Place a cushion on the chair seat. This raises the resident's body and allows for proper placement of the arms.

     If the shoulders appear to be hanging:

   - Place pillows or pads to support the resident's lower arms.

4. The back of the wheelchair or other similar chair should come to the level of the resident's shoulder blades. If the back is too high:

   - Place a cushion on the chair seat to elevate the resident's body.

     If the back is too low:

   - Ask the nurse if an extension can be placed on the back of the chair to make it higher.

(continues)

PROCEDURE 22-79
Chair Positioning (Continued)

5. The back and buttocks should be back in the chair. The back and hips form a 90-degree angle.

    - A postural support may be needed to keep the hips back in the chair. Special flat pads can be placed between the resident's clothing and the chair to prevent sliding.

6. The upper and lower leg should form a 90-degree angle. The front edge of the seat should be about two fingers' width away from the back of the knees. If the seat is touching the back of the resident's knees:

    - Place a cushion between the resident and the back of the chair. This will bring the resident forward.

7. The feet and ankles also form 90-degree angles. If the resident's feet do not touch the floor:

    - Place a footstool under the feet. This prevents plantar flexion of the ankle.
    - Place resident's feet on footrests of wheelchair.

8. Carry out each procedure completion action.

PROCEDURE 22-80
Repositioning a Resident in a Wheelchair

Residents who slide down in a wheelchair will need to be moved back and up. You will need another assistant to help you. One stands in back of the wheelchair and one stands in front of the wheelchair.

1. Carry out each beginning procedure action.
2. Use good body mechanics: separate your feet and knees, bend your knees, and keep your back straight.
3. The assistant in back places both arms around the resident's waist.

    - He crosses his own arms in front of the resident's waist.
    - He grasps the resident's left forearm with his right hand and the resident's right forearm with his left hand.

4. The assistant in front places both arms around the resident's knees (Figure 22-62).
5. On the count of three, both assistants lift and raise the resident up and back in the chair.
6. Carry out each procedure completion action.

NOTE: It is helpful to place a lifting sheet (turning sheet) in the seats of chairs for residents who are very frail or heavy. With an assistant on each side, the sheet can be grasped to move the resident.

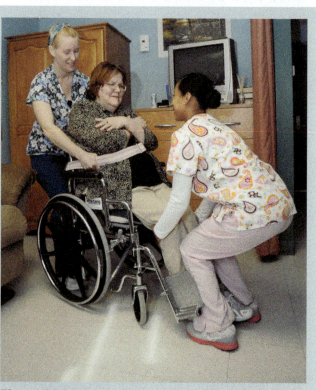

Figure 22-62 Residents may need to be repositioned in their wheelchairs.

PROCEDURE 22-81
Wheelchair Activities to Relieve Pressure

OBRA

Residents who are in a wheelchair for longer than 1 to 2 hours need to relieve the pressure on the hips and buttocks. Teach them to do these activities. You may need to help dependent residents to do these.

Leaning

1. Lock the wheels.
2. Have resident lean slightly forward. (Do not let resident fall out of chair.)
3. Have resident lean from side to side, getting as much weight as possible off each hip.

Wheelchair Pushups

1. Raise the foot pedals. Make sure the resident does not stand on the pedals. Lock the wheels.
2. Tell the resident to place the palms of the hands on the arms of the chair. Then tell the resident to flex (bend) the elbows.
3. Have the resident lean forward, put the feet back, and spread the knees.
4. Tell the resident to lift the buttocks off the chair by pushing down with the hands and straightening the knees (Figure 22-63).

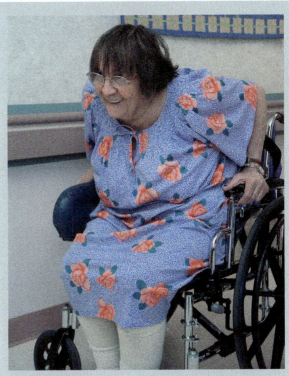

Figure 22-63 Residents in wheelchairs can relieve pressure by doing wheelchair pushups.

? EXERCISE 22-5

BRIEF ANSWERS
Briefly answer the following.

1. Describe four ways to help a resident who has had a leg amputated from developing hip flexion contractures.

   a. _____

   b. _____

   c. _____

   d. _____

2. Four areas in which bridging could be used to avoid the development of pressure areas include:

   a. _____

   b. _____

   c. _____

   d. _____

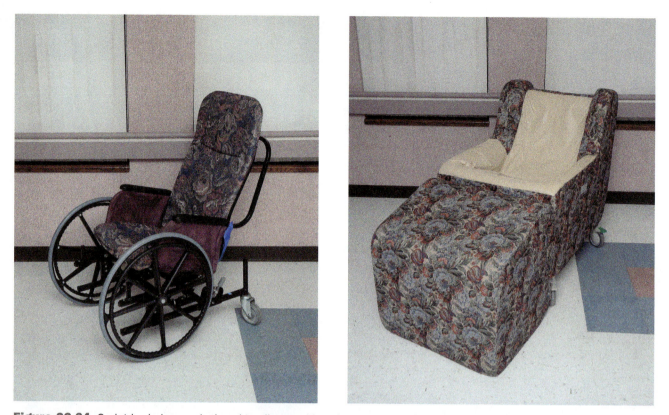

Figure 22-64 Geriatric chairs are designed to allow position changes while maintaining body alignment and comfort.

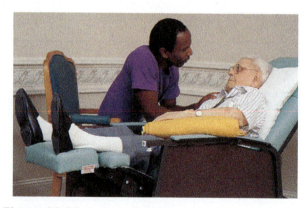

Figure 22-65 Correct positioning in a chair is just as important as positioning in bed.

Some long-term care facilities use geriatric chairs. These allow the resident's position to be changed (Figure 22-64). *Note:* If the tray on the geriatric chair is in place, this is considered to be a restraint.

Cardiac chairs are also frequently used for residents. These are similar to recliners. The resident may be placed in different positions. Pillows can be used to relieve pressure on the shoulders, arms, and hips (Figure 22-65).

INDEPENDENT BED MOVEMENT

The next step in progressive mobilization is to teach the resident how to move independently in bed. This provides exercise and prepares the resident to learn how to move into position to transfer out of bed.

The directions given in Procedure 22-73 are for residents with hemiplegia. These directions can be used with any resident. You should not implement these procedures without instructions from the physical therapist or nurse.

CONTINUING WITH PROGRESSIVE MOBILIZATION

It is important to complete passive range-of-motion exercises and positioning procedures correctly. This will prevent contractures and other complications that can prevent the resident from making progress in mobilization.

Transfer and ambulation activities are the next steps in progressive mobilization. Instructions for these procedures are given in Lesson 23.

? EXERCISE 22-6

Answer the following statements about nursing assistants' actions with A for appropriate or I for inappropriate. If the action is inappropriate, write the appropriate action in the space provided.

1. _____ Lock bed wheels before beginning. _____
_____

2. _____ Raise bed to comfortable working height. _____
_____

3. _____ Secure or tie safety devices to side rails. _____
_____

4. _____ Use fingertips to gently handle the resident's body during mobility. _____
_____

5. _____ Incorporate range of motion into positioning procedures so that range-of-motion exercises do not have to be performed. _____
_____

6. _____ Avoid overhelping residents to encourage independence. _____
_____

7. _____ Turn residents at least every 4 hours. _____
_____

8. _____ Always use a turning sheet to move dependent residents to avoid shearing the skin. _____
_____

9. _____ Allow wrists and feet to hang independently especially when there is paralysis. _____
_____

10. _____ Tighten sheets frequently to avoid wrinkles. _____
_____

11. _____ Always consider resident privacy when positioning. _____
_____

12. _____ Place a trochanter roll so that it extends from just below the hip to just below the knee. _____
_____

13. _____ Padded footboards need to extend just to the tops of toes. _____
_____

14. _____ Always check splints to be sure there are no pressure areas. _____
_____

15. _____ Rolled washcloths may be placed in the resident's hand to support its position. _____
_____

16. _____ When using a sling to support the resident's arm, be sure the fingers and hand remain below heart level. _____

? EXERCISE 22-7

TRUE OR FALSE

Indicate whether the following statements are true (T) or false (F).

1. T F One person can move a heavy resident by using a lift sheet.

2. T F A turning sheet should always be used to move dependent residents in bed.

(continues)

? EXERCISE 22-7 (Continued)

3. T F When more than one assistant is involved in a transfer, one person should give the signals to move on the count of one.

4. T F Logrolling is a technique used to turn residents whose spinal columns must be kept straight.

5. T F Special care and instruction are needed when positioning a resident in the prone position.

6. T F Residents who are hemiplegic should be encouraged to move the unaffected side during position change.

7. T F When the resident is in a lateral position, there should be no pillow under the head or between the legs.

8. T F When sitting in a chair, the resident's hips and knees should be at 45-degree angles.

9. T F Residents remaining in wheelchairs for longer than 1 to 2 hours need to relieve pressure in the hips and buttocks.

10. T F Complete passive range-of-motion exercises and positioning procedures help prevent complications.

11. T F The Residents' Rights state that residents' independence must be promoted.

12. T F Restorative care and rehabilitation are very similar and in many instances identical.

13. T F Task segmentation breaks a task down into several steps.

14. T F The prone position relieves pressure on the iliac crest and greater trochanter.

15. T F In the semiprone position, a foam block is placed under the sheepskin above and below the iliac crest.

16. T F Range-of-motion exercises is one technique used to prevent the formation of contractures.

BOWEL AND BLADDER PROGRAMS

Bowel and bladder programs are considered restorative and/or rehabilitation procedures. These programs are implemented for residents who are incontinent. Incontinence is the inability to control the bowel or the bladder (or both). Incontinence is not a disease and it is *never* a normal consequence of aging.

Some of the most common types of urinary incontinence can be categorized as follows:

- Stress incontinence, the most common type, involves leakage of urine associated with certain activities such as laughing, coughing, or sneezing. This condition also may result from weakened muscles in the bladder or muscles that support the bladder, a weakened urethral sphincter, or hormone imbalances or following multiple childbirths in women. It also may be associated with a variety of disease conditions such as stroke, Parkinson's disease, or diabetes. In men, stress incontinence may be evidence of enlargement of the prostate gland or following prostate surgery.

- Urge incontinence may occur in healthy adults and involves a sudden urge to urinate and the inability to control the flow of urine. It may be a symptom of a urinary tract infection or the result of injury, following surgery, or a spinal cord injury. Urge incontinence also may be present in persons with chronic diseases such as diabetes, Parkinson's disease, multiple sclerosis, or Alzheimer's disease.

- Overflow incontinence occurs when a person cannot fully empty the bladder; the bladder becomes over-distended and causes small, frequent voiding. This may be the result of damage to the bladder by disease conditions such as diabetes, blockage of the urethra by urinary calculi (stones), bladder tumors, or spinal cord injuries.

- Functional incontinence occurs unpredictably. A usually continent person is unable to control the flow of urine before reaching the bathroom. This may be the result of impaired mobility, medication therapy with diuretics or sedatives or other drugs that affect the nervous system, or following stroke or in persons with dementia, such as Alzheimer's disease, or the inability to unbutton clothing quickly due to arthritis of the hands.

- Mixed incontinence involves simultaneously experiencing two types of incontinence such as stress and urge incontinence. This type most often occurs in women.

Incontinence causes many physical and psychological problems. It is embarrassing and may cause the resident to withdraw from all activities. Incontinence can quickly cause skin breakdown and urinary tract infections. It is difficult to avoid unpleasant odors when residents are incontinent. It is better to prevent incontinence than to try and deal with the consequences. Many different types of programs can be used to treat incontinence.

PROCEDURE 22-82
Assisting with Independent Bed Movement

OBRA

1. Carry out each beginning procedure action.

2. Make sure the resident understands what you are going to do.

3. These directions are for moving to the head of the bed.

   - Instruct the resident to place his affected arm over his abdomen. Have resident grasp the side rail with his strong hand.

   - Have resident place his strong foot under his weak leg and then slide his strong foot down under his weak ankle. The weak leg will be supported by the stronger leg.

   - Tell the resident to flex the knee of his strong leg and push that foot against the mattress to help him lift his hips.

   - Have the resident raise his head and pull up with his strong arm and leg, pushing himself toward the head of the bed. (If resident is unable to support his weak leg, hold the leg off the bed while the resident moves. This avoids shearing and friction of the weak leg against the sheet.)

4. Moving to the foot of the bed

   - Reverse procedure in Step 3.

5. Moving toward affected side, to side of bed

   - The resident moves segments of his body in sequence; legs and hips, head and shoulders. Order may be reversed.

   - Instruct the resident to place his affected arm over his abdomen.

   - Tell the resident to place his strong foot under the knee of his affected leg and slide it down under the affected ankle. Lift his affected leg and move it toward edge of bed on affected side.

   - Have the resident remove his strong foot and flex the knee of the strong leg. Now have the resident place his foot firmly on the bed and push down, raising his hips and moving them toward his affected side.

   - Tell the resident to raise his head and shoulders and move them toward his affected side by pushing against the mattress or side rail with his strong side. The resident can use his strong arm to push against the mattress to assist in the move.

6. Moving toward strong side, to side of bed

   - Follow above procedure, moving to strong side.

   - Resident can use the strong arm to grasp side rail to assist in move.

7. Turning onto the side for lateral position.

   - If the resident is going to lie on the affected side, follow directions for moving to the strong side first.

   - Then have the resident use his strong arm to reach toward the opposite side rail to bring himself onto his side.

   - If the resident is going to lie on the strong side, follow directions for moving to affected side first. Have resident grasp his weak hand with his strong hand and raise his arms up with elbows extended. Then have resident use strong arm to "swing" body onto strong side.

8. When the procedure is completed, position the resident according to your instructions.

9. Carry out each procedure completion action.

⊘N THE JOB

Unfortunately, you may work with a person who will put forth little effort in carrying out some of these very important procedures. The resident will eventually suffer from shortcuts taken by staff. Always let your conscience be your guide and perform all tasks to the very best of your ability.

Reasons for Implementing Bowel and Bladder Management Programs

1. To avoid incontinence
2. To reduce the resident's anxiety, fear, and embarrassment related to incontinence
3. To restore self-respect and dignity, which encourages the resident to participate more fully in facility activities
4. To prevent overfilling of the bladder and complications
5. To prevent urinary tract infections and skin problems

⚠ GUIDELINES FOR... BOWEL AND BLADDER PROGRAMS

Before beginning a bowel and bladder program, the nurse will complete an assessment and then plan the program. A bladder retraining assessment form is shown in Figure 22-66. As a nursing assistant, you can help in the following ways:

1. Carry out all instructions accurately and on a timely basis.
2. Avoid the use of incontinent panties or pads during a retraining program.
3. Be consistent in carrying out the program.
4. Assist the resident to be well groomed and appropriately dressed at all times. This increases motivation to succeed.
5. Remember that comfort and privacy are important during all toileting procedures.

It may take several days for the assessment to be completed. Your responsibilities may be to:

1. Record the resident's daily fluid intake.
2. Check the resident for continence at least every 2 hours between 7:00 AM and 10:00 PM and every 4 hours during the night.
3. Record bowel eliminations and the amount of all voidings.
4. Record observations of symptoms that may indicate the reasons for the incontinence. This may

include such problems as disorientation and inability to ambulate.

After the assessment is completed, the nurse will determine the type of program best suited to that resident. Program selection is based on the cause of the incontinence and the resident's mobility skills, cognitive orientation, and motivation.

In most cases, you will need to continue with the actions you carried out during the assessment. Different methods are used for each program. The programs may:

1. Restore a normal pattern of voiding by increasing the time between voiding.
2. Avoid incontinence by taking the resident to the bathroom according to the resident's habits. Positive reinforcement (giving praise) is important.
3. Avoid incontinence by taking the resident to the bathroom on a fixed voiding schedule, usually every 2 hours.

Other techniques are incorporated into each program. Your facility will have specific procedures to follow. It is important that all team members understand the procedures and the reasons for doing them faithfully.

Incontinence is not an inevitable problem in long-term facilities. Not all residents can be "retrained" but, in most cases, incontinence can be avoided. Catheters are not an alternative to incontinence except in very rare circumstances.

(continues)

⚠ GUIDELINES FOR... BOWEL AND BLADDER PROGRAMS (Continued)

BLADDER RETRAINING ASSESSMENT
(Reference tags: F315, F316)

CURRENT RESIDENT STATUS

DIAGNOSIS_____ RESIDENT'S AGE_____

RECENT SURGERY? ☐ Yes ☐ No If Yes, date _____/_____/_____ and type_____

CURRENT MEDICATIONS (i.e., Diuretics, Psychotropics, etc.)_____

_____

Mental Status and Ability to Communicate	Mobility Status	Vision Status	Right	Left
☐ Alert	☐ Independent	Adequate	☐	☐
☐ Aphasic	☐ Transfer/standing ability	Adequate w/aid	☐	☐
☐ Oriented x_____	☐ Wheelchair bound	Poor	☐	☐
☐ Disoriented	☐ Bed rest	Blind	☐	☐
☐ Depressed	☐ Contractures	**Hearing Status**	**Right**	**Left**
☐ Cooperative	☐ Other_____	Adequate	☐	☐
☐ Uncooperative	_____	Adequate w/aid	☐	☐
☐ Slow comprehension	_____	Poor	☐	☐
☐ Other_____	_____	Deaf	☐	☐

BLADDER ASSESSMENT

1. **LENGTH OF INCONTINENCE:** _____ Days _____ Months _____ Years

2. **REASON FOR INCONTINENCE (if known):** _____

   CATHETER: ☐ Yes ☐ No If Yes, specify type and size _____

   Date inserted _____/_____/_____ Reason for catheter _____

3. **USUAL VOIDING PATTERN:** Frequency _____ Amt./voiding _____ cc: /24 hrs. _____ cc

   Pattern: ☐ Upon arising ☐ After meals ☐ No apparent pattern ☐ Night time only

   ☐ Other (specify) _____

4. **SYMPTOMS:** (Check all that apply)
   - ☐ Voids often in small amounts
   - ☐ Fills bladder/voids large amount
   - ☐ Unable to void
   - ☐ Difficulty starting stream
   - ☐ Difficulty stopping stream
   - ☐ Dribbles constantly
   - ☐ Dribbles after voiding
   - ☐ Dribbles while coughing
   - ☐ Urgency
   - ☐ Burning/Pain
   - ☐ Edema
   - ☐ Other (specify)_____

5. **HISTORY OF:** ☐ Urinary Disorders ☐ Bladder Disorders ☐ Kidney Disease ☐ Prostate Problems

   ☐ Neurological Disorders ☐ Fecal Impactions ☐ Other (specify)_____

6. **RELIEF AFTER VOIDING:** ☐ Complete ☐ Continued desire to void

7. **BLADDER DISTENDED:** ☐ Yes ☐ No **EMPTIED BY EXTERNAL STIMULI:** ☐ Yes ☐ No

   If Yes, Check: ☐ Kegel Exercises ☐ Warm water over perineum

   ☐ Other (specify) _____

8. **RESIDUAL URINE:** ☐ Yes ☐ No If Yes, Amount: _____ cc

9. **PERCEPTION OF NEED TO VOID:** ☐ Present ☐ Diminished ☐ Absent

10. **WELL HYDRATED:** ☐ Yes ☐ No **AVERAGE FLUID INTAKE (24 HRS)** _____ cc

    AVERAGE FLUID OUTPUT (24 HRS) _____ cc

    Fluids Preferred _____

Figure 22-66 Bladder retraining assessment form.

(continues)

▲ GUIDELINES FOR... BOWEL AND BLADDER PROGRAMS (Continued)

EVALUATION FOR BLADDER RETRAINING POTENTIAL

☐ ABLE TO PARTICIPATE IN RETRAINING   EVALUATION PERIOD:_____ TO _____

PLAN:_____

_____

PROVIDE FLUIDS: **FLUIDS SHOULD BE SPACED AS FOLLOWS:**

_____ cc every 24 Hrs	☐7AM	☐11	☐3PM	☐7	☐11PM	☐3
_____ cc 7-3 shift	☐8	☐12N	☐4	☐8	☐12MN	☐4
_____ cc 3-11 shift	☐9	☐1PM	☐5	☐9	☐1AM	☐5
_____ cc 11-7 shift	☐10	☐2	☐6	☐10	☐2	☐6

OFFER NO FLUIDS AFTER _____ PM   **TOILET FOR VOIDING EVERY** _____ Hrs (Day and Evening) _____ Hrs (Night)
(Except as needed for medications)
RECORD RESULTS ON BLADDER RETRAINING RECORD.

☐ UNABLE TO PARTICIPATE IN RETRAINING

REASON: _____

_____

REEVALUATION DATE: _____

COMPLETED BY: _____   _____ / _____ / _____

Signature/Title   _Date_

BLADDER RETRAINING PROGRESS NOTES OR REEVALUATION NOTES

DATE	TIME	NOTES - ALL ENTRIES MUST BE SIGNED WITH NAME AND TITLE

NAME—Last	First	Middle	Attending Physician	Chart No.

BLADDER RETRAINING NOTES

Figure 22-66 (Continued)

LESSON SYNTHESIS: Putting It All Together

You have just completed this lesson. Now go back and review the Clinical Focus. Try to see how the Clinical Focus relates to the concepts presented in this lesson. Then answer the following questions.

1. Why will you encourage Mrs. Murphy to do as much of her own care as possible?

2. If range-of-motion activities are not carefully and regularly carried out with her left arm and leg, what serious complication could develop?

3. When not being exercised, what is the proper position for Mrs. Murphy's affected arm and leg?

4. Before attempting to move Mrs. Murphy, what actions should the nursing assistant take?

Courtesy of J. T. Posey Co., Inc, Arcadia, CA

22 REVIEW

A. Select the one best answer for each of the following.

1. Restorative care is the responsibility of the

   (A) physician

   (B) nursing staff

   (C) physical therapist

   (D) occupational therapist

2. "Activity strengthens and inactivity weakens" is a principle of restorative care and means that

   (A) complications result from physical and mental inactivity

   (B) residents should receive several hours of bed rest each day

   (C) residents are not encouraged to move about

   (D) inactivity is not harmful

3. "Treat the whole person" is a principle of restorative care and means that it is important to

   (A) attend to the physical needs of the resident

   (B) attend to the emotional needs of the resident

   (C) attend to the mental needs of the resident

   (D) provide for the physical, emotional, and mental needs of the resident

4. Contractures can be prevented by all but

   (A) doing range-of-motion exercises regularly

   (B) using correct positioning techniques

   (C) correctly applying splints

   (D) encouraging bed rest

5. An example of an instrumental activity of daily living (IADLs) is

   (A) feeding oneself

   (B) managing a household

   (C) swimming

   (D) riding a bicycle

6. A self-care deficit may be due to all but

   (A) paralysis

   (B) perceptual deficits

   (C) depression

   (D) being active

7. The first step in progressive mobilization is teaching the resident to

   (A) come to a standing position

   (B) change position in bed

   (C) move in bed

   (D) move about in a wheelchair

8. Passive range of motion means

(A) the care provider moves the joints for the resident

(B) the care provider supports the joints and assists in the movements while the resident attempts independent movement

(C) the resident is able to move the joints without any assistance

(D) the resident uses the strong extremity to move the affected extremity

9. An orthosis is (a, an)

(A) artificial body part

(B) sling

(C) splint

(D) cane

10. The purpose of an orthosis is to

(A) replace a missing body part

(B) simplify an activity of daily living (ADL)

(C) help a person ambulate

(D) support a joint in correct position

11. The main purpose of bowel and bladder programs is to

(A) save time for the nursing staff so they do not have to change incontinent residents

(B) increase the resident's self-esteem and dignity

(C) save money on incontinent pads

(D) save on laundry costs

12. A predisposing factor in functional incontinence is

(A) bladder injury

(B) coughing and sneezing

(C) inability to reach call signal

(D) failure to completely empty the bladder

B. Match each term (items a–j) with the proper definition.

a. flexion

b. extension

c. abduction

d. adduction

e. rotation

f. pronation

g. supination

h. inversion

i. eversion

j. opposition

13. _____ bringing palmar surface of thumb to the finger joint

14. _____ bending a joint

15. _____ moving an extremity away from the body

16. _____ turning the forearm so the palm is facing downward

17. _____ straightening a joint

18. _____ turning inward

19. _____ moving an extremity back to the body

20. _____ turning around an axis

21. _____ turning the forearm so the palm is facing upward

22. _____ turning outward

C. Answer each statement true (T) or false (F).

23. T F It is a resident's right to have the staff do everything for him or her.

24. T F OBRA requires that restorative care be included in nursing assistant courses.

25. T F One purpose of restorative care is to help the resident adapt to limitations imposed by a disability.

26. T F Successful restorative care means that the resident always regains his or her functional abilities.

27. T F Restorative care generally involves training from physical therapists and occupational therapists.

28. T F Long-term inactivity can cause the heart to become deconditioned.

29. T F Restorative care is only important for residents who are planning to return to their homes.

30. T F Correct positioning can prevent pressure ulcers and contracture formation.

31. T F Incontinence is not considered a normal change of aging.

32. T F Incontinence is primarily a condition that affects women.

RESTORING RESIDENTS' MOBILITY

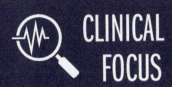

CLINICAL FOCUS

Think about the special precautions you must take to safeguard a resident during periods of mobility as you study this lesson.

OBJECTIVES

After studying this lesson, you should be able to:

- Define vocabulary words and terms.
- List the guidelines for transfer procedures.
- State the contraindications to using a transfer belt.
- Describe the factors that are considered in determining the correct method of transfer.
- List the guidelines for ambulation procedures.
- Describe the purpose of assistive devices used in ambulation.
- Describe safety measures when using assistive devices.
- Demonstrate the following:

  Procedure 23-83   Using a Transfer Belt (Gait Belt)
  Procedure 23-84   Bringing the Resident to Sitting Position at the Edge of the Bed
  Procedure 23-85   Assisted Standing Transfer
  Procedure 23-86   Transferring the Resident from Chair to Bed
  Procedure 23-87   Assisted Standing Transfer/Two Assistants
  Procedure 23-88   Wheelchair to Toilet and Toilet to Wheelchair Transfers
  Procedure 23-89   Transferring to Tub Chair or Shower Chair
  Procedure 23-90   Transferring a Non-weightbearing Resident from Wheelchair to Bed
  Procedure 23-91   Transferring Resident with a Mechanical Lift
  Procedure 23-92   Sliding Board Transfer
  Procedure 23-93   Ambulating a Resident
  Procedure 23-94   Assisting Resident to Ambulate with Cane or Walker

CASE STUDY

Ms. Peabody, although ambulatory with a walker since her hip surgery, is unsteady and needs assistance.

VOCABULARY

ambulate (AM-byou-late)
aneurysm (AN-you-rizm)
assistive device (ah-SIS-tiv dih-VICE)
colostomy (koh-LAHS-toh-mee)
gait (gayt)
gait belt (gayt belt)
gait training (gayt TRAYN-ing)
mechanical lift (mih-KAN-ih-kul lift)

non-weight bearing (NON-wayt BAIR-ing)
pacemaker (PAYS-may-ker)
paraplegia (pair-ah-PLEE-jee-ah)
partial weight bearing (PAR-shul wayt BAIR-ing)
sliding board (SLYD-ing bord)
transfer (TRANS-fer)
transfer belt (TRANS-fer belt)
weight bearing (wayt BAIR-ing)

Many residents in long-term care facilities have impaired mobility. *Mobility* means movement or the ability to move. Restorative care includes assisting dependent residents with mobility and helping residents regain independent mobility.

In Lesson 22 you learned how to help residents regain independence in activities of daily living (ADLs). You also learned how to perform procedures that will prevent the complications caused by immobility. The next step is to help residents get out of bed, to transfer, and to ambulate (walk).

TRANSFERS

The word transfer means to move a resident from one place to another. Transfers are used to:

- Move a resident out of bed and into a chair
- Move a resident from a chair and into bed
- Move a resident from a wheelchair to a toilet or commode
- Move a resident from a toilet or commode to a wheelchair
- Move a resident from a chair into a car and back
- Move a resident from a chair into a tub lift or shower chair and back into the chair

The nurse or physical therapist determines the method of transfer. The method selected depends on:

1. The resident's physical condition, including:
   - Paralysis of any extremity
   - Absence of an extremity due to amputation
   - Recent hip surgery
   - Issues with blood pressure variations
2. The resident's strength, endurance, and balance. These abilities may be affected by:
   - Respiratory disease
   - Cardiac disease

- Neurologic disease
- Ability to stand on one or both legs. This is called weight bearing. For example, a resident may not be able to bear weight on a paralyzed leg. After hip surgery the physician may order the resident to be non-weight bearing or partial weight bearing.

3. The resident's mental condition. Can the resident understand instructions?
4. The resident's size

There are two basic types of transfer: standing and sitting. For a standing transfer, the resident must be able to stand and have weight bearing on one leg. Examples of sitting transfers are those done with a mechanical lift or sliding board. Before getting the resident out of bed, it is important to correctly position the wheelchair (at a 45- to 60-degree angle) and lock the brakes (Figure 23-1). Always position the wheelchair on the resident's strong side; the resident's unaffected

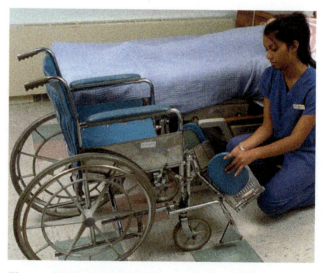

Figure 23-1 Prepare for the transfer by positioning the chair correctly at a 45- to 60-degree angle. Position the large part of the small front wheels facing forward. Lock the brakes. Move the footrests back or up and out of the way.

⚠ GUIDELINES FOR... TRANSFERS

NOTE: Always use the correct transfer method as directed by the nurse or physical therapist. Disregarding these instructions can result in injury to the resident or to you. If you have difficulty transferring a resident by the indicated method, consult with the nurse.

1. If the transfer requires two people, do not try to do it alone. You risk injuring yourself and the resident.

2. Use correct body mechanics for all transfers.

3. *Residents should not place their hands on your body during a transfer.* This is a dangerous practice. A resident who is disoriented or frightened can cause you to lose your balance. A resident who loses balance during transfer can pull you down. If a resident's arms are around your neck, any sudden movement can injure you.

4. *Hands should not be placed under a resident's arms.* Remember that residents' bones are fragile.

This practice can fracture ribs and dislocate shoulders.

5. Use a transfer belt for standing transfers unless it is contraindicated (see Procedure 23-83).

6. The resident should wear sturdy, well-fitting shoes with nonslip soles for all standing transfers and ambulation.

7. Give the resident only the assistance needed.

8. Stand close to the resident when transferring. If the resident has an affected or paralyzed leg, brace that knee with your knee or leg.

9. Always transfer toward the resident's strongest side.

10. Allow the resident to see the surface to which the resident is being transferred. Encourage the resident to keep their head up.

11. Always explain to the resident what you are doing and how the resident can help.

or strongest side should move toward the chair. Check the front, pivoting wheels of the chair. These wheels help the chair move in all directions, as well as to provide stability when you are transferring the resident. When you are wheeling the chair, the larger portion of the pivoting wheel faces the back of the chair, however, the large section of the front wheel should face forward when you are transferring the resident. Maneuver the chair so the larger portion of the wheel is facing the front in order to provide more stability during transfer. Make sure that the chair is at the correct angle and that all wheels are in alignment, then lock the brakes. You are then ready to position the resident and transfer the resident to the chair.

Several steps are involved in transferring a resident from bed to chair:

- Bringing the resident to a sitting position on the edge of the bed, raising the head of the bed to assist
- Bringing the resident to a standing position
- Moving the resident to the chair
- Seating the resident

PROCEDURE 23-83
Using a Transfer Belt (Gait Belt)

OBRA

A **transfer belt** is a webbed belt 1½ to 2 inches wide. It is 54 to 60 inches long. It is an assistive and safety device used to transfer or ambulate residents who need help. When the belt is used to assist a resident with ambulation, it is called a **gait belt**.

1. Carry out each beginning procedure action.

2. Show the resident the transfer belt and explain that it is a safety device. Assure the resident that the belt is used only for a short time during the actual transfer or ambulation exercise.

3. The belt should never be placed over bare skin. If it is used to transfer a resident to a shower seat or tub lift, place a towel around the resident's waist and then apply the belt over it.

4. Keep the belt low on the resident's waist.

5. Buckle the belt in front—not at the back or the side (Figure 23-2A).

(continues)

PROCEDURE 23-83
Using a Transfer Belt (Gait Belt) (Continued)

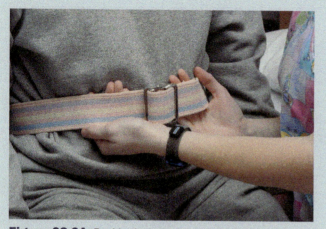

Figure 23-2A Buckle the transfer belt in the front.

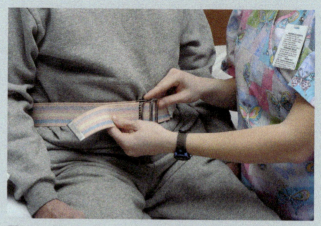

Figure 23-2B Thread the belt through the teeth side of the buckle first.

6. Thread the belt through the teeth side first and place belt through both openings to ensure a safe closure (Figure 23-2B).

7. Use an underhand grasp when holding the belt (Figure 23-3).

8. The belt should be snug but you should be able to get your fingers under it. This will prevent the belt from riding up under the breasts, rib cage, or axillae.

9. When applying the belt, check female residents to be sure breasts are not under the belt.

10. Avoid overusing the belt by pulling the resident up with force. Remember: The belt is not a lifting device—it is used for support and stability.

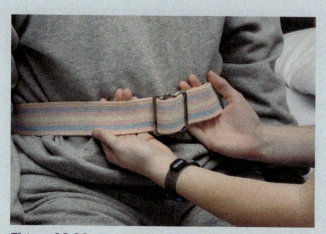

Figure 23-3A Hold transfer belt with an underhand grasp.

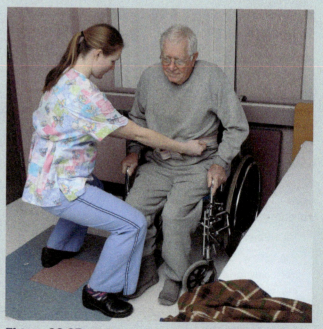

Figure 23-3B Instruct the resident to hold the chair arms with both hands.

(continues)

PROCEDURE 23-83
Using a Transfer Belt (Gait Belt) (Continued)

11. Transfer resident using the correct method.

12. Carry out each procedure completion action.

NOTE: The transfer belt may be contraindicated for these conditions:

1. **Colostomy** located in the upper abdomen. This is a surgical opening created for the evacuation of feces.

2. **Pacemaker** located in the abdomen. This is a device used to maintain a normal heart rate.

3. Gastrostomy tube or feeding tube that is surgically inserted into the resident's stomach.

4. Recent abdominal surgery or a new abdominal incision (surgical cut through the skin).

5. Fractured vertebrae or ribs.

6. Severe cardiac or respiratory disease.

7. Implanted medication pumps. Some residents may receive medications via tube from a pump that is implanted under the skin (frequently the abdomen). Check with the nurse and/or the care plan for information as to the safety of using a transfer belt for the particular resident.

8. Pregnancy.

9. Abdominal aortic aneurysms. An **aneurysm** is a weakness or an outpouching in the wall of an artery due to a structural defect in the arterial wall. If the aneurysm ruptures, the resident could die of massive hemorrhage.

10. Severe osteoporosis (brittle, porous bone structure).

NOTE: Do not use the pants/slacks belt as a transfer or gait belt when transferring or ambulating residents. Upward movement of the belt can cause male residents severe pain in the scrotum.

? EXERCISE 23-1

BRIEF ANSWERS

1. Who determines the method by which a resident will be transferred? _____
_____

2. What four factors must be considered when planning the proper method to transfer a resident?

 a. _____
 _____

 b. _____
 _____

 c. _____
 _____

 d. _____

3. What three factors can affect the resident's physical condition?

 a. _____
 _____

 b. _____
 _____

 c. _____
 _____

(continues)

4. What condition can affect a resident's weight-bearing ability?

_____

_____

5. What can happen if the correct method of transfer is not followed?

_____

_____

PROCEDURE 23-84
Bringing the Resident to Sitting Position at the Edge of the Bed

OBRA

1. Carry out each beginning procedure action.

NOTE: You may be asked to check the resident's pulse before beginning any activity. If so, take the pulse now.

2. If you will be transferring the resident into the chair:
   - Have the chair ready to receive the resident. If it is a wheelchair, lock the brakes. Put the foot pedals up or remove them if possible. If the arm of the chair is removable, it is easier to work with it off.
   - Have the resident's clothing and shoes ready.
   - Have the transfer belt ready if it is to be used.

NOTE: If the resident is to transfer out of the bed, the bed must be in the low position. Remember to use correct body mechanics.

3. Begin with the resident lying in supine position in the center of the bed.

4. Have the resident cross arms over the abdomen or chest.

5. Cross the resident's farthest leg over the leg nearest you.

6. Stand facing the bed with your thigh that is nearest the resident's head braced against the bed. Bend your knees and hips. Assume a broad base of support. Get close to the resident.

7. With one hand on the resident's far shoulder and one on the far hip, turn the resident onto the side, facing you (Figure 23-4).

8. Flex the resident's hips and knees.

9. With your arm that is closest to the resident's legs, reach across the top leg and secure both legs with your arm.

10. Place your other arm so that your forearm supports the resident's shoulders. The resident's neck and head are cradled by your elbow.

11. As you shift your weight from your front to back leg, lower the resident's legs over the edge of the bed. At the same time, bring the resident's head and shoulders to upright position (Figure 23-5).

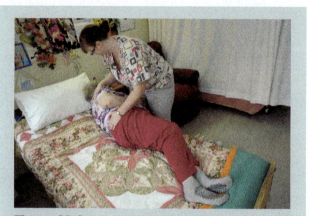

Figure 23-4 Help the resident turn to the side before sitting on the edge of the bed.

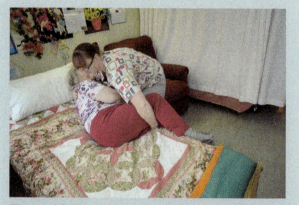

Figure 23-5 Help the resident to a sitting position on the edge of the bed.

(continues)

PROCEDURE 23-84
Bringing the Resident to Sitting Position at the Edge of the Bed (Continued)

NOTE: If the resident is able to, ask the resident to use the lower arm to support the upper body. Ask the resident to use the upper arm to push into the mattress to raise the upper body.

12. Carry out transfer as indicated in the next procedures.

13. If the resident is unable to assume a sitting position on their own, raise the head of the bed and then assist them to sit up on the side of the bed.

? EXERCISE 23-2

COMPLETION
Complete the following statements

1. Seven reasons a transfer belt may be contraindicated are:

a. _____

b. _____

c. _____

d. _____

e. _____

f. _____

g. _____

2. Four steps involved in transferring a resident from bed to a chair include:

a. _____

b. _____

c. _____

d. _____

PROCEDURE 23-85
Assisted Standing Transfer

OBRA

NOTE: The bed should be in the low position when you transfer a resident into or out of bed. You must use good body mechanics—keep your back straight, bend from the knees and hips, and maintain a broad base of support.

1. Carry out each beginning procedure action.

2. The chair is placed on the resident's strong side. Place it at the foot or the head of the bed and parallel to the bed.

3. If you are using a wheelchair, lock the brakes. The front casters of the chair should be straight. Put the foot pedals up or remove them from the chair.

4. Lock the wheels of the bed.

5. Check the resident's pulse if instructed to do so. Bring the resident to a sitting position on the edge of the bed as directed in Procedure 23-84. Allow resident to sit for a few seconds to stabilize.

6. Put a transfer belt around the resident's waist.

7. Put nonskid shoes or slippers on the resident (Figure 23-6).

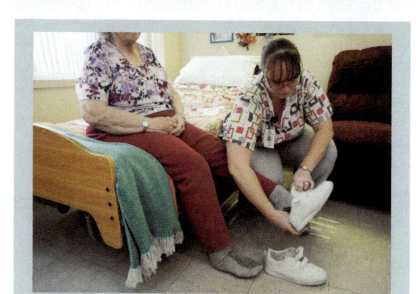

Figure 23-6 Put shoes on the resident.

NOTE: If you are unsure of the resident's balance, you can put the transfer belt on while the resident is lying down. You can also put the nonskid shoes or slippers on at that time.

8. Tell the resident what to do to help.

9. Assist the resident to assume the transfer position:

   ▪ Ask the resident to lean forward ("nose over toes").

   ▪ Have resident separate the knees for a broad base of support.

   ▪ Have resident move the feet back.

NOTE: Be sure to check the resident's feet before transferring. Some residents are unable to tell what position their feet are in.

   ▪ Ask the resident to place the palms of the hands against the edge of the mattress. This will help the resident to "push off."

10. Place yourself in front of the resident. If the resident has an affected or paralyzed leg, brace that knee with your knee.

11. Place your other leg several inches back.

12. Place your hands in the transfer belt (underhand grasp) with one hand on each side of the resident's body.

13. If the resident has an affected or paralyzed arm, do not let it hang or dangle during the transfer.

   ▪ If the resident has a sling, put this on before the transfer.

   ▪ If there is no sling, the hand can be placed in the pants pocket or the resident can cradle the affected arm with the strong arm.

14. Before moving the resident, make sure both you and the resident are ready to move.

(continues)

PROCEDURE 23-85
Assisted Standing Transfer (Continued)

15. Tell the resident that on the count of three she will:
    - Use the hands (if able) to press into the mattress.
    - Straighten the elbows.
    - Straighten the knees and come to a standing position.

16. At the same time, you will use the transfer belt to gently assist the resident to stand—do not lift the resident with the belt.
    - Remember, the resident should not grasp your neck, arms, or any part of your body. You should not use your hands and arms on the resident's body.

17. If the resident cannot take any steps:
    - Have resident pivot around to the front of the chair until the chair touches the back of the resident's legs.

18. Instruct resident to place hands on the arms of the chair and then gently lower resident into the chair (Figure 23-7).

19. If you took the resident's pulse before the activity, recheck it now. If there is a significant difference, report this to the nurse.

20. Position the resident comfortably. Place the call light within easy reach. Be sure the resident has access to drinking water and any other items that may be needed.

21. Carry out each procedure completion action.

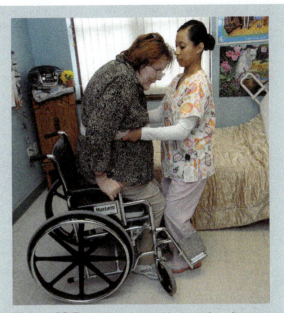

Figure 23-7 Instruct the resident to place her hands on the arms of the chair and then gently lower the resident into chair.

PROCEDURE 23-86
Transferring the Resident from Chair to Bed

OBRA

NOTE: Use good body mechanics—keep your back straight, bend from the knees and hips, and maintain a broad base of support with your feet.

1. Reverse Procedure 23-85.
2. If the resident has an affected or paralyzed side, place the wheelchair so that the resident can transfer from the strong side. Lock the brakes on the wheelchair and remove the footrests.
3. Lock the wheels on the bed.
4. Place the transfer belt around the resident's waist.
5. Have resident assume the transfer position as described in Procedure 23-85.
6. Follow Steps 10 through 14 in Procedure 23-85.
7. Tell the resident to place the hands on the arms of the wheelchair or chair.
8. On the count of three, have resident straighten both elbows and knees to come to a standing position.

(continues)

PROCEDURE 23-86
Transferring the Resident from Chair to Bed (Continued)

9. Pivot around to the bed. When the resident feels the bed against the backs of the legs, have resident slowly sit down on the edge of the bed.
10. Remove the transfer belt and the resident's shoes and socks. If balance is questionable, this can be done after the resident is lying down.
11. Place your arm closest to the head of the bed around the resident's shoulders. Place your other arm around the resident's knees (Figure 23-8).
12. Guide the resident to a supine position. Position the resident comfortably.
13. Carry out each procedure completion action.

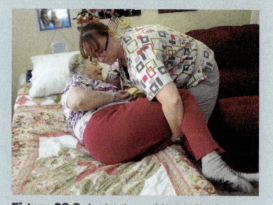

Figure 23-8 Assist the resident to lie down.

PROCEDURE 23-87
Assisted Standing Transfer/Two Assistants

OBRA

NOTE: This procedure is for a resident who is heavier or taller, or has impaired balance or only partial weight-bearing ability.

Follow your instructions when you are told that two people are required to move or transfer a resident. Disregarding instructions can result in serious injury to you and the resident.

Remember: Use good body mechanics—keep your back straight, bend from the knees and hips, and maintain a broad base of support with your feet.

1. Carry out each beginning procedure action.

This procedure is carried out the same as a one-person transfer except:

2. Both assistants stand in front of and to each side of the resident.
3. Both assistants put both hands in the transfer belt. Each assistant has one hand in the front of the belt and one in the back of the belt (Figure 23-9).

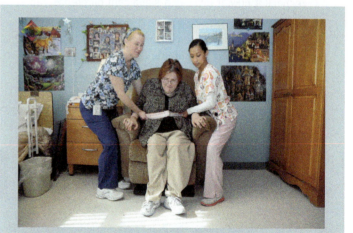

Figure 23-9 Some residents need the help of two nursing assistants. The nursing assistants have both hand on the transfer belt.

4. If the resident has a paralyzed or affected leg, one assistant blocks that leg with her knee against the resident's knee.

It is important that both assistants and the resident clearly understand the direction of the move.

5. On the count of three, both assistants and the resident pivot around to the chair.
6. Continue procedure as with one assistant.
7. Carry out each procedure completion action.

PROCEDURE 23-88
Wheelchair to Toilet and Toilet to Wheelchair Transfers

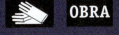 **OBRA**

Remember: Use good body mechanics—keep your back straight, bend from the hips and knees, and maintain a broad base of support with your feet.

1. Carry out each beginning procedure action.

2. You may need to adapt the procedure to the physical arrangement of the bathroom.
   - Grab bars should be placed securely on the wall or attached to the toilet seat (Figure 23-10). Towel bars are not safe to use as grab bars.

3. Most toilets are 16 inches high. Some residents may have difficulty coming to a standing position from this level. A raised toilet seat can be added, which will raise it to 20 inches.

4. Follow all the guidelines for transfers. Use the transfer belt.

5. Place wheelchair at a right angle to the toilet. Lock the brakes. Be sure the foot pedals are up or off.

6. While the resident is still sitting, loosen clothing.

7. Bring resident to a standing position as described earlier.
   - Ask the resident to lean forward.
   - Have the resident separate knees for a broad base of support.
   - Have the resident move the feet back.
   - Have resident place palms of the hands on the wheelchair arms to help "push off."
   - On the count of three, help the resident to a standing position (Figure 23-11).

8. Encourage the resident to stand erect. Pivot to toilet seat.

9. Have resident use the grab bars for support while you manipulate the clothing. If the resident's balance is questionable, you will need another assistant to do this while you help the resident stand.

10. With your hands in the transfer belt, assist the resident to sitting position on the toilet.

11. Remove transfer belt. Provide privacy, but remain close by.

    When resident is finished toileting:

12. Position wheelchair at a right angle to toilet. Lock the brakes. Be sure the foot pedals are up or off. If possible, place wheelchair on resident's strong side.

13. Have toilet tissue ready.

14. Put on gloves.

15. Bring resident to standing position. Have resident use grab bars while you clean resident's buttocks and genitalia.
    - If resident is able, provide support while the resident performs this task.

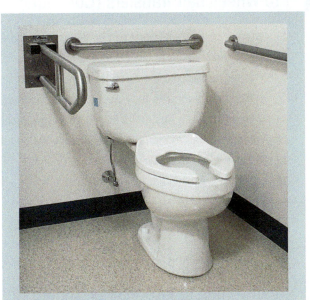

Figure 23-10 Grab bars provide safety.

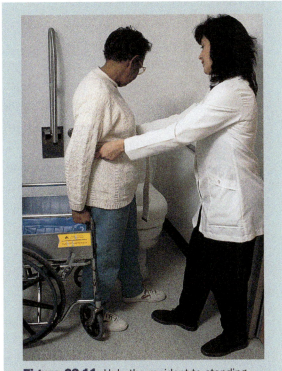

Figure 23-11 Help the resident to standing position.

(continues)

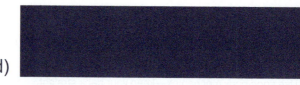

PROCEDURE 23-88
Wheelchair to Toilet and Toilet to Wheelchair Transfers (Continued)

16. Arrange clothing while resident is still using the grab bars for support.
17. Assist the resident to pivot to the wheelchair.
    - Have resident put hands on the arms of the chair.
    - When resident feels the edge of the seat against the back of the legs, have the resident slowly sit in the chair.
    - Your hands are still in the transfer belt so you can provide assistance.
18. Wheel the chair to the lavatory. Assist the resident in washing and drying hands.
19. Remove your gloves. Wash and dry your hands.
20. Carry out each procedure completion action.

PROCEDURE 23-89
Transferring to Tub Chair or Shower Chair

Remember: Use good body mechanics—keep your back straight, bend from the hips and knees, and maintain a broad base of support with your feet.

The procedure for transferring a resident from a wheelchair to a tub chair or shower chair is carried out in the same manner as a transfer from a wheelchair to toilet or chair, with added considerations.

1. Carry out each beginning procedure action.
2. Transport the resident to the shower or tub room by wheelchair.
3. Lock wheelchair. Remove footrests.
4. Remove the resident's top clothing while resident is seated in the wheelchair.
5. Leave the resident's shoes on until the resident has transferred to the shower or tub chair.
    - Place a large towel around the resident's shoulders to avoid chilling and exposure.
    - Place a towel around the resident's waist before applying transfer belt. Apply transfer belt.
    - Assist the resident to stand.
    - Have resident pivot around or take a step to the shower or tub chair.
    - Loosen and bring underwear and slacks down below resident's hips.
6. Have resident sit down in shower chair or tub chair. Place towel over resident's lap for privacy.
7. Remove underwear, slacks, shoes, and socks.
8. Remove transfer belt. When shower/bath is completed, reverse procedure.
9. Dry resident while seated in tub or shower chair.
10. Help resident put on upper body clothing while seated in tub or shower chair. Then apply transfer belt.
11. Put resident's underwear and slacks on.
    - Pull up to the hips.
    - Put on socks and shoes.
12. Assist resident to stand. Pull up underwear and slacks.

(continues)

PROCEDURE 23-89
Transferring to Tub Chair or Shower Chair (Continued)

13. Assist resident to pivot or step to wheelchair.
    - When the resident feels the wheelchair against the back of the legs, have resident place hands on arms of wheelchair.
    - Then have resident slowly seat self in wheelchair.
14. Carry out each procedure completion action.

PROCEDURE 23-90
Transferring a Non-Weightbearing Resident from Wheelchair to Bed

OBRA

This procedure is used for residents who are unable to stand. The resident must be able to follow directions. This is not an appropriate transfer for a resident who is large. The procedure requires two assistants. It should only be done when the wheelchair has removable arms and removable footrests.

Remember: Use good body mechanics—keep your back straight, bend from the hips and knees, and maintain a broad base of support with your feet.

1. Carry out each beginning procedure action.
2. Lock wheels of bed. Put bed in lowest horizontal position.
3. Remove arms from wheelchair. Remove footrests from wheelchair. Place wheelchair at head of bed facing foot of bed. Wheelchair should be parallel to bed.
4. The first assistant stands behind the wheelchair. The second assistant stands in front of the wheelchair.
5. The first assistant places arms around resident's trunk. This assistant crosses arms and grasps the resident's left forearm with assistant's right hand. The resident's right forearm is grasped with the assistant's left hand.
6. The second assistant stands beside resident's legs, facing bed. This assistant places both arms under resident's legs.
7. Remember to use good body mechanics. On the count of three, the resident is lifted out of the chair and into bed.
8. Position resident as necessary.
9. Carry out each procedure completion action.

USING MECHANICAL LIFTS

A mechanical lift may be needed to transfer certain residents. This device is used to move residents who are unable to bear weight, are heavy, or have poor trunk control. The use of the mechanical lift makes the transfer procedure safer for the resident and for the staff. A variety of types of seats or slings are available as well as adaptations for weighing the residents. In addition, mechanical lifts are designed to assist in transferring a resident into a bathtub or onto the toilet.

The most commonly used type of mechanical lift is the hydraulic lift, often called a hoyer lift. Some are manually operated; others are electric or battery operated.

Remember these precautions when using the mechanical lift:

- *Two people are required for this procedure. Never attempt to operate the hydraulic lift alone. In some states, a CNA must be 18 years of age to operate or assist with a mechanical lift.*
- Be sure both staff members have been instructed in the correct procedure before attempting to use a mechanical lift with residents. The procedure may vary depending on the manufacturer of the equipment.
- Be sure that the sling is not torn or soiled; the manufacturer should indicate the longevity of the sling. The sling must be washed according to manufacturer's directions. Monitor weight limits for the equipment.

- Check the floor under the lift. If you notice an oily substance (leaking hydraulic fluid), do not use the lift. Tag the faulty piece of equipment for repair according to facility policy because the lift may cause injury to the resident or to staff.

- Obtain safe equipment before you attempt to transfer the resident with a lift.

PROCEDURE 23-91
Transferring Resident with a Mechanical Lift

OBRA

1. Carry out each beginning procedure action.

2. Get another assistant or nurse to help you. One person operates the lift. The other person guides the sling and resident.

3. Check sling and straps for frayed areas or poorly closing clasps.

4. Place a wheelchair or other chair parallel to bed, facing the head of the bed.

5. Lock the bed. Lock the wheelchair or other chair wheels.

6. Position the sling under the resident's body by rolling him first onto his left side. Place the folded sling against his body (Figure 23-12).

7. Roll resident onto his right side and straighten the sling (Figure 23-13).

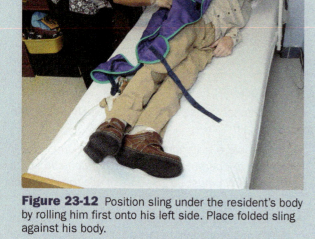

Figure 23-12 Position sling under the resident's body by rolling him first onto his left side. Place folded sling against his body.

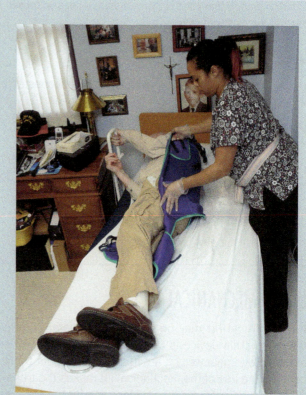

Figure 23-13 Roll resident onto his right side and straighten the sling.

8. Make sure that the sling reaches from his shoulders to his knees (Figure 23-14).

9. Position the lift over the bed and attach the hooks to the sling (Figure 23-15). Make sure that the open end of each hook is turned away from the resident's body (Figure 23-16).

10. Raise the lift following the directions for the specific type of lift used at your facility. Gently swing the resident to the chair. One nursing assistant can support the resident's legs (Figure 23-17).

(continues)

PROCEDURE 23-91
Transferring Resident with a Mechanical Lift (Continued)

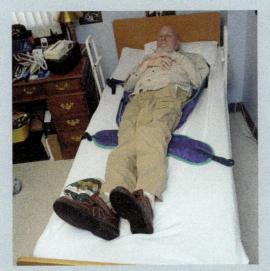

Figure 23-14 Make sure that the sling reaches from his shoulders to his knees.

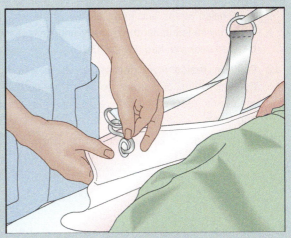

Figure 23-16 Make sure that the open end of each ("S") hook is turned away from the resident's body.

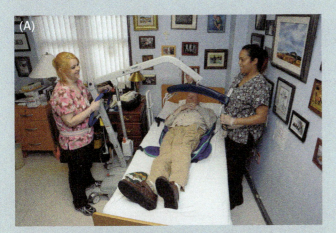

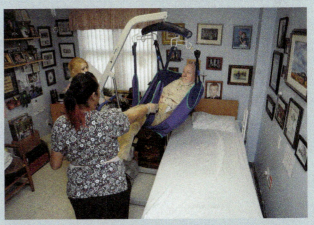

Figure 23-17A Raise the lift following the directions for the type of lift used at your facility.

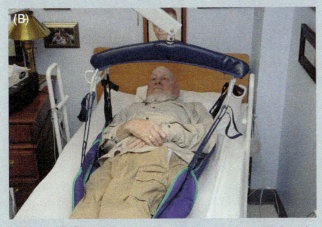

Figure 23-15 (A) Position the lift over the bed. (B) Attach the hooks to the sling.

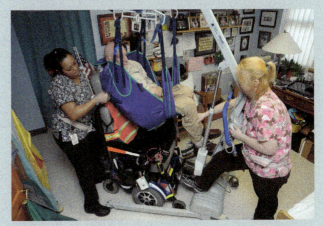

Figure 23-17B Gently swing resident into chair.

(continues)

PROCEDURE 23-91

Transferring Resident with a Mechanical Lift (Continued)

11. Lower the lift and seat the resident in the chair. Unhook suspension straps and move lift out of the way. The sling may be left under the resident until he is ready to be lifted back into bed (Figure 23-18).

12. Position resident as necessary. Place call light, drinking water, and other items as needed within resident's reach. Make sure resident is covered and warm.

13. Carry out each procedure completion action.

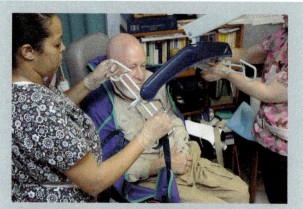

Figure 23-18 Lower the resident into the chair. Unhook suspension straps and move the lift out of the way. The sling may be left under the resident until he is ready to be lifted back into bed.

? EXERCISE 23-3

COMPLETION

Answer the following statements about nursing assistants' actions with A for appropriate or I for inappropriate. If the action is inappropriate, write the appropriate action in the space provided.

1. _____ The nursing assistant asks for help in carrying out a transfer procedure when the resident is heavy.
   _____

2. _____ Slings and straps are checked for frayed areas.
   _____

3. _____ Wheelchair or chair is placed at right angles to the bed.
   _____

4. _____ The nurse assistant leaves the sling underneath the resident until the resident is returned to bed.
   _____

5. _____ The sling should be positioned just below the shoulders.
   _____

6. _____ Fasten hooks to sling so that the hooks face away from the resident.
   _____

7. _____ As one person operates the mechanical lift, a second helper guides the sling and resident.
   _____

SLIDING BOARD TRANSFER

A **sliding board** (Figure 23-19) is used for a sitting transfer. The board should be smooth and waxed to ease movement. This procedure is used for residents who are paralyzed in both legs (**paraplegia**) or who have had both legs amputated. It can be used for other residents who are non-weight bearing as designated by the nurse or physical therapist. The resident must have stability of the upper body for this type of transfer. Some residents learn to do this transfer independently.

The sliding board can be used by two nursing assistants to transfer a dependent resident. Use a transfer belt and position one nursing assistant behind and one in

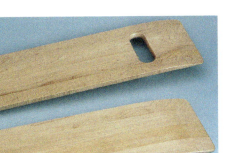

Photo courtesy of Briggs Corporation

Figure 23-19   The sliding board is used when the wheelchair has removable arms and swing-away leg rests. Make sure the resident is wearing pants that will slide easily across the surface.

front of the resident. On the count of three, one assistant stands behind the resident and guides the upper body with the use of the transfer belt; the second assistant guides the resident's legs so that they do not drop down.

AMBULATION

Ambulation is the process of walking. It is good exercise for the resident. The weight bearing on the legs helps prevent or delay the onset of disuse osteoporosis. Walking increases the resident's independence, self-esteem, and provides more opportunities for socializing and activities.

The term **gait** refers to the way in which a person walks. There are many disorders that can affect a person's gait, such as:

- Stroke—one side of the body is paralyzed (hemiplegia).
- Multiple sclerosis—one or both legs are weakened and balance may be disturbed.
- Huntington's disease—the resident has involuntary movements that disturb balance.
- Parkinson's disease—the resident has stiffness and slowness of movements, causing shuffling.
- Arthritis—resident has pain and stiffness in joints.

⚠ GUIDELINES FOR... SLIDING BOARD TRANSFERS

1. The two transfer surfaces should be at the same level.
2. The wheelchair must have removable, swing-away, or lift-off footrests and removable armrests.
3. Residents with adequate upper body strength may eventually be able to do this transfer independently.
4. The resident must be dressed for this transfer so that the buttocks and backs of the upper

legs are completely covered. Never attempt to transfer a resident across the sliding board if there is a possibility that bare skin will contact the board.

5. Position wheelchair so resident can transfer toward strong side.
6. Place a transfer belt around resident's waist.
7. Lock the wheelchair and the bed.

PROCEDURE 23-92
Sliding Board Transfer

 OBRA

1. Carry out each beginning procedure action.
2. Place wheelchair at slight angle next to bed. Remove armrest and footrest on side next to bed.
3. Bring resident to sitting position on edge of bed as described in Procedure 23-84. Apply transfer belt.
4. Position sliding board so one end is on wheelchair and the other end is just under the resident's buttocks. The beveled side of the sliding board is facing up.
5. One nursing assistant stands in front of the resident and one behind. Assume a broad base of support with your knees and hips flexed and your back straight. (If the resident is an amputee, one nursing assistant can transfer the resident by standing in the front of the resident.)
6. Using an underhand grasp, grasp the belt on each side of the resident.
7. Slide the resident across the board and into the chair.
8. Remove the board from under the resident. Remove the transfer belt.

(continues)

PROCEDURE 23-92
Sliding Board Transfer (Continued)

9. Replace the armrest and footrest.

10. Reposition resident in wheelchair if necessary. Make sure call light and any items the resident may need are within reach.

11. Carry out each procedure completion action. To return resident to bed, reverse the procedure.

Evaluation by the Nurse or Physical Therapist

Before an ambulation program is started, the nurse or physical therapist will evaluate the resident's:

- Tolerance to movement in bed
- Ability to participate in active (as opposed to passive) exercise (Figure 23-20)
- Ability to transfer safely with minimal assistance
- Ability to stand and bear weight
- Strength, endurance, and balance
- Mental state to determine if the resident can follow directions
- Ability to walk alone (or is the assistance of a person or equipment needed?)

Normal Gait Pattern

There are two phases to a normal gait (walking). The leg is on the floor during the first phase and the leg is brought forward during the second phase. Walking begins with the ankle in dorsiflexion and the heel striking the floor first (Figure 23-21), rolling onto the ball of the foot. The resident must be able to stand straight

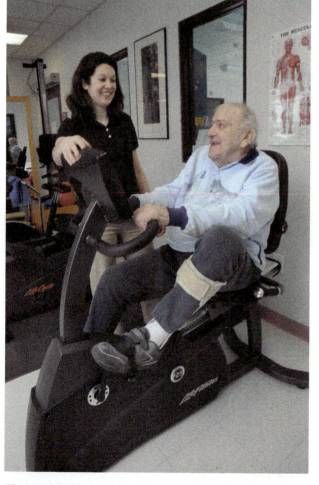

Figure 23-20 A physical therapist will evaluate the resident's ability to participate in active exercise.

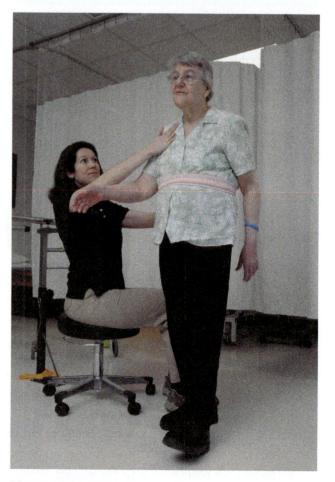

Figure 23-21 Walking begins with the ankle in dorsiflexion. The heel strikes the floor first.

on this leg while bringing the other leg forward. The arms normally have slight swinging movement during walking. Each arm moves in the same direction as the opposite leg. To walk safely, the resident must have adequate joint motion in the hips and knees and strength in the muscles of the hips, buttocks, and legs. The physical therapist may work with the resident on exercises to promote movement and strength before the resident starts walking.

Gait Training

The physical therapist may work with the resident on gait training (teaching the resident to walk).

The physical therapist will teach the resident how to:

- Walk correctly
- Walk on different surfaces, such as linoleum floors, carpet, grass, gravel
- Maneuver stairs (Figure 23-22)
- Get in and out of a chair
- Use an assistive device if one is ordered

Assistive Devices

An assistive device is often prescribed. These devices include crutches, canes, and walkers. An assistive device can help compensate for problems the resident has with walking. Several types of crutches, canes, and walkers are used. The needs of the resident and the cause of the problem are factors in selecting the device. The nurse or physical therapist will adjust the device to fit the resident. The gait used with the device is determined by the resident's abilities, the cause of the impairment, and the type of assistive device. The nurse or physical therapist will select the appropriate gait. You should know the gaits that have been selected. When you walk with the resident you can then observe to make sure the resident is using the device correctly.

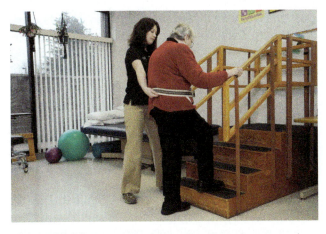

Figure 23-22 The physical therapist will teach some residents how to maneuver stairs.

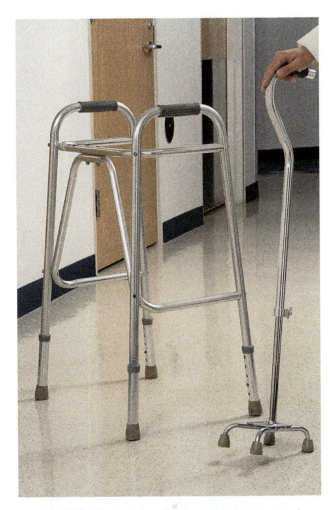

Figure 23-23 All assistive devices have rubber tips on the bottoms and rubber handgrips.

Safety Guidelines for Using Assistive Devices

All canes, crutches, and walkers have rubber tips on the bottoms and rubber handgrips (Figure 23-23). These must be replaced if the ridges are cracked, loose, or worn down. If the ridges are filled with debris, use alcohol and cotton swabs to clean them. Replace any loose or cracked handgrips. Check screws, nuts, and bolts for tightness. Do not use any device that appears unsafe. Report the problem according to facility policy.

Use of Crutches

Standard crutches (Figure 23-24) are seldom recommended for older adults. They can be hard to handle and require balance and two strong arms. Metal forearm or Canadian crutches may be used by residents who have weakness of both legs. The cuff of the crutch encloses the forearm so the resident can release that hand without dropping the crutch (Figure 23-25).

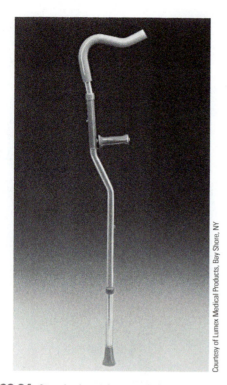

Figure 23-24 Standard crutches are seldom recommended for older adults.

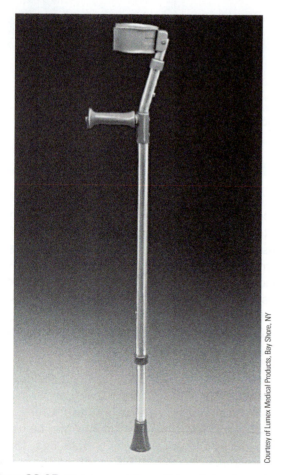

Figure 23-25 Forearm crutches will remain in place when the handle is released.

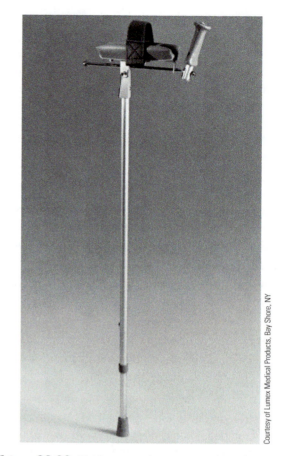

Figure 23-26 Platform crutches permit weight bearing on the forearms, creating stability.

Forearm crutches with platforms permit weight bearing on the forearms, which provides stability. During use, the elbows are in a constant 90-degree angle to the shoulder (Figure 23-26). The resident may need assistance in attaching the arm straps of the platforms. If you care for residents with crutches, you will be taught the gaits the resident is to use.

Use of Canes

Quad canes and tripod canes provide a wide base of support. Pyramid canes are four-pronged devices with a broad base and are narrower at the top. Single-prong canes with T-handles or J-handles have straight handles with a handgrip and are easier to hold than half-circle handled canes (Figure 23-27). Canes are recommended for aiding balance rather than for providing support. The cane is always held by the arm on the *strong* side of the body.

Use of Walkers

Walkers also come in a variety of styles (Figure 23-28A–G). Walkers are recommended for individuals who have general weakness of both legs, partial weight bearing on one leg, or mild balance problems.

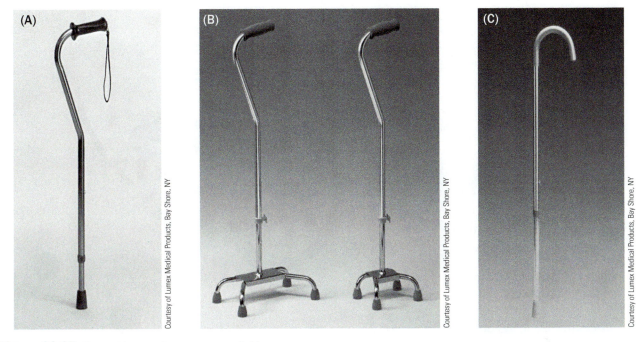

Figure 23-27 Several types of canes are available.

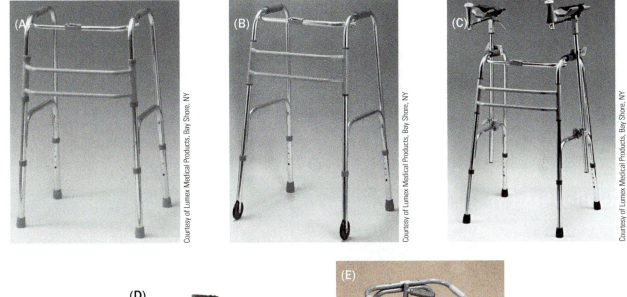

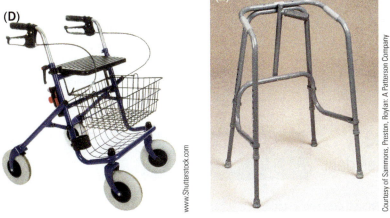

Figure 23-28 (A–E) (A) Aluminum walker. (B) Wheeled walker. (C) Handlebar walker. (D) Rollerator walker. (E) Stroke walker.

(continues)

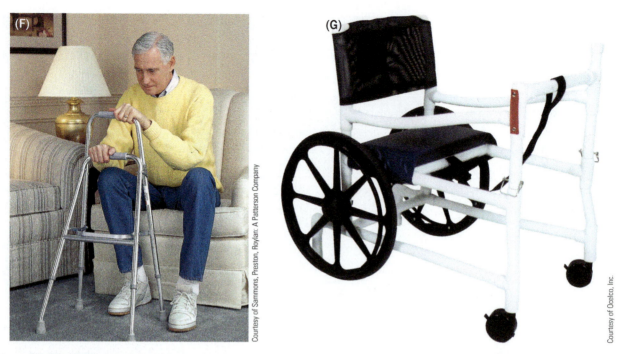

Figure 23-28 (F–G) (Continued) (F) Cane/walker or Hemi-walker. (G) Combination wheelchair/walker.

USING A WHEELCHAIR

Many residents who are unable to ambulate can gain some independence with the use of a wheelchair. A wheelchair should fit the person using it. Correct fit and body alignment will prevent contractures. An appropriate wheelchair will have:

- About 4 inches between the top of the back upholstery and the resident's axillae

- Armrests that support the arms without pushing the shoulders up or forcing them to hang
- Two to 3 inches clearance between the front edge of the seat and the back of the resident's knee
- Enough space between the resident's hip and the chair to slide your hand between the resident's hips on each side and the side of the wheelchair; the right amount of space avoids internal or external rotation of hips.

⚠ GUIDELINES FOR... AMBULATION

1. Always use a transfer (gait) belt if the resident has problems with balance, coordination, or endurance.

2. If the resident's endurance is questionable, ask another person to follow behind with a wheelchair. Have the resident sit in the chair if weakness occurs.

3. If resident has balance problems, two people should ambulate the resident to provide counterbalance.

4. The resident should wear sturdy, well-fitting shoes with nonslip soles.

5. Check clothing to be sure shoelaces or slacks are not inhibiting safe ambulation.

6. Know whether the resident needs an assistive device. An assistive device is anything the resident uses during ambulation, such as canes, walkers, and crutches.

PROCEDURE 23-93
Ambulating a Resident

OBRA

1. Carry out each beginning procedure action.

2. Place the bed in lowest position.

3. Bring the resident to a sitting position on the edge of the bed.

(continues)

PROCEDURE 23-93
Ambulating a Resident (Continued)

4. Put the gait belt around the resident's waist.

5. Using an underhand grasp on the gait belt, assist the resident to a standing position.

6. Stand on the resident's affected side. Place your hand closest to the resident in the back of the gait belt, using an underhand grasp.

7. Place your other hand in front of the resident's shoulder.

8. Walk with the resident, coordinating your steps. Watch the resident for signs of weakness, dizziness, or faintness.

9. Encourage the resident to walk erect. Encourage normal arm swing.

10. Stop the activity before the resident becomes fatigued.

11. Assist the resident back into chair or bed.

12. Carry out each procedure completion action.

PROCEDURE 23-94
Assisting Resident to Ambulate with Cane or Walker

OBRA

1. Carry out each beginning procedure action.

2. Get walker or cane as directed.

3. Check walker or cane for worn areas or loose parts. Be sure rubber tips and handgrips have adequate tread. If these are cracked or worn, they should be replaced.

4. Place bed in lowest horizontal position.

   - Assist resident to sitting position on edge of bed.
   - Apply transfer (gait) belt if needed.
   - If resident is sitting in a wheelchair, lock the brakes and be sure footrests are up or off. Apply gait belt if needed.

5. Place walker or cane within reach.

NOTE: Canes and walkers are not transfer devices. Never allow residents to use either device while they are getting up from the chair or bed.

6. Help resident to come to a standing position.

7. Place cane or walker within resident's reach.

Ambulating with a Cane

NOTE: A cane is always held on the strong side (Figure 23-29). For example, a person who has hemiplegia (paralysis on one side) on the right side would hold the cane with the left hand. A person who has had hip surgery on the right side would hold the cane on the left side.

1. For a three-point gait, resident advances the cane 10 to 18 inches. Then resident brings the affected leg forward and then the stronger leg.

2. For a two-point gait, resident advances the cane and affected leg at the same time. Then resident brings the strong leg forward.

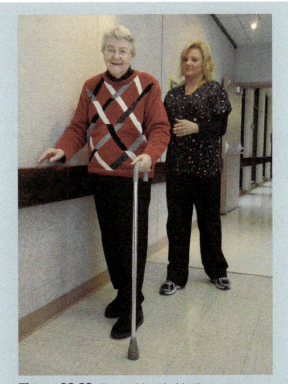

Figure 23-29 The resident holds the cane on the strong side of the body. The resident's weight should be distributed evenly between her feet and the cane before she starts to walk. Use an underhand grip on the transfer belt.

(continues)

PROCEDURE 23-94
Assisting Resident to Ambulate with Cane or Walker (Continued)

3. If resident has a gait belt on, stand slightly in back of the resident on resident's affected side, with your hand closest to resident in the gait belt.

4. After ambulating, return resident to bedside or chair.
   - Have resident walk within a step of bed or chair.
   - Place cane to one side and assist resident to turn around.
   - When resident feels the bed or chair touching the back of the legs, have resident reach for the arm of the chair or mattress of bed and lower self into chair or bed.

5. Carry out each procedure completion action.

Ambulating with a Walker

NOTE: There are many different types of walkers. The directions given here are for a standard walker.

1. Have resident advance walker 10 to 18 inches. All four points of the walker should strike the floor at the same time.

2. The resident then brings affected leg forward into walker, followed by stronger leg.

3. After ambulating, return resident to bedside or chair.
   - Have resident walk within a step of bed or chair.
   - Place walker to one side and assist resident to turn around.
   - When resident feels the bed or chair touching the back of the legs, have resident reach for arm of chair or mattress of bed and lower self into chair or bed.

4. Carry out each procedure completion action.

- Two inches between the bottom of the footrests and the floor
- The feet at 90-degree angles to the legs, whether they are on the footrests or on the floor (when the footrests have been removed) (Figure 23-30)

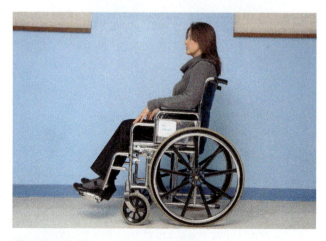

Figure 23-30 The wheelchair should fit the resident correctly.

If the wheelchair does not fit the resident, check with the nurse or physical therapist to see how you can use pads or other devices to adapt the chair to the resident.

Wheelchair Safety

Observe residents in wheelchairs. Remind them to:

- Place the casters in forward position for balance and stability. To do this, go forward and then back up so the casters swing to the forward position.
- Keep the wheelchair locked when not moving.
- Lift footrests out of the way when getting in or out of the wheelchair.
- Not attempt to pick up an object off the floor. If there is satisfactory trunk stability and balance, the resident may be taught to do so, but instruct resident to:
  - Remember to avoid shifting weight in the direction of the reach
  - Not move forward in the seat
  - Not reach down between the knees

The safest method is to ask for help in picking up an object from the floor. Otherwise, position the chair beside the object with casters in forward position. Lock the chair and reach only as far as the arm will extend. The resident may have an assistive reaching device that can be used to pick up objects.

The following procedures for wheelchair maneuvers are rarely implemented in a long-term care facility. However, residents may go outside the facility or be discharged. In these situations, the skills will be required. The caregiver should be evaluated on the ability to carry them out.

SPECIAL MANEUVERS WITH WHEELCHAIRS

Certain situations will require special maneuvers to be made with residents in wheelchairs. Do not attempt to use the following procedures unless you have been instructed to do so.

Tilting a Wheelchair Backward

1. This procedure is used for curbs, single steps, ramps, and doorsills. Do not use this procedure with an indoor wheelchair.
2. Before proceeding, make sure the resident understands what you are doing. Check to see that arms, hands, fingers, and legs are in safe position. Use good body mechanics to avoid injury. Have an assistant with you the first few times you do this.
3. The purpose of the procedure is to rotate the wheelchair around the axles of the rear wheels until it reaches the balance point.
4. With your foot on the tipping lever, apply a pushing force down and under the chair while pulling back and down on the handgrip (Figure 23-31).
5. Tilt back until little or no effort is required to stabilize the chair. This is the balance point, about 30 degrees. You can now maneuver the chair on the rear wheels (Figure 23-32).
6. To return the wheelchair to the upright position, keep your foot on the tipping lever. Lower the chair, reversing the procedure. Do this slowly and smoothly and do not let the chair drop (Figure 23-33).

Manipulating Ramps and Inclines

1. Push the resident up a ramp or incline, facing forward, with the trunk slightly forward, with or without an attendant.
2. To go down a ramp, turn the chair around and back down so that the resident is facing forward and

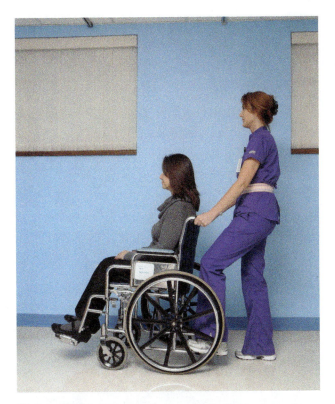

Figure 23-31 With your foot on the tipping lever, apply a pushing force down and under the chair while pulling back and down on the handgrip.

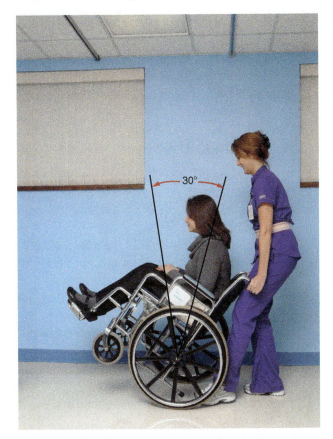

Figure 23-32 You can maneuver the chair on the rear wheels when you have reached the balance point.

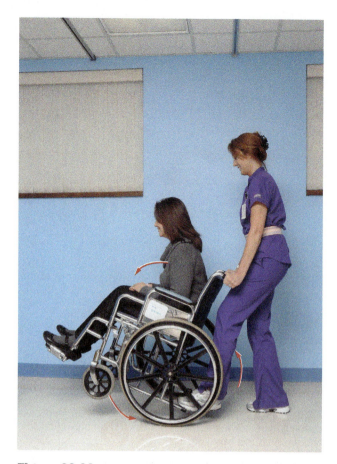

Figure 23-33 Reverse the procedure to lower the chair.

cannot fall out of the chair. Position yourself be-hind the chair and slowly move down the ramp.

3. Keep your back straight and knees bent through-out the procedure.

Manipulating Curbs

1. To go up, place the chair in balance position. Move forward until the front casters are on top of the curb and the rear wheels are touching the curb (Figure 23-34).

2. Lower the front of the chair to the sidewalk, mak-ing sure the wheelchair does not roll backward (Figure 23-35).

3. With your body close to the wheelchair, use one single smooth movement to lift the chair by the handles, rolling it up over the curb and pushing it forward (Figure 23-35).

4. After the wheelchair is safely on the sidewalk, step up onto the curb (Figure 23-36).

5. To go down, turn the wheelchair around and pull it to the edge of the curb.

6. Stand below the curb and allow the large wheels to slowly roll down onto the lower level.

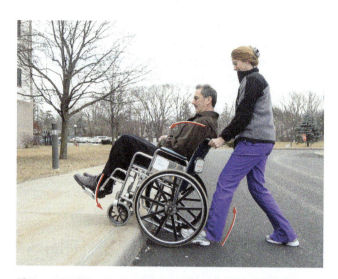

Figure 23-34 Move forward until the front casters are on the tip of the curb and the rear wheels are touching the curb.

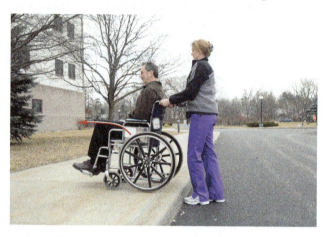

Figure 23-35 Make sure the wheelchair does not roll backward. Use one single smooth movement to lift the chair by the handles, rolling it up over the curb.

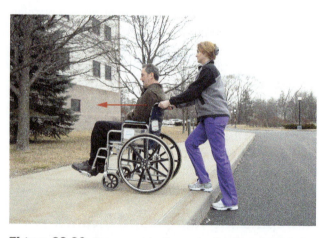

Figure 23-36 Step up onto the curb after the wheelchair is on the sidewalk.

7. After the large wheels are on the lower level, tilt the chair to its balance point while lifting the front casters off the curb.

8. When the wheelchair is on the lower level, move backward until you can safely turn the chair around. A second assistant is needed if the curb or step is high.

Going Up and Down Stairs

Attempt this procedure only in an extreme emergency and an elevator is not available. Never use a wheelchair on escalators. At least two people are needed who are strong enough to carry the procedure out to its completion. Check the position of the resident's extremities and inspect the handgrip for good fit on the chair.

1. To go upstairs, place the wheelchair in backward position with the rear wheels touching the first step. The strongest assistant is at the rear of the chair, standing on the second step.
2. The assistant in front grasps the chair frame on either side of the resident's lower legs, taking care not to grasp a removable part.
3. The rear assistant tilts the wheelchair to its balance point.
4. Working together, the assistants lift and roll the chair up onto the next step, keeping it at the balance point, moving themselves up with the chair (Figure 23-37).
5. This procedure is continued until the top step is reached.

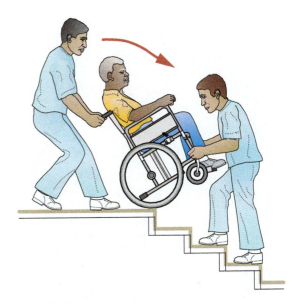

Figure 23-38 All assistants move down one step.

6. With the chair still at the balance point, the rear assistant rolls the chair back until the assistant(s) in front are off the steps.
7. The rear assistant turns the chair around and gently returns it to upright position.
8. To go downstairs, the front assistant(s) stands on the third step from the top.
9. The rear assistant tilts the chair to the balance point and rolls it to the edge of the top step. This person is in charge of the procedure.
10. With the front assistant firmly grasping the wheelchair frame, the chair is lowered one step by rolling the large wheels over the edge of the step. All assistants move down one step (Figure 23-38).
11. Repeat the process until the chair reaches the bottom of the stairs. The rear assistant gently returns the wheelchair to the upright position.

POSITIONING THE DEPENDENT RESIDENT IN THE WHEELCHAIR

The dependent person may slide down in the wheelchair, requiring assistance to regain body alignment. Several procedures can be implemented to correct the dependent resident's position in the wheelchair.

Method 1: Stand in front of the resident and make sure the feet are in alignment and arms are on the armrests. Help resident lean forward and push with the hands and legs as you push against the resident's knees (Figure 23-39).

Method 2: An alternate method is to place a soft towel or small sheet under the resident's

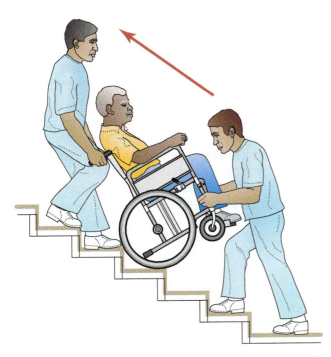

Figure 23-37 The assistants lift and roll the chair up and onto the next step, keeping it at balance point.

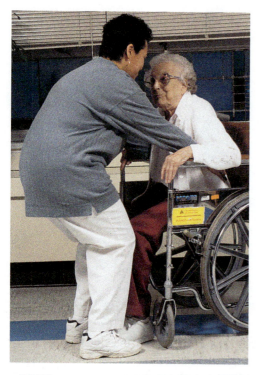

Figure 23-39 Use an underhand grip on the transfer belt. Help resident lean forward and push with the hands and legs as you push against the resident's knees.

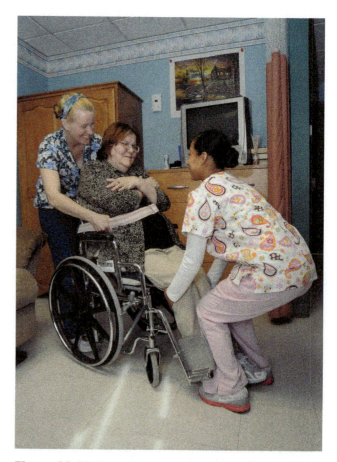

Figure 23-41 A transfer belt may be used to move a lighter resident up in the wheelchair.

buttocks. Use this as a pull sheet to move the resident up in the chair. This technique also works well when repositioning the resident in a high-backed chair such as a geri-chair; two people are required (Figure 23-40).

Method 3: This method also requires two people. Place the transfer belt around the resident's waist. One caregiver stands in back of the wheelchair and grasps the transfer belt with one hand on each side of the resident. The other one stands in front of the resident and places her hands and arms under the resident's knees. On the count of three this caregiver supports the lower extremities while the other one moves the resident back in the chair (Figure 23-41). This method is not recommended for a heavy resident.

Method 4: This method also requires two people. One assistant stands in back of the wheelchair and a second caregiver stands in front of the resident. Both caregivers work with knees and hips bent and backs straight. You are the caregiver behind the chair. Lean forward with your head over the resident's shoulder. Instruct the resident to fold the arms. Place your arms around the resident's trunk. Grasp the resident's right wrist with your left hand and grasp the resident's left wrist with your right hand. The other caregiver encircles the resident's knees with hands and arms. On the count of three, both caregivers lift and move the resident up (Figure 23-42).

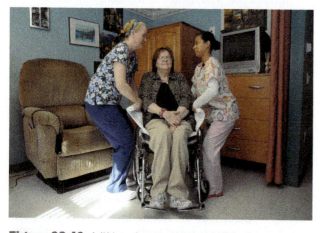

Figure 23-40 A lifting sheet may be used to move the resident up in the wheelchair.

? EXERCISE 23-4

COMPLETION

Answer the following statements about nursing assistants' actions with A for appropriate or I for inappropriate. If the action is inappropriate, write the appropriate action in the space provided.

ACTIONS RELATED TO WHEELCHAIR SAFETY

1. _____ When getting in and out of a wheelchair, the footrests must be in position of use.
   _____

2. _____ When not moving a wheelchair, the wheels should be locked.
   _____

3. _____ Residents may safely pick up articles while in a wheelchair as long as the chair wheels are locked.
   _____

4. _____ To tilt a wheelchair backward, the nursing assistant places a foot down on the tipping lever while pulling back and down on the handgrip.
   _____

5. _____ When tilting a wheelchair backward, the balance point is approximately 60 degrees.
   _____

6. _____ When using a wheelchair on a downward ramp, the resident faces and leans forward.
   _____

7. _____ When lowering a wheelchair down over a curb, the front wheels are lowered first..
   _____

8. _____ When carrying a resident in a wheelchair upstairs, the resident faces the bottom of the flight of stairs.
   _____

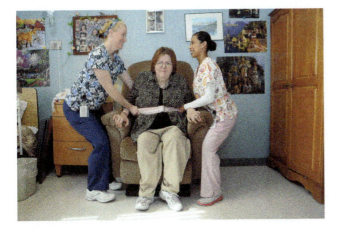

Figure 23-42 On the count of three, both assistants lift and move the resident up.

WHEELCHAIR ACTIVITY

Pressure over the ischia is greatly increased when the resident is sitting. Teach the resident (and provide assistance if necessary) to periodically relieve the pressure by shifting weight every 15 minutes. *Be sure*

wheelchair is locked before beginning any activities involving the resident's movement in the chair.

Wheelchair Pushups

1. Teach the resident to place one hand on each armrest, keeping both elbows bent.
2. Then have resident lean forward slightly, pushing on the armrests and straightening the elbows while lifting the buttocks off the seat of the wheelchair. Have resident hold this position to the count of five if possible (Figure 23-43).

Leaning

1. Teach the resident who cannot do pushups to place the hands on the armrests or thighs and lean forward slightly, and then to lean to each side to relieve pressure on buttocks (Figure 23-44). Monitor the resident with balance problems to avoid falling out of the chair.

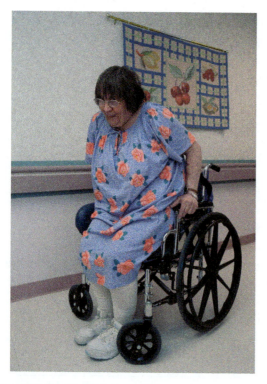

Figure 23-43 Wheelchair pushups relieve pressure from sitting.

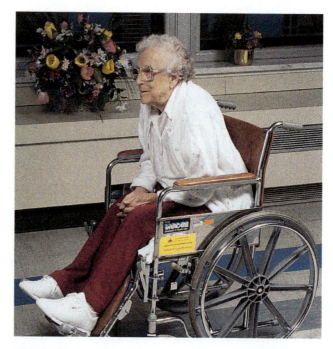

Figure 23-44 Leaning forward is another method of relieving pressure.

❓ EXERCISE 23-5

TRUE OR FALSE

Indicate whether the following statements are true (T) or false (F).

1. T F If a transfer belt is not available, the belt of a resident's pants or slacks can be used.

2. T F Residents should never place their hands on a nursing assistant's body during the transfer.

3. T F If a resident has a paralyzed leg, the nursing assistant should always brace the unaffected leg with his or her knee or leg.

4. T F When making a transfer, always transfer toward the weakest side.

5. T F A transfer belt should be snug enough so that the nursing assistant can just get the fingers under it.

6. T F Always make sure the wheels of a wheelchair are locked before making a transfer.

7. T F A transfer belt used in the tub area can be applied directly over the resident's bare skin.

8. T F A wheelchair should be used to transport a resident to the tub room.

9. T F One person can safely carry out a transfer using a mechanical lift.

10. T F A gait belt should always be used to ambulate a resident who has problems with balance or coordination.

11. T F A cane should always be held on the weak side when the resident has hemiplegia.

12. T F In the three-point gait method of cane-assisted walking, the cane is advanced approximately 10 to 18 inches and the weaker leg is brought forward.

13. T F In the two-point gait method of cane-assisted walking, advance the cane and strong leg together.

14. T F When using a walker, the front two points should strike the floor first and then the back two points should strike the floor.

15. T F When assisting a falling resident, be sure to always protect the resident's head.

16. T F Wheelchairs can safely be used on escalators.

LESSON SYNTHESIS: Putting It All Together

You have just completed this lesson. Now go back and review the Clinical Focus. Try to see how the Clinical Focus relates to the concepts presented in the lesson. Then answer the following questions.

1. Why is it important for the person doing the transfer always to maintain a wide base of support?

2. Why are *specific instructions* written about how a resident is to be transferred?

3. The person doing the transfer should never place his or her hands under the resident's arms. Explain the reasons for this.

4. Explain why a transfer should always be toward the resident's strongest side.

23 REVIEW

A. Select the one best answer for each of the following.

1. When using the transfer (gait) belt to assist the resident

(A) stand behind the resident

(B) lift from the side

(C) use an overhand grip

(D) use an underhand grip

2. A transfer belt should never be used on a resident who

(A) has a gastrostomy tube

(B) needs assistance in transferring

(C) is tall

(D) cannot walk

3. During a transfer, the resident should never

(A) be allowed to help in the move

(B) place his hands on your body

(C) wear shoes

(D) be allowed to stand

4. When transferring a resident, you should never place your hands under a resident's arms because

(A) the resident may not want you to stand so close

(B) the resident cannot see where he is going

(C) the resident's bones are fragile

(D) the resident may be ticklish

5. Using a mechanical lift requires that

(A) there always be two persons to do the procedure

(B) the resident be able to assist in the move

(C) the resident be mentally alert

(D) the resident be very small

6. A sliding board transfer is useful for residents who

(A) are paraplegic

(B) have cardiac problems

(C) have had a stroke

(D) have diabetes

7. A resident's gait may be affected by all but

(A) a stroke

(B) Parkinson's disease

(C) multiple sclerosis

(D) incontinence

8. Mrs. Romeriz has a diagnosis of osteoporosis. Which of the following would be inappropriate for her?

(A) Transfer belt

(B) Two-person transfer

(C) Dangling on the side of the bed

(D) Use of the bed protector as a lift assist

9. When transferring the resident from the wheelchair to the toilet, position the wheelchair:

(A) directly in front of the toilet.

(B) at a 30-degree angle to the toilet.

(C) at a 60-degree angle to the toilet.

(D) at a 90-degree angle to the toilet.

10. The resident is using the walker to ambulate. Which of the following is incorrect usage?

(A) Advance the walker 10 to 18 inches.

(B) Bring the weak leg forward, then the stronger leg.

(C) Have all four points on the walker on the floor at the same time.

(D) Use the walker for support when getting back into bed.

B. Answer each statement true (T) or false (F).

11. T F During a transfer, a resident should place his or her hands on the nursing assistant's shoulders.

12. T F A transfer belt should always be used when ambulating a resident, unless contraindicated.

13. T F Always transfer toward the resident's strong side.

14. T F When pushing the wheelchair you should go forward over thresholds or uneven surfaces.

15. T F Always explain what the assistant is doing and what the resident can do to help.

16. T F Towel bars are not safe to use as grab bars.

17. T F Always hold a cane on the affected side.

18. T F When using a walker, the front two tips of the walker should strike the floor first and then the back two tips should strike the floor.

8

Residents with Specific Disorders

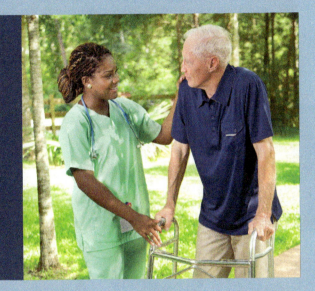

LESSON 24
CARING FOR RESIDENTS WITH CARDIOVASCULAR SYSTEM DISORDERS

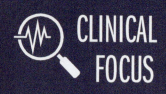

CLINICAL FOCUS

Think how you might assist a resident with cardiovascular disorders as you study this lesson.

OBJECTIVES

After studying this lesson, you should be able to:

- Define vocabulary words and terms.
- Identify the parts and function of the cardiovascular system.
- Review changes in the cardiovascular system as they relate to the aging process.
- Differentiate between the cardiovascular system and the lymphatic system.
- Describe common cardiovascular disorders affecting the long-term resident.
- List observations to make when caring for residents with cardiovascular disorders.
- Describe the care given by the nursing assistant to residents with cardiovascular disorders.
- Explain how to correctly apply elasticized stockings.
- Demonstrate the following:

  Procedure 24-95 Applying Elasticized (Support) Stockings

CASE STUDY

Walter Rabinowitz has congestive heart failure and poor circulation in his feet. He sits in a cardiac chair that supports him in an upright position comfortably. He is always complaining that his feet are cold. He has an order for elasticized stockings. During morning care, he asks for a hot water bag to put on his feet. Nursing assistants know there are safer methods of providing the comfort he needs.

VOCABULARY

anastomosed (ah-**NAS**-tah-mohzd)

anemia (ah-**NEE**-mee-ah)

angina pectoris (an-**JYE**-nah or **AN**-jih-nah **PECK**-tor-is)

aorta (ay-**OR**-tah)

arteriosclerosis (are-**ter**-ree-oh-skleh-**ROH**-sis)

artery (**ARE**-ter-ee)

ascites (ah-**SIGH**-teez)

atherosclerosis (ath-er-oh-skleh-**ROH**-sis)

atrium (plural: atria) (**AY**-tree-um; pl. **AY**-tree-ah)

capillary (**KAP**-ih-lair-ee)

cardiac cycle (**KAR**-dee-ack **SIGH**-kul)

cardiovascular (**kar**-dee-oh-**VAS**-kyou-lar)

congestive heart failure (kon-**JES**-tiv hart **FAIL**-your)

coronary artery (**KOR**-i-nair-ee **ARE**-ter-ee)

dementia (dee-**MEN**-she-ah)

deoxygenated (dee-**ock**-sih-jen-**AY**-ted)

diaphoresis (**die**-ah-foh-**REE**-sis)

diastole (die-**AS**-toh-lee)

dyspnea (**DISP**-nee-ah)

edema (eh-**DEE**-mah)

electrocardiogram (ECG or EKG) (ee-**leck**-troh-**KAR**-dee-oh-gram)

erythrocytes (eh-**RITH**-roh-sights)

heart attack (hart ah-**TACK**)

heart block (hart block)

hemoptysis (hee-**MOP**-tih-sis)

hypertension (high-per-**TEN**-shun)

hypoxia (high-**POCK**-see-ah)

infarction (in-**FARK**-shun)

inferior vena cava (in-**FEER**-ee-or **VEE**-nah **KAY**-vah)

ischemia (is-**KEE**-mee-ah)

leukemia (loo-**KEE**-mee-ah)

leukocytes (**LOO**-koh-sights)

lumen (**LOO**-men)

lymph (limf)

lymph node (limf nohd)

myocardial infarction (**my**-oh-**KAR**-dee-al in-**FARK**-shun)

nitroglycerin (**nigh**-troh-**GLIS**-er-in)

orthopnea (or-**THOP**-nee-ah)

orthopneic position (or-thop-**NEE**-ick poh-**ZISH**-un)

oxygenated (ock-sih-jen-**AT**-ted)

pacemaker (**PAYS**-may-ker)

peripheral vascular disease (peh-**RIF**-er-al **VAS**-kyou-lar dih-**ZEEZ**)

phlebitis (fleh-**BYE**-tis)

plaque (plak)

plasma (**PLAZ**-mah)

platelet (**PLAYT**-let)

pulmonary artery (**PULL**-moh-nair-ee **ARE**-ter-ee)

pulmonary veins (**PULL**-moh-nair-ee vains)

serum (**SEER**-rum)

stent

stroke (strohk)

superior vena cava (soo-**PEER**-ee-or **VEE**-nah **KAY**-vah)

syncope (**SIN**-koh-pe)

systole (**SIS**-toh-lee)

TED hose (**TED** hohs)

thrombocyte (**THROM**-boh-sight)

thrombophlebitis (throm-boh-fleh-**BYE**-tis)

transient ischemic attack (TIA) (**TRAN**-see-ent is-**KEE**-mick ah-**TACK**)

valve (valv)

varicose veins (**VAIR**-ih-kohs vains)

vasodilator (**vas**-oh-die-**LAY**-tor)

vein (vain)

ventricle (**VEN**-trih-kul)

venule (**VEN**-youl)

INTRODUCTION

The circulatory or **cardiovascular** system is the transportation system of the body. It carries substances from where they are formed to where they may be used or eliminated. The cardiovascular system (Figure 24-1) consists of the:

- Heart—a central pump
- Blood vessels—a closed circuit of arteries that lead from the heart to capillaries and then to veins that lead back to the heart
- Blood—a collection of various cells, each with a special job to perform

The bloodstream, spleen, liver, and bone marrow make some of the blood cells and destroy them when they are worn out.

Cardiovascular disease is the most common cause of death in the United States. Many residents in your care may suffer from disabilities caused by cardiovascular disease. Cardiovascular disease is responsible for changes that reduce the blood flow to the body tissues and result in

- Heart attack
- Peripheral vascular disease
- Hypertension (high blood pressure)
- Stroke

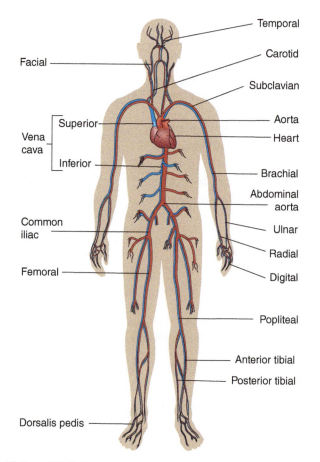

Figure 24-1 The cardiovascular system. (Red: arteries; blue: veins).

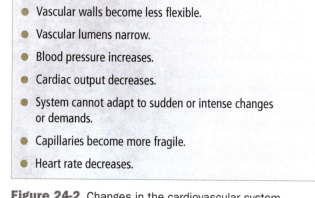

- Vascular walls become less flexible.
- Vascular lumens narrow.
- Blood pressure increases.
- Cardiac output decreases.
- System cannot adapt to sudden or intense changes or demands.
- Capillaries become more fragile.
- Heart rate decreases.

Figure 24-2 Changes in the cardiovascular system caused by aging.

Reduced blood flow is called ischemia. Ischemia means that less oxygen is delivered to tissues, leading, eventually, to death of the tissues (infarction or necrosis). Changes in the cardiovascular system caused by aging are summarized in Figure 24-2.

THE HEART

The heart is a muscular organ that pumps the blood in a continuous flow through the blood vessels of the body. It is separated into a right and left side (Figure 24-3).

Structure and Function

The *right side* of the heart:

- Receives blood from the body via vena cava
- Sends blood to the lungs where carbon dioxide is removed and oxygen is picked up (Figure 24-4)

The *left side* of the heart:

- Receives blood from the lungs by way of the pulmonary veins

- Sends blood out to the body, where the oxygen is given up to the cells and the waste product carbon dioxide is picked up

Each side of the heart is divided into upper and lower parts (chambers) by valves. The valves permit blood flow in one direction only. The *upper chambers* are called the right atrium and left atrium. The *lower chambers* are the right and left ventricles.

The two upper chambers contract first, forcing the blood through the open valves into the two lower chambers. The ventricles fill and the valves close. The ventricles then contract, squeezing the blood up through the large blood vessels.

Blood Vessels of the Heart

The major blood vessels of the heart are the:

- Superior vena cava (SVC)—returns blood to the right atrium from the upper part of the body
- Inferior vena cava (IVC)—returns blood to right atrium from the lower part of the body
- Pulmonary arteries—carry blood to the lungs from the right ventricle
- Pulmonary veins—return blood to the left atrium from the lungs
- Aorta (a large artery)—carries blood to the body from the left ventricle
- Coronary arteries—nourish the heart muscle with fresh blood

Valves at the base of the pulmonary artery and aorta close as the blood moves forward, preventing backflow of blood into the ventricles between contractions.

Cardiac Cycle

The contractions and relaxations of the heart muscle are called the cardiac cycle. The cardiac cycle is

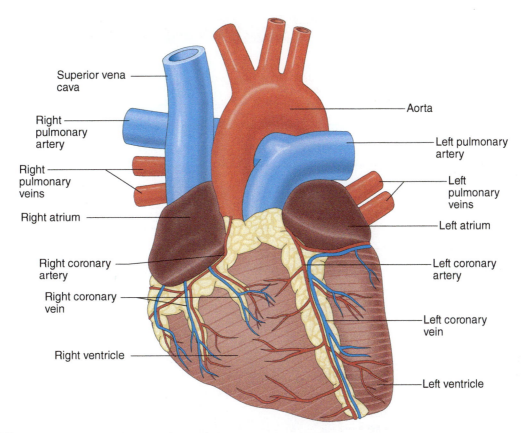

Figure 24-3 External view of the heart and vessels.

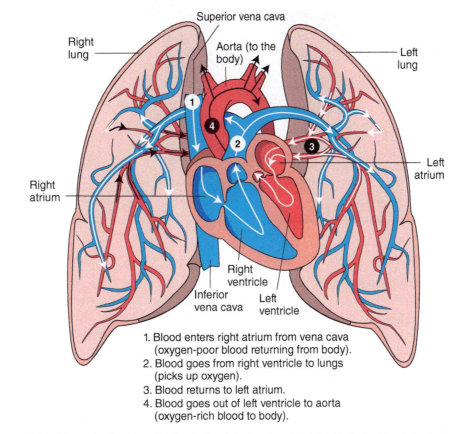

1. Blood enters right atrium from vena cava (oxygen-poor blood returning from body).
2. Blood goes from right ventricle to lungs (picks up oxygen).
3. Blood returns to left atrium.
4. Blood goes out of left ventricle to aorta (oxygen-rich blood to body).

Figure 24-4 Flow of blood from the heart to the lungs, back to the heart, to the body, and back to the heart to begin the cycle again.

? EXERCISE 24-1

SCIENTIFIC PRINCIPLES

Write the names of the structures shown in the figure below.

1. _____
2. _____
3. _____
4. _____
5. _____
6. _____
7. _____
8. _____
9. _____

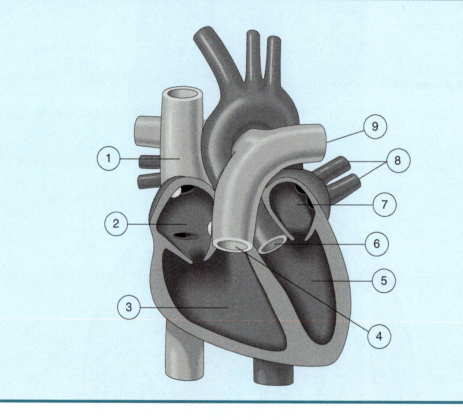

controlled by special nerve tissues within the heart and by two sets of nerves:

- One set of nerves carries messages to increase the heart rate.
- The other set of nerves carries messages to slow the heart rate.

Electrical impulses passing through the nerve tissue make the muscle contract:

- **Systole** is the term meaning heart *contraction*.
- **Diastole** is the term meaning heart *relaxation*.

For a short time, the heart rests completely between beats. The pulse you feel at the radial artery corresponds to ventricular contraction. The sounds you hear when listening to the heart and when taking a blood pressure are the sounds made by the closing of the valves during the cardiac cycle.

An **electrocardiogram**, called an ECG or an EKG, is a test that traces the electrical impulses of the heart. Heart disease may be detected with this test.

BLOOD VESSELS

There are three kinds of blood vessels:

- Arteries
- Capillaries
- Veins

Arteries

Arteries carry blood away from the heart. The blood contains oxygen picked up in the lungs. The blood is oxygenated and is needed to keep the body cells alive and functioning. The arteries get smaller (arterioles) and finally form tiny networks of vessels called capillaries.

Capillaries

Nutrients and oxygen in the blood are exchanged through the walls of the capillaries for carbon dioxide and waste products. The capillaries form small veins called venules to begin the journey back to the heart.

Veins

Many venules join to form larger vessels called veins. The largest veins, the superior vena cava and the inferior vena cava, return the blood to the right atrium. This blood has less oxygen and more carbon dioxide and is called deoxygenated blood.

The cardiovascular system is a closed system, with the gases and other substances passing into and out of the bloodstream as the blood passes throughout the body.

Blood vessels frequently take their names from bones nearby. For example, the radial artery and radial vein are found close to the radius, which is one of the forearm bones.

THE BLOOD

The blood is a red body fluid that carries blood cells, nutrients, chemicals, and waste products. The average quantity of blood in the body is about 4 to 6 liters (or 4 to 6 quarts). The blood consists of two portions:

- Plasma
- Blood cells

Plasma

The liquid part of the blood, called plasma, consists of:

- Water
- Nutrients

- Wastes
- Proteins that help blood to clot
- Proteins that fight infection and help to move materials in and out of the bloodstream

Serum is the fluid that is left after the cells and some of the proteins have been removed.

Blood Cells

Three kinds of blood cells are:

1. Erythrocytes (red blood cells)—carry oxygen and a small amount of carbon dioxide
2. Leukocytes (white blood cells)—protect the body by fighting infection
3. Platelets or thrombocytes—pieces of cells that contain a chemical important to blood clotting

DISORDERS OF THE BLOOD

Blood abnormalities commonly seen in older adults include:

- Cancer
- Anemia

Cancer

Cancers of the blood include forms of leukemia. In leukemia:

- Excessive numbers of white blood cells are formed.
- Too few platelets and red blood cells are produced.

The person with leukemia:

- Tires easily
- Is subject to infections and anemia
- Is apt to bleed

These conditions are normally treated with radiation or drugs.

Anemia

Anemias are the result of a decrease in (1) the quantity or quality of red blood cells and (2) their ability to carry oxygen. People suffering from anemia have little energy. They:

- Are usually pale or jaundiced (skin is yellow)
- Complain of light-headedness
- Feel cold
- Experience dizziness
- Have an increased respiratory rate
- Suffer from poor digestion

? EXERCISE 24-2

Identify the arteries shown in the figure below

1. _____
2. _____
3. _____
4. _____
5. _____
6. _____
7. _____
8. _____
9. _____
10. _____

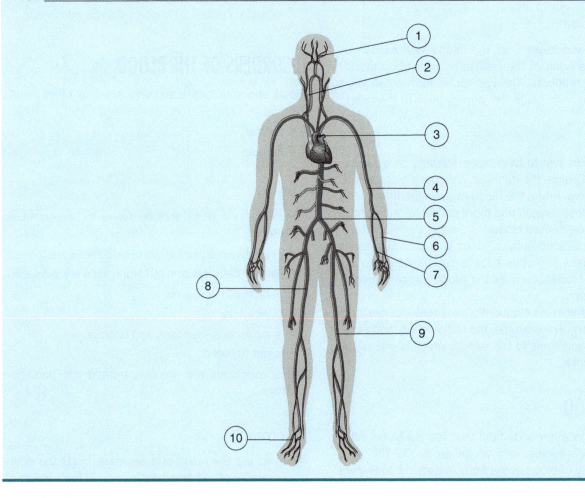

Special Care

Residents who have cancer or anemia require special care. You must:

- Check vital signs.
- Encourage rest and a good diet.
- See that resident avoids unnecessary exertion.
- Handle resident very gently.
- Give special mouth care because the mouth and tongue become sensitive.
- Be sure to report any signs of bleeding, such as bruises or discolorations, because further blood loss makes the condition worse.
- Keep resident warm.

? EXERCISE 24-3

COMPLETION

Complete the following statements by writing in the correct words.

1. Blood is a _____ composed of _____ and _____.
2. Cellular elements found as part of blood include:
   a. red blood cells or _____
   b. white blood cells or _____
   c. platelets or _____
3. Five changes in the cardiovascular system associated with the aging process are:

   a. _____
   _____

   b. _____
   _____

   c. _____
   _____

   d. _____
   _____

   e. _____
   _____

4. Two important blood disorders seen in the elderly are _____ and _____.
5. Residents who have cancer or anemia require special care. List nursing assistant interventions that may be necessary.

   _____
   _____

? EXERCISE 24-4

CLINICAL SITUATION

Read the following situation and answer the questions by selecting the correct term from the list provided.

   Mrs. Kroneberger is one of your residents. She is pale, often complaining of light-headedness and feeling cold. She has told you she is dizzy, and you note her respiratory rate is slightly increased. She has digestive problems. You report these findings because you know they are often associated with the condition when there is inadequate or poor quality of red blood cells. The nurse and doctor identify the problem.

anemia	special
avoid	two
bleeding	vital
gently	warm
rest	

1. This condition is called _____.

As a nursing assistant you should care for the person by:

2. Checking _____ signs.
3. Encouraging _____ and good diet.
4. Helping resident _____ unnecessary exertion.
5. Handling the resident very _____.
6. Providing _____ mouth care.
7. Reporting signs of _____ such as bruises or discolorations.
8. Changing the resident's position at least every _____ hours.
9. Keeping the resident _____.

- Protect resident from falls that may result from dizziness or weakness.
- Change the resident's position often—at least every 2 hours.

DISORDERS OF THE BLOOD VESSELS AND CIRCULATION

Several changes can occur in blood vessels that will affect the flow of blood (circulation) through the vessels. Arteriosclerosis means hardening of the arteries. When this happens, the arteries lose their elasticity. It is then more difficult for the blood to flow through the vessels. Atherosclerosis occurs when deposits of fatty materials and calcium form roughened areas (plaques) on the inner walls of the arteries. As the plaques thicken, the space within the arteries (the lumen) narrows (Figure 24-5). This causes the blood flow to decrease. When this happens, ischemia can occur.

Arteriosclerosis and atherosclerosis are especially dangerous when they affect the arteries of the brain, heart, and those leading from the body to the legs. When the vessels in the brain are affected, the risk is high for stroke (cerebral vascular accident, CVA, or brain attack). Stroke is discussed in Lesson 29. Before a stroke happens, the person may have a transient ischemic attack (TIA). The person may experience a form of delirium (confusion and disorientation) when the brain cells do not receive adequate oxygen. Delirium is discussed in Lesson 30.

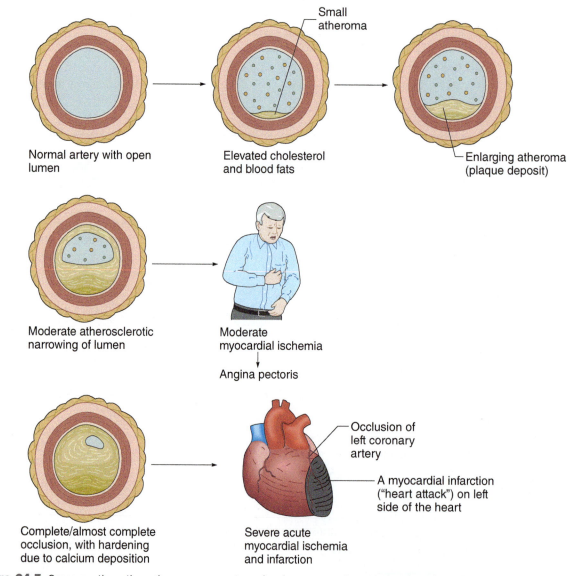

Normal artery with open lumen

Elevated cholesterol and blood fats

Small atheroma

Enlarging atheroma (plaque deposit)

Moderate atherosclerotic narrowing of lumen

Moderate myocardial ischemia

↓

Angina pectoris

Complete/almost complete occlusion, with hardening due to calcium deposition

Severe acute myocardial ischemia and infarction

Occlusion of left coronary artery

A myocardial infarction ("heart attack") on left side of the heart

Figure 24-5 Cross sections through a coronary artery showing progressive arteriosclerosis and atherosclerosis.

AFFECTED SITE   **COMPLICATION**

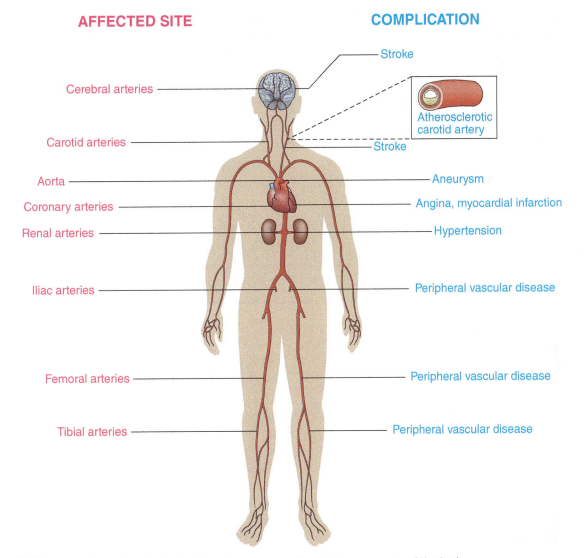

Figure 24-6 Atherosclerosis and arteriosclerosis can cause disease in many parts of the body.

When the vessels of the heart are affected, the person may have a heart attack (**myocardial infarction**). When the vessels in the legs are affected, the person has **peripheral vascular disease**. When the arteries are diseased, hypertension (high blood pressure) may occur (Figure 24-6).

The veins can also cause problems. **Varicose veins** form when the valves in the veins in the legs become weakened (Figure 24-7). This means the blood does not flow through the veins as it should. The veins then become distended and visible through the skin. The veins may become inflamed (**phlebitis**). A blood clot may form (**thrombophlebitis**). Report the signs of these disorders:

- Pain or aching in the area
- Signs of inflammation (warmth and redness)
- *Never* rub or massage the area.

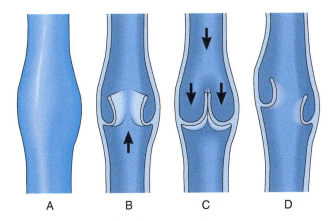

Figure 24-7 Veins contain valves to prevent the backward flow of blood. (A) External view of the vein shows wider area of valve. (B) Internal view with the valve open as blood flows through. (C) Internal view with the valve closed. (D) Vein with weakened valve causing a varicose vein.

Transient Ischemic Attack

Transient ischemic attack (TIA) is a temporary interruption of the blood flow to part of the brain. The resident may experience:

- Weakness or paralysis of any extremity or the face
- Vision problems
- Difficulty with speech
- Difficulty with swallowing

These symptoms come on quickly and may last from just a few minutes but no longer than 24 hours. There are no permanent effects. However, a TIA is usually a warning that a stroke will occur at some time. If a resident has any of these symptoms, you should report them to the nurse immediately.

Peripheral Vascular Disease

Peripheral vascular disease may be caused by:

- Diseases of the arteries (arteriosclerosis and atherosclerosis)
- Abnormalities of the veins (varicose veins)

The signs and symptoms of diminished circulation due to peripheral vascular disease include:

- Burning pain during exercise
- Hair loss over feet and toes
- Thick and rigid toenails
- Dusky red skin or cyanotic, brownish skin
- Dry and scaly or shiny skin
- Chronic edema of the feet and legs
- Cool skin temperature of feet and legs
- Difficulty with ambulation
- Diminished pulses

When the arteries are affected, the blood flow may be seriously interrupted. This condition requires immediate medical treatment. Because of severe loss of blood supply to an area, gangrene may occur (Figure 24-8). Vascular ulcers, also called stasis ulcers, may occur. These are sores that start because of the poor circulation of the blood in the legs. These ulcers are difficult to treat and may take months to heal.

When residents have peripheral vascular disease, it is important that:

- Circulation be maintained. Complications such as ulcers may then be prevented.
- The feet and legs receive excellent skin care.

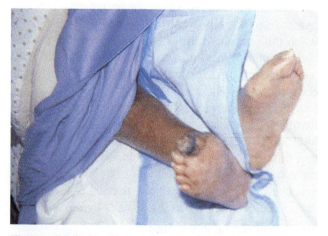

Figure 24-8 The big toe lost adequate blood supply and is gangrenous. The toe was eventually amputated, but the foot was saved.

Hypertension

Hypertension means elevated blood pressure. Hypertension may have an unknown origin or follow disease of the:

- Blood vessels
- Kidneys
- Liver

Diseases of the blood vessels increase the overall blood pressure. When blood vessels are narrowed due to disease, the heart attempts to make up for the resistance in the vessels by enlarging. Over a period of time, the heart eventually fails. Hypertension further increases the rate at which disease progresses in the vessels.

Older people usually have a somewhat higher pressure than younger people. The normal blood pressure for young adults is 120/80, but in older persons, the norm is higher, with the highest level of normal being 140/90 mmHg. Above this level, the probability of stroke and heart attack increases dramatically. Hypertension is dangerous because often there are no symptoms. It may be detected during a routine blood pressure check. Report any blood pressures when the systolic is over 140 or the diastolic is over 90.

Control of Hypertension

Control of hypertension is essential. Steps can be taken to bring the hypertension under control to avoid the serious consequences of stroke and heart attack. These steps include:

- Drugs to lower the pressure
- Weight reduction
- Dietary restrictions, such as limiting salt intake
- Discouraging smoking
- Regular exercise

Report immediately any signs or symptoms of hypertension:

- Flushed face
- Dizziness
- Nose bleeds
- Headaches
- Changes in speech patterns
- Blurred vision

⚠ GUIDELINES FOR... CARING FOR RESIDENTS WITH PERIPHERALVASCULAR DISEASE

1. Elevate the feet when the resident is sitting in a chair for prolonged periods of time. When the feet are not elevated, make sure that the resident's feet are flat on the floor. If they are not, support the feet with a footstool. Discourage the resident from crossing the legs when sitting.

2. Discourage the resident from using circular garters.

3. Discourage smoking because it interferes with circulation.

4. Avoid raising the knee gatch on the bed.

5. Avoid the use of heating pads or hot water bottles. The resident may not feel temperatures that are too hot.

6. Maintain body warmth. Make sure the resident has warm clothes, including well-fitting socks. Provide blankets for the bed, but avoid heavy quilts.

7. Prevent injury to the feet:
   - Instruct the resident to wear shoes when out of bed.
   - Check to see that the shoes are in good repair and that they fit well.
   - Avoid pressure to the legs and feet from any source.

8. Inspect the feet carefully when you bathe the resident or if the resident complains of any discomfort in the feet. Promptly report any signs of inflammation, injury, or circulatory problems (Figure 24-9).

9. Bathe the feet regularly.
   - Dry thoroughly and gently between the toes.
   - Use a moisturizing lotion to the feet and legs if the skin is dry.

10. Do not cut the toenails of residents with peripheral vascular disease without instructions from the nurse.

- Broken skin (ulcer formation)
- Coldness or heat of an extremity
- Color changes
- Diminished pulses
- Dry, brittle, or shiny skin
- Pain (more often arterial)
- Loss of function
- Swelling of extremities

Figure 24-9 Signs that may indicate peripheral vascular disease.

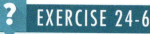

EXERCISE 24-6

1. Mrs. Hawkins has a diagnosis of peripheral vascular disease. Her toenails are thin, dry, and brittle. She complains of pain in her legs, especially at night, and her feet are cold to touch. Describe the special attention you will give to her feet.

    _____

    _____

    _____

    _____

2. What other general care will you provide for Mrs. Hawkins and other residents who have peripheral vascular disease?

    _____

    _____

    _____

    _____

EXERCISE 24-7

1. A blood clot is called a thrombophlebitis. Signs of this may include:

    a. _____

    _____

    b. _____

    _____

    c. _____

    _____

    d. _____

    _____

2. Five signs and symptoms of peripheral vascular disease to be noted are:

    a. _____

    _____

    b. _____

    _____

    c. _____

    _____

    d. _____

    _____

    e. _____

    _____

3. List three lifestyle changes an individual can make to avoid the risk factors that contribute to heart disease.

    a. _____

    _____

    b. _____

    _____

    c. _____

    _____

LYMPHATIC SYSTEM

The lymphatic system is a separate system made up of vessels, nodes, ducts, and organs. Unlike the circulatory system, it is not a closed ring with a pump (the heart). Lymph moves through the system by movements of the body muscles performing daily functions. This system is located throughout the body in close proximity to the circulatory system. It is responsible for several important functions:

- Aids the immune system by producing lymphocytes that help destroy certain bacteria and viruses and other harmful toxins. It works with the cardiovascular system in helping to deliver nutrients, oxygen, and hormones from the blood to the cells of the body via the lymph system.

- Helps to maintain fluid balance by returning excess interstitial (body) fluids back to the cardiovascular system. However, one negative effect occurs as fluids and small cells are absorbed in the lymph fluid, cancer cells may be transported and deposited to other parts of the body such as the lungs (metastasis).

The organs of the lymphatic system include the bone marrow, spleen, and lymph nodes. The tonsil, appendix, and the thymus gland also are considered to be lymphatic tissues. These tissues contain large quantities of lymphocytes. The cells that form the lymphocytes are found in the bone marrow.

Lymph nodes occur in clusters and are located throughout the body along the path of the lymph vessels and contain accumulations of lymphocytes and other substances to help protect the body from pathogens. The nodes normally range in size from a few millimeters to 1 to 2 centimeters. During an infectious process in the body, the lymph nodes may enlarge as the lymphocytes ingest the foreign materials. If the nodes are close to the surface of the body such as in the neck, underarm, or groin they may be easily palpated if they become infected and swollen.

Lymph is a fluid that flows through the lymphatic system. Fluid comes from the blood in the capillaries of the circulatory system and passes into the interstitial spaces. Pressure buildup becomes higher in the fluid in the tissues; the excess fluid then passes into the lymphatic system and is carried back to the circulatory system from the lower portion of the body through the thoracic duct to the subclavian vein. A series of valves in the lymph vessels help the fluid to return to the central portion of the body. Lymph from the area of the head and neck flows back into the circulatory system through the right lymphatic duct. Since there is no pump, muscle activity, peristalsis, and respiration are responsible for helping to move the lymph through the system.

HEART DISEASE

Many residents have some form of heart disease. Heart disease often makes self-care difficult because the resident tires easily, and residents become depressed and frustrated by their limitations. Heart disease may be due to an infection, but most heart disease develops because of narrowing of the coronary arteries. These changes make it harder for the heart to pump blood to the body.

Preventive Measures

Individuals can take positive steps in managing their own lifestyles to avoid the risk factors that contribute to heart and artery disease. These risk factors include:

- Cigarette smoking
- Obesity
- Physical inactivity
- Hypertension
- Abnormally high levels of blood cholesterol
- Excessive emotional stress and depression

These factors are especially important when there is a history of diabetes or a family history of coronary artery disease at an early age.

Cardiac Medications

Drug therapy has become an important facet in the care of residents with a variety of cardiovascular conditions. The nursing assistant can be of benefit by reporting critical observations to the nurse and by anticipating some of the events that arise because of the drug therapy.

Diuretics are drugs that increase the flow of urine by helping to remove excess fluid from the body. Residents, who may have congestive heart failure, have hypertension, or some kidney diseases, may be taking a diuretic. It is important to note that those drugs may begin to act within 30 minutes of administration. You can help the resident get to the bathroom or be alert that the resident may need to use the bedpan to void and help to keep the intake and output records accurate. Diuretics also may cause orthostatic hypotension; a fall in the blood pressure and/or dizziness associated with quick body movements.

Nitroglycerin (NTG), which is discussed in the section on angina pectoris is a **vasodilator**. It is available as a sublingual (under the tongue) tablet and a transdermal or topical (through the skin) preparation. If a transdermal preparation, patch or ointment, is used, it is applied to a hairless portion of the body. Observe the skin at the site of application; report any signs of redness, irritation, or itching to the nurse. Do not remove the patches before bathing the resident, the patches are waterproof. Notify the nurse if the patch becomes loose or dislodged. Patches are applied and removed only by the nurse. If you note any ointment that may have oozed from under the applicator pad report this to the nurse and use caution not to get any on your skin. Since NTG ointment is a vasodilator, it will react on you as well. Caution the resident to arise slowly and sit on the edge of the bed for 1 to 3 minutes before standing. NTG is a vasodilator and may cause orthostatic or postural hypotension.

Varieties of antihypertensive medications are used to treat high blood pressure and are used by a number of elderly persons. Since these drugs also are vasodilators, they may precipitate postural hypotension. Remind the resident to arise slowly from reclining or seated position. Report to the nurse any signs of dizziness or lightheadedness. Accurately record the resident's vital signs.

Heart Attack

A **heart attack** occurs when the heart is not able to function properly. There are different kinds of attacks, and some have more serious effects than others. However, every attack is serious, and each requires some form of treatment (therapy). A heart attack is often referred to as an MI (myocardial infarction).

With a myocardial infarction, the normal flow of blood to the heart is decreased. Narrowing of the coronary (heart) blood vessels that supply blood to the heart may occur slowly over a period of years, allowing some new circulation to develop. However, when the heart attack occurs, the flow of blood has diminished so much that not enough blood reaches the heart and the heart muscle may die. This lack of blood flow is known as ischemia.

Sometimes the flow of blood is cut off abruptly because a blood clot lodges in a coronary artery.

Acute Myocardial Infarction

An acute MI is a serious medical emergency. The blood flow to the myocardium is cut off suddenly. The closure of a large vessel can result in death (infarction) of that part of the heart muscle not being supplied with blood. If too much of the heart muscle dies, the resident cannot survive.

Survival depends largely on how quickly proper medical intervention occurs (Figure 24-10). You must recognize the signs and symptoms of this type of heart attack and report to the nurse immediately.

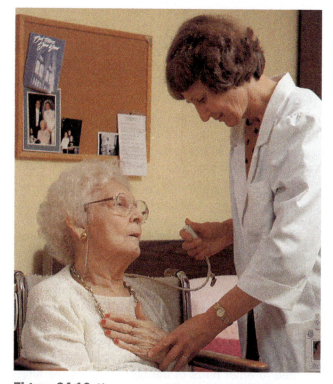

Figure 24-10 If you suspect the resident is having a heart attack, summon help immediately and do not leave the resident.

Signs and Symptoms

These include:

- Crushing chest pain, spreading down the arms and up into the neck and jaw; sometimes described as "severe indigestion"
- Clammy, ashen, or pale skin
- Excessive sweating (**diaphoresis**)
- Nausea
- Vomiting (sometimes)
- Anxiety and weakness
- Weak pulse
- Low blood pressure
- Shock
- Shortness of breath
- **Syncope** (fainting)
- Restlessness

Nursing Assistant Care

You can help by:

- Staying with the resident
- Using the intercom or call light to summon help
- Staying calm
- Provide reassurance

The resident will usually be transferred immediately to the intensive care unit (ICU) or coronary care unit (CCU) of an acute care hospital. Early treatment is designed to reverse the shock, relieve the pain, and keep the heart functioning. Choice of therapy depends on how quickly care is started and the stability of the resident's condition. Several therapies are described in Figure 24-11.

Angina Pectoris

Angina pectoris is a condition in which there is a decreased flow of blood and oxygen to the heart muscle. This may occur during times of stress, physical or mental. It may be the consequence of increased exercise, following a large, heavy meal, or receiving stressful news. Signs and symptoms of an angina attack that you should immediately report include:

- The classic signs and symptoms are a squeezing pain in the chest under the sternum (breast bone) that may radiate to the left shoulder and down the left arm.
- Others may experience pain that radiates to the right shoulder and possibly to the jaw, teeth, and up to the ear.
- Pale or flushed face
- Resident freely perspiring

The signs and symptoms each resident experiences will be similar with each attack and may increase in

---

- Bypass graft: Blood flow is diverted through an **anastomosed** graft to bypass the thrombosed arterial segment.

- Embolectomy: A balloon-tipped catheter is used to remove thrombolytic material from an artery (Figure 24-12A).

- Laser surgery: A hot-tip laser obliterates the blood clot and plaque by vaporizing it.

- Percutaneous transluminal coronary angioplasty (PTCA): The nonsurgical technique uses a tiny balloon catheter that is inserted into the narrowed vessels to open them up and allow the blood to flow. The balloon is then removed and replaced with a **stent**, a mesh device used to keep the artery open (Figure 24-12B).

- Reperfusion therapy: Medical therapy that uses blood clot-dissolving drugs or a mechanical therapy for the same purpose.

- Thromboendarterectomy: The artery is opened and the obstructing thrombus and medial layer of the arterial wall are removed.

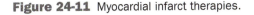

Figure 24-11 Myocardial infarct therapies.

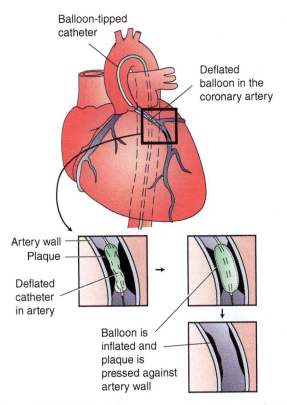

Figure 24-12A The balloon presses the plaque against the wall of the artery, making the vessel larger.

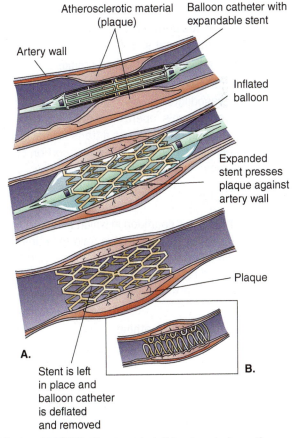

Figure 24-12B The stent is left in place to keep the artery open and the balloon is removed.

? **EXERCISE 24-8**

COMPLETION
Select the correct terms from the following list to complete each statement.

cut   myocardial infarction   strokes
elasticity   narrows   transient ischemic attacks
massaged   peripheral vascular disease

1. When atherosclerosis occurs, the arteries lose their _____.
2. The space within the arteries _____ when atherosclerosis develops.
3. When atherosclerosis affects the arteries of the brain, _____ may result.
4. Before a stroke happens a person may experience a series of TIAs or _____.
5. When the atherosclerosis affects the leg vessels, it causes _____.
6. Atherosclerosis of the heart blood vessels can lead to _____.
7. If there are signs of inflammation in a leg, the area should not be _____.
8. The toenails of a resident with peripheral vascular disease should not be _____ without instructions from the nurse.

frequency, duration, and intensity over time. The nursing assistant may help the resident with angina pectoris by:

- Immediately reporting any signs and symptoms to the nurse
- Helping the resident to avoid any unnecessary physical or emotional stress
- Encouraging the resident not to smoke

Residents with a history of angina pectoris are treated with vasodilator drugs, such as NTG to help keep the blood vessels open. In the facility you will most often see it administered as a transdermal patch. The nurse places the patch on a hairless portion of the body for the prescribed length of time each day.

Heart Failure

Many residents have a condition in which the heart functions less efficiently. The resident is said to be in heart failure (also called **congestive heart failure**). Heart failure can affect the right or left side of the heart, or both sides. Left-sided heart failure is manifested by:

- Cough
- **Dyspnea** (difficulty breathing)
- **Orthopnea** (difficulty in breathing unless sitting upright)
- Cyanosis
- **Hemoptysis** ("frothy, bright blood" from the oral cavity, larynx, trachea, bronchi, or lungs)
- Fluid retained in the lungs and throughout the body
- Jugular neck vein distension (Figure 24-13A)

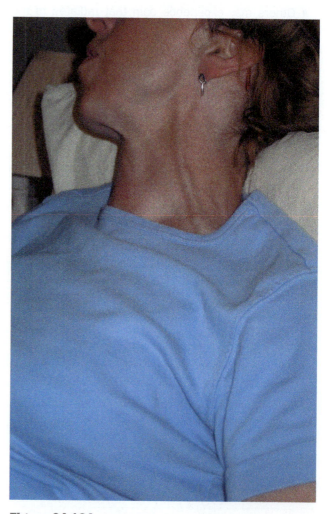

Figure 24-13A Jugular vein distension.

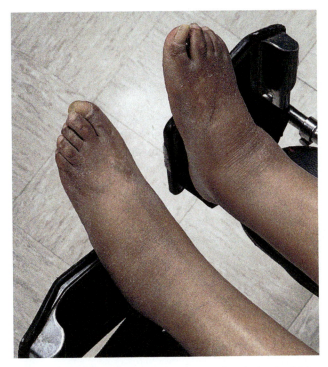

Figure 24-13B Edema is often a prominent sign in right-sided heart failure.

Signs and symptoms of right-sided heart failure may include the following:

- **Edema** (fluid in the tissue spaces) (Figure 24-13B)
- **Ascites** (fluid collecting in the abdominal cavity)
- Neck veins swell
- Fatiguing easily
- **Hypoxia** (inadequate oxygen levels)

- Confusion
- Irregular and rapid pulse
- Ultimately inadequate blood flow to the lungs may occur and then left-sided heart failure will develop

Nursing Assistant Care

Acute heart failure is an urgent situation requiring expert care. You will assist in this care. Watch the resident carefully and report any increase in signs and symptoms at once.

Nursing care may include:

- Positioning. The resident is usually more comfortable either sitting up in bed, in an **orthopneic position** or high Fowler's position, supported by pillows, or supported in a chair. The position must be changed frequently, but changes in position should be made slowly. Padded footboards help keep the weight of the bedding off the toes.

- Application of elasticized antiembolism stockings. Antiembolism stockings are not the same as support hose. T.E.D. is a common brand made by Kendall-Futuro Co.; many persons refer to antiembolism stockings as **TED hose**. Antiembolism stockings have graduated compression from the ankle to the thigh. The greatest compression is at the ankle, slightly less at the calf, and even less compression at the thigh. This design helps to keep the blood flowing in the deeper, larger vessels. Several types of stockings are made: some have an open portion over the toes that facilitates inspection of the circulation in the feet, and some have a closed toe. The circulation in the legs and feet must be checked every 6 to

---

? EXERCISE 24-9

MATCHING
Match the signs and symptoms of congestive heart failure on the right with their meanings on the left.

Meaning Signs and Symptoms

1. _____ dyspnea
2. _____ hemoptysis
3. _____ hypoxia
4. _____ edema
5. _____ orthopnea
6. _____ syncope
7. _____ cyanosis
8. _____ ascites

a. bluish discoloration of skin

b. inadequate oxygen levels

c. difficulty breathing

d. frothy, bright blood from oral cavity, larynx, bronchi, or lungs

e. fluid collecting in abdominal cavity

f. fainting

g. difficulty in breathing unless sitting upright

h. fluid in tissue spaces

8 hours. The skin should be warm and pink. Because the hose come in a variety of sizes, the nurse is responsible for measuring the resident's leg to ensure that the hose are the correct size.

- Give attention to general hygiene. Complete bathing is tiring, but partial baths can stimulate circulation and provide comfort. Special attention must be given to the skin because the combination of position, edema, and poor circulation contributes to tissue breakdown.

- Assist with oxygen therapy. Oxygen therapy may be provided either by face mask or nasal cannula. Because cardiac residents often breathe through the mouth, the mouth tends to be very dry. Special mouth care may be needed. (For oxygen safety, refer to Lesson 8.)

- Provide for elimination. A bedside commode is convenient. The use of a commode is less tiring for the resident than using a bedpan for elimination.

- Encourage adequate nutrition. Small, easily digested meals should be encouraged. You may need to assist in feeding the resident to prevent fatigue.

- Monitor and record fluid intake. Residents with acute heart failure may be given drugs that increase the output of urine and alter the heart rate. Measuring the intake and output and taking daily weights are ways of determining if fluid is being retained. These procedures are part of the care you will give.

- Regularly check vital signs. Sometimes the force of heart contraction, which propels the blood forward into the blood vessels, does not have enough strength to make the vessels expand.

Chronic Heart Failure

Residents can live for years with some level of chronic heart failure. A resident with chronic heart failure

PROCEDURE 24-95
Applying Elasticized (Support) Stockings

1. Carry out each beginning procedure action.

2. Assemble equipment:

   - Elasticized stockings of proper length and size

3. With resident lying down, expose one leg at a time.

4. Insert hand into stocking as far as heel pocket. Grasp center of heel pocket and turn stocking inside out (Figure 24-14).

5. Carefully slip the stocking over foot and heel. Center heel in heel pocket (Figure 24-15).

6. Lift the leg and pull stocking up and around ankle and calf, working up the thigh. Make sure stocking is pulled evenly up the leg (Figure 24-16).

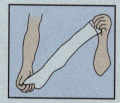

Figure 24-14 Insert hand into stocking as far as heel pocket. Grasp center of heel pocket and turn stocking inside out.

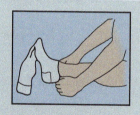

Figure 24-15 Carefully slip stocking over foot and heel.

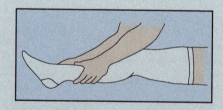

Figure 24-16 Lift leg and pull stocking up around ankle and calf, working up thigh. Make sure stocking is pulled evenly up the leg.

(continues)

PROCEDURE 24-95
Applying Elasticized (Support) Stockings (Continued)

7. Assure that stocking is not wrinkled over the ankle or behind the knee (Figure 24-17).

8. Make sure the stocking material over the toes is not stretched too tight (Figure 24-18).

9. Repeat procedure on other leg.

10. Carry out each procedure completion action.

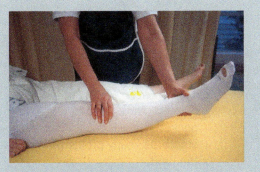

Figure 24-17 Check to be sure stocking has no wrinkles.

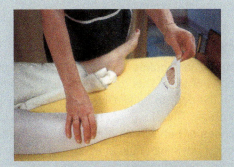

Figure 24-18 Check material on toes to be sure it is not too tight.

? EXERCISE 24-10

COMPLETE THE CHART
The resident with congestive heart failure needs special care. List nursing assistant actions for such a resident.

Technique
 1. Checking vital signs
    Nursing Assistant Actions
    _____
    _____

Technique
 2. Bathing procedure
    Nursing Assistant Actions
    _____
    _____

Technique
 3. Oxygen therapy
    Nursing Assistant Actions
    _____
    _____

Technique
 4. Elimination assistance
    Nursing Assistant Actions
    _____
    _____

needs a calm environment with planned activity that promotes mobility but not fatigue. Visiting should be limited to one or two people because too many visitors at one time can be tiring.

The basic care given to residents in chronic failure includes:

- Measuring fluid intake and output
- Assisting the nurse by taking the radial pulse while the nurse takes the apical pulse
- Assisting with ADLs when necessary to prevent fatigue and maintain mobility
- Reporting any change in signs and symptoms
- Reporting unusual behavior or responses

This condition requires the use of medications for long periods of time. This results in a tendency for drug levels in the body to build. Older people are more sensitive to drugs. Therefore, you must be alert to unusual responses or behavior that may indicate a drug reaction. Report anything unusual about the residents in your care to your supervisor.

Heart Block

Heart block is a condition that develops due to interference in the electrical current through the heart. (The flow of electrical current through the heart muscle makes the normal cardiac cycle possible.)

An electronic device called a **pacemaker** (Figure 24-19) is implanted under the chest muscles or in the abdomen. An electrode carries electrical current from the pacemaker directly into the heart muscle to replace the lost control. The electrical current signals the heart to contract. Some pacemakers send messages only if normal messages carried by the conduction system are delayed. This type of pacemaker is called a demand pacemaker. Other pacemakers send regular signals to keep the heart contracting. The rate of signals is preset.

When caring for a resident who has a pacemaker:

- Count and record the pulse rate.
- Report any irregularities or changes below the preset rate.
- Report any discoloration over the implant site.
- Report hiccoughing because this may indicate problems.
- Caution the resident not to carry a cell phone in an area near where the pacemaker has been implanted, for example, not in the shirt or blouse pocket. Newer cell phone technology does not create as many problems with pacemakers as in the past.

Residents usually function very well with pacemakers so long as they are adequately monitored.

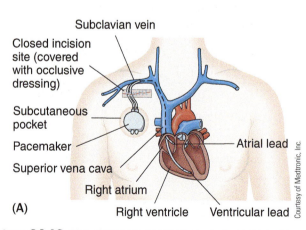

Subclavian vein

Closed incision site (covered with occlusive dressing)

Subcutaneous pocket

Pacemaker

Superior vena cava

Right atrium

Atrial lead

Right ventricle   Ventricular lead

(A)

Courtesy of Medtronic, Inc.

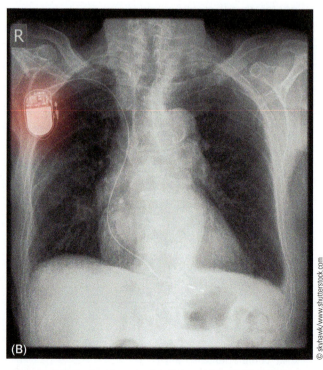

(B)

© skyhawk/www.shutterstock.com

Figure 24-19 The electronic pacemaker sends electrical impulses to the heart muscle, causing it to contract. (A) A typical pacemaker. (B) The pacemaker inserted under the skin with electrode placed inside the heart, resting on the heart muscle.

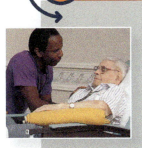

LESSON SYNTHESIS: Putting It All Together

You have just completed this lesson. Now go back and review the Clinical Focus. Try to see how the Clinical Focus relates to the concepts presented in the lesson. Then answer the following questions.

1. Explain how a cardiac chair contributes to Mr. Rabinowitz's comfort and improved functioning of his cardiovascular system.

2. What actions can you take to increase Mr. Rabinowitz's warmth without using a hot water bag?

3. How do elasticized stockings assist the circulation in the legs?

4. What precautions should be taken when applying the elasticized stockings?

24 REVIEW

A. Select the one best answer for each of the following.

1. The cardiovascular system includes the

(A) liver

(B) lungs

(C) heart, blood, and blood vessels

(D) spleen

2. Which of the following is not a possible result of an inadequate blood supply?

(A) dementia

(B) myocardial infarction

(C) pneumonia

(D) stroke

3. The structures of the heart that permit blood flow in one direction only are called

(A) valves

(B) ventricles

(C) atria

(D) myocardium

4. The major artery is called the

(A) vena cava

(B) aorta

(C) pulmonary vein

(D) pulmonary artery

5. One of the following is a function of the lymph system

(A) manufacturing new red blood cells

(B) transporting oxygen

(C) filtering out harmful substances before they reach the general circulation

(D) inhibiting bleeding

6. Red blood cells are responsible for

(A) delivery of oxygen to all body cells

(B) protecting the body by fighting infection

(C) the blood clotting process

(D) making lymph fluid

7. One effect of aging on the cardiovascular system is to

(A) increase cardiac output

(B) increase heart rate

(C) enlarge vascular lumens

(D) increase blood pressure

8. The formation of plaque on the inner walls of the arteries is called

(A) atherosclerosis

(B) arteriosclerosis

(C) varicose veins

(D) peripheral vascular disease

9. When the valves in the veins of the legs become weakened, the result is

(A) dementia

(B) stroke

(C) varicose veins

(D) heart failure

10. When caring for persons with peripheral vascular disease, all of the following are required *except*

(A) regularly inspecting the feet and legs

(B) maintaining appropriate hygiene of the feet and legs

(C) preventing injury to the feet and legs

(D) allowing person to cross legs when sitting

11. A symptom of heart attack or MI is

(A) crushing chest pain

(B) dry skin

(C) high blood pressure

(D) strong pulse

12. Persons with left-sided heart failure are more comfortable in the

(A) orthopneic position

(B) supine position

(C) side-lying position

(D) prone position

13. Which of the following actions is not appropriate when caring for a resident who has a pacemaker?

(A) counting, recording, and reporting the pulse rate

(B) reporting hiccoughing

(C) reporting any discoloration over the implant site

(D) keeping a cellular phone in the shirt pocket

14. When caring for a resident with right-sided heart failure all of the following activities are important *except*

(A) daily weight

(B) range of motion exercises

(C) increase fluid intake

(D) record intake and output

15. The lymph nodes become enlarged when there is:

(A) infection or disease present

(B) a blood clot is present

(C) increased lymph fluid

(D) oxygen levels in the blood are high

B. Match each term (items a–i) with the proper explanation.

a. edema
b. myocardial infarction
c. ventricles
d. ischemia
e. radial artery
f. atria
g. valves
h. atherosclerosis
i. arteries

16. _____   upper heart chambers

17. _____   fluid in the tissue spaces

18. _____   vessels that carry blood away from the heart

19. _____   located close to the radius

20. _____   lower heart chambers

21. _____   form of vascular disease in which plaques are formed in the walls of arteries

22. _____   diminished blood flow

C. Answer each statement true (T) or false (F).

23. T F The older heart muscle may be less effective.

24. T F The person with orthopnea has difficulty breathing in an upright position.

25. T F A person with anemia must be handled very gently.

26. T F Leukemias are an example of a blood abnormality.

27. T F Diabetes is not a risk factor for coronary artery disease.

CARING FOR RESIDENTS WITH RESPIRATORY SYSTEM DISORDERS

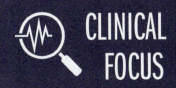

CLINICAL FOCUS

Think about the special care needed by residents with respiratory disorders as you study this lesson.

OBJECTIVES

After studying this lesson, you should be able to:

- Define vocabulary words and terms.
- Identify the parts and function of the respiratory system.
- Explain changes in the respiratory system as they relate to the aging process.
- Describe common respiratory conditions affecting the long-term care resident.
- Describe how to give proper care to residents in respiratory distress and receiving respiratory therapy.

VOCABULARY

allergen (**AL**-er-jen)
alveoli (al-**VEE**-oh-lie)
aspiration (ass-pih-**RAY**-shun)
asthma (**AZ**-mah)
bronchi (**BRONG**-kie)
bronchioles (**BRONG**-kee-ohls)
bronchitis (brong-**KEYE**-tis)
cannula (**KAN**-you-lah)
carbon dioxide (**KAR**-bon dye-**OCK**-side)

chronic obstructive pulmonary disease (COPD) (**KRON**-ick ob-**STRUCK**-tiv **PULL**-moh-nair-ee dih-**ZEEZ**)
dyspnea (disp-**NEE**-ah)
emphysema (em-fih-**SEE**-mah)
expectorate (eck-**SPECK**-toh-rayt)
high Fowler's position (high **FOW**-lerz poh-**ZISH**-un)
influenza (in-flew-**EN**-zah)
larynx (**LAR**-inks)

CASE STUDY

Mary Calcetas is 60 and has been a cigarette smoker for many years. Emphysema has made the act of breathing an effort. Walking the length of the corridor to the lounge requires two rest periods along the way. When a lung infection occurs, she requires nasal oxygen and orthopneic positioning. The nurse assigns you to care for Mrs. Calcetas this morning.

orthopneic position (or-**THOP**-nee-ick poh-**ZISH**-un)
oxygen (**OCK**-sih-jen)
oxygen mask (**OCK**-sih-jen mask)
pharynx (**FAR**-inks)
phlegm (flem)
pleura (**PLOOR**-ah)
pneumonia (new-**MOH**-nee-ah)
regurgitate (ree-**GUR**-jih-tayt)

rhinitis (ri-**NI**-tis)
sputum (**SPEW**-tum)
tachypnea (tack-**IP**-nee-ah)
thorax (**THOR**-acks)
trachea (**TRAY**-kee-ah)
tracheostomy (tray-kee-**OS**-toh-mee)
ventilation (ven-tih-**LAY**-shun)
vocal cords (**VOH**-kal kords)

INTRODUCTION

The respiratory system exchanges gases to meet the body's metabolic needs. The two gases are:

- Oxygen (O_2)
- Carbon dioxide (CO_2)

Oxygen is brought into the lungs and carried to the cells to produce energy. Carbon dioxide is a waste product that is carried to the lungs from the cells for excretion.

There is a close connection between the respiratory and circulatory systems. Cells depend on the bloodstream to carry gases to and from the lungs.

THE RESPIRATORY STRUCTURES

The respiratory structures are shown in Figure 25-1.

Upper Respiratory Tract

The upper respiratory tract consists of the:
- Nose (nostrils)
- Pharynx (throat)
- Larynx (voice box)
- Upper trachea (windpipe)
- Mouth

The lower respiratory tract consists of the structures inside the chest cavity, the:
- Lower trachea
- Bronchi
- Bronchioles
- Alveoli

The Lungs

There are two lungs, each surrounded by a double-walled membrane called the pleura. Between the layers of the pleura is a small amount of fluid that

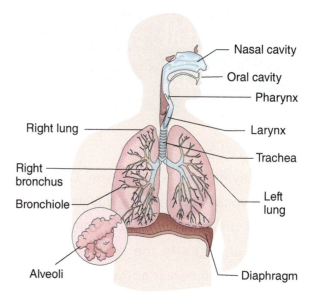

Figure 25-1 The respiratory system.

reduces friction as the lungs alternately expand and contract, filling with and then expelling air. The air is warmed, filtered, and moistened as it passes over the vascular mucous membrane that lines the respiratory tract, from nose to alveoli.

The bronchi join the upper respiratory tract to the lungs. Within the lungs, the bronchi branch into smaller and smaller divisions called bronchioles. The alveoli are tiny air sacs that extend from the bronchioles. The alveoli, bronchioles, and the important pulmonary blood vessels form the lungs (Figure 25-2). The way in which oxygen and carbon dioxide are exchanged between the alveoli and the capillaries is shown in Figure 25-3.

The Act of Respiration

The lungs are located in the thorax (chest). The size of the thorax depends on the contraction of the diaphragm and intercostal muscles. As the muscles contract, the thorax enlarges, expanding the lungs.

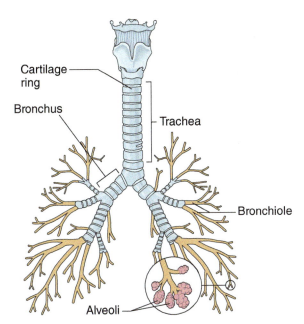

Figure 25-2 Ventral (front) view of the structures of the lower respiratory tract.

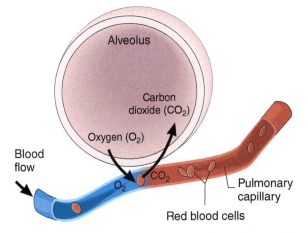

Figure 25-3 Oxygen and carbon dioxide are exchanged between the capillaries and each alveoli.

Air carrying oxygen enters the lungs. When the muscles relax, the thorax resumes its normal size and the lungs recoil. Air carrying carbon dioxide leaves the lungs and is breathed out.

- *Inspiration* is the act of drawing air into the lungs.
- *Expiration* is the act of expelling air.
- **Ventilation** is the combination of these two actions.

VOICE PRODUCTION

The larynx, or voice box, is part of the respiratory tract. It is important in voice production. Two membranes called the **vocal cords** stretch across the inside of the larynx. As air passes upward through the larynx, it moves through an opening in the vocal cords. Changes in the shape of the vocal cords and the size of the opening permit controlled amounts of air to reach the mouth, nasal cavities, and sinuses, where—formed by the teeth, lips, and tongue—specific speech sounds are made.

? EXERCISE 25-1

IMAGE LABELING

Identify the organs of the respiratory system shown in the accompanying figure by selecting the correct terms from the list provided.

bronchus (left)	lung (left)
bronchus (right)	nasal cavity
diaphragm	pharynx
larynx	trachea

1. _____
2. _____
3. _____
4. _____
5. _____
6. _____
7. _____

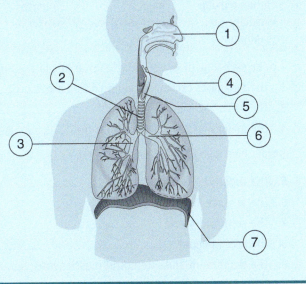

CHANGES CAUSED BY AGING

Refer to Figure 25-4. With aging, the following changes occur gradually:

- Breathing capacity drops by one-half.
- The alveoli enlarge and lose elasticity, making recoil less effective.
- The respiratory rate increases.
- The diaphragm and intercostal muscles lose strength, so gaseous exchange is less efficient.
- Changes in the larynx make the voice higher pitched and weaker.
- Cough mechanism is less effective.
- Lower resistance to infection.

- Lung tissue loses elasticity
- Slower rate of gas exchange
- Breathing capacity diminished
- Diaphragm less efficient
- Rate of breathing increases
- Larynx changes make voice weaker and higher pitched
- Less efficient cough

Figure 25-4 Changes in the respiratory system as a result of aging.

INTRODUCTION TO PATHOLOGY

The respiratory system is affected by the same kinds of pathologies as other systems. Two of the most common disease conditions are:

- Malignancies
- Infections

Malignancies

Malignant tumors can develop in any part of the respiratory tract. Although the exact causes of malignancy are not fully understood, cigarette smoking and exposure to other cancer-producing agents in the environment are known to be contributing factors. Lung cancers are treated by surgery, radiation, chemotherapy, or a combination of all three therapies.

Cancer of the Larynx

Cancer of the larynx may require removal of the larynx, resulting in loss of the voice. The resident breathes through an artificial opening in the neck and trachea. The permanent opening is called a tracheostomy or stoma.

Loss of voice is a major trauma for anyone. Just think for a moment of how frustrated you would feel if you could no longer use your voice to communicate your thoughts, feelings, wants, and needs to others.

? EXERCISE 25-2

COMPLETION
Select the correct term from the following list to complete each statement.

alveoli · drops · oxygen
carbon dioxide · higher · strength
elasticity · increases · weaker
diaphragm · larynx

1. The exchange of gases in the lungs occurs in the tiny air sacs called _____
2. The two gases exchanged in respiration are _____ and _____
3. The voice box is properly called the _____
4. The major muscle of respiration is the _____

Consider how aging impacts the following:

5. The breathing capacity _____
6. The air sacs lose _____
7. The respiratory rate _____
8. The voice becomes _____ and _____
9. The diaphragm and intercostal muscles lose _____

Postsurgical care is given in the acute care hospital. At this time, writing is the major form of communication available to patients. Later, the resident may be taught new ways to speak through:

- Esophageal speech
- Electronic speech

Esophageal Speech

The resident learns to swallow air and then bring it back up (**regurgitate**) through the esophagus into the mouth. Here it is formed by the teeth and tongue into words as it would be if it were being exhaled from the lungs. Esophageal speech is difficult to learn, but motivated residents can succeed.

Electronic Speech

Residents who cannot use esophageal speech may be able to use an electronic artificial larynx to create speech. Some residents may use a combination of both techniques.

Residents with laryngectomies (removal of larynx) need patience and understanding from all health care providers. Communication is possible, but the voice does not sound normal. More time is needed by the resident to formulate the sounds. A difficult psychological adjustment must be made by the resident. The loss of one's voice requires an adjustment similar to that experienced when grieving for the loss of a loved one. Periods of depression, anger, and hostility are frequently noted with residents who have had a laryngectomy.

Infections

The respiratory tract is exposed to many pathogens in the environment. Respiratory infections are common in older persons because of reduced resistance and can be life-threatening.

Common Cold

The common cold, also called viral **rhinitis**, is a viral infection that is easily spread from the secretions in the upper respiratory tract. More than 100 viruses may be responsible for the cold, but the rhinovirus is the most common.

The mucosal surfaces of the nose and throat become inflamed. This inflammation causes the most common symptoms: nasal congestion, increased mucous secretion (runny nose), and sneezing. Some persons also will complain of a scratchy or sore throat.

There is no specific treatment but the person is encouraged to drink a lot of fluids and get plenty of rest. Some persons may take a decongestant and antihistamine to help ease the symptoms related to the nasal congestion and drainage. Antibiotics and sulfonamides are not used to treat a cold because they

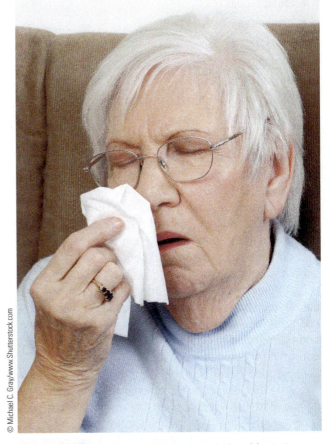

© Michael C. Gray/www.Shutterstock.com

Figure 25-5 For infection control remind residents to use a tissue when sneezing or coughing.

are not effective against viruses. The duration of most colds is 1 to 2 weeks. Because they are spread so easily, persons with a cold should be encouraged to cover their mouth and nose with a tissue when coughing or sneezing (Figure 25-5). In addition to frequent handwashing, persons should try to keep their hands away from their eyes, nose, and mouth. A cold is sometimes accompanied by a low-grade fever (under 102°F). The person may complain of fatigue and should be encouraged to rest as much as possible.

Notify the nurse if the resident who has had a cold, manifests a fever over 102°F, and/or is accompanied by increased perspiration and chills, persistent cough with green or yellow sputum or sever sinus pain. These may be signs of a more serious infection. Two common infections are influenza and pneumonia. Both can be life-threatening to older persons and those with compromised immune systems.

Influenza

Influenza (flu) is a viral respiratory infection. There is usually a sudden onset of signs and symptoms, including:

- Chills
- Fever

- Muscle pain
- Weakness
- Fatigue
- Laryngitis
- Hoarseness
- Nonproductive cough
- Runny nose and eyes

The symptoms usually last 3 to 5 days. In older persons, however, the fatigue and cough may last for several weeks. Influenza can also lead to pneumonia. Older people and those with chronic illness are encouraged to receive a yearly flu vaccine. There are two flu vaccines that do not contain egg proteins, approved for use in adults age 18 and older. Even flu vaccines that do have egg proteins can be given safely to most people with egg allergy.

Influenza can be very dangerous to elderly people. This disease is caused by a virus and therefore is not treatable with antibiotics. New medications have been developed to fight the virus, but it is too early to determine their effectiveness.

Vaccines are available to prevent the disease. The virus that causes influenza changes each year. This means that the vaccine must be modified each year. Long-term care facilities give the vaccine annually to residents unless a resident refuses or there are other reasons not to administer it. Employees working in health care should also receive the vaccine annually. Employers cannot charge employees for the flu shot. Many states mandate all employees receive an annual flu shot and require a mask be worn if the vaccine is declined.

Pneumonia

Pneumonia is a serious infection of the lungs that causes the alveoli to fill with fluid, affecting the exchange of gases. Pneumonia is the fifth leading cause of death in the United States. Older persons and persons with a chronic disease are at greater risk for developing pneumonia. There also is higher prevalence among men. Each year in the United States, about 1 million people seek care in a hospital due to pneumonia. Unfortunately, about 50,000 die from the disease. It is difficult to determine the exact cause. Possible causes of pneumonia include:

- Viruses
- Bacteria
- Fungi
- **Aspiration** of food and liquids (accidentally taking food and liquids into the trachea instead of the esophagus)
- Immobility, which allows fluid to accumulate in the lungs

The resident may have chills, fever, chest pain, and a productive cough (produces sputum). **Phlegm** is matter that is brought up (**expectorated**) as **sputum** from the lungs. Sputum varies in color and character. Respiration may be labored and cyanosis may be present. Treatment includes bed rest, oxygen, and positioning to relieve breathing. Antibiotics are given for bacterial pneumonia. Drugs are also given to relieve chest pain. Residents are encouraged to take fluids. A pneumonia vaccine has been available for a number of years. Older persons and those at risk should be offered the vaccine. The vaccine is usually effective for more than 5 years.

Residents are better able to resist respiratory tract infections when they eat a nutritious diet, take in adequate fluids, and remain active. The nursing assistant can help prevent infections by strict adherence to Standard Precautions.

Effect of Age on the Response to Infections

As people age, their bodies may not respond as strongly to infections as those of younger people. The signs and symptoms of infection may not be as pronounced. Be sure to report:

- Changes in rate or rhythm of respirations
- Cough
- Elevated temperature
- Persistent fatigue
- Difficulty breathing (**dyspnea**)
- Rapid, shallow, or noisy breathing (**tachypnea**)
- Confusion
- Restlessness
- Changes in color of secretions
- Cyanosis
- Pallor
- Shortness of breath (SOB)

Infections are treated vigorously with:

- Rest
- Antibiotics (for bacterial infections)
- Oxygen therapy
- Drugs to keep air passageways clear
- Supportive care

Always practice standard precautions when caring for residents with respiratory infections. Remember that these infectious organisms are often airborne and found in droplets of respiratory secretions. Transmission-based precautions may be required in addition to standard precautions.

? EXERCISE 25-3

VOCABULARY EXERCISE
Complete the puzzle by matching the terms and definitions.

Terms:
a. allergen   h. larynx
b. aspiration   i. oxygen
c. bronchitis   j. pleura
d. emphysema   k. sputum
e. expectorate   l. trachea
f. influenza   m. tracheostomy
g. inspiration

Definitions:

1. _____ gas needed for life
2. _____ inflammation of the bronchi
3. _____ matter brought up from deep in the lungs
4. _____ another name for the windpipe
5. _____ condition in which there is chronic obstruction of air flow out of the alveoli
6. _____ called the voice box
7. _____ a viral respiratory infection
8. _____ accidentally drawing foreign materials into trachea
9. _____ serous membrane covering lungs
10. _____ artificial opening into the trachea

CHRONIC OBSTRUCTIVE PULMONARY DISEASE

Chronic obstructive pulmonary disease (COPD) is also called chronic obstructive lung disease (COLD). This term refers to conditions resulting from a prolonged impairment in the exchange of gases in the respiratory system. Several conditions can lead to COPD, including:

- Chronic asthma
- Chronic bronchitis
- Emphysema

Asthma

Asthma is a breathing disorder resulting from:
- Constriction of the muscles of the bronchioles
- Swelling of the respiratory membranes
- Production of large amounts of mucus that fill the narrowed passageways

A person having an asthma attack has labored breathing and frequent coughing. An attack may result when the person contacts an allergen or is under emotional stress. Common allergens are:

- Tobacco smoke
- Pollens and molds
- Medications
- Dust
- Feathers and animal dander
- Foods
- Perfumes

If a resident has known allergies (hypersensitivity to specific items), the allergy should be marked boldly in the resident's health record. Long-term treatment consists of determining the allergen and eliminating it. To relieve the attack, the resident is given medication to decrease the swelling and dilate the bronchioles. Low levels of oxygen are also given.

Chronic Bronchitis

Chronic bronchitis is prolonged inflammation in the bronchi due to infection or irritants. Signs and symptoms include:

- Swollen and red bronchial tissues, resulting in narrowed bronchial passageways
- Persistent, productive cough

- Respiratory distress
- Increased production of mucus

Treatment, in general, includes:

- Antibiotics to fight the infection
- Drugs to loosen the phlegm (secretions) deep in the respiratory tract
- Techniques to improve ventilation and drainage
- Adequate fluid intake to thin secretions

Emphysema

Emphysema develops after chronic obstruction of the airflow to the alveoli. The damage is irreversible. The air sacs:

- Become distended
- Lose their elasticity and recoil ability
- Finally become nonfunctional
- Lose ability to exchange gases

The resident can bring air into the lungs, but it becomes more difficult to expel air from the lungs. As a result, there is less and less room for air to reenter.

Several factors contribute to emphysema, including:

- Air pollutants, such as cigarette smoke, auto exhaust fumes, and insecticides
- Genetic predisposition to emphysema
- Recurrent infections, such as pneumonia and bronchitis
- Chronic asthma

People with emphysema are at greater risk for infections such as pneumonia. They experience:

- Chronic oxygen shortage and fatigue
- Increased breathing difficulty (requires greater and greater effort)
- Productive coughing that may bring up large amounts of heavy mucous secretions (phlegm), or nonproductive coughing
- Dizziness and restlessness as carbon dioxide levels rise in the bloodstream
- Loss of appetite and weight loss
- Strain on the heart and blood vessels

CLINICAL FOCUS

Compare Mrs. Calcetas's symptoms with the changes in the respiratory system that are a result of aging. Think about how one condition affects the other.

TREATMENT AND CARE OF RESIDENTS WITH COPD

The goals of treatment of the resident with COPD are to:

- Stay hydrated
- Loosen and thin phlegm
- Improve ventilation
- Improve gaseous exchange
- Prevent infections

Special techniques are used to loosen the phlegm and make it easier to bring up. Removing secretions from the passageways makes breathing easier. Some procedures will be carried out by the nurse or respiratory therapist. You may assist in:

- Positioning the resident for better ventilation
- Breathing exercises to improve respiratory efficiency
- Caring for the resident during oxygen therapy to improve gaseous exchange

Positioning for Better Ventilation

Two positions are used to improve ventilation:

- High Fowler's position
- Orthopneic position

In the **high Fowler's position**, the resident is sitting almost upright, with the knees flexed. The resident must be supported in proper alignment with pillows.

In the **orthopneic position**, an overbed table is positioned in front of the resident (Figure 25-6). The resident leans forward with arms on the table. A pillow on the overbed table supports the head. The arms may be positioned on or around the pillow. Additional pillows are used to support the resident's body and maintain proper alignment.

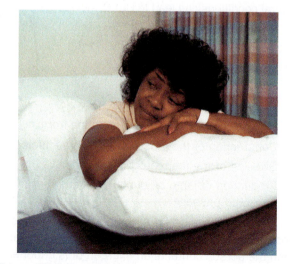

Figure 25-6 The orthopneic position.

Most residents with COPD who are ambulatory breathe best when sitting in a chair and leaning forward with the elbows on the arms of the chair or on their legs.

Exercises

Residents can be taught breathing exercises that improve respiration and general respiratory muscle tone. Breathing exercises stress the expiration phase of respiration. The resident is first taught the basic breathing pattern, which is to:

- Breathe in through the nose to the count of one, allowing the abdomen to rise.
- Purse the lips to the count of two and three as the abdominal wall is contracted and air is forced out of the lungs.

Oxygen Therapy

Residents with COPD benefit by breathing low-dose oxygen. Too high a concentration of oxygen can cause death for these persons. Oxygen therapy may be administered by:

- Cannulas—small tubes placed in the resident's nostril and held in place by elastic straps (Figure 25-7).

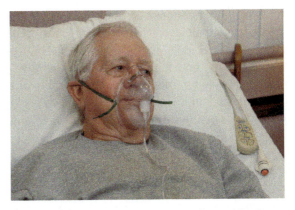

Figure 25-8 The mask is placed over the resident's nose and mouth to deliver oxygen.

- Oxygen mask—placed over the resident's nose and mouth and secured in place with elastic straps (Figure 25-8).
- Nasal catheter—small plastic or latex tube that is inserted several inches into the nose. (**Nasal catheters are rarely used because they cause injury to the mucous membranes of the nose.**)

The nurse is responsible for setting up the oxygen equipment and will start the oxygen flow according to the doctor's orders. The nursing assistant should never start, stop, or change the flow of the oxygen. The nursing assistant's responsibilities include:

- Knowing the flow rate of oxygen for the resident (check each time you enter the room). Note the amount of oxygen in the tank (Figure 25-9).
- Implementing the necessary safety precautions (see Lesson 8).
- Elevating the head of the bed to facilitate ease of breathing (usually semi-Fowler's or high Fowler's position). Use the information on the resident's care plan.

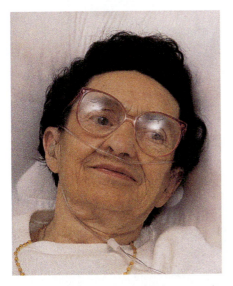

Figure 25-7 This resident is receiving oxygen through a cannula attached to the oxygen source.

Liter flow meter   Amount of O$_2$ in tank

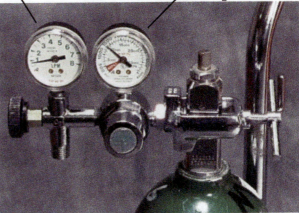

Figure 25-9 One gauge shows the liter flow the resident receives. The other indicates how much oxygen is in the tank.

- Noting the proper position of the cannula or mask. Make sure the elastic is snug but not constricting.
- Checking the skin of the nostrils, skin over the cheekbones, and the skin behind the ears to assure there is no irritation from the cannula or tubing. Noting that there are no secretions on the face.
- Making sure the oxygen tubing is not kinked, pinched, or restricted in any way.
- Noting the humidifier fluid level and changing the canister per agency protocol (Figure 25-10).
- Knowing where oxygen supplies are stored in your facility.
- Knowing the facility policy for cleaning oxygen equipment.

Source of Oxygen

Oxygen is present in the air we breathe. Sometimes residents will have conditions and diseases that cause the resident to need supplemental oxygen. The doctor will order additional oxygen to be given to a resident, as well as the way the oxygen is to be administered and the length of time it is to be delivered. In most long-term care facilities, tanks of oxygen or oxygen concentrators are used (see Figure 25-10). If a tank is to be used, be sure that:

- "No Smoking" signs are in place.
- There is sufficient oxygen in the tank. Check the gauge each time you visit the resident. Notify the nurse if the supply is low.
- An additional tank is available.

- Empty tanks are marked and stored according to facility policy.
- The tank is upright and secured on the carrier or in the stand.
- The oxygen is moisturized.

Oxygen does not explode, but when it is concentrated, burning is more intense and rapid. Everyone must follow oxygen safety measures. If there is a fire, sound the alarm and move the resident to safety, following facility policy.

Oxygen Concentrator

An oxygen concentrator takes in room air and removes impurities and gases other than oxygen, allowing the oxygen to become concentrated in the unit. The air delivered to the resident from the concentrator is more than 90% oxygen. It is delivered by tubing attached to a nasal cannula or mask. The flow rate is usually 2 liters per minute (L/min). A humidifier bottle may be attached to the concentrator to offset the drying effect of the oxygen.

General Oxygen Concentrator Precautions

Be sure to follow these precautions when a concentrator is used to supply oxygen to a resident:

- Concentrator is placed at least 5 feet away from a heat source and at least 4 inches from the wall.
- Smoking or open flames are not permitted in the same room.

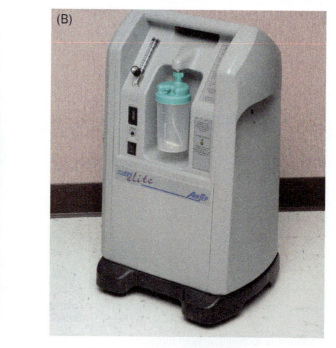

Figure 25-10 Most long-term care facilities use oxygen in (A) tanks and (B) concentrators.

- Be sure the unit is plugged in and grounded.
- Do not use an extension cord with the concentrator.
- Never change the flowmeter setting.
- Notify the nurse if the alarm sounds.
- Be sure the fluid level in the humidifier (if used) is adequate.
- Wipe cannula or mask daily with a damp cloth (do not use alcohol or oil-based products).
- Clean concentrator surfaces using a damp cloth only.
- Remove filter weekly. Wash in warm soapy water, rinse, squeeze dry, and replace.

Special Care Needs

Breathing through the mouth and breathing oxygen are drying to the mucous membranes of the mouth and the nasal passages. The resident may complain that their sputum has a bad taste. Make sure that the resident rinses his or her mouth frequently and that you provide special mouth care. This attention adds greatly to the resident's comfort. During oxygen therapy, the resident may have an adequate oral intake of fluid, but the mouth may still be dry. Residents who need oxygen may be too sick to use a mouth rinse. Commercially prepared artificial saliva products may be of benefit. These products are available in sprays, gels, and rinses. Check the resident's care plan to note if these products are being used. The sprays are the most effective and the easiest to use. Take care not to touch the spray nozzle on the inside of the mouth or lips or your hands, to ensure it is kept clean. Apply the gel with a clean, gloved finger to the roof of the mouth, cheeks, gums, tongue, and the inside of the lips. Dispose of the glove in the appropriate manner. Nasal gels also are available to help soothe the nasal mucous membranes.

Do not use petroleum-based products like Vaseline or other products like Chapstick as oral or nasal lubricants. These products may cause deterioration of the oxygen delivery tubing or cannula and have been determined to be a fire hazard in the presence of oxygen.

? EXERCISE 25-4

CLINICAL SITUATION
Read the following situations. Complete the following statements related to each clinical situation.

Mrs. Smith has asthma and is not breathing easily this morning. She had a distressing argument with her son when he visited yesterday. She is known to be allergic to chicken.

1. Five substances people are commonly allergic to are:
   a. _____
   b. _____
   c. _____
   d. _____
   e. _____
2. The staff is alerted to Mrs. Smith's hypersensitivity by placing _____.
3. No _____ should be served as food to this resident.
4. Chronic asthma can lead to _____.
5. Mrs. McDonnell is a mouth breather and coughs up thick sputum. Mouth breathing is _____ to the mucous membranes.
6. Sputum often leaves a _____ taste in the mouth.
7. Three things a nursing assistant can do to add to Mrs. McDonnell's comfort include:
   a. _____
   b. _____
   c. _____

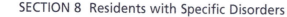

LESSON SYNTHESIS: Putting It All Together

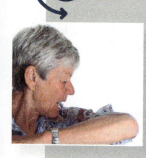

You have just completed this lesson. Now go back and review the Clinical Focus. Try to see how the Clinical Focus relates to the concepts presented in the lesson. Then answer the following questions.

1. Why does Mrs. Calcetas have to rest so often when she tries to walk to the day room?

2. Why did smoking make Mrs. Calcetas's condition more difficult?

3. What nursing care techniques could you use to help improve Mrs. Calcetas's breathing?

4. Why is it important to keep Mrs. Calcetas well hydrated?

25 REVIEW

A. Select the correctly spelled word and then write its definition using the word in the definition.

1.	xpectorate	expectorate	espectarate
2.	expiration	xpiration	expiration
3.	thorax	tharox	thori
4.	flegm	flem	phlegm

B. Complete each statement by filling in the missing information.

5. Another name for the windpipe is the _____.

6. As a person ages, breathing capacity diminishes by _____.

7. Changes in the larynx make the voice _____ and _____.

8. List three changes that occur in the respiratory system as a person ages _____.

9. When the resident is receiving oxygen, the cannula may irritate the skin of the _____, the _____, or _____.

10. State the two positions used to assist a resident in respiratory distress. _____ _____

C. Select the one best answer for each of the following.

11. Rapid and shallow breathing is known as
    (A) apnea   (C) pleura
    (B) emphysema   (D) tachypnea

12. The technique of swallowing air, regurgitating it, and forming words with the teeth and tongue is called
    (A) nasal speech
    (B) esophageal speech
    (C) electronic speech
    (D) sinus speech

13. Sputum is matter from the
    (A) lungs   (C) mouth
    (B) nose   (D) sinuses

14. An asthma attack may occur when a sensitive person
    (A) contacts an allergen
    (B) washes hands regularly
    (C) sleeps soundly
    (D) eats nonallergenic foods

15. When your resident is receiving oxygen therapy, you should

(A) monitor intake and output

(B) check the flow rate once each shift

(C) check the flow rate every 4 hours

(D) know the ordered flow rate

16. Breathing exercises for residents with COPD stress

(A) inspiratory phase

(B) expiratory phase

(C) resting phase

(D) inhalation phase

17. When a resident receives oxygen from a tank through a nasal cannula, the nursing assistant must be sure that

(A) the flowmeter registers the proper moisture content

(B) oxygen is being administered with humidification

(C) there is no irritation from the strap or cannula

(D) tank leans against the wall

18. When the resident has a cold, all but *one* of the following is important.

(A) Encourage increased fluid intake

(B) Antibiotic therapy

(C) Promote naps

(D) Frequent handwashing

D. Identify and write the name of each structure shown in the figure.

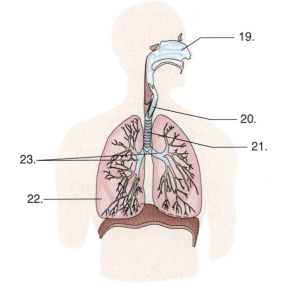

19. _____

20. _____

21. _____

22. _____

23. _____

E. Clinical experience fill in the blanks by selecting the correct word from the list.

adjustment	gloves
anger	normal
burned	patience
common	report
cover	sputum
depression	strongly

24. Mr. Drummond had a laryngectomy. He is new to your unit. He uses esophageal speech. What characteristics might you expect of him?

a. His speech will not sound _____.

b. He had to make a great psychological _____ to his condition.

c. He will experience periods of _____ _____ and _____.

d. His care will require much _____ _____ from staff members.

25. Mrs. Burton, who is 87, is one of the residents you care for. She said she does not have "much energy" this morning. She seems a little confused and has a slight cough. Her temperature is elevated only slightly.

a. You know that influenza and pneumonia are _____ complications of the aging process.

b. You also remember that as people age, they do not respond to infection as _____ as younger people.

c. You will _____ your findings promptly.

26. Mr. Ornsteen has a respiratory infection and is confined to bed. You are assigned to care for him. What do you need to remember to protect yourself?

a. Use _____ when handling respiratory or nasal secretions.

b. Instruct him to _____ his nose and mouth when coughing or sneezing.

CARING FOR RESIDENTS WITH ENDOCRINE SYSTEM DISORDERS

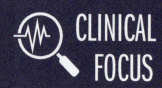

CLINICAL FOCUS

Think about the special observations and care residents with endocrine disorders need as you study this lesson.

OBJECTIVES

After studying this lesson, you should be able to:

• Define vocabulary words and terms.

• Identify the parts and function of the endocrine system.

• Explain changes in the endocrine system as they relate to the aging process.

• Discuss reportable signs and symptoms of hypoglycemia and hyperglycemia.

VOCABULARY

adrenal glands (ah-DREE-nal glands)
adrenaline (ah-DREN-ah-lin)
cortisone (KOR-tih-sohn)
diabetes mellitus (die-ah-BEE-teez MEL-ih-tus)
diabetic coma (die-ah-BET-ick KOH-mah)
diabetic ketoacidosis (DKA) (dye-ah-BET-ick kee-toh-ah-sih-DOH-sis)
endocrine gland (EN-doh-krin gland)
estrogen (ES-troh-jen)
gangrene (GANG-green)
glucagon (GLOO-kah-gon)
glucose (GLOO-kohs)

glycosuria (gligh-koh-SOO-ree-ah)
goiter (GOY-ter)
gonad (GOH-nad)
hormone (HOR-mohn)
hyperglycemia (high-per-gly-SEE-mee-ah)
hyperthyroidism (high-per-THIGH-roy-dizm)
hypoglycemia (high-poh-gly-SEE-mee-ah)
hypothyroidism (high-poh-THIGH-roy-dizm)
insulin (IN-soo-lin)
insulin-dependent diabetes mellitus (IDDM) (IN-soo-lin dee-PEN-dent die-ah-BEE-teez MEL-ih-tus)
insulin shock (IN-soo-lin shock)

CASE STUDY

John Begay is an insulin-dependent diabetic assigned to your care. He has had a cold. This morning he seems very restless and less responsive than usual. He grows increasingly confused. His 11:00 AM glucometer reading shows hyperglycemia. Certain actions must be taken immediately.

islets of Langerhans (EYE-lets of LANG-ger-hans)
ketones (KEE-tohns)
metabolism (meh-TAB-oh-lizm)
non–insulin-dependent diabetes mellitus (NIDDM)
(non–IN-soo-lin dee-PEN-dent die-ah-BEE-teez
MEL-ih-tus)
ovaries (OH-vah-rees)
pancreas (PAN-kree-as)
parathormone (pair-ah-THOR-mohn)
parathyroid glands (pair-ah-THIGH-royd glands)
pineal gland (PIN-ee-al gland)

pituitary gland (pih-TOO-ih-tair-ee gland)
polydipsia (pol-ee-DIP-see-ah)
polyphagia (pol-ee-FAY-jee-ah)
polyuria (pol-ee-YOU-ree-ah)
progesterone (proh-JES-teh-rohn)
scrotum (SKROH-tum)
testes (TES-teez)
testosterone (tes-TOS-teh-rohn)
thyroid gland (THIGH-royd gland)
thyroxine (thigh-ROCK-sin)

INTRODUCTION

The endocrine system (Figure 26-1) consists of duct-less glands. Seven distinct **endocrine glands** are:

- Pituitary gland
- Pineal body
- Adrenal glands
- Gonads—ovaries (women); testes (men)

- Thyroid gland
- Parathyroid glands
- Islets of Langerhans (pancreas)

The endocrine tissues are located throughout the body. They have the following functions and properties:

- Produce chemical messengers (**hormones**)
- Directly enter the bloodstream (no ducts)
- Regulate body activities and body chemistry

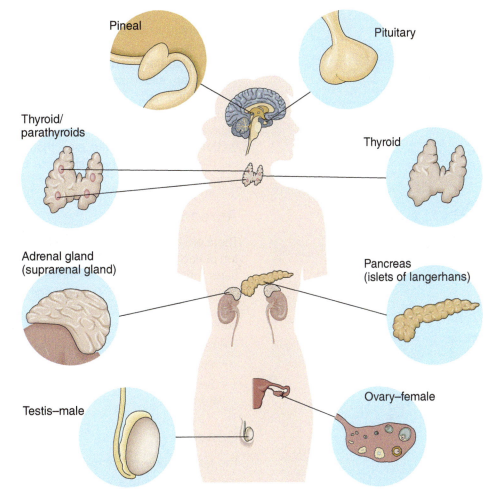

Figure 26-1 The endocrine system.

Some endocrine glands secrete more than one hormone. Hormone-producing cells may be found as part of organs that carry on other functions. For example:

- The thyroid gland produces two hormones:
  - Thyrocalcitonin (also known as calcitonin)
  - Thyroxine

IMAGE LABELING

Identify the endocrine glands that are indicated in the accompanying figure.

Use the terms provided to make your selection.

Adrenal glands
Ovaries
Pancreas
Parathyroid glands
Pituitary gland
Testes
Thyroid gland

1. _____
2. _____
3. _____
4. _____
5. _____
6. _____
7. _____

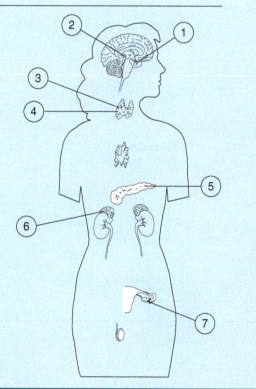

- The **pancreas** produces two hormones:
  - Glucagon
  - Insulin

The pancreas also produces enzymes that are important in the digestive process.

ENDOCRINE GLANDS

Pituitary Gland

The **pituitary gland** is found under the brain and secretes more than one hormone. It is sometimes called the master gland. The hormones secreted by this gland control:

- Growth
- Urine production
- Activity of most of the other glands
- Reproductive activity
- Blood chemistry

Pineal Gland

The **pineal gland** is a small gland that is located deep in the brain. It is especially important because it secretes serotonin and melatonin. The gland is sometimes called the "third eye" because it communicates information about environmental lighting to various parts of the body. Typically, melatonin levels are low during the day and elevate at night. This is important because it helps regulate sleep-wake cycles. The secretions of the gland are also thought to delay sexual maturation until the rest of the body is ready for reproduction.

Adrenal Glands

There are two **adrenal glands**. One gland is located on top of each of the two kidneys. Each gland has two portions that secrete separate hormones. Two of these hormones, **adrenaline** (epinephrine) and **cortisone**, are often prescribed medications. In general, the adrenal hormones:

- Control the release of energy to meet emergencies
- Control water and electrolyte balance in the body
- Secrete small amounts of male and female sex hormones

Gonads

The term **gonads** refers to the sex glands.

- Female gonads = ovaries
- Male gonads = testes

Symbols are used to indicate the different sexes:

- ♀indicates female (woman)
- ♂indicates male (man)

Ovaries (♀)

The paired **ovaries** are located within the pelvis on either side of the uterus. When stimulated by the pituitary gland, they produce the hormones:

- **Progesterone**—helps to maintain pregnancy
- **Estrogen**—responsible for the development of female characteristics such as:
  - Enlargement of the female reproductive organs
  - Appearance of pubic and axillary hair
  - Enlargement of the breasts
  - Onset and regulation of menstruation

Testes (♂)

The paired **testes** are located outside of the body in a pouch called the **scrotum**. They produce the hormone **testosterone**, which regulates the development of male secondary characteristics, including:

- Muscular development
- Deepening voice
- Growth of hair on body and face
- Growth and maturity of the reproductive organs

The male and female gonads also produce special cells, the female ovum and the male sperm, that unite during conception to form a human embryo.

Thyroid Gland

The **thyroid gland** is located in the neck, in front of the larynx. The thyroid gland produces two hormones:

- **Thyroxine**—helps regulate the metabolic rate of all body cells
- Thyrocalcitonin—helps regulate the levels of calcium and phosphates in the blood. These are two of the electrolyte minerals involved in electrolyte balance.

Metabolism is the production of heat and energy by the cells. Energy production is related to the ability of the cells to take up and use oxygen.

Disorders of the thyroid gland include:

- **Hyperthyroidism** (exophthalmic **goiter** or toxic goiter) results from overproduction of thyroxine. The resident shows:
  - Irritability and restlessness
  - Nervousness
  - Rapid pulse
  - Increased appetite
  - Weight loss
  - Sensitivity to heat

- **Hypothyroidism** results from underproduction of thyroxine. The lack of iodine can result in a low thyroxine production. This is known as simple goiter. A severe lack of thyroxine results in a condition called myxedema. The resident with hypothyroidism shows:
  - Slow responses
  - Lethargy
  - Weight gain
  - Slow pulse

Parathyroid Glands

The **parathyroid glands** are several tiny glands embedded in the back of the thyroid gland. They produce the hormone **parathormone** that also helps control the use of calcium and phosphorus by the body.

Islets of Langerhans

The **islets of Langerhans** are small groups of cells found within the pancreas. Two very important hormones produced by these cells are insulin and glucagon. These hormones help regulate blood sugar.

Blood sugar is called **glucose**. Glucose is needed by all cells for *all* body work. Glucose metabolism is discussed later in this lesson.

AGING CHANGES

Changes in the endocrine system caused by aging include:

- Decreased glucose tolerance
- Increased levels of parathormone
- Decreased vaginal secretions
- Increased blood sugar level
- Decreased metabolic rate resulting from changes in the thyroid
- Decreased sensitivity of body tissues to insulin (body ignores insulin)

GLUCOSE METABOLISM

Glucose is the primary energy source for all of the work done by the body. The level of glucose is an important factor in proper functioning. Various hormones and enzymes maintain this level and help the body to use (metabolize) glucose for energy. Two of these hormones are:

- **Glucagon**—raises the blood sugar level by converting stored sugar (glycogen) to glucose.

?　**EXERCISE 26-2**

MATCHING

Match the gland on the right with the hormone on the left.

HORMONE GLAND

1. _____ progesterone
2. _____ testosterone
3. _____ insulin
4. _____ thyroxine
5. _____ parathormone
6. _____ adrenaline
7. _____ estrogen
8. _____ glucagon

a. thyroid
b. parathyroid
c. pancreas
d. adrenal
e. ovary
f. testes

- **Insulin**—lowers the blood sugar level by causing glucose to move from the bloodstream into the cells. It also helps to convert glucose to glycogen (stored sugar).

  Abnormal blood sugar levels are called:

- **Hyperglycemia**—the blood sugar level is too high.
- **Hypoglycemia**—the blood sugar level is too low.

DIABETES MELLITUS

Diabetes mellitus is a major disorder of carbohydrate, fat, and protein metabolism. It is usually caused by inability of the cells to use the available insulin or decreased sensitivity of body tissues to insulin (body ignores insulin).

In diabetes mellitus, the body cannot use glucose normally to meet the energy needs of the body. This disease is common in older people. In fact, in people older than age 65, one of every 20 requires treatment for diabetes.

The two forms of diabetes are:

- **Insulin-dependent diabetes mellitus (IDDM)** (Type 1). Insulin is produced by beta cells in the pancreas. In Type 1 diabetes, the beta cells are damaged, resulting in decreased or no production of insulin. Insulin is required for the metabolism of glucose. With too little insulin released by the pancreas, abnormal amounts of glucose accumulate in the bloodstream, because it cannot be absorbed by body cells where it is used for energy.

- **Non–insulin-dependent diabetes mellitus (NIDDM)** (Type 2). In Type 2 diabetes, insufficient insulin is produced or the body ignores the insulin. As a result, glucose builds up in the bloodstream and is not absorbed by body cells.

  Both forms may be seen in older people, but the non–insulin-dependent (Type 2) form is more common.

Insulin-Dependent Diabetes Mellitus (Type 1)

Insulin-dependent diabetes mellitus (IDDM) is more often seen in younger people. Signs and symptoms include:

- Abrupt onset
- Excess thirst (**polydipsia**)
- Excess urine elimination (**polyuria**)
- Excessive hunger (**polyphagia**)
- Sugar in the urine (**glycosuria**)
- Excess blood sugar (hyperglycemia)

This form of diabetes is more difficult to control. Diabetic persons may experience periods of hypoglycemia (**insulin shock**) or hyperglycemia (**diabetic coma**). People with Type 1 diabetes require:

- Regular injections of insulin to balance their blood sugar
- Regulation of food intake
- Planned exercise (which uses sugar for energy) as part of the treatment program

Non–Insulin-Dependent Diabetes Mellitus (Type 2)

Non–insulin-dependent diabetes mellitus (NIDDM) has been known as "old-age" diabetes. However, Type 2 diabetes is now found to be present in younger populations as well. The older the person, the more likely that diabetes will develop. This form of diabetes is more stable than IDDM, with fewer incidents of diabetic coma or insulin shock.

Signs and Symptoms

Often only one or two symptoms appear in the older person. The person is usually overweight and may have constant fatigue or a sore or infection that takes an unusually long time to heal. About half of those with diabetes show the obvious signs (Figure 26-2).

Therapy consists of:

- Diet control
- Weight reduction
- Exercise
- Oral hypoglycemic agents (sometimes combined with insulin injections)

Complications of Diabetes

Complications of diabetes, especially uncontrolled diabetes, may result in the following:

- Renal disease
- Vision changes

- Polyuria (excessive urine)
- Polydipsia (excessive thirst)
- Polyphagia (excessive hunger)
- Weight loss
- Weakness and fatigue
- Blurring of vision
- Skin infections
- Slow healing of infections or injuries
- Complaints of itching (vulvar itching in women)
- Numbness and tingling (mouth, tongue, fingers, distal extremities)

Figure 26-2 Signs of diabetes mellitus.

- Cardiovascular damage
- Hyperglycemia
- Hypoglycemia

Vision Changes

This is particularly common in long-term diabetes. Serious vision changes are often thought to be due to general aging. However, they may really be related to diabetes. Complications include:

- Glaucoma
- Cataracts
- Blindness

? EXERCISE 26-3

VOCABULARY EXERCISE

Select the correct term(s) from the following list to complete each statement.

diabetes	IDDM	pineal
estrogen	insulin	polydipsia
gangrene	pancreas	testes

1. The male gonads are also referred to as _____.

2. _____ is the name of a diabetic condition that is treated with insulin.

3. Excessive thirst, or _____, is a symptom of IDDM.

4. The _____ is the tiny gland under the brain.

5. Amputation as a result of _____ is a common problem for the older resident with diabetes.

6. The hormone that lowers blood sugar is _____.

7. Insulin is produced by the _____.

8. _____ is a major disorder caused by breakdown in glucose metabolism.

9. The hormone _____ is responsible for the development of female characteristics.

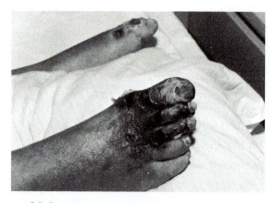

Figure 26-3 Gangrene of the toes and feet often results in amputation.

Diabetic coma (Hyperglycemia)	Insulin shock (Hypoglycemia)
Gradual onset	Sudden onset
Drowsiness	Nervousness
Deep, difficult breathing	Shallow breathing
Nausea	Hunger
Hot, flushed, dry skin	Moist, pale skin
Mental confusion	Mental confusion
Loss of consciousness	Vision disturbance
Sweet odor to breath	Loss of consciousness

Figure 26-4 Signs and symptoms to be reported for diabetes coma and insulin shock.

Cardiovascular Damage

The consequences of hyperglycemia to the cardiovascular system can be severe in the older resident and may include:

- Heart attacks
- Strokes
- Peripheral vascular disease
- Amputation

Because injuries heal poorly, an ingrown toenail or improperly cut nails can lead to serious problems. Vascular changes can interfere with the normal circulation to the legs and feet. Damage may be so extensive that the tissues of the toes, feet, and legs may die. As a result, they have to be removed (amputated). **Gangrene** (death of tissue) (Figure 26-3) followed by amputation is a common problem for the older resident with diabetes. Careful observations and care can help prevent this serious condition.

Hyperglycemia

This condition occurs when too little insulin is available for metabolic needs. Sugar and acid compounds (**ketones**) build up in the blood. The condition is known as **diabetic ketoacidosis (DKA)** and can lead to death. Sugar and ketones then spill over into the urine.

A sudden, unexpected need for insulin brought about by stress, illness, injury, or curtailed activity may bring on DKA. It usually develops slowly, sometimes over a 24-hour period. The first symptoms may be headache, drowsiness, and confusion. The resident seems less responsive, irritable, confused, and drowsy and may slip slowly into unconsciousness (coma).

Signs and symptoms of hyperglycemia include:

- Thirst
- Blurred vision
- Nausea and vomiting

- A sweet odor to the breath
- Dry, flushed skin

It is important to note these signs early so that treatment can begin right away. Learn the signs and symptoms of diabetic coma (Figure 26-4). If these signs are noted in a resident, report them immediately. The treatment for hyperglycemia is insulin and fluids, which will be given intravenously by the nurse.

Hypoglycemia

Hypoglycemia or low blood sugar is less common when oral antidiabetic agents are given than when insulin is given by injection. When hypoglycemia results from an overdose of insulin, it is known as *insulin reaction* or insulin shock. Hypoglycemia can be brought on by:

- Not eating planned snacks or eating less food (as a result of decreased appetite)
- Unusual activity
- Stress
- Vomiting
- Diarrhea
- Interaction of oral drugs with other medications being taken

In contrast to DKA, which develops slowly, hypoglycemia may occur rapidly. Signs and symptoms of hypoglycemia include:

- Hunger
- Sweating
- Dizziness
- Drowsiness
- Blurred vision
- Erratic behavior

- Staggering gait
- Mental confusion
- Disorientation
- Pale and moist skin

Learn the signs and symptoms of hypoglycemia (see Figure 26-4). Report immediately to the nurse if you observe them in a resident.

The resident with hypoglycemia is treated with sugar in some form. A food containing sugar is given orally if the resident is conscious. If the resident is unconscious, glucagon (a hormone) may be given by injection. Orange juice or other easily absorbed sources of sugar are usually kept on the unit where they are easily accessible for the nurse to use in an emergency. Every staff member should be aware of the storage location.

Treatment of Diabetes

For people with diabetes living independently, control of the disease depends on self-care. For a resident with diabetes, self-care is assisted. Residents should be encouraged to take part in their own care as much as possible.

The goals for the care of the person with diabetes, whether at home or in a facility, are the same:

- Maintain a proper metabolic balance
- Prevent complications

Although uncommon, the less stable form of diabetes (IDDM) may appear in later years. If you notice any of the acute signs, they should be reported at once. Some elderly diabetic residents are insulin dependent. The treatment is then the same as for any insulin-dependent person. Most people who have had diabetes since youth will continue to require regular insulin injections.

Three factors must be balanced in each diabetic's life:

- Diet
- Exercise
- Drugs

Note that some people with diabetes are able to manage the disease by diet and exercise and do not require drug therapy, including daily injections.

Diet

Nutritional management is an important component of the treatment of diabetes. The physician will determine the calorie count for the day for the resident. The dietitian will then plan a diet based on the resident's likes and dislikes. The amount of carbohydrate, fat,

and protein is calculated to meet the person's need. Many persons in long-term care have a regular diet with no concentrated sweets. It is important for the person to have consistent amounts of nutrients; meals and snacks are given at regular times. The meals and snacks help to regulate the blood sugar levels in the body. Your responsibilities include:

- Checking trays carefully to be sure the correct diet is given
- Serving the trays and snacks on time
- Assisting in feeding
- Noticing and recording how much and what food was eaten
- Returning trays after meals
- Informing the nurse if food is not eaten
- Giving supplemental foods as ordered

If concentrated sugars such as jellies or jams are on the tray, be sure to check with the nurse before feeding the resident (concentrated sugars usually are limited in a diabetic diet). You must know what is allowed for each resident with diabetes in your care.

Exercise

The more a person exercises, the more sugar is needed for energy. The increased need for sugar usage increases the need for insulin. Less exercise decreases the need. A resident's activity will influence the need for both food and insulin. Be sure to report unusual activity or unusual inactivity.

Drugs

Drugs used in the treatment of diabetes are called antidiabetic drugs. Some of these may be taken by mouth (oral hypoglycemics). Insulin must be injected. The nurse will administer the drugs, but you also have some responsibilities. For oral hypoglycemics, be sure to report if the drugs are not taken. For example, if a pill is given to the resident and then is spit out after the nurse leaves the room, report this to the nurse immediately.

If the resident is receiving insulin, check the injection site and report:

- Redness
- Pain
- Itching

Nursing Assistant Responsibilities

Residents who experience emotional stress or have an infection of any kind are at greater risk for imbalance.

They need to be monitored with extra care and attention. When providing routine care for the resident with diabetes you must:

- Know the signs of insulin shock and diabetic coma.
- Be alert for the signs of diabetic coma or insulin shock and report them immediately to the nurse.
- Know the storage location of juice or other easily absorbed carbohydrates.
- When food trays are delivered, check that the resident receives the proper diet.
- Give extra nourishments only as ordered.
- Keep a record of the food consumed on the resident's chart.
- Report uneaten meals to the nurse.
- Give special attention to the feet of a diabetic resident to prevent infections.
  - Wash daily, carefully drying between toes.
  - Inspect feet closely for any breaks or signs of irritation.
  - Report any abnormalities to the nurse.

- Do not allow moisture to collect between toes.
- Apply lotion to dry feet, but not between the toes.
- Toenails of a diabetic are cut only by a podiatrist or an RN who is a specialist in foot care.
- Shoes and stockings should be clean, free of holes, and fit well. Anything that might injure the feet or interfere with the circulation must be avoided.
- Do not allow the resident to go barefoot.
- Prevent pressure over the toes and feet by not tucking in bedding tightly.
- Inspect the skin regularly for signs of infection.
- Avoid very warm or cold applications to the skin.

Testing to Monitor Control of Diabetes

Oral hypoglycemic drugs and insulin are prescribed according to how well the body uses glucose for energy. For this reason, blood tests for glucose are performed regularly and treatment is adjusted as necessary. This is a licensed nursing procedure.

? EXERCISE 26-4

COMPLETE THE CHART
Place the signs or symptoms that are listed under the proper column.

Diabetic Coma (Hyperglycemia)	Insulin Shock (Hypoglycemia)

SIGNS/SYMPTOMS

a. drowsiness	f. deep, difficult breathing
b. pale, moist skin	g. sweet odor to breath
c. nervousness	h. vision disturbances
d. nausea	i. hot, dry, flushed skin
e. shallow breathing	j. mental confusion

1. What actions should a nursing assistant first take when any of these signs and symptoms are noted?

_____

LESSON SYNTHESIS: Putting It All Together

You have just completed this lesson. Now go back and review the Clinical Focus. Try to see how the Clinical Focus relates to the concepts presented in the lesson. Then answer the following questions.

1. How might Mr. Begay's cold have affected his condition?
2. Explain what is meant by the fact that the resident is demonstrating hyperglycemia.
3. What action should the nursing assistant take after noting the change in Mr. Begay's behavior?
4. What actions might the nurse decide would be appropriate?
5. What general actions should the nursing assistant take when caring for the resident with diabetes mellitus?

26 REVIEW

A. Match each term (items a–j) with the proper definition.

a. thyroxine
b. hypoglycemia
c. gonads
d. polyuria
e. glycosuria
f. hormone
g. obesity
h. hyperglycemia
i. glucose
j. gangrene

1. _____ internal secretion produced by glands
2. _____ death of tissue
3. _____ low blood sugar
4. _____ sugar in the urine
5. _____ reproductive glands
6. _____ blood sugar
7. _____ produced by the thyroid gland
8. _____ excessive urine output
9. _____ overweight
10. _____ excessive blood sugar

B. Provide brief answers for each of the following.

11. List three changes in the endocrine system due to aging.
12. Describe the role of thyroxine in the body.
13. What two chemical elements are influenced by the levels of parathormone?
14. List the names of the two forms of diabetes mellitus.
15. What is the most common form of diabetes mellitus?
16. List four signs of insulin-dependent diabetes mellitus.
17. List four signs of non–insulin-dependent diabetes mellitus.
18. List three factors that must be balanced for the resident with diabetes.

C. Select the one best answer for each of the following.

19. Endocrine glands

(A) release secretions into tubes that reach the body surface

(B) are all located in the abdomen

(C) each secrete one hormone only

(D) release secretions directly into the bloodstream

20. Hormones produced by the ovaries help

(A) urine production

(B) enlarge breasts

(C) control electrolyte balance

(D) regulate the levels of calcium

21. Which of the following is the male gonad?

(A) pituitary gland

(B) ovary

(C) testes

(D) thyroid

22. Hypoglycemia can be brought on by

(A) eating less dinner

(B) resting

(C) watching television

(D) listening to jazz music

23. Signs of hypoglycemia include all but one of the following

(A) hunger

(B) dry, flushed skin

(C) dizziness

(D) staggering gait

24. The nursing assistant entered Mr. Lanzo's room and noted that he did not look well. His skin was dry and flushed and he said he was thirsty. She reported to the nurse right away. What other symptom did she note that made her suspect the resident was hyperglycemic?

(A) complaint of hunger

(B) disorientation

(C) sweet odor to his breath

(D) pale, moist skin

25. When taking care of residents who have diabetes mellitus, the nursing assistant must remember to

(A) administer insulin on time

(B) wash the feet only occasionally so they will not get too dry

(C) avoid applying lotion to the feet

(D) make sure to serve the proper diet

26. If a resident with diabetes is receiving insulin, the nursing assistant should check the injection site for

(A) redness or itching

(B) blueness

(C) coldness

(D) puncture marks

27. The nursing assistant notices that a resident with diabetes has long toenails. Her proper action is to

(A) cut the nails

(B) let the resident cut his own nails

(C) report to the nurse so the podiatrist can be called to cut the nails

(D) ignore the matter because the resident wears shoes to protect his feet

D. Clinical Experience

28. Mrs. Barker, a diabetic, has not eaten all the food on her tray. She is on a diabetic diet. What action should the nursing assistant take?

(A) Ignore it because it is not important.

(B) Insist the resident eat every spoonful.

(C) Report and record the amount of food eaten.

(D) Throw the food away so no one knows.

29. Mr. Samuels, a diabetic, has a darkened area on the little toe of his left foot. The nursing assistant reports this because she knows that a complication of diabetes is

(A) glaucoma

(B) renal disease

(C) cataracts

(D) gangrene

30. Mr. Lorenzo, who has IDDM, has an unpleasant visit with his daughter and her husband and now seems very upset. The nursing assistant will watch him closely for signs of hyperglycemia including all but one of the following

(A) sweet breath odor

(B) moist, pale skin

(C) nausea

(D) deep, difficult breathing

CARING FOR RESIDENTS WITH REPRODUCTIVE SYSTEM DISORDERS

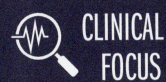

CLINICAL FOCUS

Think about the special care required by residents with disorders of the reproductive system as you study this lesson.

OBJECTIVES

After studying this lesson, you should be able to:

- Define vocabulary words and terms.
- Identify the parts and functions of the male and female reproductive systems.
- Discuss changes in the reproductive systems of men and women caused by aging.
- Describe conditions of the reproductive tract affecting long-term residents.
- Identify and describe common sexually transmitted infections.

VOCABULARY

benign prostatic hypertrophy (bee-NINE pros-TAT-ick high-PER-troh-fee)
chlamydia (klah-MID-ee-ah)
climacteric (kligh-MACK-ter-ick)
clitoris (KLIT-or-is)
Cowper's glands (KOW-perz glands)
ejaculatory duct (ee-JACK-you-lah-toh-ree dukt)
endometrium (en-doh-MEE-tree-um)
estrogen (ES-troh-jen)
foreskin (FOR-skin)
genitalia (jen-ih-TAY-lee-ah)
gonorrhea (gon-or-REE-ah)
hysterectomy (his-teh-RECK-toh-mee)

labia majora (LAY-bee-ah mah-JOR-ah)
labia minora (LAY-bee-ah mih-NOR-ah)
menopause (MEN-oh-pawz)
menstruation (men-stroo-AY-shun)
ovulation (oh-vyou-LAY-shun)
ovum (plural: ova) (OH-vum; plural: OH-vah)
papilloma (pap-i-LO-ma)
penis (PEE-nis)
perineum (pair-ih-NEE-um)
progesterone (proh-JES-ter-ohn)
prostate (PROS-tayt)
pruritus (prew-RYE-tus)
puberty (PYOU-ber-tee)

CASE STUDY

Bessie Shutt is the mother of seven and grandmother to 23 children and 14 great-grandchildren. She suffers from congestive heart failure and chronic obstructive pulmonary disease. She has a prolapsed uterus and complains of itching in the vaginal area. She is also occasionally incontinent of urine.

scrotum (SKROH-tum)
seminal vesicles (SEM-ih-nal VES-ih-kuls)
sperm (spurm)
syphilis (SIF-ih-lis)
testes (TES-teez)
testicles (TES-tih-kuls)
testosterone (tes-TOS-teh-rohn)
transurethral prostatectomy (trans-you-REE-thral
   pros-tah-TECK-toh-mee)

trichomonas vaginitis (trick-oh-MOH-nas
   vaj-ih-NIGH-tis)
urethra (you-REE-thrah)
uterine tubes (YOU-ter-in toobs)
uterus (YOU-ter-us)
vagina (vah-JYE-nah)
vaginitis (vaj-ih-NIGH-tis)
vas deferens (vas DEF-er-ens)
vulva (VUL-vah)

INTRODUCTION

The male and female reproductive systems share some features. They:

- Consist of gonads, tubes, and accessory structures
- Contribute to the reproductive process
- Provide the sex hormones
- Bring pleasure

Remember, human sexuality is the interaction between the physical and emotional needs of an individual. Sexuality is intimately involved with the individual's sense of identity. You may wish to return to Lesson 13 and review human sexuality.

THE MALE REPRODUCTIVE SYSTEM

The male reproductive system consists of the genitalia and the accessory glands (Figure 27-1).

The primary structures are the:

- Penis
- Testes
- Epididymis

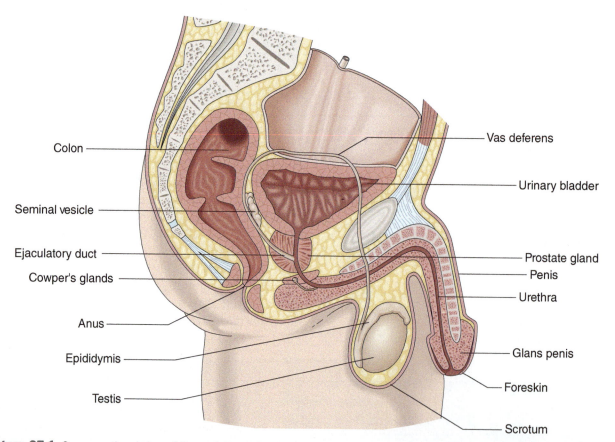

Figure 27-1 Cross-sectional view of the male reproductive system.

- Vas deferens
- Ejaculatory duct

    The accessory glands include the:

- Seminal vesicles
- Prostate
- Cowper's glands

Penis

The male penis is the organ used for sexual intercourse (also called coitus or copulation). When the special tissues of which the penis is made become filled with blood, the penis becomes enlarged and firm. The outer portion of the glans of the penis is covered by a loose skin fold called the foreskin.

    The male urethra passes through the penis and serves two purposes. It carries:

- Reproductive fluid during intercourse
- Urine during voiding

    The two activities cannot occur at the same time because they are under the control of different parts of the nervous system.

Testes

The testes (testicles) are found in a pouch-like structure called the scrotum, which is located outside the body. The testes produce sperm throughout life and the male hormone testosterone. Testosterone is responsible for the male characteristics.

Epididymis

The epididymis is a tube 20 feet long coiled on the back of each testis, which stores the sperm. The epididymis is the beginning of a pathway that moves the sperm upward and out of the body. This pathway includes the:

- Epididymis
- Vas deferens
- Ejaculatory duct
- Urethra

Vas Deferens

The vas deferens that transports the sperm passes behind the urinary bladder, joining with the ejaculatory duct and entering the urethra.

Ejaculatory Duct

The ejaculatory duct carries the fluid produced in the seminal vesicles. Fluids are added as the sperm are propelled forward. The sperm and fluid form the seminal fluid or ejaculate. The fluid contains nutrients and other substances needed by the sperm.

    Glands that contribute to the seminal fluid are the:

- Seminal vesicles—the ejaculatory duct carries the fluid from the vesicles into the urethra.
- Prostate gland—surrounds the urethra just below the neck of the urinary bladder. The gland secretes a fluid that enhances the sperm motility through the seminal vesicles.
- Cowper's glands—two small glands located beside the urethra. They produce mucus for lubrication.

Accessory Glands

The seminal fluid or ejaculate is released as the result of a rhythmic series of muscular contractions. These force the fluid through the urethra to the outside. The process is called ejaculation and occurs during sexual intercourse. Ejaculation may also occur spontaneously at other times.

THE FEMALE REPRODUCTIVE SYSTEM

The female reproductive system consists of the internal structures (Figure 27-2A and B) and the external genitalia (the vulva) (Figure 27-3). The internal structures are the:

- Ovaries
- Fallopian (uterine) tubes
- Uterus
- Cervix
- Vagina

Vulva

The outside of the vulva is made up of two folds called the labia majora (see Figure 27-3). The labia majora:

- Is covered with hair
- Surround the openings of the female urethra and vagina
- Enclose two hairless lips, the labia minora

    The area between the vagina and anus is called the perineum.

Clitoris

The clitoris is an organ similar to the male penis. It:

- Is found near the union of the labia
- Is a sensitive structure
- Functions during sexual stimulation to begin the rhythmic series of contractions associated with female climax, or orgasm

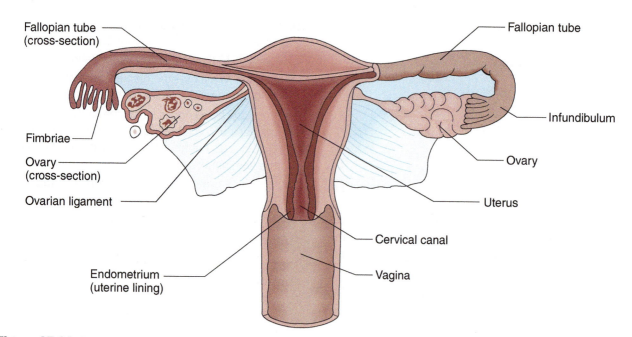

Fallopian tube (cross-section)

Fallopian tube

Fimbriae

Infundibulum

Ovary (cross-section)

Ovary

Ovarian ligament

Uterus

Cervical canal

Endometrium (uterine lining)

Vagina

Figure 27-2A Female internal reproductive structures (anterior view).

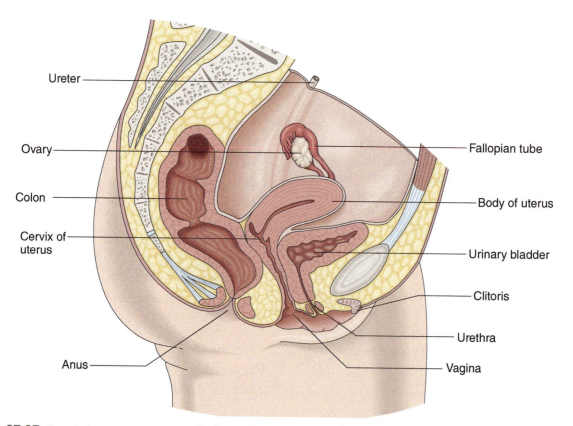

Ureter

Ovary

Fallopian tube

Colon

Body of uterus

Cervix of uterus

Urinary bladder

Clitoris

Urethra

Anus

Vagina

Figure 27-2B Female internal reproductive system (lateral view).

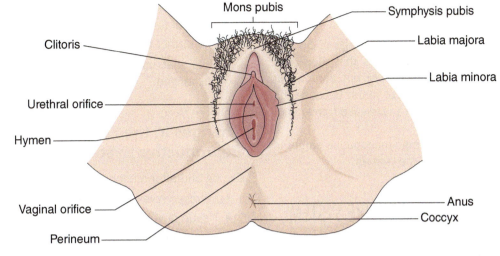

Figure 27-3 External female genitalia.

Ovaries

The two ovaries, which are the female gonads, produce the egg (ovum) and the hormones progesterone and estrogen. Estrogen is needed in the development of female characteristics. Progesterone is the hormone that maintains pregnancy.

Fallopian Tubes

The fallopian tubes (uterine tubes or oviducts) carry the ovum toward the uterus.

Uterus

The uterus (or womb) is a hollow muscular organ about 3 inches long, 2 inches wide, weighs about 6 ounces, and resembles an upside down pear. It is the organ of menstruation and carries the growing fetus. The uterine lining is a special membrane called the endometrium, that:

- Is shed periodically unless pregnancy occurs
- Nourishes the growing fetus (unborn infant in the uterus) during pregnancy

Vagina

The vagina is muscular, hollow tube that stretches during labor to facilitate delivery and also serves as the outlet for the menstrual flow, and is about 3 to 5 inches long in an adult female. It receives the penis during sexual intercourse.

MENSTRUAL CYCLE

The menstrual cycle (female sexual cycle) begins at puberty. Puberty occurs in girls between the ages of 9 and 17. The cycle varies in length, usually between 25 and 30 days. The average is 28 days, which is why it is considered a monthly cycle.

During the menstrual cycle, a mature egg, or ovum (plural, ova):

- Is released from one of the ovaries
- Travels from the ovary to one of the fallopian tubes
- May be fertilized by a male sperm

At the same time that the ovum is being matured and expelled from the ovary (ovulation), the lining of the uterus (endometrium) is:

- Being built up
- Made ready to receive the fertilized ovum

    If fertilization does not occur, the endometrium is:

- No longer needed
- Carried out of the body as the menstrual flow

This process is known as menstruation.

It is interesting that, unlike the sperm cells, all the special cells that will become the ova exist at the time a woman is born. When the last ova are released, the menstrual cycle ceases and menopause begins.

MENOPAUSE

As women age, the menstrual cycle becomes irregular and gradually ceases altogether. This is called:

- Menopause

- **Climacteric**
- Change of life

Menopause usually occurs around the age of 55 and involves a natural series of changes that stops the menstrual cycle. These changes are not abrupt, but usually take place over a period of years. Because the ova are no longer being matured and released, pregnancy cannot occur.

Some women may undergo menopause earlier in life after surgical removal of the ovaries.

CHANGES IN THE REPRODUCTIVE SYSTEM AS A RESULT OF AGING

Changes occur in both male and female reproductive organs with aging. However, the need for sexual pleasure and sensual satisfaction does not stop.

Changes in the Male Reproductive System

As men age, these changes occur:

- Sexual response is slower.
- Ejaculation is delayed.
- The number of sperm decreases (but number is still adequate for reproduction).
- Testosterone levels gradually decrease.
- The prostate gland may enlarge causing difficult urination.
- The scrotum becomes less firm.
- Seminal fluid thins.
- The size of the testes decreases.
- Note that usually the sex drive (libido) remains unchanged.

Changes in the Female Reproductive System

During and after menopause, these changes occur:

- Estrogen levels decrease.
- Tissue of vulva and vaginal walls thins.
- Lubrication of vagina decreases (because of this, older women are more prone to vaginal infections).
- Breast tissues and muscles weaken (sagging of breasts).
- Maturation of the ovum ceases.
- Ovulation and the menstrual cycle cease.
- Again, the libido remains unchanged.

RELATED CONDITIONS

Malignancy

Malignancies of the male and female reproductive organs are common. Be sure to report any bleeding or discharge from the reproductive tract.

? EXERCISE 27-1

COMPLETE THE CHART
Complete the chart indicating signs of aging by placing an X in the appropriate column.

Decreased estrogen levels	Male	Female
Delayed ejaculation		
Enlargement of the prostate		
Unchanged libido		
Decrease in size of testes		
Thinning of vaginal walls		
Loss of egg production		
Sagging of breasts		
Cessation of menstruation		
Thinning of seminal fluid		

In women, frequent sites for cancer development include the:

- Uterine wall
- Ovaries
- Cervix
- Breasts

In men, malignancies are often found in the:

- Prostate gland
- Testes

Radiation, surgery, and chemotherapy may be used alone or in combination to treat malignancies.

Any condition that affects the reproductive organs threatens the individual's self-concept and sense of sexual identity. In addition to the fear resulting from the diagnosis of a malignancy, the resident also fears that he or she will lose the ability to function fully as a sexual human being.

You must provide emotional support to those who are diagnosed with a malignancy of the reproductive system.

Breast tumors develop in men and women, both old and young. They are most common among mature women.

Breast tumors are often first found during self-examination or through *mammography* (x-ray examination). Most of these masses are benign tumors. The self-examination procedure should be:

- Performed by all adult women
- Carried out each month on the last day of the menstrual flow
- Carried out on one selected day of the month, after menopause
- Carried out using a procedure recommended by the American Cancer Society

Prolapsed Uterus

Prolapsed uterus is a condition that may be experienced by women who have had:

- Repeated pregnancies
- Injuries to the pelvic organs
- Injury to the muscles of the pelvic floor
- Weakening of the supportive pelvic structure due to aging

When prolapsed uterus occurs:

- The uterus drops down from its normal position, causing pressure in the vagina.
- There is a feeling of weight in the pelvic area.
- Urinary incontinence or retention occurs.
- The person is predisposed to urinary infections.

Prolapsed uterus is treated by repositioning the uterus or removing it (**hysterectomy**). Both treatments require surgery in a hospital.

Rectocele and Cystocele

Rectoceles and cystoceles are hernias. They usually occur at the same time and are frequently seen in older women.

- A rectocele is a weakening of the wall between the vagina and rectum. This hernia frequently causes

---

? EXERCISE 27-2

BRIEF ANSWERS
Briefly answer the following:

1. Common sites for cancer of the male and female reproductive tracts include:

   Female: Male:

   _____   _____

   _____   _____

   _____

   _____

2. Three ways malignancies are usually treated include:

   a. _____

   b. _____

   c. _____

3. Breast self-examination can be lifesaving. The procedure should be:

   _____

   _____

   _____

constipation and hemorrhoids (varicose veins of the rectum).

- A cystocele is a weakening of the muscles between the bladder and vagina. Cystoceles cause urinary incontinence.

These conditions are corrected by a surgical procedure that tightens the vaginal walls. It is performed in a hospital.

Vaginitis

Vaginitis is a fairly common condition in older women because of the decrease in protection resulting from the thinner vaginal wall. This type of infection tends to be chronic and difficult to control.

A fungus infection caused by *Candida albicans* often results in vulvovaginitis. When infection is present:

- There may be a thick, white, cheesy vaginal discharge.
- Inflammation and itching are intense.
- Douches are not given for this condition.
- Special drugs and creams are prescribed to fight the infection.

Senile vaginitis responds to estrogen therapy, vaginal suppositories, and mild douches to wash out the canal. Each treatment requires a physician's order.

Pruritus

Itching (**pruritus**) of the vulva and anus is a common complaint of older women. Continual irritation can cause tissue breakdown and permit bacteria to enter and cause infection. Many factors can contribute to pruritus. A search must be made for the cause and steps taken to correct the condition. For example:

- If soaps are irritating, they should not be used.
- If incontinence allows acid urine to irritate the tissues, regular perineal care can often eliminate the problem.
- Some medications can cause vaginal itching.

Benign Prostatic Hypertrophy

Benign prostatic hypertrophy (BPH) is a common problem for elderly men. It is a nonmalignant enlargement of the prostate gland. Recall that the urethra passes through the center of this gland. Thus, as the gland enlarges it closes off the flow of urine (Figure 27-4).

Residents with this condition may have difficulty starting and stopping the stream of urine. They may

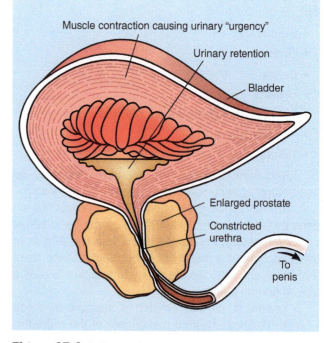

Figure 27-4 Cell growth causes the prostate to enlarge, constricting the urethra. The bladder may not empty completely, causing discomfort and increasing the risk of infection.

not be able to empty their bladder completely, leading to bladder infections. Observe for the following:

- Frequency of urination
- Nocturia
- Poor urinary control such as dribbling

Mild to moderate BPH may be treated with medication. The drugs do not reduce the size of the prostate but relax the muscles of the neck of the bladder and allow for better emptying of the bladder. These medications may cause orthostatic hypotension. Caution the resident to change positions slowly and sit on the edge of the bed for several minutes before standing up.

To release the obstruction, a surgical procedure can be performed by entering through the urethra. This is called a **transurethral prostatectomy** (TURP). Although some surgical procedures on the prostate gland can cause impotence, this is not a complication of the transurethral approach.

An alternative procedure to the TURP is the transurethral microwave procedure (TUMP). This procedure is done on an out-patient basis and takes about an hour to complete. This procedure is not a complete cure; it helps to reduce the symptoms of BPH and improves the flow of urine. Another new surgical procedure is the transurethral needle ablation (TUNA). This procedure also helps to improve the flow of urine from

? EXERCISE 27-3

COMPLETION
Select the best answer and either circle it or write it in the space provided to complete each statement.

1. A weakening of the area between the vagina and rectum is called _____.
   (rectocele) (cystocele)

2. A prolapsed uterus causes a feeling of weight in the _____.
   (breasts) (pelvis)

3. A mammogram is an x-ray film of the _____.
   (stomach) (breasts)

4. The foreskin is part of the _____.
   (vulva) (penis)

5. The endometrium is periodically lost during _____.
   (intercourse) (menstruation)

6. A rectocele often causes _____.
   (constipation) (bleeding)

7. Transurethral prostatectomy (TURP) is a surgical procedure often done to remove the

   _____.
   (prostate gland) (womb)

? EXERCISE 27-4

MATCHING
Match the terms to the definitions

Term	Definition
Menopause	age of sexual maturity
Pruritus	climacteric
Endometrium	external reproductive organs
Genitalia	gland surrounding neck of male bladder, contributes to seminal fluid
Testes	itching
Prostate gland	lining of the uterus
Puberty	male organs that produce sperm
Menstruation	the periodic loss of endometrium

the bladder. Twin needles are inserted through the urethra into the enlarged prostatic tissue. Low-level radiofrequency energy burns away some of the prostatic tissue that is occluding the urethra creating a channel for the flow of urine from the bladder.

SEXUALLY TRANSMITTED INFECTIONS

Sexually transmitted infections (STIs), also known as sexually transmitted diseases (STDs), affect both men and women. Although most STIs can be treated and cured, people do not develop immunity to repeated infections. In older persons, an STI may indicate sexual abuse. The organisms causing STIs can be transmitted from:

- Mucous membrane to mucous membrane such as from genitals to mouth or genitals
- Mucous membrane to skin, such as genitals to hands
- Skin to mucous membrane, such as hands to genitals

Any disease that is transmitted mainly in this way is an STI. There are many STIs. Some are seen more commonly than others. Contact precautions should be used when caring for residents with STIs. In addition, the nursing assistant should:

- Observe for signs of redness of the genitalia
- Note any unusual drainage (color and odor): green, yellow, fishy odor
- Note any complaints of burning on urination
- Observe for sores (lesions) on the penis, vulva, or vagina

A complete discussion of STIs is presented here for your protection because these diseases pose a risk for health care workers as well as the people being cared for.

The most common STIs are gonorrhea, herpes simplex II, and syphilis. Other STIs are caused by chlamydia, human papillomavirus, human immunodeficiency virus, and the *Trichomonas* parasite.

It is important to realize that people may:

- Not always be aware that they have been infected
- Be too embarrassed to talk about the problem
- Not realize the serious damage these infectious diseases can do to the body

STIs are as easily transmitted between older persons as between younger.

Trichomonas Vaginitis

Trichomonas vaginitis is caused by a parasite, *Trichomonas vaginalis*. This condition:

- Is sexually transmitted
- May affect the male reproductive tract with no signs and symptoms
- In women, causes a large amount of white, foul-smelling vaginal discharge called leukorrhea
- Can be controlled with medication
- Requires that both sex partners receive treatment

Gonorrhea

Gonorrhea is a serious STI caused by the bacterium *Neisseria gonorrhoeae*. The disease causes an acute inflammation.

- In men:
  - Greenish yellow discharge appears from the penis within 2 to 5 days after contact.
  - There is a burning on urination.
  - The disease can spread throughout the reproductive tract, causing sterility (inability to reproduce).
- In women:
  - Eighty percent of women infected may have no signs or symptoms until after the disease spreads.

- Pelvic inflammatory disease can lead to formation of abscesses and sterility.
- The disease can be spread before a woman is aware of being infected.
- All sex partners must be treated with antibiotics.
- When a pregnant woman has gonorrhea, her baby's eyes may be permanently damaged if they are contaminated by the disease during birth. As a preventive measure, all babies' eyes are routinely treated with antibiotics shortly after birth.

Syphilis

Syphilis is caused by the microorganism *Treponema pallidum*. Both sexes show the same effects of the disease. It is treated with antibiotics. If untreated, the disease may pass through three stages.

1. First stage—a sore (chancre) develops within 90 days of exposure. The chancre heals without treatment. Because it is not painful, it may go entirely unnoticed.
2. Second stage—a rash, sore throat, or other mild symptoms suggestive of a viral infection may occur. Again, the signs and symptoms disappear without treatment. The disease is infectious during the first and second stages and may be transmitted to a sexual partner. By this time, the microorganisms have entered vital organs such as the heart, liver, brain, and spinal cord.
3. Third stage—the stage in which permanent damage is done to vital organs. It may not appear for many years or at all.

If an infected woman is pregnant the microorganisms can attack the fetus, causing it to die or be seriously deformed.

Herpes

Herpes simplex II (genital herpes) is an infectious disease caused by the herpes simplex virus. It is transmitted primarily through direct sexual contact. The person who has herpes:

- May develop red, blister-like sores on the reproductive organs
- Has sores that are associated with a burning sensation
- Usually has sores that heal in about 2 weeks
- Must remember that the fluid in the blisters is infectious
- May shed organisms even when an outbreak is not present

People infected with herpes may have only one episode or repeated attacks. In many cases, repeated attacks are milder. Other consequences of a herpes infection include:

- A greater incidence of cancer of the cervix and miscarriages in infected women compared to women who are not infected.
- Newborn children can be infected during the birth process.
- The mother with an active case of herpes simplex II usually delivers by cesarean section.

Treatment with the drug acyclovir reduces the discomfort and degree of communicability. There is no cure at the present time.

Genital Warts

Genital warts are a type of STI. According to the CDC, they are most often caused by 1 of more than 70 strains of human papillomavirus (HPV), HPV 6 and 11 strains are most common. Vaccines may help to prevent against certain strains of the virus.

Characteristics of the infection include:

- Lesions on the genitals on both skin and mucous membranes
- Cauliflower-shaped, raised, and darkened warts

- Warts may be removed by ointments or surgery but often recur.
- HPV may cause discomfort during intercourse and may cause bleeding when dislodged.
- They predispose to development of cancer of the cervix in women.
- The infection rate for HPV is the most rapidly growing for all STIs.

Chlamydia Infection

Chlamydia are small infectious organisms that invade mucous membranes of the body. These organisms are:

- Introduced into the eyes infecting the conjunctiva. This causes inflammation (conjunctivitis) and a more serious condition called trachoma. Trachoma can lead to blindness.
- Sexually transmitted and commonly cause infections of the reproductive tract
- The cause of pelvic inflammatory disease with scarring and systemic infections. The scarring can result in sterility.
- Responsible for signs and symptoms similar to those of gonorrhea, except that the discharge is usually yellow to whitish in color
- Treated with antibiotics

? EXERCISE 27-5

Complete the chart about sexually transmitted diseases.

Disease	Cause	Signs and Symptoms
1. Trichomonas vaginitis	_____	_____
2. Gonorrhea	_____	_____
3. Syphilis	_____	_____
4. Herpes simplex II	_____	_____
5. Genital warts	_____	_____
6. Chlamydia infection	_____	_____

People with pelvic infections are usually checked for gonorrhea. If they test negative for gonorrhea, they are frequently diagnosed with nonspecified urethritis because many different organisms may cause the infection. However, chlamydia organisms are the most common cause.

Personal Precautions

An individual can practice certain actions to lessen the risk of contracting STIs. These include:

- Abstaining from sex
- Knowing your sexual partner well before engaging in sexual activity

- Limiting the number of sexual partners
- Using a latex condom throughout sexual contact
- Washing well following sexual intercourse
- Using approved germicides that can be applied to the vagina, penis, and condom
- Providing to your partner and being provided with a negative test result covering the 3-month period before sexual activity
- All caregivers should institute strict adherence to Standard Precautions. Thorough handwashing is essential.

LESSON SYNTHESIS: Putting It All Together

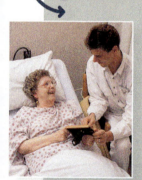

You have just completed this lesson. Now go back and review the Clinical Focus. Try to see how the Clinical Focus relates to the concepts presented in the lesson. Then answer the following questions.

1. What change occurs in the lubrication of the vagina in the aging woman?
2. What increased risk does this change pose for Mrs. Shutt?
3. Do Mrs. Shutt's periods of incontinence contribute to her pruritus?
4. What special care can you give to make Mrs. Shutt more comfortable?
5. If Mrs. Shutt does not tell you of her discomfort, how may you be alerted to her problem?
6. Which of Mrs. Shutt's diagnoses might contribute to her incontinence?

27 REVIEW

A. Match each term (items a–e) with the proper definition.

(A) chlamydia

(B) climacteric

(C) hysterectomy

(D) pruritus

(E) vaginitis

1. _____   itching

2. _____   small infectious organisms

3. _____   menopause

4. _____   inflammation of the vagina

5. _____   removal of the uterus

B. Select the one best answer for each of the following.

6. The male organ used for intercourse is the

(A) vas deferens

(B) testis

(C) penis

(D) prostate

(E) vagina

(F) perineum

7. The male gland that may become enlarged and obstruct the flow of urine is the

(A) prostate

(B) seminal vesicles

(C) Cowper's glands

(D) penis

8. The female gonads are the

(A) uterus

(B) ovaries

9. As men age,

(A) ejaculation is more rapid

(B) sperm count increases

(C) testosterone levels decrease

(D) sexual response is more rapid

10. One characteristic of female menopause is

(A) loss of egg production

(B) reduced libido

(C) regular menstrual periods

(D) thickening of vaginal walls

C. Fill in the blanks by selecting the correct word or phrase from the list.

abuse

cystocele

genitalia

testes

vulva

11. The primary sexual organs are known as the _____.

12. An STI in the elderly may be a sign of sexual _____.

13. The female external genitalia are called the _____.

14. The male glands that produce the sperm are called the _____.

15. A weakening of the wall between the vagina and bladder is called a _____.

D. Brief answers

16. List three functions of both the male and female reproductive systems.

17. List three changes resulting from aging for the male reproductive system and three changes for the female reproductive system.

18. List five common STIs.

19. List four precautions to take to avoid getting an STI when caring for residents with an STI.

E. Clinical experience

20. Mr. Fazzio is acting very withdrawn this morning. When Starr, the nursing assistant, reports to her supervisor she learns that the physician has told Mr. Fazzio that he has a "lump" in his prostate gland that must be treated.

a. Could this knowledge explain Mr. Fazzio's behavior?

b. What fears may Mr. Fazzio be feeling?

c. How can you help Mr. Fazzio at this time?

21. Mrs. Wells was admitted to your facility this morning. She has a diagnosis of mild confusion, malnutrition, congestive heart failure, and pelvic inflammatory disease. A culture was ordered to determine the cause of her infection. What type of precautions should be used with this resident?

CARING FOR RESIDENTS WITH MUSCULOSKELETAL SYSTEM DISORDERS

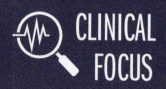

CLINICAL FOCUS

Think of the special challenges in providing nursing assistant care to a resident with disorders of the musculoskeletal system as you study this lesson.

OBJECTIVES

After studying this lesson, you should be able to:

• Define vocabulary words and terms.

• List the functions of the voluntary muscles.

• List the functions of the bones.

• Describe the changes of aging that affect the musculoskeletal system.

• Identify the symptoms related to common musculoskeletal system disorders.

• Describe the appropriate nursing care for residents with musculoskeletal disorders.

VOCABULARY

amputation (am-pyou-TAY-shun)
arthritis (are-THRY-tis)
atrophy (AT-roh-fee)
bursae (BUR-see)
bursitis (bur-SIGH-tis)
cartilage (KAR-tih-lij)
cast (kast)
contracture (kuhn-TRAK-tyoor)
fracture (FRACK-shur)

gout (Gout)
joint (joynt)
kyphosis (kigh-FOH-sis)
ligament (LIG-ah-ment)
open reduction/internal fixation (ORIF)—(OH-pen ree-DUCK-shun/in-TER-nal fiks-AY-shun)
osteoarthritis (os-tee-oh-are-THRY-tis)
osteoporosis (os-tee-oh-poor-OH-sis)
phantom pain (FAN-tom payn)

CASE STUDY

Essie Branch suffers from osteoarthritis and osteoporosis. These conditions affect both her ability to provide self-care and to enjoy full mobility. Her osteoporosis has caused compression fractures of her spine so she is no longer able to hold her head erect easily.

podiatrist (poh-DYE-ah-trist)
prosthesis (pros-THEE-sis)
rheumatoid arthritis (REW-mah-toyd are- THRY-tis)

tendon (TEN-don)
traction (TRACK-shun)

THE MUSCULOSKELETAL SYSTEM

The musculoskeletal system is composed of:

- Bones
- Skeletal muscles
- Joints
- Tendons
- Ligaments
- Bursae

The bones form a framework for the body that is called a *skeleton*. The muscles are formed of tissue that has the ability to contract and relax and allow movement. The muscles lie over the bones. Together, the bones and muscles have many functions, including:

- Giving shape and form to the body
- Protecting and supporting vital body organs such as the brain and heart
- Permitting movement
- Producing some of the red blood cells
- Storing calcium and phosphorus

Bones

The human body has 206 bones (Figure 28-1). We are born with 270 bones but the number decreases to 206 by adulthood after some bones fuse together. All of the bones are not alike. Some are:

- Longer bones—bones of the arms and legs
- Short bones—bones of the fingers and toes
- Irregular bones—bones that form the spinal column
- Flat bones—pelvic bones and shoulder blades

Each bone has a name. Many other body structures take their names from that of the nearby bone.

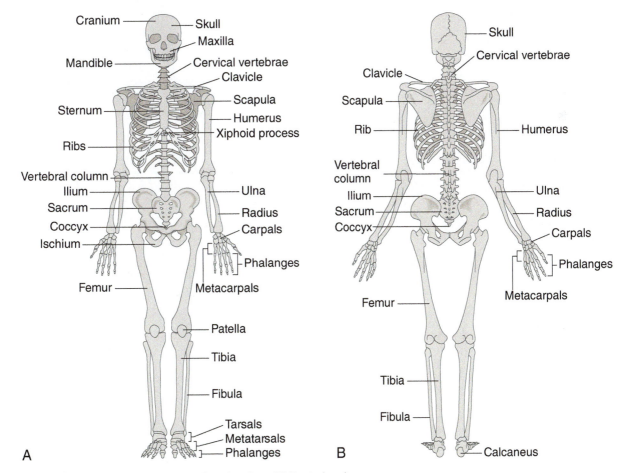

Figure 28-1 The human skeleton. (A) Anterior view. (B) Posterior view.

For example, the radius is a bone in the forearm. Close by are the:

- Radial nerve
- Radial artery
- Radial vein

Learning the names of the bones is not difficult. Draw a line down the center of the skeleton in Figure 28-1, dividing it in half. Note that the bones on one side of the line are matched by bones on the other side.

Muscles

The body contains over 650 named skeletal muscles (Figure 28-2). They work in groups to bring about body movement. There are three types of muscles:

- Cardiac muscle—found only in the heart wall
- Skeletal muscles—also called voluntary muscles because you can control their actions of contraction and relaxation

- Visceral or smooth muscles—also called involuntary muscles because we do not usually control them consciously

Involuntary muscles make up the walls of organs like the stomach and guard body openings like those of the digestive and urinary tracts. A special part of the brain controls involuntary muscles automatically.

Muscles are named by location, shape, or action. The quadriceps femoris, for example, is located near the femur (thigh bone). Muscles have three parts:

- Origin, or beginning
- Body, or middle part
- Insertion, or ending

The origin and body of a muscle are found on one side of a joint and the insertion is attached to the other side. Skeletal muscles are attached to the bones by tough, fibrous bands called **tendons**.

When the muscle shortens (contracts), it pulls the point of insertion toward the point of origin, changing

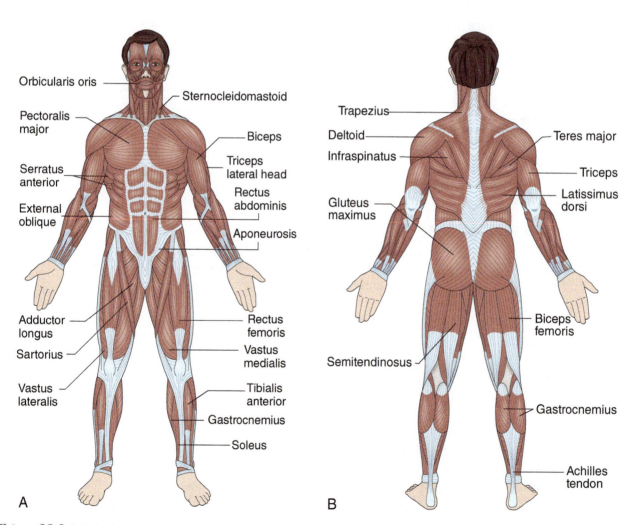

A   B

Figure 28-2 Principal skeletal muscles of the body. (A) Anterior view. (B) Posterior view.

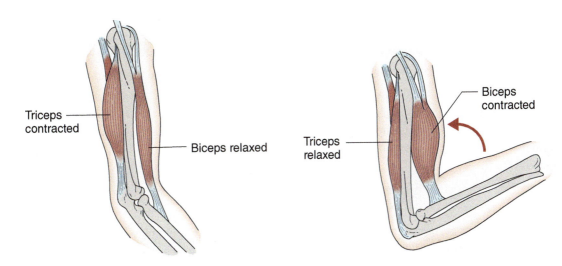

Figure 28-3 Coordination of muscles.

the position of the bone (Figure 28-3). This relationship between muscles and bones permits movements such as walking, sitting, or holding a pencil.

Muscles that are not used will **atrophy**. This means they become weaker and smaller. Lack of joint movement may cause a **contracture** to form. The muscle shortens, causing the joint to become fixed, making further movement difficult or impossible.

Joints

Two bones meet or come together (articulate) at a **joint**. The elbows, knees, and hips are joints. **Ligaments** are fibrous bands that help support the points of articulation.

The ends of movable bones are covered with a protective substance called **cartilage**. The bones of the skull are not movable. The joints of the skull bones are called suture lines.

Joint movements depend on the way in which the joint is formed. Elbows and knees, for example, are hinge joints. The hip and shoulder are ball joints (Figure 28-4).

Joints are enclosed in a capsule lined with synovial membrane. The membrane secretes small amounts of fluid called synovial fluid. Small sacs of synovial fluid called **bursae** are located around joints and help reduce friction during joint movement.

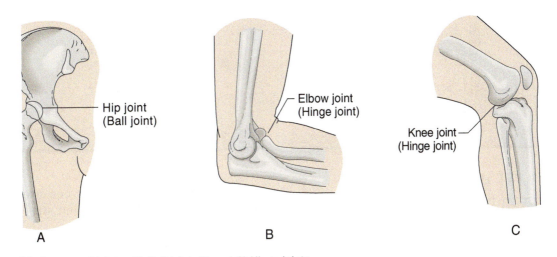

Figure 28-4 Types of joints. (A) Ball joint. (B and C) Hinge joints.

? EXERCISE 28-1

Refer to the figures below and name the muscles indicated using the terms provided. Write the names in the space provided.

biceps   pectoralis major
external oblique   rectus abdominis
gastrocnemius   rectus femoris
gluteus maximus   trapezius
latissimus dorsi   triceps

1. _____   6. _____
2. _____   7. _____
3. _____   8. _____
4. _____   9. _____
5. _____   10. _____

A   B

CHANGES IN THE MUSCULOSKELETAL SYSTEM CAUSED BY AGING

The aging process causes several changes in the musculoskeletal system:

- The bones become more brittle because of calcium loss.
- The joints become less flexible. The range through which the joints can be moved (range of motion) decreases.
- Muscles may become smaller because of less regular exercise. This may limit the person's strength and endurance.
- The body tends to become more flexed with age, thus the posture becomes stooped. In addition, discs between the vertebrae thin, causing the trunk to shorten. When placing the resident in the bed or chair, assure that the body is in good alignment to avoid flexion. Flexion, or stooping of the body, makes walking more difficult.

Because of these changes, older adults are at risk for falling. Maintain a safe environment to prevent falls. Closely monitor residents who have a history of falling. When an older person falls, the bones may easily fracture because they are more brittle.

CONDITIONS AFFECTING THE MUSCULOSKELETAL SYSTEM

Residents with diseases or problems of the musculo-skeletal system receive special care that is known as orthopedic care.

Bursitis

Sometimes a bursa becomes inflamed. This is called bursitis. The bursa is painful and movement may be reduced. Bursitis may be due to infection or excessive pressure or movement placed on the area.

OSTEOPOROSIS

Osteoporosis may develop because of a lack of mobility or as a result of aging. It affects primarily women due to lack of the hormone estrogen following meno-pause. As osteoporosis develops, the bones lose calcium and become brittle (Figure 28-5). The vertebrae in the spine of a person with osteoporosis may collapse without warning, resulting in a curvature of the spine called kyphosis (hunched back).

Osteoporosis

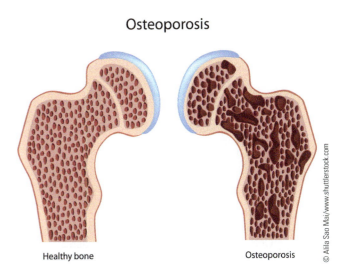

Healthy bone   Osteoporosis

© Alila Sao Mai/www.shutterstock.com

Figure 28-5 Bone loss from osteoporosis causes pain and disabling fractures in both sexes. Note the differences between a healthy femur and one with osteoporosis.

Fractures are common in people with osteoporosis because the bones lack strength and density. It is important to carry out all safety measures to prevent falls. Care must be used when moving and lifting the residents. Unsafe handling can damage the resident's joints and bones. The casting material may be applied over a cotton stockinette and/or padding.

Fractures

A fracture is a break or loss of continuity in a bone (Figure 28-6). The break may be completely through the bone (*complete fracture*) or only partially through

---

? EXERCISE 28-2

TRUE OR FALSE
Indicate whether the following statements are true (T) or false (F).

1. T F In addition to movement, muscles give shape and form to the body.

2. T F There are 500 bones in the body.

3. T F Unused muscles begin to atrophy.

4. T F As aging occurs, bones become more brittle.

5. T F Extension of the body increases with age.

6. T F Osteoporosis can affect both men and women.

7. T F There is only one type of arthritis that affects the elderly.

8. T F Foot problems interfere with a person's ability to ambulate.

9. T F Arthritis is an unusual problem in the elderly.

10. T F It is important to avoid hitting or bumping the resident's feet.

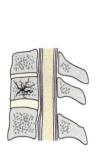
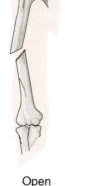
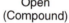
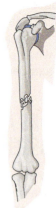

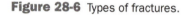

Compression   Closed   Open   Comminuted
                     (Simple, Complete)   (Compound)

Figure 28-6 Types of fractures.

the bone (*incomplete fracture*). All fractures are either closed or open:

- Closed fracture
  - The bones do not protrude through the skin and are in good alignment after the fracture.
- Open fracture
  - Fragments of broken bone protrude through the skin.

Fractures are also identified according to the type of break in the bone:

- Comminuted fracture
  - The bone is broken into many pieces.
- Compression fracture
  - The internal spongy part of the bone is crushed but the hard outer covering of the bone is not broken. This type of fracture occurs most often in the vertebrae.

- Spiral fracture
  - The bone is broken in a twisted manner.

To promote the healing of fractures, the bone must be:

- In correct alignment
- Kept immobile

CLINICAL FOCUS

Review safety measures for Mrs. Branch that are most important for preventing fractures.

Treatment of Fractures with a Cast

If a resident in the facility breaks a bone, the resident may be taken to the hospital to have the cast applied and then return to the facility. A **cast** or splint

? EXERCISE 28-3

MATCHING
Match the fracture on the right with the description on the left.

DESCRIPTION FRACTURE

1. _____ bones broken in many places   a. closed
2. _____ bones are crushed   b. open
3. _____ bone is broken in a twisted manner   c. comminuted
4. _____ bones do not protrude through skin   d. compression
5. _____ fragments of bone protrude through skin e. spiral

to support the area may be all that is needed to treat a closed fracture of the arm or lower leg. A cast is made by applying a wet substance to the extremity, in layers. The substance is molded and shaped as it is applied so it will fit the extremity. Two types of cast materials are commonly used:

- Plaster of Paris or plaster cast, which can take up to 48 hours to dry completely (because it dries from the inside to the outside), is frequently used as an initial cast for approximately a week after a fracture. The material is inexpensive and can be easily removed if the cast becomes too tight due to edema (swelling) of the extremity. However, plaster is heavy and bulky. Plaster casts must remain dry because water or drainage from a wound can distort the shape of the cast.

- Fiberglass, which dries rapidly (in approximately 15 to 20 minutes and allows for weight bearing in approximately 24 hours), is a lighter weight material that can be used as an initial cast, but frequently is used as a secondary cast that is applied to the extremity after the physician is sure no more edema is present. Fiberglass has a number of advantages as a cast material. It is lightweight, less bulky, and less likely to have rough edges. These casts are usually covered with stockinette to prevent snagging of clothing because they have a rougher surface than plaster.

Cast Material Is Wet when It Is Applied

During the drying period, the cast gives off heat. When the resident returns to the facility, special precautions are required to care for the resident who has a new cast:

- Allow the cast to air dry; keep it uncovered until it is dry. Turn the resident frequently to expose all cast surfaces to the air. Turning will promote even drying of the cast.

- Support the cast and the body in good alignment with pillows covered by cloth pillowcases. Avoid placing plastic under a wet cast. Do not place the new cast on a hard surface until it is completely dry to prevent denting the cast, which may cause skin trauma or loss of skin integrity.

- Elevate the casted extremity on a pillow as instructed. If the resident has a leg cast, elevate the foot higher than the hip; if the arm is in a cast, the fingers should be higher than the elbow.

- Put no pressure on the wet cast. Any pressure can leave permanent indentations that can press against the resident's skin, causing it to break

down. Use the *palms of your hands*, not your fingers, to move the casted extremity. Ensure that the cast is not touching the footboard or any type of turning device.

- Observe the uncasted areas of the extremities, such as the fingers and toes, for signs of decreased circulation: blue color (cyanosis), cold to touch, edema, and/or complaints of pain or tingling in the area. Also, note any signs of odor or drainage that may be coming from or through the cast. Immediately report any of these signs to the nurse.

- Note any signs of drainage through the cast. Immediately report this to the nurse because this may be a sign of infection or ulceration under the cast.

- Observe the skin areas around the cast edges for signs of irritation. Rough edges of the cast should be covered with strips of adhesive tape to prevent abrasion and irritation. Always report the irritation before the skin becomes broken and infected.

- Use a sling for an arm cast as directed (after it is thoroughly dry) to help support the weight of the cast and to keep the extremity elevated and in alignment. A resident with a leg cast may need to use a wheelchair to help support the leg.

- Keep the cast dry during bathing. The cast is usually protected with a plastic bag applied with waterproof tape to ensure there is no leakage of water under the bag. Follow your agency protocols. When using a handheld showerhead, always direct the spray of water away from the cast. Do not allow a plaster cast to become wet; the plaster will soften the cast, which will become damaged and need to be replaced.

- Follow agency protocols in case a fiberglass cast becomes wet. A blow-dryer set on the lowest temperature setting is frequently used to dry the cast thoroughly. The padding inside the cast *must* be completely dry to prevent irritation of the skin under the cast.

- Report any resident complaints of itching under the cast. The physician may need to prescribe a medication to alleviate the problem. Also, observe the resident's unit for signs of any type of device that might be used to "scratch" under the cast. These devices may injure the skin and predispose the resident to infection under the cast.

Immobilizers

An immobilizer is a conservative, but effective way to treat acute injuries such as minor, hairline fractures of the long bones, chronic conditions such as osteo-arthritis, and following surgery such as for rotator cuff (shoulder surgery) or fracture of the elbow. The immobilizer is worn to prevent injury to a joint or allow for healing of a fracture or the surgical incision. The immobilizer may sometimes be referred to a brace or a splint, as well. This discussion will focus on the frequently used knee and shoulder immobilizers.

Prior to applying an immobilizer on a resident's extremity, you must be educated by the physical therapist or the nurse on proper placement of the device. Before applying the immobilizer, always check for irritation or skin breakdown on the extremity, and in the armpit if a shoulder immobilizer is worn. The immobilizer is worn over lightweight clothing to limit irritation. If the immobilizer is equipped with pads to prevent irritation, make sure these are clean and available for use. Never send the pads for the immobilizer to the laundry; these must be washed by hand.

When applying the knee immobilizer, while in bed, ask the resident to place the leg in a horizontal position. Keep the leg straight and lift and swing the leg over the brace, center the patellar (knee cap) opening in line with the knee cap. The physical therapist will have molded the metal stays to fit the curves of the resident's leg. Place the pad under the knee (if the brace comes with one). Begin attaching the straps at the ankle; feed the straps through the D-rings and secure. Next secure the straps at the thigh, then at the knee and all remaining straps or per agency protocol. Ensure the immobilizer is not too tight, as it can compromise circulation. After the immobilizer is in place, check the positioning in a standing position (if possible). Adjust the straps as needed; the brace should not slip.

The shoulder immobilizer is designed to support the arm and keep the resident from performing incorrect movements. At night the immobilizer keeps the arm protected from involuntary movements and prevents the resident from sleeping on it. The immobilizer is worn at all times except when bathing or dressing; always assist the resident to keep the arm in the correct position during these times.

The immobilizer should never be in direct contact with bare skin. The resident should wear a soft T-shirt or cotton button down shirt, as preferred. Some therapists advise keeping a small, cotton washcloth or towel in the armpit to keep the area dry and free from irritation and fungal infections. If the immobilizer encloses the elbow, check for signs of irritation to the elbow because of the seam that runs down the center of the arm support. Pad the elbow area if necessary. The hand should rest comfortably in the sling; the level of the hand should be above the level of the elbow to prevent the blood from pooling and edema from forming in the hand. The over-the-shoulder support strap should be placed over the nonaffected shoulder. It should be comfortable and not impair circulation.

Treatment of Fractures with Traction

Traction is used to treat some fractures. This means the broken ends of the bone are pulled into normal alignment. In *skin traction* a belt or strap is applied to the body and weights are attached to the ropes (Figure 28-7). *Skeletal traction* involves the insertion of a metal pin into the bone. Weights are then attached by ropes to the pin (Figure 28-8). Traction may be used until the bone heals or it may be used only until surgery is performed or a cast is applied. When caring for a resident in traction:

- Review the placement of pulleys, ropes, and weights with the nurse so you know the purpose and correct placement of each.

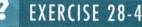

? EXERCISE 28-4

1. When caring for the resident with a cast, a nursing assistant should:

_____

_____

_____

_____

_____

_____

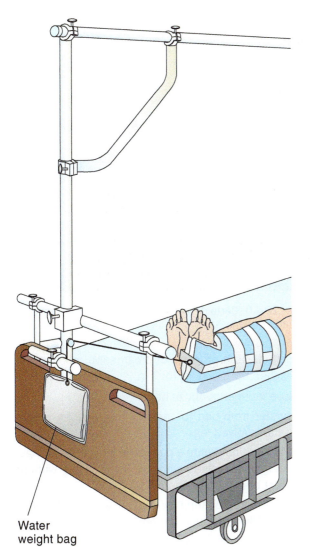

Water
weight bag

Figure 28-7 Buck's traction is an example of skin traction sometimes used for a fractured hip.

- Do not disturb the weights or permit them to swing, drop, or rest on any surface.
- Keep the resident in good alignment and ensure that the body is acting properly as countertraction.

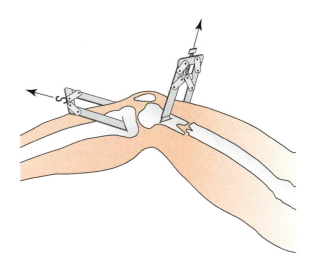

Figure 28-8 Skeletal traction immobilizes a body part by attaching weights directly to the resident's bones with pins, screws, wires, or tongs.

- Check under belts or straps for areas of pressure or irritation.
- Make sure that straps and belts are smooth, straight, and properly secured.
- Do not touch the metal pins (skeletal traction) where they come through the skin.

Fractured Hip

The most common fracture seen in residents of long-term care facilities is a fractured hip. This term refers to any break involving the upper third of the femur (upper leg bone) (Figure 28-9). A fractured hip may occur spontaneously as a result of osteoporosis. The resident is walking and, without warning, the bone breaks, causing the resident to fall. In other cases, the resident falls, causing the bone to break. Signs and symptoms of a fractured hip include:

- Pain in the hip or groin sometimes radiating to the knee

? EXERCISE 28-5

1. Five areas the nursing assistant should check when caring for a resident in traction are:

   a. _____

   b. _____

   c. _____

   d. _____

   e. _____

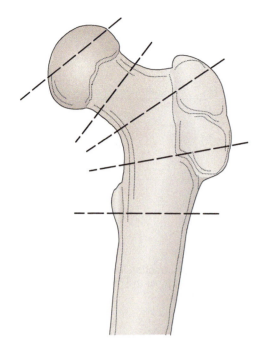

Figure 28-9 The lines indicate where fractures usually occur in the femur.

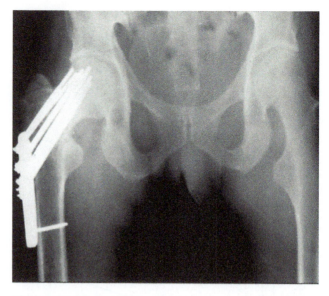

Figure 28-10 Certain fractures are repaired using plates, pins, nails, or screws.

- Feeling of pressure on the hip
- Shortening and turning outward of the leg on the injured side
- Bruising and swelling of the hip, groin, and thigh
- The resident may have heard a "snap or crack" just before or after the fall.

If you suspect a fractured hip, *never* attempt to move the resident without instructions from the nurse. The resident will be taken by ambulance to the hospital for x-rays of the affected joint and bones. If a fracture has occurred, the resident will be admitted to the hospital for repair of the fracture.

Open Reduction/Internal Fixation

Fractured hips are usually repaired by **open reduction/ internal fixation (ORIF)**. This method may also be used for fractures of other large bones. The resident is given a general anesthetic and is asleep during surgery. An incision is made, the surgeon aligns the broken ends of the bone, and a nail, pin, screw, and a metal plate are inserted to maintain alignment (Figure 28-10). The device is usually permanent. The resident will stay in the hospital for several days and then recover in the long-term care facility.

Caring for Residents with ORIF

Residents who have had an ORIF usually have physical therapy for several weeks after the repair. The physical therapist starts a program of progressive mobilization and teaches the resident to:

- Move independently in bed
- Transfer from bed to chair without bearing weight on the involved leg
- Stand and hold onto a bar while doing active range-of-motion exercises with the involved leg without weight bearing (Figure 28-11).
- Start weight bearing by standing and balancing, then walking through the parallel bars
- Walk with cane or walker

When you care for a resident with ORIF, you must:

- Know whether there are any restrictions for positioning the resident in bed
- Know whether the resident is allowed to bear weight on the affected leg
- Know how to transfer the resident if the resident is non-weight bearing or partial weight bearing
- Know whether you should do passive range-of-motion exercises on the affected leg
- Encourage the resident to do activities of daily living (ADLs) as independently as possible
- Encourage involvement in activities away from the nursing unit
- Report:
  - Complaints of pain
  - Changes in vital signs
  - Signs of bleeding, inflammation (redness, heat, swelling), or drainage from the incision
  - Signs of disorientation or confusion (common after hip surgery and usually temporary)

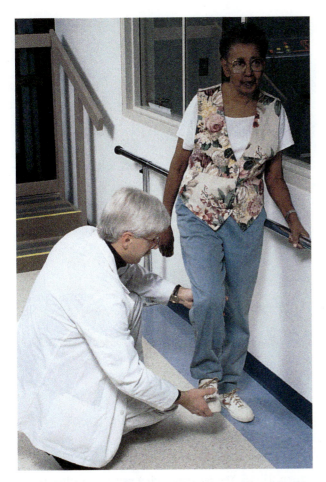

Figure 28-11 The resident is doing active range of motion exercises without weight bearing on the affected side.

Arthritis

Arthritis is a common problem in older persons. The conditions and care are described in Figure 28-12. Many forms of arthritis exist, but the most common forms are:

- Osteoarthritis (OA)
- Rheumatoid arthritis (RA)
- Gout (gouty arthritis)
- Psoriatic arthritis (PsA)
- Fibromyalgia

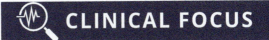

CLINICAL FOCUS

Think of how the osteoarthritis affects Ms. Branch's ability to carry out ADL. How can you help her without increasing her dependency?

Osteoarthritis is due to the "wear and tear" of the joints. The cartilage at the ends of the bones wears away with movement. It begins during middle age and can be very painful. This form of arthritis does not usually cause severe disability. However, for some individuals, it can limit their mobility. Residents may feel more stiff in the morning or after prolonged periods of immobility. This is why encouraging movement is so important and should not be overlooked. The joints, especially hip joints, may require replacement with an artificial joint (**prosthesis**) (Figure 28-13).

Condition	Disease Process	Treatment	Special Care
Osteoarthritis	Breakdown (degeneration) of joints. Weight-bearing joints such as ankles, knees, and hips are most commonly involved. Movement is painful and condition is progressive.	Medication to relieve pain; physiotherapy to maintain mobility; light massage and heat; ambulatory aids to reduce pressure in joints; weight reduction; surgery in selected cases.	Give positive, emotional support; carry out heat treatments, massage, and ROM exercises, as ordered.
Osteoporosis	Defective bone formation and maintenance. Bones become brittle and are easily broken. Complications: fractures, kidney stones, and loss of height and posture. More common in females than males.	Keep resident as active as possible; diet adequate in protein and vitamins C and D, and calcium; maintain adequate fluid intake; hormone therapy.	Encourage food and fluid intake. Assist in exercise. Report pain; apply support as needed. Emotional support must not be overlooked.
Rheumatoid Arthritis	Inflammation of joint lining (synovium). Joint changes cause painful muscle spasms, flexion, and deformities. Signs and symptoms may temporarily disappear (remission). Flareups may be related to emotional stress.	Drugs to reduce pain and inflammation; heat treatments for comfort; exercise when inflammation subsides; surgery in selected cases.	Provide emotional support. Provide self-help devices such as long shoe horns and grab bars. Carry out heat treatments and ROM exercises, as ordered.

Figure 28-12 Orthopedic problems in older adults.

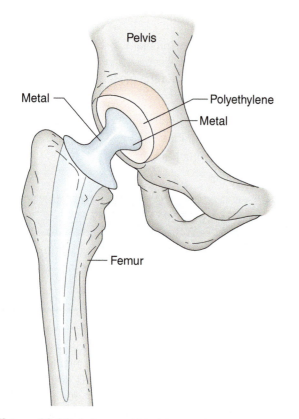

Figure 28-13 A damaged hip joint can be replaced with an artificial joint (prosthesis).

Caring for Residents with a Hip Prosthesis

The physician usually places the resident on hip precautions for a minimum of 6 weeks after surgery. These precautions may include:

- Turn to back and unaffected hip only.
- Keep affected leg in neutral position when in bed and during activities.
- Place abductor splint (Figure 28-14) or at least two pillows between the legs when turning. Keep hips abducted when in wheelchair.
- Use an elevated toilet seat to avoid hip flexion when rising.
- Report any signs or symptoms of:
  - Swelling of affected leg
  - Redness or discoloration of hip
  - Pain at the hip, groin, or thigh
  - Drainage or bleeding from incision
  - Chest pain (a blood clot in the lungs is sometimes a complication of hip surgery)
- Do not allow the resident to:
  - Adduct the legs (cross affected leg over midline) (Figure 28-15)

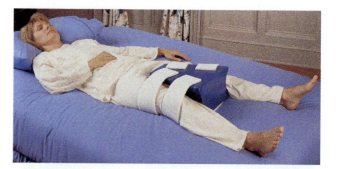

Figure 28-14 Residents often use the abduction pillow upon their return to the facility following hip surgery. The pillow prevents the resident from crossing the ankles, and holds the hip in proper alignment, preventing contractures.

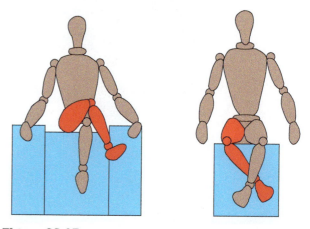

Figure 28-15 The resident with a new hip prosthesis should never cross the affected leg (in red) over the midline of the body.

- Flex legs past 90 degrees
- Flex hip when in side-lying position
- Bend forward at hip during transfers or other activities or when sitting up in bed (Figure 28-16)
  - Sit for long periods of time
  - Internally rotate affected leg (Figure 28-17)

Rheumatoid arthritis can begin at any age and sometimes occurs in children. This disease can be mild or progressive until it destroys the joints. In either case, severe pain is a symptom. Hand deformities from rRA are shown in Figure 28-18A.

The most important aspect of care for residents with arthritis is to balance activity with rest. Too much activity at one time may increase the pain. Too much rest results in stiffness and can lead to contractures (Figure 28-18B). When you touch the resident's body, remember to be gentle.

Gout (Gouty Arthritis)

Gout is a metabolic disorder that is caused by an increase in uric acid in the bloodstream or a failure of the body to

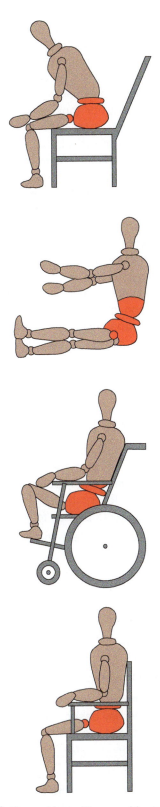

Figure 28-16 The resident with a new hip prosthesis should never flex the affected hip (in red) more than 90 degrees.

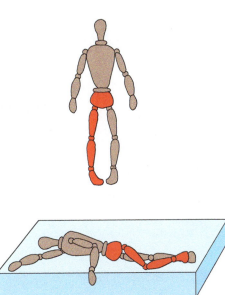

Figure 28-17 The resident with a new hip prosthesis should never internally rotate the hip on the affected side (in red).

seems to be an inherited tendency to the disorder. Gout can also occur or recur in a resident following a period of dehydration. The uric acid crystals are deposited in the affected joints, which become inflamed (red, hot, and swollen); the associated pain is severe. The resident may also have a low-grade fever. In order to help relieve the pain, reduce the uric acid levels in the body, and aid in excretion of the uric acid in the urine, the physician may order certain medications for the resident. Gout goes into periods of remission but then may recur more severely. After many years, some persons can develop chronic gout; other body systems are also affected at that time.

Dietary treatment is important for persons with gout. The dietitian will plan the diet to restrict foods rich in purines (organ meats like liver and kidney, meat soups, and broths). Alcohol intake is restricted. The resident should be encouraged to drink liberal amounts of fluid to prevent dehydration.

Psoriatic Arthritis

A chronic autoimmune disease, psoriatic arthritis is characterized by inflammation of the skin (psoriasis) and joints (inflammatory arthritis). This type of arthritis is a condition that features red patches of skin topped with silvery scales. The disease may lay dormant in the body until triggered by an outside influence such as a common throat infection. There are five types of PsA, most of which are triggered by injury, an infection, sunlight, or certain types of medication. Treatment usually consists of alternating warm and cool cloths, exercises, and nonsteroidal anti-inflammatory drugs (NSAIDs). In severe cases, antirheumatic drugs may be given to help prevent long-term joint damage.

excrete the uric acid. The concentrated uric acid forms crystals that are deposited in and around the joints. Men are more often affected and the most common site is the joint of the great toe. The cause is unknown but there

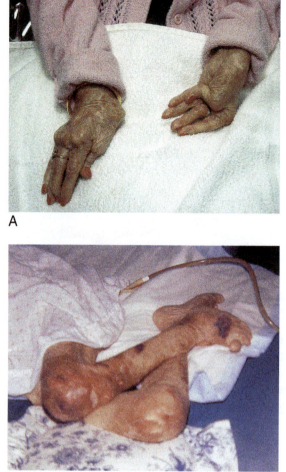

A

B

Figure 28-18 (A) These deformities, caused by rheumatoid arthritis, make hand movements difficult. (B) This resident has many problems with her legs, including arthritic deformities and contractures.

Fibromyalgia

A disorder characterized by widespread musculoskeletal pain and accompanied by fatigue, sleep, and memory issues, fibromyalgia amplifies painful sensations by affecting the way your brain processes pain signals. Treatment consists of self-care (talk therapy), physical exercise, stress management, and relaxation techniques. Massage therapy, acupuncture, hydrotherapy, and NSAIDs can be effective treatments as well.

Lower Extremity Amputation

You may care for residents who have had parts of one or both feet or legs surgically removed (amputated). When an older person has an amputation, it is usually because of circulatory problems. These problems may be due to changes in the blood vessels or because of complications of diabetes. Gangrene may develop (the tissues die) and amputation is needed.

It is common for people to experience **phantom pain** after the removal of a limb. Residents may feel pain or tingling where the limb used to be. These feelings may persist for months. The pain or sensation is real, although it is difficult to explain.

As a CNA caring for those with amputations, it is important to believe a resident when they say their toes itch on the foot of the leg that is no longer present. Offer to listen and allow them to vent or describe the pain. Report the situation to the charge nurse who may offer an over-the-counter analgesic for discomfort.

After an amputation, some people are fitted with a prosthesis (an artificial limb). They have to learn how to walk and sit when the prosthesis is worn. If you are responsible for helping a resident put on a prosthesis, be sure you know how to attach and secure it. The loss of all or part of a limb is traumatic. Following amputation the person is likely to experience depression, anxiety, fear, grief, and anger. The resident needs emotional support in adapting to the changes in the body image and changes in function of the limb and ADL.

Residents who have had amputations need to be positioned correctly. This is explained in Lesson 22.

Foot Problems

As people age, foot and toenail problems develop. If these problems are not corrected, they may affect the person's ability to walk. Many people require the services of a **podiatrist** for treatment of the feet and toenails. Nursing assistants provide foot care as follows:

1. Clean the resident's feet thoroughly during the bathing procedure.
   - Wash, rinse, and dry carefully between each toe.
   - Clean the toenails.

2. Observe the feet for:
   - Bluish color
   - Swelling
   - Breaks in the skin

3. Report any changes to the nurse. Changes may vary during the day based on positioning, time of day, or response to medications.

4. Protect the resident's feet.
   - Be sure the resident wears properly fitting wide, box toed shoes and socks when up.
   - Avoid bumping or hitting the resident's feet as you do positioning and range-of-motion procedures.
   - Loosen the covers over the resident's feet.

5. Do not allow the resident's feet to dangle. If the feet do not touch the floor when sitting in a chair, provide a footstool.

6. Know your facility's policy for cutting toenails.

? EXERCISE 28-6

Read the following situations and answer the questions.

1. You notice that Ms. Thompson is up and wandering barefoot in her room. What action should you take?

   _____

   _____

   _____

2. When caring for a resident's feet, the nursing assistant should _____

   _____

   _____

   _____

? EXERCISE 28-7

COMPLETION

Select the correct term(s) from the following list to complete each statement.

air   phantom pain
bursitis   podiatrist
contractures   rest
correct   rheumatoid arthritis
fractures   shoes
open reduction and   stiffness
internal fixation   to balance rest with activity
osteoarthritis

1. Inflammation of the bursa is called _____.

2. The person with osteoporosis is at greater risk for _____.

3. Wet casts should be allowed to _____ dry.

4. For fractures to heal, they must be kept in _____ alignment.

5. When referring to a resident who has a fractured hip, the letters ORIF mean _____.

6. With any form of arthritis, it is important to balance activity with _____.

7. Too much rest for an arthritic person's joints will result in _____ and _____.

8. Pain experienced by a person in a limb that has been amputated is called _____.

9. Many elderly people require the services of a(an) _____ for treatment of the feet and toenails.

10. Residents should always wear properly fitting _____ when up and ambulating.

11. The two most common forms of arthritis are: _____

    _____

    _____

12. What is the most important aspect of care when a resident suffers from arthritis?

    _____

    _____

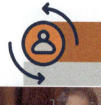

LESSON SYNTHESIS: Putting It All Together

You have just completed this lesson. Now go back and review the Clinical Focus. Try to see how the Clinical Focus relates to the concepts presented in this lesson. Then answer the following questions.

1. What factors contribute to Essie Branch's flexed posture?
2. Why are women more prone to osteoporosis in later years compared to men?
3. Because the bones of this resident have less strength, what special precautions must be included in her care?

28 REVIEW

A. Select the one best answer for each of the following.

1. The musculoskeletal system performs all of the following, except

(A) gives shape and form to the body

(B) produces hormones

(C) produces red blood cells

(D) permits movement

2. Skeletal muscles are attached to the bones by

(A) ligaments

(B) tendons

(C) cartilage

(D) bursae

3. Small sacs of synovial fluid are located around joints. They sometimes become inflamed, causing

(A) bursitis

(B) arthritis

(C) tendinitis

(D) osteoporosis

4. When a resident develops osteoporosis, all of the following occur, except

(A) the bones become brittle and porous

(B) the bones fracture easily

(C) kyphosis may develop

(D) the bones become stronger

5. When a resident has a new cast, signs and symptoms indicating circulatory impairment include all of the following, except

(A) pink toes

(B) cold to touch

(C) complaints of pain and tingling

(D) swelling

6. Skin traction involves

(A) application of a belt or strap to the body and attachment of weights

(B) insertion of a metal pin into the bones and attachment of weights

(C) application of a splint

(D) application of an external fixation device

7. When a resident has had an ORIF, you must know

(A) whether the resident can bear weight

(B) what type of device was installed

(C) how long the surgery took

(D) how the fracture occurred

8. When a resident has had a hip prosthesis inserted, you must discourage the resident from

(A) doing ADLs independently

(B) being out of bed

(C) adducting the legs

(D) participating in activities

9. A resident with rheumatoid arthritis may have all of the following, *except*

   (A) no joint deformity

   (B) inflammation of the joint lining

   (C) painful muscle spasms and flexion

   (D) temporary remissions

10. Osteoarthritis is

    (A) due to wear and tear of the joints

    (B) common in children

    (C) a cause of severe disability

    (D) not painful

11. With any type of arthritis, the most important aspect of care is to

    (A) encourage the resident to remain in bed as much as possible

    (B) encourage the resident to exercise as much as possible

    (C) balance rest and activity

    (D) perform all ADLs for the resident

12. Amputation of a lower extremity may cause phantom pain. Phantom pain is

    (A) due to the resident's imagination

    (B) due to the resident's need for attention

    (C) a type of surgical pain

    (D) real and may persist for months

13. A diabetic resident who has a severe infection and develops gangrene of the foot may require:

    (A) gout

    (B) osteoporosis

    (C) atrophy

    (D) amputation

14. Phantom leg pain:

    (A) is real

    (B) may be imagined

    (C) lasts approximately 2 months

    (D) is permanent

B. Answer each statement true (T) or false (F).

15. T F As one ages, the joints become more flexible.

16. T F Movements in a joint depend on the way in which the joint is formed.

17. T F When a person has osteoporosis, the vertebrae may collapse without warning.

18. T F Gangrene can be treated successfully with medication.

19. T F A fracture is a break in a bone.

20. T F Gout is caused by increased uric acid levels in the bloodstream.

21. T F Inflammation of the joints is called arthritis.

22. T F Cover a leg cast tightly while it is drying.

CARING FOR RESIDENTS WITH NERVOUS SYSTEM DISORDERS

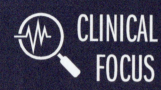

CLINICAL FOCUS

Think of the special challenge presented in providing nursing assistant care to a resident with neurologic disorders as you study this lesson.

OBJECTIVES

After studying this lesson, you should be able to:

• Define vocabulary words and terms.

• List the functions of the nervous system.

• List the structures of the nervous system.

• Discuss the changes of aging that affect the nervous system.

• Describe the sensory deficits caused by disease.

• Identify the symptoms related to common nervous system disorders.

• Describe the nursing care for residents with nervous system disorders.

• Demonstrate the following:

Procedure 29-96   Care of Eyeglasses
Procedure 29-97   Applying and Removing In-the-Ear or Behind-the-Ear Hearing Aids

VOCABULARY

age-related macular degeneration (ayj-ree-LAY-ted MAH-kyou-lar dee-jen-er-AY-shun)
amyotrophic lateral sclerosis (a-MY-o-TRO-fic LAT-er-al sk-le-RO-sis)

aneurysm (AN-you-rizm)
aphasia (ah-FAY-zee-ah)
atherosclerosis (ath-er-oh-skleh-ROH-sis)
audiogram

CASE STUDY

Thomas Raye suffers from Parkinson's disease. This is a neurologic disorder that affects his ability to control and coordinate his voluntary movements. Although able to move, Mr. Raye cannot stop and start activities smoothly. He walks with small, shuffling steps and stands with a characteristic bent frame.

audiologist
auditory nerve (awe-dih-TOH-ree nurv)
autonomic dysreflexia (aw-to-NOM-ik did-re-FLEX-si-a)
autoimmune
brain stem (brayn stem)
cataract (KAT-ah-ract)
central nervous system (SEN-tral NUR-vus SIS-tem)
cerebellum (ser-eh-BELL-um)
cerebrospinal fluid (ser-eh-broh-SPY-nal FLEW-id)
cerebrovascular accident (CVA) (ser-eh-broh-VASS-kyou-lar ACK-sih-dent)
cerebrum (SER-eh-brum)
choroid (KOH-royd)
conjunctiva (kon-junk-TIGH-vah)
cornea (KOR-nee-ah)
dementia (dee-MEN-she-ah)
diabetic retinopathy (die-ah-BET-ick ret-ih-NOP-ah-thee)
embolus (EM-boh-lus)
emotional lability (ee-MOH-shun-al lah-BILL-ih-tee)
equilibrium (ee-kwih-LIB-ree-um)
genetic disease (jeh-NET-ick dih-ZEEZ)
glaucoma (glaw-KOH-mah)
hemianopsia (hem-ee-an-OP-see-ah)
hemiplegia (hem-ee-PLEE-jee-ah)
Huntington's disease (HUNT-ing-tonz dih-ZEEZ)
intention tremor (in-TEN-shun TREM-or)
iris (EYE-riss)
lens (lenz)
magnetic resonance imaging (MRI) (mag-NET-ick REZ-oh-nans IM-aj-ing)
meninges (meh-NIN-jeez)
motor nerve (MOH-tor nerv)

multiple sclerosis (MS) (MULL-tih-pul skle-ROH-sis)
myasthenia gravis (MG) (my-as-THEE-nee-ah GRAH-vis)
nerve impulses (nurv IM-pul-ses)
nerves (nurvs)
neurons (NEW-ronz)
neurotransmitter (new-roh-TRANS-mit-er)
nystagmus (nis-TAG-mus)
ophthalmologist (of-thal-MOL-oh-jist)
optic nerve (OP-tick nurv)
paralysis (pah-RAL-ih-sis)
paraplegia (pair-ah-PLEE-jee-ah)
Parkinson's disease (PARK-in-sons dih-ZEEZ)
peripheral nervous system (peh-RIF-er-al NUR-vus SIS-tem)
position sense (poh-ZISH-un sens)
presbycusis (pres-beh-KYOU-sis)
presbyopia (pres-bee-OH-pee-ah)
pupil (PYOU-pil)
quadriplegia (kwahd-rih-PLEE-jee-ah)
reflex (REE-flex)
retina (RET-ih-nah)
sclera (SKLEH-rah)
sensory nerve (SEN-sor-ee nurv)
spatial-perceptual deficit (SPAY-shul-per-SEP-tyou-al DEF-ih-sit)
stroke (strohk)
thrombus (THROM-bus)
transient ischemic attack (TIA) (TRAN-see-ent is-KEE-mick ah-TACK)
traumatic brain injury (TBI)
unilateral neglect (you-nih-LAT-er-al neh-GLECT)

COMPONENTS OF THE NERVOUS SYSTEM

The nervous system is the center for control and communication for all body functions and activities. Electrical messages called nerve impulses are sent throughout the body. The two major parts of the nervous system are the (Figure 29-1):

- Central nervous system (CNS)—the brain and spinal cord
- Peripheral nervous system (PNS)—the cranial nerves and spinal nerves

Special sense organs and receptors receive information from the environment. The information travels along the cranial or spinal nerves to reach the brain and spinal cord, where the sensation is interpreted. Information is received by the:

- Eyes
- Ears
- Taste buds
- Receptors in the nose for smell
- Nerve endings (receptors) in the skin, muscles, joints, and tendons
- Receptors in body organs

The nerve endings in the skin pick up sensations of pain, pressure, and variations in temperature. Receptors in muscles, tendons, and joints carry information about the degree of muscle contraction and position of body parts. Receptors in the walls of body

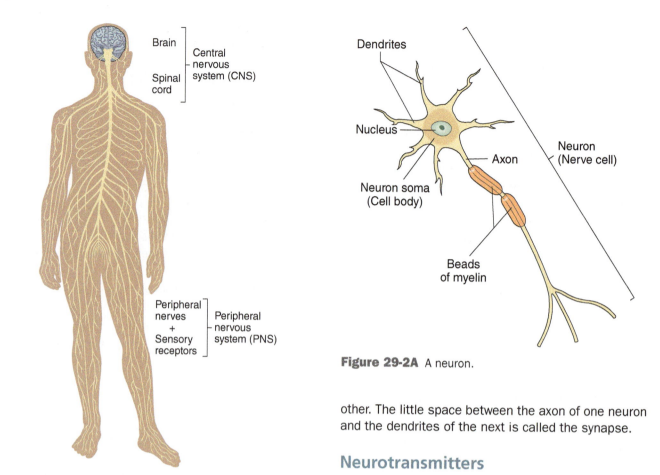

Figure 29-1 The peripheral nervous system connects the central nervous system to the various structures of the body. Messages are relayed from these structures back to the brain through the spinal cord.

Figure 29-2A A neuron.

organs carry information related to hunger, thirst, and visceral (organ) pain.

Neurons

Neurons are special cells that carry messages (Figure 29-2A). The neurons and other cells make up the nervous tissue of the brain, spinal cord, and peripheral nerves. Neurons are composed of:

- A central area, called the body
- One or more dendrites—structures that receive messages and carry them toward the cell body
- An axon—the structure that carries messages away from the cell body

Axons and dendrites are called nerve fibers. A message or nerve impulse begins in the dendrites and is carried along the cell body and then to the axon. It takes more than one neuron to carry the message from where it begins to where it can be carried out or interpreted. The neurons do not actually touch each other. The little space between the axon of one neuron and the dendrites of the next is called the synapse.

Neurotransmitters

Neurotransmitters are chemicals that enable messages (nerve impulses) to pass from one cell to another (Figure 29-2B). If the chemicals are not produced in adequate amounts, the message pathway becomes confused or blocked.

Nerves

Nerves are bundles of nerve fibers (axons and dendrites) that connect the body with the CNS. Nerves are named according to the type of message they carry and the direction in which they carry the message. The two general types of nerves are:

- Sensory nerves
- Motor nerves

Sensory nerves carry messages about pain, temperature change, changes in body position, taste, touch, sound, and sight. They carry messages toward the brain and spinal cord. When sensory nerves are damaged, the ability to receive messages and interpret sensations is impaired or lost.

Motor nerves carry messages from the brain and spinal cord to muscles and glands to bring about responses. When motor nerves are damaged, the person loses the ability to voluntarily control body movement. This condition is called **paralysis**. Paralysis may be

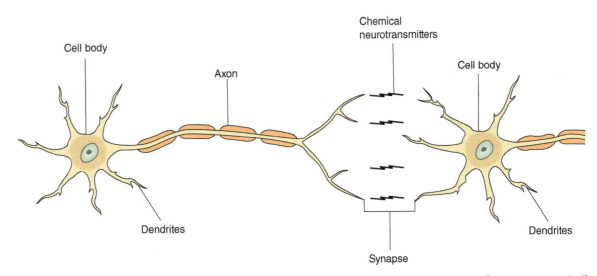

Figure 29-2B Chemicals called neurotransmitters help pass the nerve message across the synapse from one neuron to the next.

complete, with no movement possible, or partial with a weaker than normal response.

Peripheral nerves carry both incoming and outgoing information. These are mixed bundles of nerves carrying both sensory and motor fibers throughout the body.

CENTRAL NERVOUS SYSTEM

The CNS is made up of the brain and spinal cord. These organs are protected by the bones of the skull and vertebral column. A triple-layered membrane, the meninges, surrounds the brain and spinal column, providing additional protection. The system is cushioned by cerebrospinal fluid.

The Brain

The brain is the most complex organ in the body (Figure 29-3). The neurons of the brain carry out many complex functions, including:

- Reasoning
- Thinking
- Forming and recalling memories
- Making judgments
- Controlling body functions
- Interpreting the sensations that are brought in by the nerves

Twelve pairs of cranial nerves carry messages into and out of the brain.

The cerebrum is the largest part of the brain. It is divided into two halves or hemispheres. The surface of the cerebrum forms lobes that have the same names as the bones under which they are located. They are the:

- Frontal lobes
- Parietal lobes
- Temporal lobes
- Occipital lobes

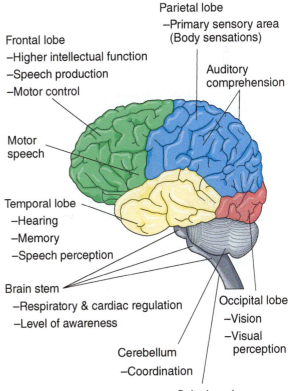

Figure 29-3 Functional areas of the brain.

- Refer to Figure 29-3. Different parts of the cerebrum carry out specific activities:
- Motor control of one side of the body is managed by cells in the opposite side of the frontal lobe.
- Sensations originating on one side of the body are interpreted on the opposite side of the parietal lobe.
- Vision is interpreted in the occipital lobe.
- Hearing is in the temporal lobe.

The cerebellum is called the little brain. It lies beneath the occipital lobes of the cerebrum. This part of the brain coordinates muscular activities and maintains balance.

The brain stem is the portion of the brain that is connected to the spinal cord. It is composed of special groups of nerve cells that control the vital (living) functions of the body. These vital functions include:

- Respiration
- Heart rate and rhythm
- Size of the blood vessels
- Functioning of internal body organs such as the organs of the digestive tract

Most of the 12 pairs of cranial nerves are attached to the brain stem.

Spinal Cord

The spinal cord is about 18 inches long and extends from the brain to just above the small of the back. Thirty-one pairs of spinal nerves enter and leave the spinal cord, carrying messages to and from the body. The spinal cord:

- Carries messages to and from the brain and relays them to the body through the spinal nerves (Figure 29-4).
- Handles certain special responses called reflexes.

A reflex occurs when an incoming message becomes an outgoing command without needing to go to a higher conscious level. For example, if you touch something hot, you immediately pull your hand back. You may then realize what you have done, but pulling back your hand was a reflex response handled by the spinal column.

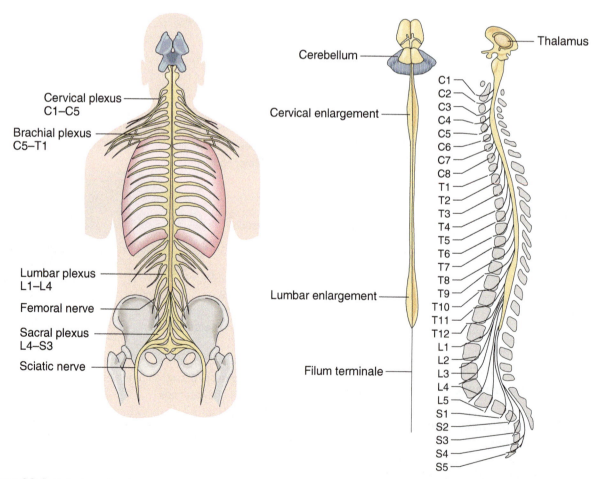

Figure 29-4 Spinal cord and nerves.

Cerebrospinal Fluid

The **cerebrospinal fluid** (CSF) is a clear, colorless fluid derived from the plasma of the blood. It fills cavities in the brain called ventricles and circulates in the central canal of the spinal cord. It acts as a watery cushion around both the brain and spinal cord. CSF is continuously produced. It is also reabsorbed at the same rate back into the bloodstream.

AUTONOMIC NERVOUS SYSTEM

The autonomic nervous system is part of the PNS. It controls heart rate, the secretions of glandular cells, and the contraction of the smooth muscular walls of organs.

SENSE ORGANS

The sense organs carry messages about the external world to the brain. Sense organs carry messages about:

- Touch
- Temperature
- Pain
- Vision
- Hearing
- Taste
- Smell
- Equilibrium

The Eye

Each eye is located in a bony cavity of the skull. Muscles move the eyes in a coordinated way. The eyelids and eye are covered by a clear mucous membrane called the **conjunctiva**. Mucus and tears from the lacrimal gland keep the eye moist (Figure 29-5). Excess tears drain into the nose and sometimes from the outside of the eyes.

The eye is a ball-shaped, fluid-filled organ made up of three layers:

- **Sclera**—the outer white protective cover. The front of the sclera forms the transparent **cornea**.
- **Choroid**—the middle layer that contains the **iris** (the colored part of the eye). The iris lies behind the cornea. The center of the iris is the **pupil**, which is an opening that changes size to control the amount of light entering the eye. The **lens** behind the iris bends and directs light rays.
- **Retina**—the innermost layer containing nerve receptors (Figure 29-6).

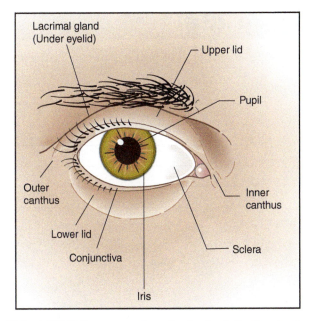

Figure 29-5 Tears come from the lacrimal gland and exit from the eye through the nasolacrimal duct.

Vision

Light rays are reflected from the object being seen. The rays pass through the cornea and pupil and are bent to focus on the retina. The image on the retina is then transmitted by the **optic nerve** to the brain for vision interpretation. (The optic nerve is one of the cranial nerves.)

The Ear

The ear enables us to hear and also assists in controlling **equilibrium**. This allows us to maintain our sense of balance. The ear is made up of the:

- Outer ear
- Middle ear
- Inner ear (Figure 29-7)

Hearing

Sound waves enter the ear and are carried toward the eardrum (tympanic membrane). This structure separates the outer and middle ear. The sound waves make the eardrum vibrate. Three tiny bones stretch across the middle ear. The first bone is attached to the eardrum. It begins to vibrate as the eardrum moves. The second bone is attached to the first and the third to the second. Each little bone vibrates in turn at the same rate as the eardrum moves. The third bone attaches to the membranous opening of the inner ear. Vibrations against this membrane set up fluid vibrations in the inner ear. The inner ear is made up of the:

- Semicircular canals
- Vestibule
- Cochlea

? EXERCISE 29-1

1. Identify the parts of the eye shown in the figure below:

A. _____

B. _____

C. _____

D. _____

E. _____

F. _____

G. _____

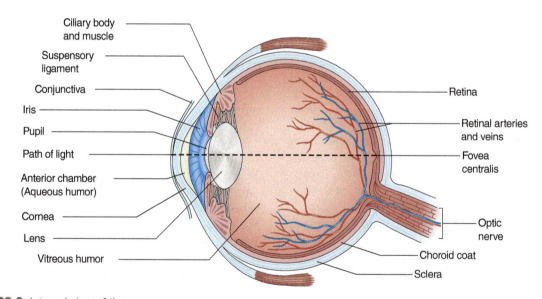

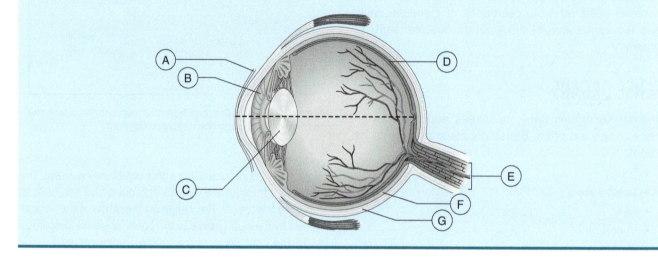

Figure 29-6 Internal view of the eye.

The three semicircular canals pick up information about starting and stopping movements. The vestibule picks up information about the position of the head. Deep within the snail-shaped cochlea are the special hearing receptors that are stimulated by the fluid vibrations. When these receptors are stimulated, the message is picked up and transmitted to the **auditory nerve** and then to the brain for interpretation of sounds that are heard.

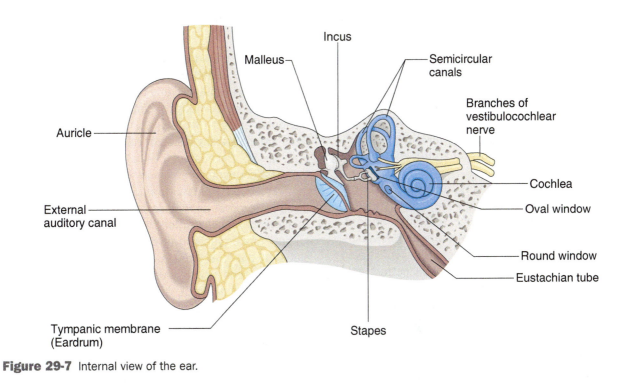

Incus

Malleus

Semicircular canals

Branches of vestibulocochlear nerve

Auricle

Cochlea

Oval window

External auditory canal

Round window

Eustachian tube

Tympanic membrane (Eardrum)

Stapes

Figure 29-7 Internal view of the ear.

? EXERCISE 29-2

1. Identify the parts of the ear shown in Figure 29-7.

A. _____

B. _____

C. _____

D. _____

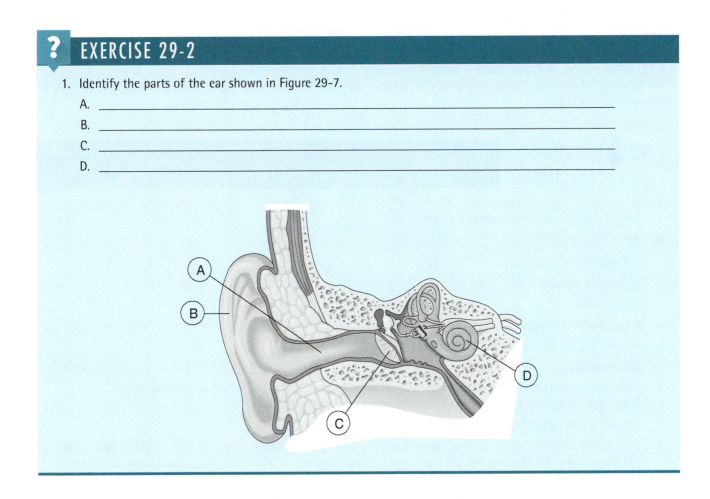

CHANGES IN THE NERVOUS SYSTEM CAUSED BY AGING

The effects of aging on the nervous system are not as noticeable as they are on some of the other body systems. It is important to remember that intelligence does not decrease, although it may take longer to perform tasks. Any change in mental status is an indication of a disease process.

Aging affects the senses of vision, hearing, taste, and smell. Most people have visual changes that make it difficult to read and see close objects. This is because the elasticity of the lens decreases with age. This condition is called **presbyopia** (also called farsightedness). Eyeglasses will correct this problem. Many older people have glasses with *bifocal* or *trifocal* lenses. These lenses correct more than one visual impairments. Some residents are not able to care for their own glasses. You must remember to do this for them.

CAUSES OF SEVERE VISION IMPAIRMENT

Several disorders of the eye may result in severely impaired vision or blindness. These changes are not due to normal aging. Some of these disorders can be treated and are reversible. Others lead to severe vision impairment or blindness.

Cataracts

The lens is normally clear. Sometimes the lens becomes cloudy and is called a cataract. The cataract causes vision to become blurred and hazy. A person with a cataract has problems judging distance. Color vision may disappear and glare from bright lights is annoying. Cataracts are the leading cause of vision loss in adults older than age 55. Because of this, cataract surgery is one of the most common surgeries in the United States.

Eyedrops are used to numb the eye. The surgery involves removal or replacement of the lens in order to allow light rays to enter the eye. Until recently, most surgery for cataracts involved removing the center (nucleus) of the lens through a larger incision. Currently, most surgeons use a small incision and ultrasound to remove the cataract. A plastic, silicone, or hydrogel lens is usually implanted, and the incision is naturally sealed. Stitches are not used.

Some residents may have cataract surgery while they are in the long-term care facility. Because the procedure is performed either as an outpatient procedure or in a day surgery center, the residents may return to the facility immediately after surgery when their condition is stabilized.

Care for the resident who has had cataract surgery includes:

- Checking vital signs when the resident returns to the facility and until stable

PROCEDURE 29-96
Care of Eyeglasses

1. Carry out each beginning procedure action.

2. Assemble equipment:

   - Resident's eyeglasses
   - Cleaning solution
   - Clear water
   - Soft cleaning tissues

3. Provide only the assistance that the resident needs.

4. Handle glasses only by the frames.

5. Clean lenses with cleaning solution or clear water. Check the condition of the frames and lenses. Report any damage to the frames and earpieces and serious scratching of the lenses.

6. Dry with a soft cotton towel.

7. Help resident put glasses on or return glasses to case and place in drawer of bedside table. If the resident puts the glasses on, note how well the glasses fit. Report any looseness or slipping. If the glasses have nosepieces, check that they are not irritating the resident's skin; also note any irritation behind the ears.

8. Carry out each procedure completion action.

⚠ GUIDELINES FOR... ASSISTING VISUALLY IMPAIRED RESIDENTS

1. Make sure the resident knows the location of all personal articles in the room. If the resident has a system for organizing belongings, do not attempt to make changes.

2. Always put things back where they were.

3. Do not rearrange furniture unless it is absolutely necessary. Then tell the resident what changes have been made.

4. Help orient the resident to a new room by teaching the resident to locate various objects from a point of reference. Just inside the door may be the reference point. Then say, for example, "The bathroom is to your right."

5. When providing walking assistance to a resident with a visual impairment, have the resident hold your arm. Walk beside and slightly ahead of the resident (Figure 29-8). Walk at the resident's pace; the resident can sense a great deal by feeling your body movements. Always tell the resident when you are going to be turning to the right or left. Notify the resident that there may be steps, a curb, or any other obstacle ahead. Pause slightly before proceeding after giving the warning. Always alert the resident when you are stopping.

6. To help the person locate a chair, place the person's hand on the chair's back or arm. The seat should be located before sitting.

7. The floor should be dry and free of clutter and throw rugs.

8. Never leave doors partially open.

9. At mealtime, the resident's dishes should always be arranged in the same way. Describe the location and type of food using a clock system. For example. "The roast beef is at 12:00, mashed potatoes and gravy are at 3:00, and there are peas at 9:00."

10. Offer to cut meat, pour beverages, butter bread, and open cartons. Some residents may be able to do this.

11. Advise the resident to sprinkle salt and pepper into the hand rather than directly on the food. It is easier to know how much is being used.

12. Advise the resident to use a small piece of bread in one hand to help push food on the fork. This also prevents the food from being pushed off the plate.

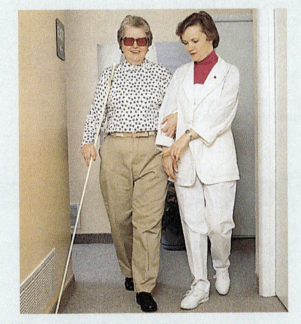

Figure 29-8 Have the resident hold your upper arm lightly while you walk at the resident's pace.

- Minimizing light for the first 48 hours
- Reminding the resident to avoid bending over to minimize pressure on the eye.
- Being sure all needed items, such as signal cords are within easy reach
- Taking extra precautions if the resident is confused or restless
- Helping the resident adapt to temporarily blurred vision caused by the eyedrops that were used to dilate the eyes during surgery

- Protecting the eye from injury for the first 4 weeks postoperatively; instruct the resident not to rub or squeeze the eye
- Ensuring that the resident avoids activities that involve straining, such as bending over, strenuous coughing, or excessive physical activity. These actions may cause an increase in pressure in the eye
- Noting that the resident wears an eye shield at night, as prescribed by the physician, to protect the eye from injury

- Immediately notifying the nurse if the resident complains of sudden, sharp pain or unrelieved pain, flashes of light or floaters, decreased or sudden vision loss, or nausea with or without vomiting; also note any signs of increased redness in the eye
- Assisting with ambulation as necessary

Glaucoma

Glaucoma exists when the pressure in the eyeball is higher than normal. This occurs when the meshwork between the iris and cornea thickens, obstructing the flow of the fluid in the eyeball. If not treated, the pressure eventually damages the optic nerve, causing blindness.

Glaucoma has few symptoms. Everyone older than 35 years should be tested for eye pressure routinely. The disease process can be stopped by using eyedrops prescribed by the ophthalmologist (eye physician).

Age-Related Macular Degeneration

Age-related macular degeneration is the leading cause of visual loss in the United States. Millions of older people are affected. The cause is unknown. The macula is located on the retina. The macula is damaged when abnormal blood vessels form and leak fluid. Laser treatments may help some people with this condition.

Diabetic Retinopathy

People with diabetes are at risk for diabetic retinopathy. It is caused by the deterioration of small blood vessels that nourish the retina. Laser treatments may interrupt the disease process. However, vision loss that has already occurred cannot be restored.

There are many things nursing assistants can do to improve the quality of life for residents with severe visual impairments.

Review Lesson 4 for communicating with persons with vision and hearing loss.

HEARING LOSS

Hearing loss is common in later years. It usually results from progressive deterioration of the cochlea. This condition is called presbycusis. Some residents

? EXERCISE 29-3

MATCHING

Match the condition on the right with the description on the left.

Description Condition

1. _____ deterioration of small blood vessels that nourish the retina
2. _____ blood clot
3. _____ genetic disorder that affects mind, body, and emotions
4. _____ excessive pressure within the eyeball
5. _____ neurologic disorder caused by lack of brain neurotransmitters
6. _____ cloudy lens
7. _____ CNS disorder thought to be an autoimmune disorder
8. _____ leading cause of visual loss in the United States
9. _____ stroke
10. _____ farsightedness
11. _____ inability to express or understand speech

a. cataract
b. presbyopia
c. glaucoma
d. macular degeneration
e. diabetic retinopathy
f. Parkinson's disease
g. cerebrovascular accident
h. multiple sclerosis
i. thrombus
j. aphasia
k. Huntington's disease

12. Four techniques to assist visually impaired residents at mealtime include:

   a. _____

   b. _____

   c. _____

   d. _____

will wear hearing aids. The devices are expensive, so they must receive proper care.

Hearing Aids

Hearing aids now have either analog or digital circuits or a combination of both. The settings for any hearing aid are determined by the hearing test (audiogram). The audiologist gives the information to the hearing aid manufacturer so the needed settings can be installed. In the past all hearing aids were analog; like a microphone and loud speaker, they used continuous, varying electrical signals provided by a battery to convey sound (speech and noise). A programmable analog hearing aid is also now available that contains a microchip that can be programmed for different listening environments (quiet conversation or, noisy situations like dining rooms).

Digital hearing aids also have a battery, microphone, and a computer chip that help to create the sound. The sound can be modified to meet the resident's individual hearing needs. The computer chip analyzes the sound a person hears and distinguishes whether the sound is noise or speech. It then makes the necessary modifications to produce undistorted speech. Digital hearing aids are usually self-adjusting and are designed for the needs of a specific resident. These devices are usually more expensive but have a longer life span than analog models.

Hearing aids come in a variety of styles, the small, in-the-canal (ITC) aids, in-the-ear (ITE) aids, or behind-the-ear (BTE) aids (Figure 29-9). The ITE variety fills the outer part of the ear; they are larger than those that fit only in the ear canal. This type may be easier for some persons to handle. The BTE type has a small plastic case (contains the mechanism and battery) that rests behind the ear. A thin, clear plastic tube runs into the ear canal and is connected to a soft, molded ear piece. This type is becoming more popular since it comes in a variety of colors and is programmable. The BTE may be easier to manipulate for the older resident.

Care for Hearing Aids

- Turn the hearing aid off before removing it and store at room temperature when not in use. Always *store the hearing aid in the off position* and open the door to the battery compartment to allow air to circulate and help to dry it out. Keep the battery in its housing so that is not lost or damaged.

- Keep hearing aids dry. If an aid is worn accidently in the shower ask the nurse how to dry it. Never try to dry the aid with a hair dryer.

- Store the extra batteries in a cool, dry, safe place. The battery will have a longer life.

- Avoid temperature extremes: Do not store hearing aids in direct sunlight, on a radiator, or on a cold windowsill.

- Keep the hearing aid in a safe place. Store in its container and place in the drawer of the bedside stand. Hearing aids are easily broken if dropped on a hard floor or bumped against a hard surface. Report lost or damaged hearing aids to the nurse at once.

- Remove hearing aid before using a hairdryer and whenever hairspray is being used. The spray may clog the microphone and cause damage.

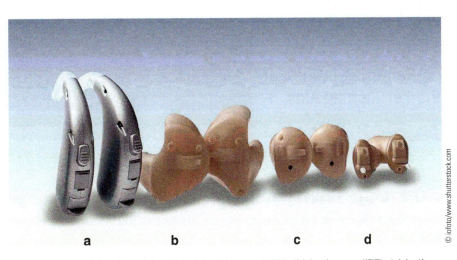

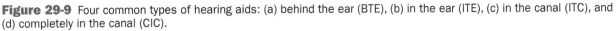

Figure 29-9 Four common types of hearing aids: (a) behind the ear (BTE), (b) in the ear (ITE), (c) in the canal (ITC), and (d) completely in the canal (CIC).

- Turn hearing aid off or remove from the ear prior to shaving a male resident with an electric razor.
- Wipe the ear molds daily with a dry tissue or soft cloth.
- Clean the hearing aid according to the manufacturer's directions. Check regularly to make sure the opening of the aid or ear mold is free of wax. The ITE types come with a cleaning tool. This should be used only by someone who has been instructed in the use of the tool.
- When taking an aural temperature, remove the hearing aid for several minutes before inserting the tympanic thermometer.
- Check with the family or audiologist before changing the programmable settings on any hearing aid.
- Observe for earwax buildup or irritation to the ear canal and report your finding to the nurse.
- Look for ways to minimize background sounds and noise.
- Always check linens before putting in the laundry for the resident who wears a hearing aid to be assured the hearing aid has not been discarded in the laundry. Hearing aids are expensive.

Troubleshooting for Hearing Aids

If the aid is not producing sound, before inserting in resident's ear:

- Check to make sure that the "+" (positive) side of the battery is next to the "+" inside the hearing aid battery case or compartment.
- Try a new battery—the old one may be dead.
- Check the earmold to see if it is plugged with wax.

- Make sure the hearing aid is set on "M" (microphone) not "T" (telephone switch).

  If the hearing aid is making squealing sounds:

- Determine if the earmold fits properly. It should be completely in the ear. If it does not fit well, report it to the nurse.
- Check the volume on the aid. If it is too high, turn it down until the squealing stops.
- Check the plastic tubing on a behind-the-ear aid. If it is cracked or split, it must be replaced.

Additional Hearing Devices

A number of different devices are available to those with hearing problems. Amplifiers are available already equipped in a telephone system or a portable amplifier may be strapped to the telephone receiver. Adaptations may be made to the ringtone on the telephone to make it more audible. Television viewing and listening to the radio has been made more accessible for the hearing impaired through the use of listening devices such as "TV-Ears," which allow personal control of the sound level without increasing the sound levels for others in the same room. The Closed Caption system is available on television sets so the hearing impaired person can read the dialog as the program is aired. Some persons find the use of "Pocket Talkers" help to improve communication. These devices amplify sound in different types of listening situations and can be adjusted by the individual user. Optimal use is in a 1 to 1 situation or in small group settings. This type of device can be worn in the pocket of a garment or placed in basket on a walker. The "Pocket Talker" also may be equipped with an extension for television viewing.

PROCEDURE 29-97
Applying and Removing In-the-Ear or Behind-the-Ear Hearing Aids

1. Carry out each beginning procedure action.
2. Assist resident to comfortable position with head turned so that the ear needing the hearing aid is closest to you.
3. Turn the hearing aid off and turn the volume down.
4. Make sure you insert the aid in the correct ear.
5. Turn on the control switch. To adjust the volume, talk to the resident as you increase the volume. Stop when the resident can hear you.

(continues)

PROCEDURE 29-97
Applying and Removing In-the-Ear or Behind-the-Ear Hearing Aids (Continued)

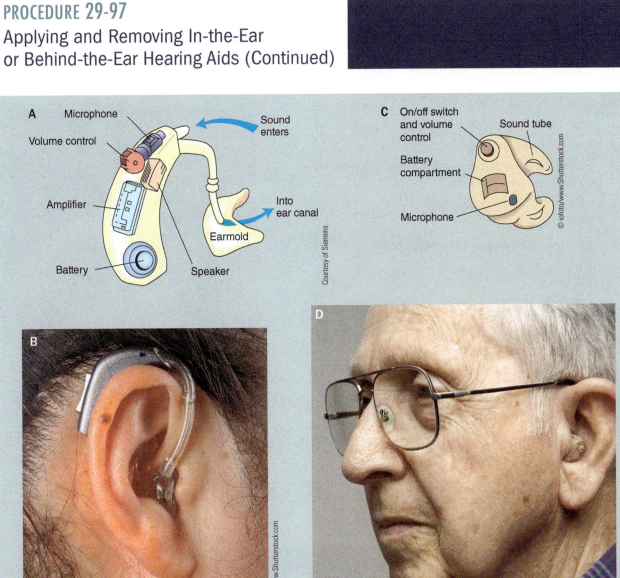

Figure 29-10 A and B: Behind-the-ear hearing aid placement. C and D: In-the-ear hearing aid placement.

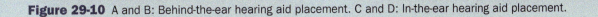

Behind-the-Ear Hearing Aid

- Place the aid over the resident's ear, allowing the earmold to hang free.
- Adjust the hearing aid behind the resident's ear (Figure 29-10A and B).

Behind-the-Ear Hearing Aid and In-the-Ear Hearing Aid

- Grasp the earmold and gently insert the tapered end into the ear canal.
- Gently twist the earmold into the curve of the ear while gently pulling on the earlobe with the other hand. The hearing aid should fit snugly but comfortably, flush with the ear (Figure 29-11 A and B).

(continues)

PROCEDURE 29-97
Applying and Removing In-the-Ear
or Behind-the-Ear Hearing Aids (Continued)

Removing the Hearing Aid

1. Wash hands and explain to resident what you plan to do.
2. Turn off hearing aid.
3. Loosen the outer portion of the earmold by gently pulling on the upper part of the ear.
4. Lift earmold upward and outward.
5. Store in safe area.
6. Carry out each procedure completion action.

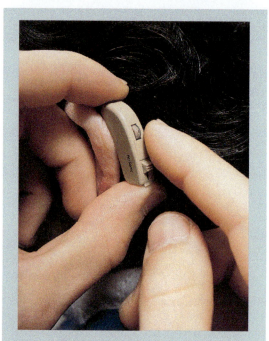

Figure 29-11 Adjust the hearing aid behind the resident's ear.

? EXERCISE 29-4

Mr. Connally uses a hearing aid. As part of his morning care you assist him to apply it. The following activities will review your understanding.

1. Which part of the hearing aid fits into the ear canal? _____
2. Always store the hearing aid in the _____ position.
3. Wipe the _____ daily with a dry tissue or soft cloth.
4. Earmolds should be checked to see if they are plugged with _____.
5. To remove a hearing aid, lift the earmold _____ and _____.

NERVOUS SYSTEM DISORDERS

Several diseases can affect the nervous system. Some of these are due to an imbalance in neurotransmitters. Other neurologic problems are caused by damage to brain cells or the spinal cord.

Diseases affecting the nervous system often have different signs and symptoms. Some common problems that may exist with these diseases include:

- Impaired mobility because of damage to the brain, spinal cord, or nerves in the legs

- Difficulty swallowing due to damage to the brain or damage to the nerves of the face and mouth
- Communication disorders due to damage to the brain or damage to the nerves of the face and mouth

Parkinson's Disease

Parkinson's disease is a chronic illness that is progressive. It is due to a decrease in a neurotransmitter that passes messages between cells in the cerebrum and the gray matter of the brain. These cells affect movement, balance, and walking (Figure 29-12).

The signs and symptoms of Parkinson's disease include:

- Tremors
- Muscular rigidity
- Difficulty and slowness in carrying out voluntary activities
- Difficulty with gait and/or balance
- Mask-like expression

Tremors of the hands commonly affect the fingers and thumbs so that the resident appears to be rolling a pill between them. The tremors begin in the fingers, then involve the entire hand and arm, and finally affect the entire side of the body. Starting on one side, the tremors eventually involve both sides of the body. The tremors cause the resident to be slow with movement and with activities of daily living (ADLs).

The muscular rigidity makes the person more prone to falls and injury. The joints may develop contractures if appropriate care and treatment are not given. The rigidity also affects muscles used in breathing. This increases the risk of respiratory infections.

Persons with advanced Parkinson's typically have a shuffling walk and difficulty starting the process. Once started, they may have episodes of "freezing" when they appear unable to move.

Speech is affected, causing words to be slurred. The tone of voice is low and the sound is monotone. Rigid facial muscles cause the face to look expressionless. The resident may not be able to smile or blink.

The resident with Parkinson's may drool and become incontinent or constipated. Depression is a common problem. Some residents with Parkinson's may experience mental changes which can lead to a type of **dementia**.

There is no specific diagnostic test for Parkinson's disease. The physician will take a history and make thorough neurologic examination to rule out other problems.

Parkinson's disease has no cure. In some cases the disease can be controlled with medications. In other cases, the disease may be progressive, causing severe disability.

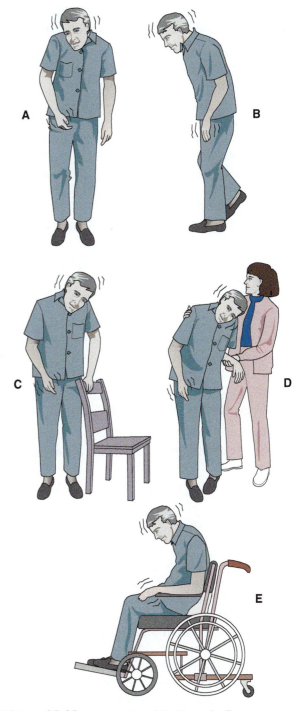

Figure 29-12 Progression of Parkinson's disease: (A) Flexion of affected arm; (B) shuffling gait; (C) need for sources of support to prevent falling; (D) progression of weakness to point of needing assistance for ambulation; (E) profound weakness.

Stroke

Stroke (also called brain attack) is the fourth most common cause of death in the United States. Two-thirds of stroke victims are older than 65 years. Stroke is also called **cerebrovascular accident** or **CVA**. The

⚠ GUIDELINES FOR... CARING FOR RESIDENTS WITH PARKINSON'S DISEASE

1. Give passive range-of-motion exercises at least twice a day. Encourage participation in active exercise if the resident is able to do so.

2. Improve walking by encouraging the resident to:
   - Bring the toes up with every step.
   - Put the foot down, heel first then toes.
   - Swing the arms.
   - Ambulate—assist by using a gait belt and walking with the resident.
   - Use good posture.

3. Reposition dependent residents frequently and avoid flexion as much as possible.

4. Observe the resident closely and report:
   - Signs of respiratory infection
   - Problems with urinary elimination
   - Constipation

   - Falls; side effects of medication may cause decrease in blood pressure

5. Give at least 2,000 mL fluid by mouth every day unless contraindicated.

6. Assist with ADLs only to the extent necessary. Encourage the use of assistive devices.

7. Observe for drooling. Residents who are unable to control saliva may also have trouble swallowing. Watch for any problems during eating.

8. Be patient. Allow adequate time to complete tasks independently.

9. Give emotional support and encouragement. The disease usually affects the facial muscles. Because of this, the resident may have no facial expression. This lack of expression is not a true indication of what the resident is feeling.

---

word *cerebrovascular* refers to blood vessels in the brain. Major risk factors for a stroke include:

- Hypertension (high blood pressure)
- **Atherosclerosis** (buildup of fatty deposits in arteries)
- History of **transient ischemic attack (TIA)**
- Smoking
- Lack of exercise
- Obesity

A TIA is not a stroke, but may be a warning that a stroke is likely to occur. During a TIA, the resident may experience speech disturbances and paralysis because of diminished blood flow to the brain. These symptoms may last from a few minutes to 24 hours. They are never permanent.

A stroke may be the result of a hemorrhage or a partial or complete blockage of one or more cerebral blood vessels caused by a thrombus or an embolus:

- Hemorrhage—For example, hemorrhage occurs when hypertension causes a blood vessel in the brain to rupture, or when an **aneurysm** in the brain ruptures. A hemorrhage also can occur following traumatic brain injury.

- Thrombus—A **thrombus** is a blood clot. It forms when fatty deposits on the artery walls cause the walls to become roughened. This causes platelets in the blood to form a clot. When the thrombus interrupts blood flow to the brain, a stroke occurs.

- Embolus—An **embolus** is a thrombus that develops in an artery in one part of the body, breaks loose, and travels to another part of the body. In the case of a stroke, the embolus travels to an artery in the brain and blocks the flow of blood.

Symptoms of Stroke

The symptoms of stroke depend on the part of the brain that is damaged. If the left side of the brain is damaged, these symptoms may be noted:

- Paralysis on the right side of the body. This is called right **hemiplegia**.
- **Aphasia**—an inability to express or understand speech
- Change in personality. The individual with left brain damage becomes very slow, anxious, and cautious.

If the right side of the brain is damaged, these symptoms may be noted:

- Paralysis on the left side of the body. This is called left hemiplegia (Figure 29-13).
- **Spatial-perceptual deficits**. This means it is difficult to distinguish between left and right, up and down. The world may appear "tilted" to the person with right-brain damage. The resident will have problems propelling a wheelchair, setting down items, and carrying out ADLs.
- Change in personality. The individual with right brain damage becomes very quick and impulsive.

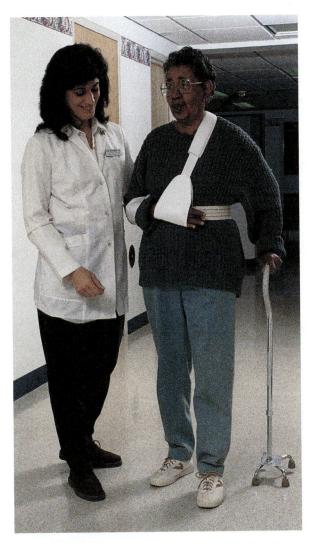

Figure 29-13 The resident had a stroke, resulting in paralysis of one side of the body.

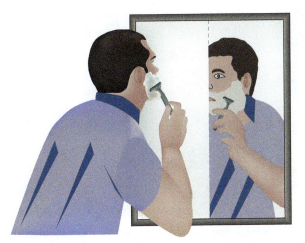

Figure 29-14 Hemianopsia causes a person to see only part of the visual field.

Other symptoms may be present with either right or left brain damage. These include:

- Sensory-perceptual deficits.
  - Loss of **position sense**. The individual cannot tell where the affected foot is or what position it is in.
  - The inability to identify common objects. The person who has had a stroke may not recognize a comb, a fork, a pencil, or other common items.
  - The inability to use common objects. The person may know what the object is, such as a comb, but be unable to pick it up and use it appropriately even with the unaffected arm. This is not a result of paralysis but of damage to certain cells in the brain.
- **Unilateral neglect**. The resident ignores the paralyzed side of the body. For example, the affected arm may hang over the side of the wheelchair without the resident realizing where the arm is.
- **Hemianopsia**. This is impaired vision. Both eyes only have half vision. For example, if the resident has left hemiplegia, the left half of both eyes is blind (Figure 29-14).
- **Emotional lability**. Residents who have had strokes may start to cry or laugh for no apparent reason. They have very little control over this and may be embarrassed.

Goals of Poststroke Care

Three major nursing goals for a resident who has had a stroke are:

1. Maintain the skills and abilities that the individual has left.
2. Prevent complications caused by immobility.
   - Contractures
   - Pressure ulcers
   - Pneumonia
   - Blood clots
3. Regain functional abilities (Figure 29-15).
   - ADL
   - Bowel and bladder control
   - Mobility
   - Communication skills

Communicating with persons with aphasia is presented in Lesson 4.

The recovery from stroke is different for each person. Some individuals recover with a minimal degree of disability. Others may have a greater degree of disability but learn to adapt and regain some independence. A few individuals are severely impaired and will regain very little, if any, ability for self-care.

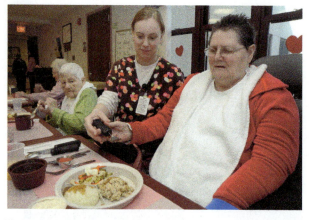

Figure 29-15 The resident who has had a stroke must be retrained in activities of daily living.

Traumatic Brain Injury

Traumatic brain injury (TBI) occurs from a sudden, severe trauma to the head that damages the brain. TBI can result from an object piercing the skull and brain or when the head hits an object with great force. The extent and location of the damage determines whether the injury is mild, moderate, or severe. The symptoms will vary depending upon the extent of the injury. The person may remain conscious or experience loss of consciousness varying from a few seconds to minutes to a permanent comatose state.

Signs and symptoms may include physical symptoms such as headache, blurred vision, dizziness, nausea and vomiting, sensitivity to light, balance problems,

---

? EXERCISE 29-5

1. Complete the chart related to two residents who have suffered from strokes.

   Mrs. Gallardo   Mrs. Dimonico
   (right-side brain   (left-side brain
   damage)   damage)

   _____   _____
   _____   _____
   _____   _____
   _____   _____
   _____   _____
   _____   _____

   Problems
   a. right hemiplegia
   b. loss of position sense
   c. slow, anxious, cautious personality change
   d. spatial–perceptual deficits
   e. quick, impulsive personality changes
   f. aphasia
   g. hemianopsia
   h. left hemiplegia
   i. emotional lability
   j. unilateral neglect

2. Three reasons a stroke may occur include:

   a. _____

   b. _____

   c. _____

3. The three major goals for a person who has had a stroke include:

   a. _____

   b. _____

   c. _____

and feeling tired. The person may have difficulty thinking clearly, concentrating, and/or remembering new information. Emotionally, the person may be irritable, nervous, anxious, or sad. Sleep patterns may be altered. They may sleep more or less than usual or have difficulty falling asleep. Symptoms may develop immediately or over time.

If the person experiences slurred speech, headache that intensifies, weakness, numbness, or lack of coordination, and repeated vomiting it is important to seek help immediately. Emergency treatment is required for a person having seizures, enlarged or unequal pupil size, those who cannot recognize people, show increased confusion and agitation, or are so drowsy they cannot be aroused.

Treatment concerns include making sure there is adequate blood flow and oxygen to the brain and the rest of the body, controlling blood pressure, and determining the cause of the TBI. Long-term treatment includes rehabilitation: physical and occupational, tailored to the needs of the individual. Speech therapy may be another important component, as well as psychological and social support.

Disabilities that result from TBI depend on a number of factors: location of the injury and the age and general health of the person. The most serious injuries may result in a vegetative state (unconscious but aware of surroundings with periods of awareness), stupor (an unresponsive state where a person may be briefly aroused by painful stimuli), and coma (unconscious, unresponsive, unaware, and unarousable state).

Multiple Sclerosis

Multiple sclerosis (MS) is another CNS disorder. The cause is unknown, but it is thought to be an autoimmune disorder. In this type of condition, the person produces antibodies that damage his or her own body cells. Researchers are looking at the possible link between viruses like those that cause diseases such as measles, mumps, and chickenpox and the part they play in persons who develop MS.

MS is usually diagnosed before the age of 50. Many persons with MS have an average life span even though they have this chronic, progressive disorder. Therefore, it is not uncommon to see elderly residents in long-term care with this diagnosis. In fact, most facilities have young residents in their twenties and thirties with MS (Figure 29-16).

The symptoms vary and may not be the same for all persons. Common symptoms include:

- Muscle weakness (primarily of the lower extremities)
- Fatigue

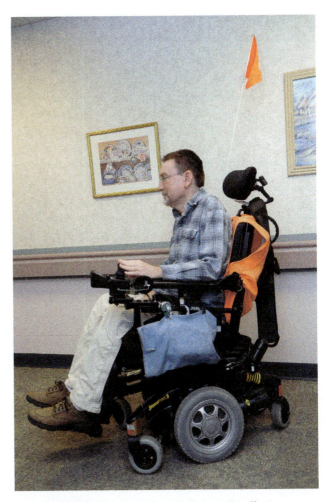

Figure 29-16 Multiple sclerosis frequently affects young people.

- Feelings of numbness or tingling in one or more extremity
- Coordination and balance difficulties
- Problems with the bowel (constipation or diarrhea)
- Problems with the bladder (urinary incontinence or retention)

Problems with vision occur in almost half of the people who have MS. This problem may be permanent or temporary. Sometimes it is the first symptom that is noted. Symptoms may include:

- Blurriness, color blindness, or difficulty seeing objects in bright light
- Double vision
- Nystagmus (jerky eye movements)

Mobility is usually affected:

- Pain in the legs that disappears with rest
- Paraplegia (paralysis of both legs)
- Spasticity

⚠ GUIDELINES FOR... CARING FOR RESIDENTS WHO HAVE HAD A STROKE

Complications following stroke can be prevented by several measures.

1. Proper positioning. Lesson 22 gives instructions for positioning residents with hemiplegia. Remember to support the paralyzed arm so that the shoulder does not become dislocated. Check the paralyzed leg and arm frequently. The resident may be unaware of injury to the extremities.

2. Passive range-of-motion exercises twice a day (see Lesson 22). The resident may learn to do self range-of-motion exercises. This also provides exercise for the unaffected arm.

3. Intake of an adequate amount of fluids each shift

4. Implementation of bowel and bladder programs

5. Maintenance of nutritional status

6. Encouraging and supporting the resident at all times

7. You can help the resident regain functional abilities by encouraging and allowing the resident to do as much as possible. Provide the help that is necessary for completing ADLs but avoid "over-helping." You can carry out restorative programs under the direction of the physical therapist, occupational therapist, and restorative nurse.

8. You can help the resident regain mobility skills by increasing the resident's mobility as directed by the nurse or physical therapist (Lessons 22 and 23).

⚠ GUIDELINES FOR... CARING FOR RESIDENTS WITH MULTIPLE SCLEROSIS

1. Prevent complications.
   - Contractures can occur rapidly because of the spasticity. Range-of-motion exercises and position changes are important. The resident may also perform muscle-stretching exercises with the help of the rehabilitation nurse or physical therapist.
   - Spasticity affects the bladder and causes incontinence. For this reason, residents with severe MS may have indwelling catheters. Excellent catheter care is necessary to prevent bladder infections. Make sure the resident has adequate fluid intake.
   - Residents with MS are at risk for pressure ulcers. Follow all directions for pressure ulcer prevention. Because of lack of sensation, ulcers may develop without the resident feeling discomfort or pain.

2. Encourage independence.
   - The use of adaptive devices for ADLs may help maintain independence for a longer period of time.
   - Mobility may be prolonged if assistive devices such as canes or walkers are used. Leg braces

   are helpful for some people. Many individuals (even in the facility) may use motorized scooters. This increases independence for people who are no longer able to walk.

3. Maintain a balanced schedule of rest and activity.
   - Residents with MS need exercise and activity. However, they also need rest periods to avoid becoming overtired.
   - Remember that fatigue can be a major problem. Help residents set priorities for their available energy. If a resident expects the family to visit in the evening for example, allow more rest periods during the day.

4. Provide emotional support and encouragement.
   - Residents in long-term care facilities may have access to MS support groups. Some people find these groups very helpful.
   - Not all residents with MS will be elderly. Remember the developmental stages of the residents in your care. This will allow you to be more empathic and give better care.

- **Intention tremor** (shaking of the hands that gets worse as the individual tries to touch or pick up an object)

In severe MS, speech is affected because of the weakness of the muscles in the chest, face, and lips. The speech may be slow with poor articulation. The mind usually remains alert. Incontinence of bowel and bladder is also common.

One of the most disabling features of MS is fatigue. This very real physical symptom, not psychological, makes it impossible for the person to move about.

The diagnosis of MS is not based on a specific test. The physician takes a thorough history and performs a complete neurologic examination. **Magnetic resonance imaging (MRI)** is a test that may reveal lesions in the neurons in the brain. The person conducting the test records pictures (scans) of brain tissue beneath the bone.

MS may eventually lead to **quadriplegia** (paralysis of all four extremities). Residents with quadriplegia require total care. However, not all persons who have MS are severely impaired. At the time of diagnosis, it is seldom known what course the disease will take. It is difficult for the person to deal with this uncertainty for the future. The disease may follow one of four courses:

- *Benign course:* Mild attacks with long periods of no symptoms
- *Exacerbating-remitting:* Severe attacks (exacerbations) followed by periods of partial or complete recovery (remissions). Often the periods of exacerbation get longer with shorter periods of remission.
- *Slowly progressive:* Slow, steady deterioration
- *Rapidly progressive:* Deterioration is rapid and progressive and may be life-threatening

Huntington's Disease

Huntington's disease, or **Huntington's chorea**, is a rare hereditary disease. This means it is a **genetic disease** because it is passed from one generation to another through a defective gene. Either parent carrying the gene can transmit the disease to either sons or daughters. Each child of a parent with the defective gene for Huntington's has a 50% chance of receiving the defective gene from the parent.

The disease is progressive and affects the CNS as well as the mind and the emotions. There is no cure. Symptoms may become evident between the ages of 20 and 60 years. The most evident symptom is the body movements called choreiform movements. These begin early in the disease with fidgeting, twitching, clumsiness, and falling. As the disease progresses, the extremities are in constant movement during waking hours. Eventually it becomes impossible for the individual to walk or perform any activities independently.

The mind is also affected, resulting in a form of dementia. The capacity to plan and organize is lost. Impulsiveness and loss of judgment are also common. Emotional disorders such as depression, antisocial behavior, and seclusion may also develop.

The disease is always chronic and progressive. There may be periods of stability. As the disease progresses, the symptoms become more severe. Eventually, death occurs, usually as a result of pneumonia or another type of infection.

Many residents with Huntington's disease are young people. Some of them may have young children. This is a difficult situation for families as children watch a parent become progressively worse. Whether or not the children will develop the disease is a major concern for all family members. Each family deals with this in its own way. Avoid passing judgment on families and the way they choose to cope with this problem. Referral for professional counseling should be made by

---

? EXERCISE 29-6

Mrs. Walters has multiple sclerosis (MS). She was diagnosed when she was 55 years old and first reported double vision to her doctor. She is 72 years old now and has been diagnosed as having a slowly progressive disease. The following questions relate to this resident.

1. Multiple sclerosis usually is diagnosed before the age of _____.

2. Many persons live the _____ life span even though they have MS.

3. Multiple sclerosis usually involves symptoms related to vision such as _____, color blindness, double vision, and _____ (jerky eye movements).

4. Multiple sclerosis affects mobility because of pain that disappears with _____.

5. In MS, the shaking of hands that gets worse with effort is called _____.

6. The tight contraction of skeletal muscles in MS is called _____.

7. The inability to control the legs in MS is called _____.

8. Nursing care in MS focuses on:

   _____

   _____

   _____

the social services staff to all family members as well as the resident. It is the individual's decision whether to participate in the counseling.

Amyotrophic Lateral Sclerosis

This disease is also known as ALS or Lou Gehrig's disease. Mr. Gehrig was a famous baseball player who died of ALS. Amyotrophic lateral sclerosis generally affects persons between the ages of 50 and 70. The nerve cells in the brain and spinal cord gradually deteriorate. The disease is chronic and progressive. There is no cure. The muscles under their control weaken and waste away. The disease eventually affects all voluntary muscles. The mind stays alert and the person is able to think clearly. The first signs and symptoms include:

- Trouble with walking—stumbling and falling
- Trouble picking up objects and frequently dropping them
- Trouble completing ADLs, for example, lacing shoes, buttoning, or cutting meat

    Persons with ALS eventually have:

- Difficulty speaking
- Difficulty swallowing (may need a feeding tube)
- Disabling fatigue
- Shortness of breath (may need a ventilator)
- Inability to move arms or legs independently

Myasthenia Gravis

Myasthenia gravis (MG) is also a chronic disease that affects the muscles. This is due to incomplete transmission of nerve impulses where the nerves and muscle join. The cause is unknown. The same muscles are not affected in all people. Signs and symptoms always involve the muscles and may include:

- Weakness of the eye muscles, causing double vision and drooping of the eyelid
- Inability to smile, frown, or pucker the lips if facial muscles are involved
- Voice weaker if larynx is involved
- Generalized muscle weakness:
  - Difficulty putting arms above head
  - Difficulty rising from chair or toilet and difficulty walking up stairs
  - Difficulty managing saliva
  - Mouth hangs open due to inability to close mouth

Spinal Cord Injuries

Residents with damage to the spinal cord have a loss of function and sensation below the level of the injury (see Figure 29-4). Most often the damage is the result of trauma, but may be the result of birth defects. For example, if the level of damage occurs in the area of the neck, the injury may result in quadriplegia (paralysis of both the arms and legs) and also may cause lack

---

⚠ GUIDELINES FOR... CARING FOR RESIDENTS WITH HUNTINGTON'S DISEASE

Safety is a major concern because of the constant body movements.

1. Prevent injuries by:
   - Limiting side rails to quarter rails to avoid injury to the arms and legs
   - Using padded clothing and shoes without laces
   - Using a gait belt and having two assistants walk with the resident—providing stability and counteracting the jerky movements
   - Positioning bed in lowest position in case of a fall
2. Prevent choking by:
   - Ensuring that all who are responsible for feeding residents are knowledgeable about the resident's abilities, if possible
   - Having all persons who feed know how to do abdominal thrusts for an obstructed airway
   - Providing a diet as tolerated

Other concerns for residents with Huntington's disease include:

3. Incontinence
   - Assist the resident to the bathroom every 2 hours or as needed. As the disease progresses, this becomes impossible with the loss of ambulatory skills.
   - Catheters usually pose a danger because of the resident's involuntary movements, which may cause tearing of the urethra.
   - Incontinent pads may be necessary.
   - Careful attention to skin care is essential.
4. Nutrition
   - Additional calories may be needed because of the energy used in the involuntary movements.
5. Independence
   - Allow the resident as much independence as possible for as long as possible.

⚠ GUIDELINES FOR... CARING FOR RESIDENTS WHO HAVE AMYOTROPHIC LATERAL SCLEROSIS

1. Keep the resident upright as much as possible to avoid aspiration and to increase lung expansion. When lying down, position the resident on either side, turning at least every 2 hours. Place a cloth beneath the mouth to absorb saliva from the mouth.

2. Encourage coughing and deep breathing to prevent respiratory infections.

3. Encourage the resident to take frequent rest periods. Encourage the use of a wheelchair to save energy.

4. Use methods of communication as directed by the nurse or speech therapist. The resident may eventually have to communicate by blinking the eyes. Remember that even though the resident cannot speak, he can understand others.

5. Observe food and fluid intake. Residents with ALS may be too weak or too tired to eat. Try to have the resident rest for a half hour before meals and for 2 hours after meals. If the resident has to be fed, allow frequent breaks during the meal.

6. Report any signs of potential pressure ulcers.

⚠ GUIDELINES FOR... CARING FOR RESIDENTS WHO HAVE MYASTHENIA GRAVIS

Medications can help most people with myasthenia gravis to live productive lives. The disease affects each person differently. It is important to know for a specific resident which muscles are affected and how much activity the resident can tolerate.

1. Pace the resident's activity and allow adequate time for rest between activities.

2. Use alternative methods of communication according to the care plan.

3. Review Lesson 17 for feeding residents who have swallowing problems.

4. Encourage the resident's independence but provide assistance as needed.

of respirations. Any damage that is the result of injury to the spinal cord at the level of the thoracic vertebrae (T1 or lower) will result in paraplegia (paralysis of the lower half of the body).

Nursing care will depend on the site of the injury. For all residents with paralysis who are prone to pressure ulcers and contracture, nursing assistants should:

- Give careful skin care (incontinence, and lack of feeling and mobility can predispose to skin breakdown).
- Pay attention to the resident's elimination needs (no bowel or bladder control).
- Position the resident to avoid contractures.
- Perform range-of-motion exercises as prescribed.
- Prevent infections (respiratory and urinary).
- Listen carefully; the resident may be able to give you directions for carrying out his or her care.
- Accept the anger, fear, frustration, and depression that the resident may exhibit.

Autonomic Dysreflexia

Autonomic dysreflexia (AD) or hyperreflexia is a syndrome that may occur in persons who have had an injury to the spinal cord below the level of T-5 or T-6 (see Figure 29-16). The portion of the nervous system that is intact sends out signals causing constriction of the blood vessels that result in increased blood pressure and decreased pulse rate. If untreated, this may lead to stroke, heart attack, and death.

AD may be triggered by an irritating or painful stimulus in the area of the body below the level of injury. Bladder distention is one of the most common causes. This might be precipitated by a bladder infection, blockage to the flow of urine by a kink in the Foley catheter drainage tubing, or other obstruction (urinary stones). Distention of the bowel is another common cause. The bowel may be distended by flatus (gas), fecal material (constipation or fecal impaction). Digital stimulation associated with removal of an impaction may precipitate an attack. Other irritating stimuli that may trigger AD include pressure ulcers, ingrown toenails, cuts, burns (hot water or sunburn), cuts and abrasions, fractures, tight or restrictive clothing.

When you are caring for a resident who has had a spinal cord injury, *immediately report* any of the following signs and symptoms:

- High blood pressure, greater than 200/100
- Sudden, severe pounding headache
- Decreased pulse rate, below 60 beats per minute
- Flushed face

- Nasal congestion
- Sweating above the level of the injury
- Cold, clammy skin and/or "goose bumps" below the level of the injury
- Blurred vision
- Nausea and restlessness

When caring for a resident who may be predisposed to AD, watch for any of the triggers mentioned above and try to prevent it from occurring. If you note any signs or symptoms notify the nurse. Immediately raise the head of the bed at least 45 degrees.

LESSON SYNTHESIS: Putting It All Together

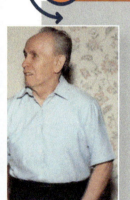

You have just completed this lesson. Now go back and review the Clinical Focus. Try to see how the Clinical Focus relates to the concepts presented in the lesson. Then answer the following questions.

1. Why might self-feeding be difficult for Mr. Raye?
2. Why is it important to carry out range of motion regularly with Mr. Raye?
3. How can ambulation be encouraged and made safer?
4. Nursing assistants must be alert to the possibility of which serious complications that could affect Mr. Raye?
5. Why do Mr. Raye and his family need the emotional support of the staff?

29 REVIEW

A. Select the one best answer for each of the following:

1. The brain and spinal cord make up the

(A) central nervous system

(B) peripheral nervous system

(C) sensory organs

(D) reception system

2. Neurotransmitters are

(A) neurons

(B) special nerves

(C) chemicals that help pass messages from one cell to another

(D) brain cells

3. The brain stem controls

(A) voluntary movements

(B) thinking

(C) vital functions of the body

(D) emotions

4. When the lens of the eye becomes cloudy and impairs vision, it is called

(A) glaucoma

(B) macular degeneration

(C) diabetic retinopathy

(D) cataract

5. Hearing aids should be kept as follows, *except*

(A) at room temperature

(B) on at all times

(C) free of wax

(D) dry

6. Parkinson's disease is due to

(A) a decrease in a neurotransmitter

(B) brain injury

(C) changes in the myelin sheath of the neuron

(D) decreased blood flow to the brain

7. Persons with Parkinson's generally have all of these symptoms, *except*

(A) tremors

(B) rigidity

(C) slowness of movement

(D) high fever

8. Nursing care for persons with Parkinson's disease does not include

(A) instructions for walking

(B) restricting self-care

(C) giving adequate fluids

(D) positioning to avoid flexion

9. A person who has had a stroke on the left side of the brain will

(A) have left hemiplegia

(B) become quick and impulsive

(C) have aphasia

(D) not experience sensory changes

10. The person who has had a stroke on the right side of the brain will

(A) have left hemiplegia

(B) have aphasia

(C) become slow and cautious

(D) not experience sensory changes

11. Residents with stroke

(A) need no support of the arm on the affected side

(B) need passive range-of-motion exercises at least twice a day

(C) should be encouraged to do as little as possible

(D) do not require restorative care

12. Multiple sclerosis occurs because

(A) the myelin sheath of the neuron is damaged

(B) of a hemorrhage in the brain

(C) of a lack of a certain neurotransmitter

(D) muscle damage

13. Residents with multiple sclerosis may experience all of the following, *except*

(A) numbness or tingling in extremities

(B) visual impairments

(C) fatigue

(D) chest pain

14. Spasticity of the muscles in multiple sclerosis may cause

(A) respiratory tract infections

(B) choking

(C) urinary tract infections

(D) urinary incontinence

15. Nursing care for residents with multiple sclerosis does not include

(A) preventing contractures

(B) preventing pressure ulcers

(C) restricting fluids

(D) maintaining mobility as long as possible

16. Huntington's disease is characterized by

(A) hemiplegia

(B) aphasia

(C) chorea

(D) slowness of movements

17. Amyotrophic lateral sclerosis (ALS) causes all of the following, *except*

(A) inability to move independently

(B) disabling fatigue

(C) difficulty speaking

(D) no change in swallowing ability

18. The person with ALS usually has

(A) mental impairment

(B) vision impairment

(C) shortness of breath

(D) hearing impairment

19. Residents with ALS should

(A) be positioned upright as much as possible

(B) be kept as active as possible through the day

(C) be positioned in supine position for several hours a day

(D) communicate by writing

20. Signs and symptoms of myasthenia gravis include all of the following, *except*

(A) weakness of the eye muscles

(B) inability to keep the mouth closed

(C) drooling

(D) unaffected speech

21. One of the most common causes of autonomic dysreflexia is

(A) increased urination

(B) decreased perspiration

(C) distended bladder

(D) low blood pressure

22. The resident with a spinal cord injury is closely monitored for autonomic dysreflexia. This life-threatening condition may cause

(A) severe high blood pressure

(B) severe anemia

(C) chest pain and heart attack

(D) encephalitis and seizures

A. Fill in the blanks by selecting the correct word or phrase from the list.

age-related	glaucoma
macular	hemianopsia
degeneration	hemiplegia
amyotrophic	neurotransmitters
lateral sclerosis	nystagmus
aphasia	paraplegia
autonomic dysreflexia	position sense
cataract	presbycusis
central nervous	presbyopia
system	quadriplegia
dementia	thrombus
equilibrium	unilateral neglect
genetic	

23. Chemicals that help pass nerve impulses from one cell to another are called

_____ .

24. The brain and spinal cord make up the

_____ .

25. The ear is responsible for hearing and for

_____ .

26. Older adults often develop a vision problem called

_____ .

27. A condition in which the pressure within the eyeball is higher than normal is called

_____ .

28. The leading cause of visual loss in this country is

_____ .

29. Many older adults suffer hearing loss called

_____ .

30. Persons with Parkinson's disease may undergo mental changes referred to as

_____ .

31. Stroke may be caused by a blood clot called a

_____ .

32. Paralysis on one side of the body is called

_____ .

33. The inability to express or understand speech is

_____ .

34. If a resident with a stroke cannot tell where the affected foot is, the resident has loss of

_____ .

35. _____ is loss of vision of one-half of the eye in both eyes.

36. _____ means the resident ignores the paralyzed side of the body.

37. Clouding of the lens of the eye is called

_____ .

38. Paralysis of both legs is _____ .

39. Paralysis of all four extremities is

_____ .

40. Jerky eye movements seen in multiple sclerosis are called _____ .

41. Huntington's disease is _____ .

42. The disease also known as Lou Gehrig's disease is

_____ .

43. A syndrome caused by bladder distention in persons with spinal cord injury is known as

_____ .

Residents with Special Needs

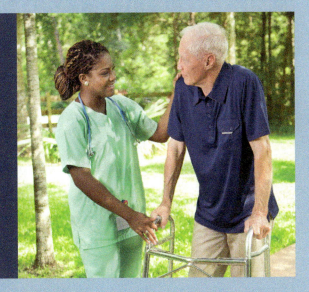

ALZHEIMER'S DISEASE AND RELATED DISORDERS (CARING FOR THE COGNITIVELY IMPAIRED RESIDENT)

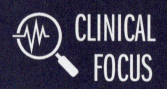

CLINICAL FOCUS

Think about the nursing care required by the resident who suffers from Alzheimer's disease and related disorders as you study this lesson.

OBJECTIVES

After studying this lesson, you should be able to:

- Define vocabulary words and terms.

- List four symptoms of Alzheimer's disease.

- Identify the concerns associated with caring for people with dementia.

- Identify three approaches that are effective when working with residents with Alzheimer's disease or other dementias.

- Describe the differences between an Alzheimer's unit and a general unit.

- State three guidelines for assisting residents with dementia with the activities of daily living (ADLs).

- Describe four effective techniques for communicating with residents with dementia.

VOCABULARY

Alzheimer's disease (ALTZ-high-mers dih-ZEEZ)
antecedent (an-ti-SEED-nt)
aphasia (ah-FAY-zee-ah)
aspiration (ass-pih-RAY-shun)

catastrophic reaction (kat-ah-STROH-fick ree-ACK-shun)
cognitive impairment (KOG-nih-tiv im-PAIR-ment)
delusion (dee-LEW-zhun)

CASE STUDY

Grace McGinnis, who has Alzheimer's disease (stage 2), has been a resident in your facility for almost 2 years. About 10 years ago, she realized that she could not remember details as well as she once had. Gradually, her mental and emotional status declined. Her husband employed a housekeeper to stay with her. Four years later, Mr. McGinnis had a heart attack and died. Family members felt admission to a long-term care facility was the only answer.

dementia (dee-MEN-she-ah)
depression (dee-PRESH-un)
disorientation (dis-oh-ree-en-TAY-shun)
hallucination (hah-loo-sih-NAY-shun)
neurotransmitter (new-roh-TRANS-mit-er)
pacing (PAYS-ing)
perseveration (per-sev-er-AY-shun)
pet therapy (pet THER-ah-pee)

reality orientation (ree-AL-ih-tee oh-ree-en-TAY-shun)
reminiscing (reh-mih-NISS-ing)
sensory-perceptual changes (SEN-sor-ee-per-SEP-tyou-al CHAIN-jes)
sundowning (SUN-down-ing)
validation therapy (val-ih-DAY-shun THER-ah-pee)
wandering (WAN-der-ing)

DEFINITION OF ALZHEIMER'S DISEASE

You will care for residents who have **Alzheimer's disease** or related dementias. **Alzheimer's disease** is a disorder of the brain that involves thinking, central memory, behavior, and personality caused by nerve cell damage and ultimately nerve cell death. As these brain cells die, the person loses mental abilities as well as other bodily functions. Organic brain disease is a general term that is used to describe physical conditions in the body that may cause mental changes (**dementias**) and is commonly found in the elderly population. Examples of physical conditions that may precipitate dementias include conditions such as strokes, breathing problems that may reduce the amount of oxygen to the brain, degenerative disorders such as Parkinson's disease, infections such as meningitis or encephalitis, or other disorders such as kidney disease and vitamin B_{12} deficiencies. The term **cognitive impairment** means that the mental or intellectual abilities of the individual are damaged (Figure 30-1).

The information in this lesson refers to Alzheimer's disease because it is the most common form of dementia. Remember that other dementias have many of the same signs and symptoms. The treatment and care are similar regardless of the medical diagnosis.

Alzheimer's disease can begin during middle age but is more common in older persons. The disease affects people of all races, intelligence levels, education, and financial status. It is progressive and has been called a "slow death" of the mind. In the past, the term *senility* was used to describe these symptoms. We now know that it is a disease of the brain cells and is not normal aging (Figure 30-2).

Research continues into the cause of Alzheimer's disease. The only specific test to confirm the diagnosis of Alzheimer's disease is through an autopsy of the brain. Currently there is no cure for Alzheimer's disease. When symptoms appear, the individual should have a complete medical diagnostic workup.

It is important to rule out other conditions such as diabetes and other endocrine problems, vitamin deficiencies, malnutrition, brain tumors, impaired

Disease	Features	Course
Alzheimer's	Lack of chemical in brain causing neurofibrillary tangles, neuritic plaques	Onset age: 60–80; slowly progressive
Multi-infarct dementia	Interference with blood circulation in brain cells due to arteriosclerosis, atherosclerosis	Onset age: 55–70; outcome depends on rate of damage to brain cells
Huntington's	Inherited from either parent who has gene for the disease	Onset age: 25–45; average duration 15 years
Parkinson's	Deficiency of chemical in brain (dopamine)	Onset age: 55–60; several years duration
Lewy body	Protein deposits inside nerve cells of the brain that control aspects of memory and motor control; displays symptoms of Parkinson's and Alzheimer's disease.	Onset age: 50–85, more predominant in males. Varying length of progression.
Creutzfeldt-Jacob	Noninflammatory virus, changes in brain	Onset age: 50–60; rapidly progressive
Syphilis	Spirochete (bacteria) causes brain damage	Occurs 15–20 years after primary infection
AIDS dementia	HIV-1 infection	Symptoms sometimes precede diagnosis of AIDS

Figure 30-1 Descriptions of major forms of dementia.

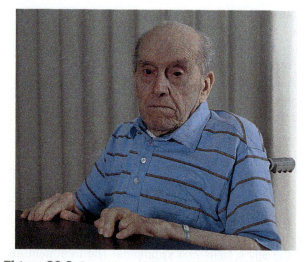

Figure 30-2 Symptoms of Alzheimer's disease are not normal aging. People with dementia exhibit indifference and lack of spontaneity.

circulation, epilepsy, depression, and medication interactions. Unlike Alzheimer's disease, these conditions may be treatable and curable. The diagnostic tests commonly include:

- Blood tests
- Electroencephalogram (EEG), a study of brain waves
- Magnetic resonance imaging (MRI)
- Brain scan
- Psychological evaluation to rule out depression
- Evaluation of all medications being taken including over-the-counter drugs
- Mental status examination

The mental status examination assesses the person's:

- Orientation to time and place
- Attention span
- Ability to recall information
- Ability to use language
- Ability to follow directions
- Ability to read and write
- Ability to copy a design

Changes in the Brain Leading to Alzheimer's Disease

Messages are normally passed between nerve cells (neurons) in the brain by chemicals called **neurotransmitters**. People with Alzheimer's lack one of these chemicals. If an autopsy of the brain is performed after death, distinctive changes are noted.

In normal aging, few brain cells are lost. However, in Alzheimer's disease the neurons (nerve cells) that control memory are destroyed and some lose connections with other nerve cells and die. Consequently, the brain becomes smaller. Cellular changes are noted in the brain. These changes include the formation of neuritic plaques and neurofibrillary tangles, indications that damage has occurred to the brain (Figure 30-3). All of these changes can be confirmed on autopsy after death.

STAGES AND SYMPTOMS OF ALZHEIMER'S DISEASE

Little is certain about Alzheimer's disease. It is believed that changes in the brain may occur for several years before symptoms appear. The most common system, developed by Dr Barry Reisberg of New York University, breaks the progression of Alzheimer's disease into seven stages. The framework for understanding the progression of Alzheimer's disease has been adopted and used by a number of health care providers as well as the Alzheimer's Association.

Stage 1—No Impairment

In the first stage, there is no detection of the disease and memory problems are hardly evident.

Stage 2—Very Mild Decline

The person may notice minor memory problems or lose things around the house. If a memory test is taken during Stage 2, the person will still do well and the disease is unlikely to be detected by physicians or family members.

Stage 3—Mild Decline

At this stage, friends and family may begin to notice memory and cognitive problems. Performance on memory and cognitive tests are affected and physicians will be able to detect impaired cognitive function. The most evident findings include:

- Remembering names of new acquaintances
- Planning and organizing
- Finding the right word during conversations

Stage 4—Moderate Decline

In this stage, clear cut symptoms are apparent:

- Have difficulty with simple arithmetic
- May forget details about their life history

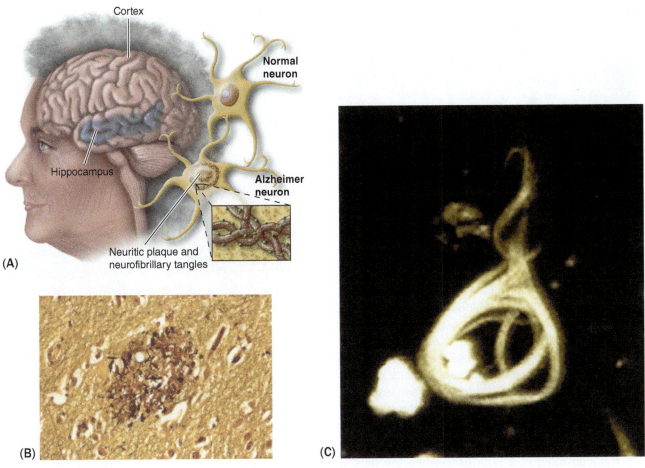

Figure 30-3 (A) Neurofibrillary tangling and neuritic plaques that occur in Alzheimer's disease (AD). (B) An actual AD plaque. (C) An actual AD tangle.

Source B & C: Courtesy of the Alzheimer's Disease Education and Referral Center, a service of the National Institute on Aging.

- Have poor short-term memory (can't remember what was for breakfast)
- Inability to manage finances or pay bills

Stage 5—Moderately Severe Decline

During the fifth stage of Alzheimer's disease, patients begin to require help with day-to-day activities. People experience:

- Significant confusion
- Inability to recall simple details about themselves such as their own phone number
- Difficulty dressing appropriately

On the other hand, patients in stage 5, a modicum of functionality. They can bathe and toilet independently and still know who family members are. During this stage, patients may recall details of their personal histories, especially their childhood and young adult life.

Stage 6—Severe Decline

Patients in this stage usually require constant supervision and professional care. Symptoms include:

- Confusion or unawareness of environment and surroundings
- Major personality changes and potential behavior problems
- The need for assistance with all ADLs
- Inability to recognize faces
- Loss of bowel and bladder control
- Wandering

Stage 7—Very Severe Decline

The final stage of Alzheimer's disease usually leads to death in a fairly short amount of time. During this stage, patients lose the ability to respond to their environment or communicate. They may be able to utter

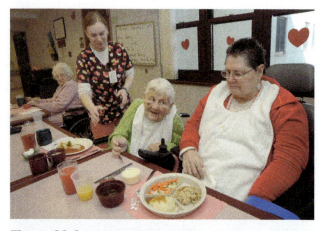

Figure 30-4 Persons with Alzheimer's disease exhibit poor judgment.

words, they have no insight into their condition or realize the extent of their limitations. In the final stage, patients may lose their ability to swallow.

Every person suffering from Alzheimer's disease or a related disorder will progress through the stages at different paces and for different periods of time. This fact alone is one of the reasons families find it difficult to understand or deal with Alzheimer's disease. No two people's journey is the same.

- Sundowning
  - Sundowning is a term used when the person has increased disorientation in the late afternoon, evening, or during the night. Sleeplessness is often accompanied by wandering. The person may go outside and wander in the middle of the night.

⊕〰 CLINICAL FOCUS

Mrs. McGinnis is in stage 2 Alzheimer's disease. Think of specific problems that might occur if she lived alone.

- Sensory-perceptual changes
  - The person with sensory-perceptual changes is unable to recognize an object and use it appropriately. This includes common objects such as eating utensils, combs, and pencils (Figure 30-5). The person is unable to distinguish right from left, up from down, left from right, hot from cold.
- Perseveration
  - Perseveration refers to repeating an action over and over. Examples are repeating the same word or phrase, lip licking, chewing, or finger tapping.

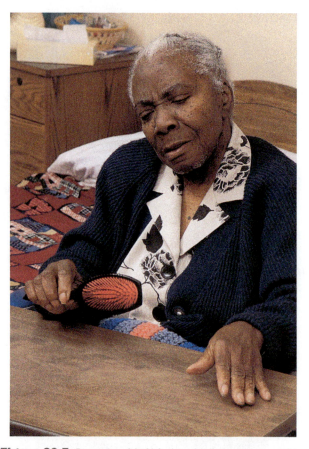

Figure 30-5 Persons with Alzheimer's disease are unable to recognize and use common items appropriately.

- Catastrophic reactions
  - Catastrophic reactions are characterized by increased agitation and anxiety. They may be noted by increased pacing, verbalization, and restlessness or they may result in violent behavior (Figure 30-6).

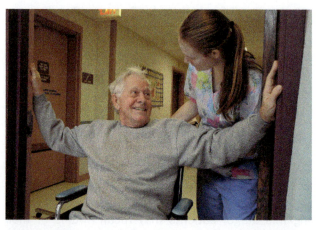

Figure 30-6 Catastrophic reactions may result in violent behavior.

- **Hallucinations**
  - **Hallucinations** are false perceptions of sensory information (seeing, hearing, smelling) that is not real.
- **Gait difficulties**
  - Walking becomes more difficult. The hips may appear to be internally rotated and a shuffling type gait is present.

- **Aphasia**
  - Problems with verbal communication occur. The person is unable to understand others and is unable to express speech. The person may have perseveration of speech or use words inappropriately. Aphasia also affects the ability to read and to write.
- Bowel and bladder incontinence

? EXERCISE 30-1

MATCHING
Match each behavior on the right with the description on the left.

Description Behavior

1. _____ false perceptions of something that is not really there
2. _____ term used when a person has increased disorientation at night
3. _____ fixed false beliefs
4. _____ hiding things that are difficult to find
5. _____ increased and uncontrolled agitation and anxiety
6. _____ collecting items from other residents' rooms
7. _____ repeating actions

a. Delusions
b. Sundowning
c. Hoarding
d. Hallucinations
e. Perseveration
f. Catastrophic reaction
g. Pillaging

? EXERCISE 30-2

MATCHING
Alzheimer's disease is progressive. Signs and symptoms seen in stage I will also be seen in the other stages as well. In this exercise, identify the specific behaviors that identify each stage.

Behavior Stage

1. _____ has seizures
2. _____ more restless during evening hours
3. _____ unable to recognize comb
4. _____ unable to remember eating breakfast
5. _____ verbally unresponsive
6. _____ wanders and paces
7. _____ decreased ability to concentrate
8. _____ careless about appearance
9. _____ totally dependent
10. _____ incontinent of bladder/bowels
11. _____ experiences hallucinations
12. _____ repeats the same word

I

II

III

CARING FOR RESIDENTS WITH DEMENTIA

Caring for a resident with a dementia is challenging, rewarding, and gratifying. Caregivers must be compassionate, patient, and calm and have a sense of humor.

Providing quality care to residents with Alzheimer's disease revolves around the ability of staff members to manage the behaviors of the residents. When caring for residents with Alzheimer's disease or other dementias, it is helpful to remember:

- Residents with Alzheimer's have the same needs as anyone else—physical needs, the need to feel safe and secure, and a need for love and self-esteem. They are dependent on the caregivers to meet these needs (Figure 30-7).

- All behavior has meaning, even though we may not always know what the reason is.

- Behavior is neither good nor bad—it just is. Avoid using negative terms such as uncooperative, rebellious, or hostile to describe behavior.

- Realize that residents with a dementia are not responsible for what they do or say.
  - Their behavior is not intentional and they cannot change.
  - They are not aware of what they are doing.
  - They lose the ability to control their impulses. They may say or do whatever comes into their minds, whether or not it is appropriate (Figure 30-8).

- Avoid confrontation. Always allow them to "save face" and not feel belittled or embarrassed.

- Residents with Alzheimer's disease can "read" us. They respond to nonverbal communication. Their behaviors tend to reflect the behaviors of those around

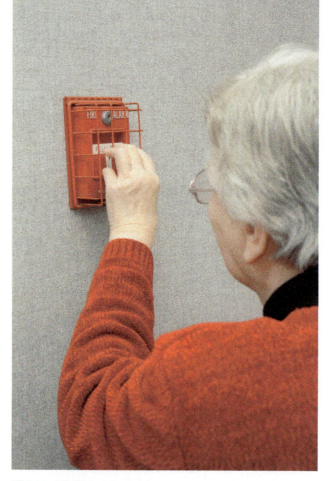

Figure 30-8 People with Alzheimer's disease lose the ability to control their impulses.

them. If staff members are anxious and abrupt, residents will tend to become anxious and agitated.

- Even though both short-term and long-term memory are eventually lost, "affective" memory tends to remain. This means that the resident may not remember certain individuals but will sense feelings of discomfort if that person was unpleasant, rude, or abusive to the resident. This may be reflected in increased verbalization or anxiety or attempts to hit that person.

- If a new behavior occurs, investigate the cause. The resident may have a physical illness or be agitated by the environment.

- Reconsider behaviors. Before attempting to modify a behavior, ask the questions:
  - "Is it interfering with the health or safety of the resident?"
  - "Is it interfering with the health or safety of others?"

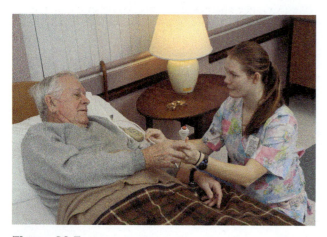

Figure 30-7 People with Alzheimer's disease need love and attention.

- "Is it infringing on the rights of other residents?"
- "Is it causing the resident to be anxious or agitated?"

If the answer to these questions is "no," then the behavior probably does not need modifying.

- No one really knows what is happening in the minds of people with dementia. Never assume that they are unaware of the environment and the people around them.

Goals for Caregiving

Always keep in mind the following goals when caring for residents with Alzheimer's disease or other dementias:

1. Protect the resident from physical injury.
2. Maintain the resident's independence as long as possible.
3. Focus on what the resident is still able to do.
4. Provide physical and mental activities within the resident's capabilities.
5. Support the resident's dignity and self-esteem at all times.

To meet these goals:

1. The care must be consistent. Procedures should be carried out in the same way, all the time. All caregivers should use the same approach.

2. The routine of care should be structured but flexible to accommodate residents when they are more responsive or less responsive.
3. The care must be given in a peaceful, quiet environment that is simple, uncluttered, and unchanged.
4. Staff members must be educated to the needs of the residents with dementia and must learn how to meet these needs.

Alzheimer's Units

Many facilities have established special Alzheimer care units. These units differ from general units in several ways:

- There is a higher staff-to-resident ratio.
- The staff has received special training in Alzheimer's care.
- Cross-training of staff may be done. For example, nursing assistants may help with activities and activity staff or social service staff may help with meals.
- The unit is a "dedicated" unit. This means that the same staff work on the unit all the time. New staff are assigned to the unit only when there is an opening that has to be filled.

⚠ GUIDELINES FOR. . . CARING FOR RESIDENTS WITH ALZHEIMER'S DISEASE

1. Call the person by name. Use eye contact with residents, if culturally appropriate (Figure 30-9). Make sure you have their attention.

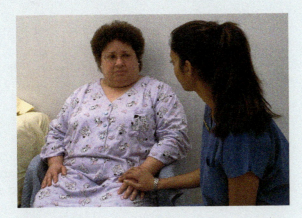

Figure 30-9 Use eye contact, if culturally appropriate.

2. Use appropriate body language.
3. Accept residents as they are without being judgmental or critical.
4. Use touch appropriately. This can be soothing, but if a resident is surprised by the body contact, it can result in a catastrophic reaction.
5. Use simple words and short sentences. Avoid using logic, reasoning, or lengthy explanations. This will only increase the resident's agitation.
6. Allow enough time for a response; do not interrupt.
7. Remember that when the ability to use speech is lost, communication can still occur through non-verbal means.
   - Biting, scratching, and kicking may be the only way the resident can express displeasure.

(continues)

▲ GUIDELINES FOR. . . PREPARING TO MEASURE BLOOD PRESSURE (Continued)

- Facial expressions, body language, and the resident's eyes may give clues to feelings and moods (Figure 30-10).
- Learn what triggers agitation or anger and work on preventing these situations.

8. Use techniques of diversion and distraction. These work well because of the resident's shortened attention span. Calmly take the resident by the hand and walk together or direct the resident's attention to another activity.

9. Remember that the most important qualities for caregivers are to:
   - Be creative. Be willing to look beyond the usual procedures and routines for solutions to giving care.
   - Be able to laugh with the resident (Figure 30-11). Many of them retain a keen sense of humor for a long time. Laughter is beneficial for residents and staff.
   - Be able to go back in time with the resident. If the resident is living in 1950, think of what life was like then.

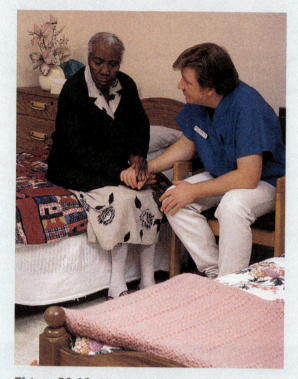

Figure 30-10 Observe facial expressions and body language for clues to the resident's feelings.

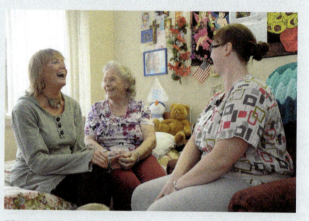

Figure 30-11 A sense of humor is beneficial for staff and residents.

This type of staffing results in:
- Staff who have a special interest in Alzheimer's residents.
- Staff who know each resident, their strengths, and their weaknesses.
- Staff who better understand the need to facilitate an interdisciplinary support system.
- Staff who can provide valuable input for the plan of care.

The environment is specially designed to:
- Provide calmness and serenity through the use of color and design.
- Avoid disturbing noises. For example, there is no loudspeaker system, telephones do not ring, and televisions are turned on only when appropriate.

- Be secure, so that residents may wander at will without threat of danger.
- Most activities can take place on the unit. The dining room and activities areas are incorporated into the unit.
- Families are encouraged to take part in the care and activities if they wish.

Residents must meet certain pre-established criteria before being admitted to the special unit. This is to ensure that placement will benefit the resident and also the other residents.

Resident's Rights

Residents with dementia have the same rights as other residents. They may need assistance to ensure that these rights are protected. It is important to remember that:

- Making decisions and having choices is a resident's right. However, residents with dementia may be unable to make decisions and may become overwhelmed with too many choices. This can cause the resident to become very upset.
- Staff must protect residents with dementia. Do not allow them to be taken advantage of or abused by other people.
- The rights of residents with dementia do not have priority over the rights of other residents. For example, it is upsetting to other residents to have confused residents wandering into their rooms. The resident with dementia is not aware of this. It is the staff's responsibility to resolve these issues without infringing on the rights of either resident.
- Residents with dementia have the right to have possessions that give them pleasure as long as these do not impair the health or safety of the resident or other people. For example, if a resident receives pleasure from a doll or stuffed animal, do not take it away. Above all, do not tease or make fun of the situation. The resident deserves to be treated with dignity (Figure 30-12).

Family Members

In most cases, family members have cared for the resident with a dementia for months or years before admission to the long-term care facility. By the time the decision is made to admit the individual, the family is often physically and emotionally drained. The admission is a traumatic experience. As you work with the residents with Alzheimer's or other dementias, remember:

1. The family remembers the resident as a vital family member. Acknowledge the family's presence.
2. Listen to the family's suggestions. They often know what will work and what will not be effective in caring for the new resident.
3. Allow the family to participate in the care, if they choose to and if it is appropriate. For example, many family members like to assist the resident at mealtime.
4. The spouse of the resident may have no other support system. If they have children, they may be many miles away. It can be very upsetting not to be recognized by a spouse of many years. Some facilities have support groups for families. In addition, the local Alzheimer's Association (800-272-3900) sponsors support groups. The National Institute on Aging is studying how computers can be used to provide information and support to family caregivers. Computer-based chat rooms and bulletin boards are being established. Interested persons can ask questions and have them answered in the privacy of their homes. Medical advice forums are also available. Computer use is convenient and available around the clock and it can reach many people at one time.

Recreational Activities

- Residents with dementia need activities that match their level of ability.
- Avoid large groups or competitive activities.
- In later stages, use sensory stimulation with soft touching, quiet talk, familiar odors, or old time pictures.
- Puppies or kittens (**pet therapy**) bring pleasure to severely impaired residents.
- Activities with children may also be satisfying to the residents with dementia.
- Music is an appropriate activity. Residents with dementia respond to soft music from their past. Many of them like to dance. Old hymns are also a favorite.
- "Normalizing" activities are beneficial. Consider the resident's past and provide opportunities for:
  - Folding towels and washcloths
  - Dusting
  - A hand craft such as knitting (Figure 30-13)
  - Baking (with supervision)
  - Using a manual carpet sweeper
  - "Tinkering" with familiar tools (with supervision)

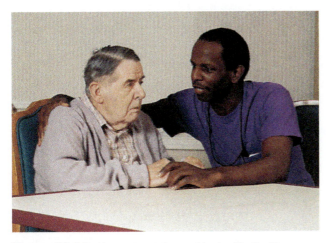

Figure 30-12 Always treat the resident with dignity.

⚠ GUIDELINES FOR. . . ACTIVITIES OF DAILY LIVING (ADLs)

1. Allow the resident to do as much as possible.
   - Use hand-over-hand techniques for personal care and eating.
   - Give only one short, simple direction at a time.

2. Assist the resident to maintain a dignified, attractive appearance by helping with grooming, dressing, and hygiene. Residents may be unaware of soiled or torn clothing.
   - Help them change when necessary.
   - Pick out clothing for the resident or hold out two outfits for the resident to choose from. Residents with a dementia are unable to make decisions. If you ask the resident, "What do you want to wear today?" the resident may become agitated. She cannot remember what is in her closet. Showing the resident all of the clothing is overwhelming and will also cause agitation.

3. Residents with dementia may not want to bathe.
   - Consider the resident's previous habits. Did the resident prefer a tub bath or shower? How often did the resident bathe? Was bathing done in the morning or evening?
   - Check the environment. Is the room warm enough? Is it light enough? Is there adequate privacy?
   - Do not ask the resident "Do you want to take a bath now?" The resident may say "no" every time you ask. Calmly walk with the resident to the bathroom. When you get there say, "I am going to help you with your bath now" and begin the bath procedure calmly and slowly. If the resident refuses, try again later.
   - Do not attempt to remove the resident's clothes right away. Many residents feel unsafe when they are nude. When the resident realizes he is going to get wet, he will usually be willing to undress.

4. Monitor food and fluid intake.
   - Too many foods at once are confusing.
   - Place one food at a time in front of the resident.

   - Use a bowl rather than a plate.
   - Do not use plastic utensils that can break in the resident's mouth.
   - Provide nutritious finger foods when the resident is unable to use utensils.
   - Offer four to six smaller meals rather than three larger ones. Check the resident's plan of care.
   - Avoid pureed foods as long as possible.
   - Check food temperatures before serving.
   - Prepare foods for eating by buttering the bread, cutting meat, opening cartons.
   - If you are feeding the resident, watch for swallowing. Sometimes they will appear to be chewing long after they have swallowed (perseveration).
   - Check the resident's mouth after eating. Pocketing or retaining food in the cheeks can cause **aspiration** (the food goes into the trachea or windpipe).
   - Maintain adequate fluid intake. Residents with dementia may not realize when they are thirsty.
   - Weigh the resident regularly to detect patterns of weight gain or loss.
   - Maintain a quiet and calm environment for eating.

5. Residents with dementia eventually lose bowel and bladder control. Taking residents to the bathroom every 2 hours keeps them dry and prevents skin breakdown. For successful toileting:
   - Toilet regularly. Do not wait for the person to ask.
   - Evaluate wandering and pacing behavior for possible need to toilet.
   - Provide privacy.
   - Make sure the bathroom is warm, quiet, and calm.
   - Allow the resident ample time to eliminate urine or stool.
   - Provide comfort. A commode may work better than the toilet.
   - Praise success.

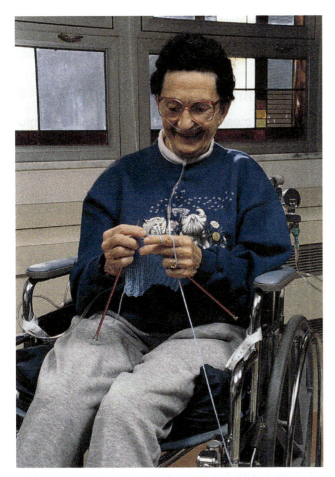

Figure 30-13 Familiar tasks bring enjoyment.

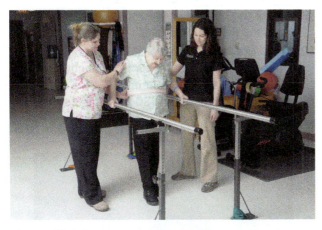

Figure 30-14 Daily exercise is important.

Daily exercise must be planned according to the resident's habits and abilities (Figure 30-14).

- The resident who wanders or paces throughout the day may need only range-of-motion exercises. Note signs of overexertion and weight loss.
- Residents in the final stage will need passive range-of-motion exercises at least twice a day.

- Many recreational activities can be directed to the abilities of the resident:
  - Shooting baskets
  - Bowling
  - Volleyball
  - Hitting a ball with a bat
  - Video game systems such as the Nintendo Wii®, Sony PlayStation 3, Move®, Microsoft X-Box 360, and Kinect® have proved to be valuable assets for physical and occupational as well as recreational therapy.

Community outings may also be enjoyable. Plan outings carefully and be sure that:

- There will be no excessive sensory stimulation. This will agitate many of the residents.
- The residents will not be fearful of wide, open spaces.
- Public places can accommodate residents with mobility problems.
- The residents will not be mistreated by others if they exhibit unusual behaviors in public.

SPECIAL PROBLEMS

Wandering and Pacing

Residents with Alzheimer's disease may wander or pace for hours at a time. No one knows why this occurs. Some reasons may be:

- They are looking for companionship, security, or loved ones.
- It is a way to handle stress.
- They realize they are in a strange environment and are looking for home.

When this behavior occurs:

1. Allow them to wander. The use of restraints increases their anxiety and frustration, resulting in other problems.
2. Adapt the environment to the residents, making it safe and secure. There are many types of security systems available. Getting lost, rather than falling, may be a problem. When the resident walks off, walk with the resident, gradually returning to the direction of the facility.
3. Watch wandering residents for signs of fatigue. They may have forgotten how to sit down and will need reminders and demonstrations of how to get into the chair or bed. Encourage rest periods.
4. Special chairs for residents with Alzheimer's disease allow the residents to rock without tipping over.

the behavior is exhibited. The "B" signifies the behavior itself, such as agitation, wandering, or confusion. The "C" stands for consequences or the result of the behavior.

When the nursing assistant is caring for the resident with dementia, it is helpful to be observant as to the causes or antecedents of the behavior. It may be possible through your observations to help the nurse identify and record the causes and possibly alter the situation(s) that have precipitated the behavior. You may note that a person becomes very agitated when there is a lot of noise, possibly every time the resident enters the dining room. That particular resident may do better in a less stressful environment. As a consequence, the resident's meals could be served in a quiet room with several other residents rather than in the communal dining room. It is important to evaluate the results of this action to note if the solution yields positive results.

SPECIAL MANAGEMENT TECHNIQUES

Reality Orientation

Reality Orientation (RO) is used for helping disoriented residents remain oriented to the environment, to time, and to themselves. When used appropriately, it decreases anxiety in the resident. RO may be effective in the first stages of dementia. In later stages, it is meaningless and increases agitation. Follow these basic guidelines for RO:

1. Always treat residents as adults, with respect and dignity, no matter how confused they may be.
2. Speak clearly and directly. Avoid the temptation to speak louder when they do not understand.
3. Give simple, brief instructions and responses.
4. Set and maintain a structured, flexible routine.
5. Be polite and sincere.
6. Allow residents to be independent as long as possible.
7. Give residents adequate time to respond.
8. Set residents' watches to the correct time.
9. Make sure they have clean eyeglasses and hearing aids if they need them.
10. Place large-numbered calendars in rooms and cross off the days as they pass.
11. Placement of large-numbered clocks around the facility helps orient residents to the time of day.
12. Call residents by name. Disoriented residents usually respond more quickly to their first names.
13. Tell residents your name, but do not expect them to remember you.
14. Use RO in conversation with residents—"It's only March fifth today, but it is very warm outside."

When using RO:

1. Do not put residents on the spot. For example, do not ask, "Do you remember who I am?" or "Do you know what day this is?" If you need to verify their orientation, ask them, "What are your plans for today?" The answer usually will tell you if the resident is oriented.
2. Answer questions honestly but avoid giving the residents information they are unable to handle. A resident whose husband is deceased may ask, "Is my husband coming today?" It is cruel to answer by saying, "Remember, your husband died 2 years ago." This response is likely to trigger a catastrophic reaction. It is better to answer by asking another question: "Emma, will you tell me about your husband?" She will receive pleasure from reminiscing and may work up to the present time on her own.
3. Never argue with a resident's reality. When a resident has a delusion, arguing increases anxiety and agitation. Many delusions are based on past life experiences. Because the resident is disoriented, the experience seems to be happening in the present. Some residents may be much happier if they are living in the past. If this is true, do not force reality on them.
4. Residents with some forms of dementia may have moments of orientation from time to time. Do not assume the resident is disoriented because you do not understand what the resident is saying.
5. Do not reinforce the resident's confusion or tease the resident about the confusion.
6. Remember that a pleasant facial expression, relaxed body language, and caring touch are the most important aspects of caring for disoriented residents.

Reminiscing

Reminiscing is a natural activity for people of all ages. We tend to reminisce when we see old friends or get together with families.

1. Pleasant times from the past are remembered and enjoyed.
2. As people age, the tendency to reminisce increases and is more important.

? EXERCISE 30-4

In each of the following situations, determine if the nursing assistant remembered the guidelines of reality orientation by answering yes (Y) or no (N).

1. _____ The nursing assistant calls Mrs. Paclat "honey" and "granny."

2. _____ The nursing assistant asks questions such as "Do you know who I am?"

3. _____ When the resident asked the whereabouts of her dead husband, the nursing assistant said "Don't you remember, he died before you came to live here."

4. _____ The nursing assistant keeps a large calendar and clock in full view of the resident.

5. _____ The nursing assistant tells the resident that her daughter did not visit today even though the resident insists that she did.

---

3. It is an appropriate activity for residents in early stages of dementia if long-term memory is still intact.

4. Reminiscing may serve as a life review as past life experiences are remembered. This process can also bring back unpleasant memories. If this occurs, the situation must be handled skillfully and tactfully. If these experiences are resolved, peace of mind can be found. The recall of happy memories can confirm the worth and value of the individual's life (Figure 30-16).

5. Reminiscing can help people adapt to old age. It helps to maintain self-esteem and allows them to work through personal losses.

6. When we listen to residents reminisce, we understand them better.

7. Reminiscing therapy can be a group activity. The leader must be skillful and sensitive to the feelings of the members.

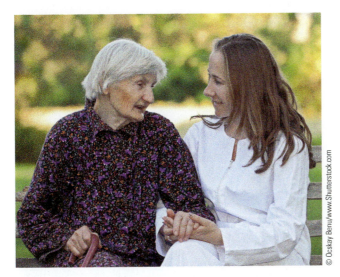

Figure 30-16 Reminiscing can help recall happy times.

Validation Therapy

Validation therapy was developed by Naomi Feil. It is based on the following assumptions:

1. The identity and dignity of the residents must be maintained.

2. We can help disoriented people with dementia feel good about themselves.

3. There is a reason for all behavior. What seems like disoriented behavior may be an acting out of memories.

4. Feelings and memories can be acknowledged.

5. Disoriented people have the right to express feelings when they are no longer able to be oriented to reality.

6. Living must be resolved to prepare for dying.

7. Elderly persons may have experienced so many losses during a lifetime that they have no coping abilities left.

8. To live in reality is not the only way to live.

9. Disoriented people have worth. We can give them joy by allowing them to express themselves.

10. Within each disoriented person is a human being who was once a child and later an adult with hopes, joys, sadness, failures, and successes. They deserve to be cared for and loved in their final years.

Validation therapy employs the use of conversation with a person who has dementia. The caregiver accepts the values and beliefs of the resident, even though they may differ from reality. Residents with dementia are apt to perceive events as being different from the actual situation. Allow the residents to express their feelings and emotions. Use a calm, nonthreatening manner in your response. When possible, draw on the residents own words to redirect the conversation. If, for example, the person is looking for their car keys, say something like, "What kind of car do you have?" This can potentially lead to a discussion about the color of the car, how long they owned the car, and how they liked the car. You may know the person has not driven a car in 25 years but you will be able to change the direction of the discussion without upsetting the resident and eventually move off the subject of cars. This form of therapy can help residents regain feelings of dignity and self-control. You will be trained in the use of this technique if your facility incorporates this form of therapy into the residents' plans of care.

? EXERCISE 30-5

COMPLETION

Answer the following statements about nursing assistants' actions with A for appropriate or I for inappropriate. If the action is inappropriate, write the appropriate action in the space provided.

1. _____ Avoid looking directly at the resident when speaking to him or her.
   _____

2. _____ Act annoyed if you feel like it because the resident does not know what is going on anyway.
   _____

3. _____ Carefully explain each of your actions in detail.
   _____

4. _____ Quickly correct inappropriate resident behavior so that the action does not become a habit.
   _____

5. _____ Touch residents gently and not abruptly.
   _____

6. _____ Watch the resident for body language to gain clues about his or her behavior._
   _____

7. _____ Recognize that residents can change behaviors if they try hard enough.
   _____

8. _____ Allow residents to always save face.
   _____

9. _____ Listen to family members but do not follow their suggestions because they usually have no medical knowledge.
   _____

LESSON SYNTHESIS: Putting It All Together

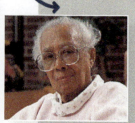

You have just completed this lesson. Now go back and review the Clinical Focus. Try to see how the Clinical Focus relates to the concepts presented in the lesson. Then answer the following questions.

1. Why do people think of Alzheimer's disease as a "slow death of the mind?"

2. Why do the families of residents with Alzheimer's disease need special understanding and support?

3. Because Mrs. McGinnis is in stage 3, what special safety precautions must be observed?

4. What special characteristics are needed in a nursing assistant who cares for residents suffering from Alzheimer's disease?

30 REVIEW

A. Select the one best answer for each of the following.

1. Alzheimer's disease is

(A) curable

(B) preventable

(C) progressive

(D) congenital

2. Alzheimer's disease is more common in

(A) young people

(B) older people

(C) middle-aged people

(D) the white race

3. One of the first symptoms of Alzheimer's disease is

(A) short-term memory loss

(B) long-term memory loss

(C) aphasia

(D) sundowning

4. Delusions are

(A) false perceptions of sensory information

(B) an example of sensory-perceptual changes

(C) false, fixed ideas

(D) the result of catastrophic reactions

5. Goals for giving care to residents with Alzheimer's include all but

(A) protecting the resident from physical injury

(B) maintaining the resident's independence as long as possible

(C) focusing on what the resident can do

(D) limiting activities for safety reasons

6. Sundowning refers to

(A) improved sleep behavior at night.

(B) increased restlessness in the late afternoon, evening, and night.

(C) going to bed as the sun sets.

(D) becoming sleepy at dusk.

7. Reminiscing is used to help residents

(A) forget problems

(B) orient the person to reality

(C) remember past experiences

(D) regain dignity

8. The resident repeatedly attempts to get out the front door of the facility. Which of the following is *not* an appropriate response by the staff?

(A) Remind him to stay indoors.

(B) Make sure he is wearing the sensor bracelet.

(C) Talk in a calm voice.

(D) Restrain him in his room.

9. When a resident with Alzheimer's disease takes something from another resident's room, this is considered to be

(A) stealing

(B) pillaging

(C) collecting

(D) hoarding

10. Validation therapy is based on all of the following, *except*

(A) helping persons who are disoriented feel good about themselves.

(B) acknowledging feelings and memories.

(C) there are reasons behind all behavior.

(D) living in reality is the only way to live.

B. Answer each statement true (T) or false (F).

11. T F There are many types of dementia.

12. T F There is no specific test for diagnosing Alzheimer's disease.

13. T F Alzheimer's disease is the result of poor circulation in the brain.

14. T F Residents who wander should be restrained.

15. T F Catastrophic reactions may result from too much stimulation in the environment.

16. T F Residents with Alzheimer's disease are unable to feel emotion.

17. T F Residents with Alzheimer's disease frequently exhibit bad behavior.

18. T F The best way to manage behavior is to use logic to reason with the resident.

19. T F Many residents with Alzheimer's disease have a keen sense of humor.

20. T F Reminiscing is healthy and beneficial.

21. T F Residents' rights do not apply to residents with Alzheimer's disease.

22. T F A dignified, attractive appearance is important for residents with Alzheimer's disease.

23. T F Residents with Alzheimer's disease enjoy large group activities.

24. T F Baking is an example of a "normalizing" activity.

25. T F Some residents are happier if they are living in the past.

CARING FOR RESIDENTS WITH DEVELOPMENTAL DISABILITIES

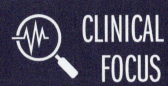

CLINICAL FOCUS Think about the special care needs of the resident who is developmentally disabled as you study this lesson.

OBJECTIVES

After studying this lesson, you should be able to:

- Define vocabulary words and terms.
- List the characteristics present in a developmental disability.
- List four examples of developmental disabilities.
- Describe three possible causes of a developmental disability.
- Define the classifications of intellectual disability.
- Describe different types of seizures.

VOCABULARY

adaptive behavior (ah-DAP-tiv bee-HAYV-yur)
anoxia (ah-NOX-ee-ah)
ataxic cerebral palsy (ah-TACK-sick SER-ew-bral PAWL-zee)
athetoid cerebral palsy (ATH-eh-toyd SER-ew-bral PAWL-zee)
behavior modification (bee-HAYV-yur mod-ih-fih-KAY-shun)
cerebral palsy (SER-ew-bral PAWL-zee)
developmental disability (dee-vel-op-MEN-tal dis-ah-BILL-ih-tee)
diplegia (die-PLEE-jee-ah)
electroencephalogram (EEG) (ee-leck-troh-en-SEF-ah-loh-gram)

epilepsy (EP-ih-lep-see)
grand mal seizure (grand mahl SEE-zhur)
hemiplegia (hem-ee-PLEE-jee-ah)
hyperbilirubinemia (high-per-bil-e-roo-bin-E-me-a)
intelligence quotient (IQ) (in-TELL-ih-jens KWOH-shent)
mental retardation (MEN-tal ree-tar-DAY-shun)
petit mal seizure (peh-TEE mahl SEE-zhur)
quadriplegia (kwahd-rih-PLEE-jee-ah)
Reye's syndrome (RISE SIN-drome)
seizure (SEE-zhur)
spastic cerebral palsy (SPAS-tick SER-ew-bral PAWL-zee)

CASE STUDY Teresa Michaels is developmentally disabled and unable to care for herself. Her mind is bright and keen. She is unable to use her hands for self-care because of the spastic paralysis related to her cerebral palsy.

CHARACTERISTICS OF A DEVELOPMENTAL DISABILITY

Long-term care facilities often provide care for residents with **developmental disabilities**. Developmental disabilities are a distinct and varied group of severe chronic conditions that are due to mental and/or physical impairments such as:

- Cerebral palsy
- Mental retardation
- Autism spectrum disorders
- Attention deficit hypersensitivity disorder
- Hearing impairment
- Vision impairment

A developmental disability has specific characteristics. It is:

- Caused by a mental or physical impairment or a combination of both
- Apparent before 22 years of age (some states indicate before 18 years of age)
- Likely to continue indefinitely

In addition, the disability must result in functional limitations in three or more of these life activities:

- Self-care
- Use of receptive and expressive language
- Learning
- Mobility
- Self-direction
- Independent living
- Economic self-sufficiency

Because of these limitations, the person who is developmentally disabled requires lifelong care, treatment, or services (Figure 31-1).

Some residents in your facility who have developmental disabilities did not acquire these as adults. Federal legislation forbids the admission of persons with developmental disabilities to skilled nursing facilities unless the facilities are licensed to care for them. However, there may be residents who were in the facility before this law was implemented. They may also be admitted if they have another medical problem that requires skilled nursing care.

A developmental disability may be caused by:

- A condition that impairs the development of the brain or body before birth (Figure 31-2)
- A condition that causes damage to the newborn infant during the birth process
- A disease or injury that causes damage to the brain or body after birth, before the age of 22 years, or the age specified by state regulations

At one time, people with developmental disabilities often died before reaching adulthood. Today they frequently live a normal life span. During childhood they go to school and attend classes that meet their needs and abilities. After graduating, they may work in a sheltered workshop or obtain a job that they are capable of doing. They may be able to

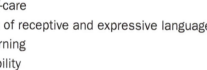

Figure 31-1 The resident on the right has needed assistance with activities of daily living throughout his life.

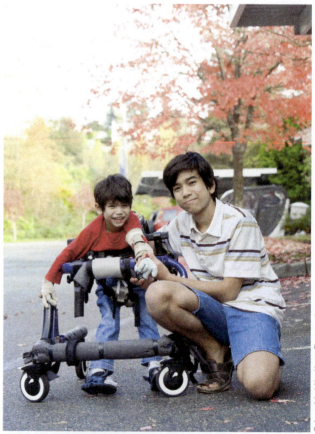

Figure 31-2 A child with a developmental disability.

live independently with assistance or in supervised group homes. Some people with milder disabilities may marry and have children.

People with developmental disabilities also experience the aging process. Sometimes the changes of aging combined with the disability make it increasingly difficult for them to function.

Of the many types of developmental disabilities, some affect physical function, some affect mental function, and some affect both. Persons with mental retardation are developmentally disabled. However, not all persons who are developmentally disabled are mentally retarded (Figure 31-3).

Legislation has been in effect for nearly 50 years to assure that individuals with developmental disabilities and their families receive the services and support that they need. Persons with developmental disabilities are encouraged to be independent and productive, to be integrated into the community in which they live, and to reside in the least restrictive environment possible. For some, this environment will be their own home; for others, it may be the long-term care setting.

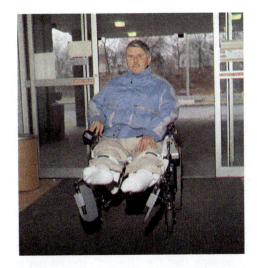

Figure 31-3 This man is developmentally disabled but not mentally impaired.

Each state is responsible for ensuring that needed services are provided. Every few years the Developmental Disabilities Assistance Act (DD Act) is reviewed and updated; the latest revision occurred in 2000.

? EXERCISE 31-1

COMPLETION

Complete the following statements by writing in the correct words.

1. The three characteristics of a developmental disorder are that it is:

    a. _____

    b. _____

    c. _____

2. The disorder must result in functional limitations in three or more of six life activities. These six activities include:

    a. _____

    b. _____

    c. _____

    d. _____

    e. _____

    f. _____

3. The individual who is developmentally disabled requires care that is

    _____

    _____

4. Three causes of developmental disabilities include:

    a. _____

    b. _____

    c. _____

5. People with developmental disabilities may have a _____ life span.

INTELLECTUAL DISABILITY (MENTAL RETARDATION)

The result of Rosa's Law, which was signed in October 2010, removes the terms "mental retardation" and "mentally retarded" from federal health, education, and labor policy and replaces it with the language, "individual with an intellectual disability" and "intellectual disability." The change in terminology reflects respect, value, and dignity for persons with intellectual disabilities (Figure 31-4).

Originally, *mental retardation* was a clinical term but it has come to be used widely in today's society to degrade and insult people with intellectual disabilities. By changing the terminology, the federal government is sending a strong message that the "R-word" should not be used to refer to any citizens. The Special Olympics (SE) has long been dedicated to promoting this respect. "Spread the Word to End the Word" is an ongoing effort by SE Best Buddies International to raise awareness about the hurtful and dehumanizing effects of the word "retard(ed)."

The definition did not change. **Mental retardation** or intellectual disability is a condition diagnosed before the age of 18 that includes below-average intellectual function, and a lack of skills needed for everyday living. Symptoms include continued infant-like behavior, decreased ability to learn, failure to meet the markers of intellectual development, inability to meet educational demands at school, and lack of curiosity. Behavior may vary from mild to very severe.

Causes of Intellectual Disability

Causes of mental impairment can be divided into several categories:

- Infections (present at birth or occurring after birth): such as congenital rubella–measles, encephalitis, HIV infection, and meningitis.

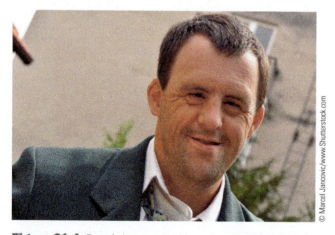

Figure 31-4 Rosa's law resulted in a change of terminology that reflects respect and dignity for persons with intellectual disabilities.

- Abnormalities in the chromosomes; deletions, defects in, or error in numbers such as with Down syndrome.
- Environmental factors such as deprivation.
- Genetic abnormalities and inherited metabolic disorders.
- Metabolic: such as hypoglycemia (poorly regulated diabetes), **Reye's syndrome**, or **hyperbilirubinemia** (very high levels of bilirubin in babies).
- Nutritional: malnutrition
- Toxic: intrauterine exposure to alcohol, cocaine, amphetamines, and other drugs; lead poisoning
- Trauma (before and after birth), intracranial hemorrhage, lack of oxygen to the brain (before during or after birth), and severe head injury.
- Unexplained: There are still a number of unexplained reasons for the development of mental disabilities.

Diagnosing Intellectual Disabilities

Intellectual disabilities are diagnosed, ideally by an interdisciplinary team. They use a number of tools in testing and examining two main areas. The person must have:

- The ability to learn, think, solve problems, and understand how to get along in the world. (This is called **intelligence quotient** or **IQ**.)
- The skills needed to live independently, also referred to as **adaptive behavior**.

Testing for Level of Impairment

People with mental impairment do not all have the same degree of disability. Screening tests may be performed during infancy if a delay in development is noted. The Denver Development Screening Test (DDST) is an important tool that is used to detect developmental problems in very young children. Another test referred to as an Adaptive Behavior Scale also is used. This scale measures a person's behaviors as they relate to ADLs, self-help skills, physical and social development, language ability, and time and number concepts. In addition, this scale examines inappropriate behaviors and violence and self-abuse. The results are compared to the expected behavior of people of the same chronological age. The IQ test is another measure; however, the results of the IQ test *alone* do not confirm absence or presence of mental retardation. Intelligence is not a constant. It is variable and is influenced by emotions and the environment. The IQ level used for classification can vary depending upon the test being used, but a score below 70 on a standardized IQ test may be a sign of mental retardation.

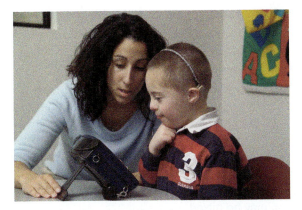

Figure 31-5 Early intervention is important for children with developmental disabilities.

The key to helping to work with a person with an intellectual disability is early intervention (Figure 31-5).

Persons with moderate mental impairment can be taught activities of daily living (ADLs). These persons need a sheltered environment and support. Severely retarded persons may have impairments in motor development, speech, and language. They may be physically challenged and need assistance with self-care. A controlled environment and supervision are needed. Profoundly retarded persons require constant care and supervision. All areas of development are impaired. Refer to Figure 31-6 for a listing of the levels of severity of intellectual disability.

Many services are available to meet the needs of persons with mental retardation. Children can benefit from special education and training. A program that is started early and is consistent is most effective in meeting their special needs and helping them to enjoy a good quality of life. Remember that individuals with mental impairment have all the needs of another person of the same chronological age. They need affection, discipline, and acceptance just as all humans do. They are less able, however, to handle rejection or confusion or the demands of too high expectations.

Families, too, need support and empathy because they may be dealing with personal feelings of guilt and frustration.

If people with mental impairment are living in your facility, the care you give depends on the:

- Specific problems of the individual
- Age of the individual

Levels	IQ
Mild	50–55 to 70
Moderate	35–40 to 50–55
Severe	20–25 to 35–40
Profound	Less than 20–25

Figure 31-6 Intellectual disability levels of severity.

- Degree of impairment
- Presence of other physical problems

Even the most profoundly mentally impaired person responds favorably to:

- Pleasant, colorful, personalized surroundings
- The healing and comforting effect of caring persons

OTHER FORMS OF DEVELOPMENTAL DISABILITIES

Cerebral Palsy

The National Institute of Neurological Disorders and Stroke define cerebral palsy as an encompassing term used to describe a group of chronic disorders that impair movement and posture in the first few years of life (usually before age 3) and generally do not worsen over time (Figure 31-7). *Cerebral* refers to the brain and *palsy* means weakness or poor muscle control. The damage is thought to be caused by a lack of oxygen,

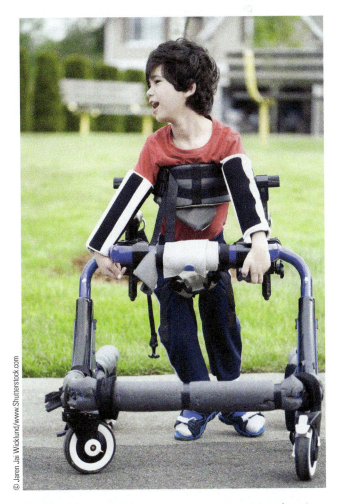

© Jaren Jai Wicklund/www.Shutterstock.com

Figure 31-7 Cerebral palsy impairs movement and posture in the first few years of life. While not curable, therapy can help improve mobility and function.

- Premature birth (leading cause)
- Maternal infection (German measles or other infections early in pregnancy)
- Cerebral anoxia
- Cord around infant's neck
- Jaundice (Rh or blood type incompatibility)
- Difficult delivery
- Head injury
- Meningitis or encephalitis

Figure 31-8 Risk factors for cerebral palsy.

during the developmental stage, to the areas of the brain that are responsible for controlling movement and posture. Cerebral palsy is not communicable and it should not be referred to as a disease. Even though it is not "curable," training and therapy can help to improve function. Figure 31-8 lists several risk factors for cerebral palsy. These risk factors include potential injuries to the baby before, during, or shortly after birth that result in damage to the nervous system.

There are several types of cerebral palsy:

- **Spastic cerebral palsy** (affects 70%–80% of cases)
  - The muscles are tense, contracted, and resistant to movement.
  - The lower legs may turn in and cross at the ankle.
  - The movements of the legs are stiff and resemble the crossed blades of a pair of scissors (scissors gait).

- **Athetoid cerebral palsy**
  - Involuntary, slow, and incessant movements (athetosis) of the parts of the body that are affected.
  - Facial grimacing and drooling may be present.
  - Movements can increase during times of stress.

- **Ataxic cerebral palsy**
  - The principal movement disturbance is a lack of balance and coordination (ataxia).
- Mixed forms
  - It is not uncommon for a person to have symptoms of more than one form of cerebral palsy. They may have problems with speaking, chewing, and swallowing, as well as the inability to focus their eyes, drooling, and loss of bladder or bowel control.
  - Most commonly the spastic and athetoid forms may be mixed.

The terms *diplegia*, *hemiplegia*, and *quadriplegia* may also be used to describe the areas of the body affected by cerebral palsy:

- **Diplegia**—the legs are primarily affected.
- **Hemiplegia**—both the arm and leg on one side are affected.
- **Quadriplegia**—both arms and both legs are affected.

In some cases, symptoms of each type of palsy may be mixed. Persons with cerebral palsy may also have problems in speaking, chewing, and swallowing. They may be unable to focus their eyes. Drooling and loss of bowel or bladder control also occur.

Caring for the Resident with Cerebral Palsy

Care may include:

- Assisting with transport to special education classes or recreation/leisure programs or employment
- Caring for and applying splints and braces
- Performing range-of-motion exercises
- Providing emotional support
- Assisting with ADLs

Other problems associated with cerebral palsy are seizure disorders, mental or emotional impairment, hearing loss, and visual handicaps.

? EXERCISE 31-2

CLINICAL SITUATION
Read the following situation and answer the questions.

Peter Drake is 17 years of age and has a diagnosis of athetoid cerebral palsy. His right arm and hand move constantly in slow involuntary movements. He makes strange facial expressions and drools and sometimes has seizures. His IQ is measured at 33. He makes his home in your facility. Answer the following questions relating to this resident.

emotional   seizures
complete care   severe

(continues)

EXERCISE 31-2 (Continued)

controlled   supervision
personalized   speech
colorful

1. Peter's level of intelligence is described as a _____ intellectual disability.

2. He will require _____ and _____ with his activities of daily living.

3. It is important that he live in a _____ environment.

4. Communication with this resident may be difficult because of his _____ impairment.

5. Peter will have to be guarded against injury during _____.

6. The nursing assistant should maintain a constant pleasant, _____, and _____ surroundings.

7. In addition to meeting Peter's physical needs, the staff must also consider the level of _____ development that is associated with being 17 years old.

Seizure Disorder (Epilepsy)

Epilepsy may be considered a developmental disability if it meets the criteria described at the beginning of this lesson. It is not a disease with a single cause. It is a set of symptoms that arise from abnormal nerve cell activity in the brain. Normally, the nerve cells (neurons) generate small bursts of electrical impulses. These impulses move between neurons, communicating with muscles, sense organs, and glands. In epilepsy, the nerve cell activity is disturbed. This may result in a seizure (convulsion). Sudden bursts of excessive electrical activity are sent from the "disturbed" nerve cells. These bursts may produce unconscious and convulsive movement as well as changes in sensation, behavior, or other muscular activities. If these episodes are recurrent (minutes, hours, days, weeks), then the syndrome is termed epilepsy. The type of seizure that occurs depends on the part of the brain that is affected by the disrupted nerve cell activity. Some causes of seizures are listed in Figure 31-9.

- Neoplasms
- Trauma
- Cerebral anoxia
- Fluid and electrolyte imbalances
- Congenital malformations
- High temperature
- Genetic trait
- Exposure to toxins and chemicals

Figure 31-9 Some causes of seizures.

Partial or generalized seizures may occur. Partial seizures arise from a localized area in the brain and are classified as follows:

1. Simple partial (also known as Jacksonian) seizure
   - Feelings are distorted
   - Seeing flashing lights, hallucinations
   - Smelling foul odors
   - Dizziness
   - Tingling sensations
   - Localized motor seizure
   - Tingling, jerking in one extremity
   - No loss of consciousness
   - May progress to generalized tonic-clonic convulsions

2. Complex partial (psychomotor or temporal lobe) seizure
   - Signs and symptoms vary
   - Purposeless behavior such as chewing movements and uncontrolled speech
   - Glassy stare
   - Aimless wandering
   - Mental confusion
   - Loss of memory following episode

Generalized seizures involve both hemispheres of the brain and are classified as follows, with general symptoms listed:

1. Generalized tonic-clonic seizure (grand mal seizure) (Figure 31-10)
   - Early changes in sensation (aura)
   - Entire body involved
   - Sudden cry

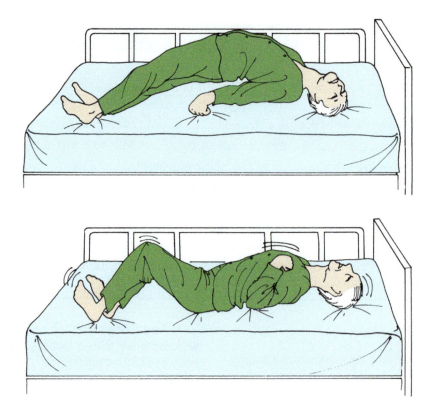

Figure 31-10 Generalized seizures may be accompanied by rigid posturing (A) or uncontrolled movements (B).

- Loss of consciousness
- Involuntary contraction of the muscles producing contortions of body and limbs
- Saliva forms around the mouth causing the appearance of "foaming at the mouth"
- Incontinence of bowel or bladder or both may occur during the seizure
- Lasts 2 to 5 minutes
- Person generally sleeps after the seizure

2. Absence seizure (petit mal seizure)
   - No convulsion
   - Occurs most often in children without warning
   - Lasts 1 to 10 seconds
   - Vacant facial expression, staring eyes
   - No recall of episode

3. Myoclonic seizure
   - Brief involuntary jerking movements of body and extremities (1–2 seconds)
   - Convulsions may occur in rhythmic waves
   - No loss of consciousness

4. Atonic or akinetic seizure
   - Split-second loss of consciousness

- Drop attacks (drooping of the jaw or an extremity or suddenly falling to the floor)
- Lasts 1 to 2 minutes

When seizure activity occurs so frequently that consciousness is not gained between seizures, it is called status epilepticus.

In some people, epilepsy begins during adulthood. This may be the result of:

- An accident causing brain injury
- Brain tumor
- Stroke
- Dementia

The diagnosis of epilepsy is made by performing an electroencephalogram (EEG). A computed tomography (CT) scan or magnetic resonance imaging (MRI) is also performed during the EEG. Electrodes are attached to the scalp to record the brain's electrical activity. The test can determine the presence and type of seizures. The test is painless. The CT scan and MRI permit visualization of the brain structures.

Many medications are able to control seizures. Sometimes the medication dosage has to be readjusted. *Care of the resident who is experiencing a seizure is covered in Lesson 9.*

? EXERCISE 31-3

TRUE OR FALSE

Indicate whether the following statements are true (T) or false (F).

1. T F A seizure disorder may be considered a developmental disability if it also meets the standard criteria of developmental disabilities.

2. T F Seizure disorder has only a single cause.

3. T F In seizures there is abnormal nerve cell activity in the brain.

4. T F Another name for a seizure is a tantrum.

5. T F The type of seizure relates to the part of the brain affected.

6. T F Seizures always involve movement of the entire body.

7. T F In status epilepticus the resident has seizures that occur once each day.

8. T F Children more often experience petit mal seizures, which last 1 to 10 seconds.

9. T F Some seizures may result from strokes.

CARING FOR RESIDENTS WITH DEVELOPMENTAL DISABILITIES

Residents with developmental disabilities may be placed in a long-term care facility for the following reasons:

- The resident may have lived in a facility most of his or her life because family members were not able to provide care.

- The resident may have been admitted as an adult to the facility when the parent(s) became elderly or died (before federal laws were changed).

- The resident may have a medical problem that cannot be treated in the resident's home.

Young adult residents are often admitted for medical problems. Their parents may have devoted all their energies to the lifelong care of their child. It is difficult in these situations for the parents to "turn over" the care of the resident to staff members. It is important to:

- Acknowledge that the parents have learned much about how to care for their child in the years they have provided care.

- Listen to the parents' suggestions and their concerns.

- Answer their questions.

- Allow the parents to participate in the care as much as possible and as much as they wish.

In some cases, the resident may be admitted after one parent has died and the other is no longer able to provide total care. In these situations, the remaining parent may be suffering from guilt for placing the child in the facility. Feelings of anger at the deceased spouse may exist for "leaving" them with this problem. Attempt to understand what the parent is going through. Be kind, considerate, and nonjudgmental.

The care you give depends on the types of problems experienced by the residents with developmental disabilities. These residents are at risk for many physical complications:

- Respiratory tract infections

- Urinary tract infections

- Contractures

- Pressure ulcers

You must study the care plan to learn exactly what approach and procedures you must use. Physical therapy and occupational therapy may be a part of the plan of care (Figure 31-11).

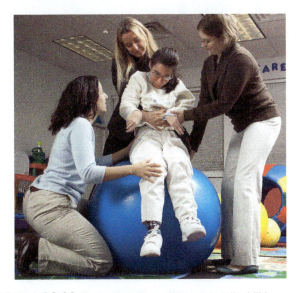

Figure 31-11 Resident with developmental disabilities may need physical therapy.

You may have residents who go out of the facility every day to attend a sheltered workshop. These workshops:

- Train persons with a developmental disability to acquire job skills within their abilities
- Train persons with developmental disabilities to get around in the community by adapting their abilities to the situation
- Provide opportunities for socializing with other people of the same age

Behavior problems may occur. **Behavior modification** is an approach to overcoming these problems that is based on:

- Rewarding positive behaviors
- Initiating corrective actions for negative behaviors

The care plan provides specific approaches and directions regarding the se of behavior modification. Behavior modification will succeed only if all staff members are consistent and follow the plan exactly as it is written.

Persons with developmental disabilities have the same physical and emotional needs as everyone else. When they are in the long-term care facility, it is the responsibility of the staff to provide for these needs so that persons with developmental disabilities will enjoy a life of quality.

LESSON SYNTHESIS: Putting It All Together

© fotaluminate/www.Shutterstock.com

You have just completed this lesson. Now go back and review the Clinical Focus. Try to see how the Clinical Focus relates to the concepts presented in the lesson. Then answer the following questions.

1. **How do you think Teresa's disability affects the way people view her until they get to talk with her and know her?**
2. **Do all people with cerebral palsy have a low IQ?**
3. **What parts of Teresa's body are affected by her condition?**
4. **How are Teresa's special needs being met?**

31 REVIEW

A. Fill in the blanks by selecting the correct word or phrase from the list.

cerebral palsy

developmental disability

diplegia

hemiplegia

mental retardation

twenty-two

1. A severe, chronic disorder present before the age of _____ best describes a _____.

2. When a person has mental function that is significantly below average, with deficits in adaptive behavior, he is said to have _____.

3. A person with mild _____ may be only a little awkward with movements but otherwise be mentally and physically capable.

4. _____ describes the fact that the legs of a person with cerebral palsy are affected.

5. A person with cerebral palsy whose arm and leg on one side are affected has _____.

B. Provide brief answers for each of the following.

6. List three characteristics a disorder must have to be classified as a developmental disability.

7. List seven functional limitations, three of which must be present in addition to those characteristics listed in question 6.

8. Name three possible causes of developmental disabilities.

9. Name four examples of developmental disabilities.

10. List the IQ values for each level of mental retardation: mild, moderate, severe, profound.

11. Describe five activities that may occur during a grand mal seizure.

C. Select the one best answer for each of the following.

12. Children and adults with mental retardation may be

(A) socially mature

(B) emotionally secure

(C) persons over 25 years of age when the disability developed

(D) limited in their ability to learn

13. Mental retardation is not likely to be associated with

(A) Down syndrome

(B) Reye's syndrome

(C) encephalitis

(D) normal physical development

14. A person with mild mental retardation

(A) may need support during stress periods

(B) requires constant care and attention

(C) is always physically challenged

(D) is not able to be educated

15. During a generalized tonic-clonic seizure, the resident

(A) loses consciousness

(B) remains conscious

(C) may wander aimlessly

(D) remembers the event clearly

16. The law that has been responsible for removing the terms *mental retardation* and *mentally retarded* from federal health, education, and labor policies is (the):

(A) Developmental Disability Assistance Act

(B) Medicaid

(C) Rosa's Law

(D) Social Security Act

D. Clinical experience

17. Rachel is 37, has spastic paralysis, and an IQ of 20. She has been a resident in your facility since her mother died. Her father visits infrequently and seems very upset when he sees her. What can you do to help reduce his stress?

18. Lea is a teenage girl who is acting out her frustration with the staff who are following the care plan. The team decides that a behavior modification approach is the way to handle the situation. On what principles is this approach based?

19. Brett is 14 and recently admitted to your facility. His mother, his primary caregiver, died and his father is unable to provide care. Brett was injured when hit by a car 11 years ago. What can you do to ease the anxiety expressed by Brett's father?

CARING FOR THE DYING RESIDENT

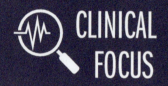

CLINICAL FOCUS

Think about the very special sensitivity the nursing assistant needs as he or she assists residents and their families during the period when death is drawing near as you study this lesson.

OBJECTIVES

After studying this lesson, you should be able to:

- Define vocabulary words and terms.
- Describe hospice and hospice care.
- Define a terminal diagnosis.
- Identify the stages of grieving as described by Elizabeth Kübler-Ross.
- Describe how different people handle the death/dying process.
- Explain how respect to the resident's cultural and religious practices during the dying process is shown.
- Discuss at least five signs of approaching death.
- Demonstrate the following:

  Procedure 32-98   Giving Postmortem Care

VOCABULARY

acceptance (ack-SEP-tans)
anger (AYN-ger)
bargaining (BAR-gan-ing)
code blue (kohd bloo)

comatose (KOH-mah-tohs)
denial (dih-NIGH-al)
depression (dee-PRESH-shun)
do not resuscitate (DNR) (do not re-sus-r-TATE)

CASE STUDY

Ernie Sperling, a Roman Catholic, suffers from terminal cancer. His malignancy originated in his prostate gland and spread throughout his pelvis and into his vertebral column. Despite surgery, radiation, and chemotherapy, the disease progressed. Mrs. Sperling had been separated from her husband for several years, but since his illness has visited him regularly. Mr. Sperling is often angry and uncooperative with the staff and his wife.

hospice (HAHS-piss)
last rites (last rights)
mottling (MOT-ling)
palliative (PAL-ee-uh-tihv)
postmortem (post-MOR-tem)
postmortem care (post-MOR-tem kair)

resuscitation (ree-sus-eh-TAY-shun)
rigor mortis (RIH-gor MOR-tis)
Sacrament of the Sick (SACK-rah-ment of the sick)
terminal illness (TER-mih-nal ILL-ness)
trajectory (tra-JEK-ta-ree)

INTRODUCTION

Death is a universal experience that we all share, yet we find it very difficult to talk about it or even to think about its possibility for ourselves or those we know or love. Our attitudes toward death and dying are influenced by our culture, religion, experience, age, and the support systems we have available to us. The grieving process and how to cope with death and dying are learned through experience.

Young children before the age of 5 years may see death as a punishment. By the age of 7, children know that death is final, although they do not believe that they themselves will die. They may also associate death with punishment and body mutilation. Adults have more fears related to pain, suffering, and invasion of their privacy and final abandonment. They also fear the loss of relationships and experience concerns about the welfare of those who will be left behind. Older people, for the most part, have fewer fears. They may even look forward to release from pain and to joining those who have gone on before (if that is part of their belief system).

The residents you care for may live in the long-term care facility for several months or years. As you get to know them, you may develop special relationships and friendships. Losing a friend through death is a sad experience.

Death, however, is a universal experience. As a nursing assistant in long-term care, you will often work with dying residents and their families. For the elderly with significant health problems, death is not unexpected. The death of younger residents may be more difficult to accept because they are closer in age to the caregivers. It is especially difficult when a young child dies. The role you play in providing care to dying residents is important and one you can perform with dignity.

Death occurs in various ways:

- A resident may be unresponsive for a long time before dying.
- Some residents develop an acute illness and are unable to recover and die suddenly.
- Others die quietly in their sleep.

HOSPICE CARE

The philosophy of **hospice** care recognizes that death is a natural process not to be hastened or delayed, and the dying person should be kept comfortable physically, emotionally, and socially. Hospice incorporates the principle of **palliative** care (relief of symptoms such as pain), not of cure. The care is usually provided to persons who are **terminally ill**, that is, those who have a life expectancy of 6 months or less. This time frame is variable, however, because no one can accurately predict the exact time of death.

Goals of hospice care include:

- Management of pain so the client can be comfortable and yet alert and in control of his or her life
- Coordinating care by providing physical, psychological, spiritual, and social support services as needed by the person or family
- Making financial and legal counseling available for the client or family members

It would be impossible to carry out these goals without a dedicated team of professionals who plan for the client's needs. Each team member contributes special skills and expertise to assure the comfort of the client and family (Figure 32-1).

You may hear the nurses and physicians refer to the Trajectory Model when caring for residents who may have a chronic illness or are near death. This model was developed by Juliet Corbin, a nurse researcher and a sociologist, Anselm Strauss. The term **trajectory** in this sense refers to the course of a disease in its varying stages. The Trajectory Model is a form of holistic care that is based on the Nursing Process and deals with the care of the chronically ill.

The model can be used as a tool to manage the care of the resident. Emphasis is on continuous, comprehensive care. This concept emphasizes that the resident and family member can help to maintain a sense of control and maintain dignity in their lives while receiving relief from symptoms (such as pain), coming to peace with spiritual issues, or helping with family burdens all from the perspective of the resident's wishes.

- Registered nurse: develops the care plan and coordinates client's care
- Home health aide/nursing assistant: provides direct personal care and emotional support to both family and client
- Medical director: co-certifies terminal prognosis, leads interdisciplinary team, and provides consultation to attending physicians
- Physician: certifies prognosis as terminal, manages symptoms, prescribes treatments, and works closely with interdisciplinary team
- Social worker: assists family and client with financial and social needs, makes referrals to appropriate community agencies, and provides bereavement support
- Spiritual advisor: assists client and family in meeting their spiritual and religious needs and provides consultation with community clergy
- Trained volunteers: offer companionship and support to the client and family by providing nonmedical services such as running errands, respite care for short periods of time, letter writing, and support during bereavement

Figure 32-1 Interdisciplinary hospice team.

Hospice care may be provided in a variety of settings: in a long-term care facility, hospital, private hospice facility, or in the person's own home. In the United States, most hospice care takes place in the home; a family member becomes the primary caregiver. A multi-disciplinary team provides strong support to the client and family members through direct personal care, family conferences, respite care (up to 5-day rest periods for caregivers), as well as bereavement counseling following the death of a loved one. Funding for hospice services is made possible through Medicare (Part A), Medicaid, or other insurance.

Palliative Care

Palliative care programs are new additions to the range of services available in the nation's health care system. These programs are similar to hospice care, but incorporate acute care to prolong life, as well as end-of-life care. Palliative care programs focus on early identification of a problem, improving the quality of life, and relieving suffering for persons with life-threatening illnesses at any time during that illness. Life expectancy for these clients may extend over several years. The emphasis of this type of care is on the resident being in control. It incorporates the wishes of the resident as outlined in their Durable Power of Attorney for Health Care document.

THE DYING PROCESS

Nursing assistants provide continuing care to residents through the dying period and into the after-death period (**postmortem**). Accepting the idea that death is the natural result of the life process may help you respond to the resident's and family's needs more generously.

Each person will have a different response to the dying process and death (Figures 32-2 and 32-3). Reactions to the diagnosis of a terminal (life-ending) illness include the following:

- Some residents may have had time to prepare psychologically for death. They may accept or be resigned to it (Figure 32-4).
- Some may look forward to relief from the pain and emotional burden of a long illness. They may await death calmly.
- Some may be fearful or angry and demonstrate behavior that swings from denial to depression (Figure 32-5).
- Others may reach out, trying to verbalize feelings and thoughts of an uncertain future.

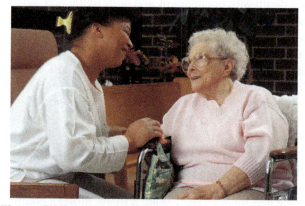

Figure 32-2 People react differently as they deal with approaching death.

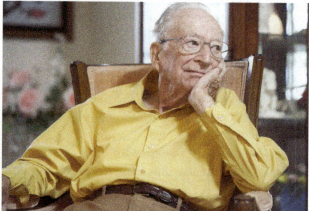

Figure 32-3 Some residents are unable to talk about their feelings and prefer to be left alone to work things out.

© Monkey Business Images/www.Shutterstock.com

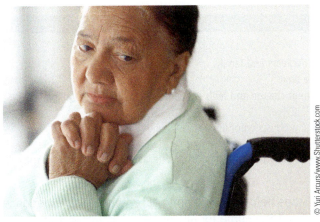

Figure 32-4 Even though the resident seems to have accepted her diagnosis, she still needs support and caring.

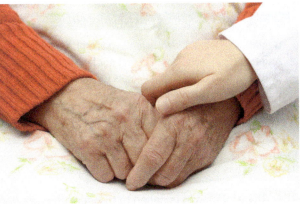

Figure 32-6 When coming to terms with the diagnosis of a terminal illness, the resident needs the support and understanding of the nursing assistant.

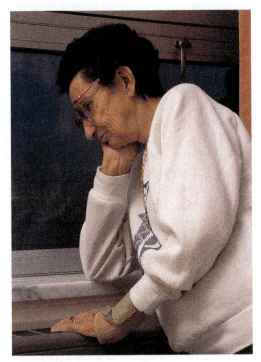

Figure 32-5 Depression and withdrawal are a natural part of the grieving process.

- In others, despair and anxiety may give way to moments of active hostility or periods of searching questions.
- Many residents experience these feelings repeatedly, especially when they are actively dying.
- Family members also may go through these same stages and experience the same type of feelings.

The residents will not all react in the same way to the prospect of death. They will not all follow the same progression of steps in the grieving process. You must accept the resident's behavior with understanding (Figure 32-6). You must also understand the dying resident's need for support, both from caregivers and

family. Finally, you will need to support the family in meeting their own needs during the adjustment period.

All staff members should know what the resident has been told about his or her condition. The amount of information given to the resident is a medical decision, with family input where possible. All staff members must abide by it.

Resuscitation

Unless otherwise ordered, every reasonable effort must be made to keep the resident alive. Be prepared to assist with cardiopulmonary **resuscitation** (CPR). In some facilities, nursing assistants who have had appropriate training are permitted to start this technique.

A resident may specify through a living will or durable power of attorney that resuscitation efforts are not to be made. If a resident does have a **do not resuscitate (DNR)** order, no CPR is performed when the person ceases breathing or the heart stops. If there is no DNR order, CPR will be performed. Each agency has a code to designate a cardiac arrest; in some agencies it is called **code blue**. This code is announced over the public address system to alert team members to respond to the call for emergency help. CPR and other aggressive measures will be instituted to save the resident's life. Unless you have specific responsibilities in the efforts to resuscitate the resident, nursing assistants should:

- Stay out of the way
- Be prepared to assist, if asked
- Help keep other residents calm and out of the way

The POLST (Physician Orders for Life Sustaining Treatment) form may be in the resident's chart in addition to the advanced directives. This form, on brightly colored paper, identifies specifically which life sustaining treatments are to be performed. Refer to Lesson 7 for more discussion of this topic.

Stages of Grief	
Denial	Resident refuses to accept the truth.
Anger	Resident may act out feelings, directing anger to caregivers and family.
Bargaining	Resident attempts to "make deals" for more livable time.
Depression	Resident comes to full realization that situation cannot change and feels saddened over things that will be left unfinished.
Acceptance	Resident recognizes that death is part of the natural progression of life.

Figure 32-7 Remember that residents with a terminal diagnosis move back and forth from one stage to another and may never progress to final acceptance before death.

The ambulance is called to transport the resident to the hospital. The paramedics will use advanced life support devices in an attempt to save the person's life both at the facility and while en route to the hospital.

Stages of Grieving

After a terminal diagnosis is made and the resident and the family are advised of the diagnosis, they will usually progress through a series of steps known as the stages of grieving* (Figure 32-7). These are:

- Denial
- Anger
- Bargaining
- Depression
- Acceptance

Both the resident and family members will experience the grieving process. Some people will progress through all steps and reach an acceptance of death as a natural part of the life experience. Other people will not reach acceptance but will stop at some intermediate step. Some people may go back and forth between

*Elizabeth Kübler-Ross has done much of the pioneer work in the understanding of the grieving process. See her book *On Death and Dying*, published by Macmillan.

steps before moving on to acceptance. The experience is not the same for all people.

As an example of the grieving process, Mrs. Bloomberg has been told of her terminal diagnosis. In the beginning she refuses to accept it. She seems cheerful and says, "I know that there are other therapies that could help. I'm too young to die. I still have much to accomplish." She may even tell you about her future plans. She is in the stage of denial.

As time passes and her health does not improve, she says, "It's all so unfair. I don't deserve this!" In anger Mrs. Bloomberg strikes out verbally at you and her family. Then, the anger gives way to bargaining. She spends time in prayer and visiting the chapel. You hear her say, "If only God (nature, or the doctors) can do something, I will be a better person from now on."

When the bargaining fails, then depression sets in. Mrs. Bloomberg speaks of past errors and says how sorry she is that there was not time to do or say certain things. She reviews her life, mourns the losses, and is saddened by things that will be left unfinished. The last step is acceptance. She seems calmer and more in control. She starts to put her affairs in order and may begin giving personal possessions away.

Residents at any stage of the grieving process need the emotional support of a caring, understanding staff.

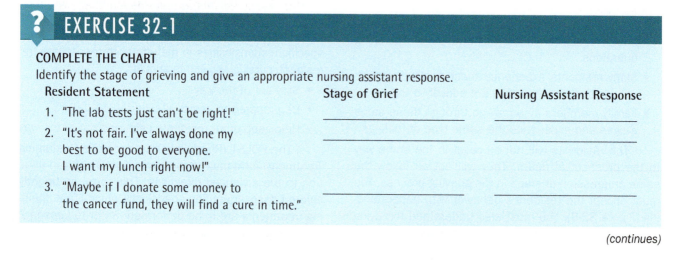

? **EXERCISE 32-1**

COMPLETE THE CHART
Identify the stage of grieving and give an appropriate nursing assistant response.

Resident Statement	Stage of Grief	Nursing Assistant Response
1. "The lab tests just can't be right!"	_____	_____
2. "It's not fair. I've always done my best to be good to everyone. I want my lunch right now!"	_____	_____
3. "Maybe if I donate some money to the cancer fund, they will find a cure in time."	_____	_____

(continues)

? EXERCISE 32-1 (Continued)

4. "What's the use of even trying anymore—no one really cares."   _____   _____

5. "I need to talk with my nephew. We haven't spoken for years."   _____   _____

6. What was the name of the person who did so much pioneering work in the field of death and dying?
_____

7. What are the stages of grieving that this person described?

a. _____
b. _____
c. _____
d. _____
e. _____

Family Dynamics

Remember that the family and friends of the resident are also going through a grieving process of their own. The relationships that exist between them and the resident are strained by the recognition that little time is left to enjoy each other or to resolve problems.

Each person may have feelings of guilt, anger, frustration, and powerlessness over the inability to avoid the final separation. Feelings that were hidden in everyday activities escape when people must also deal with the stress of terminal illness and death (Figure 32-8).

The death of a partner can result in profound grief. The remaining partner may lose the will to live, attempt suicide, and experience serious mental and physical problems. Bereaved persons experience initial feelings of shock and numbness as they go through a period of yearning for the lost loved one. Depression follows and then a final resolution and acceptance that life must go on. There is no timetable for grieving. Some people may work through their grief in a matter of weeks or months. Others may take much longer to move beyond their grief.

As a nursing assistant, you must:

- Read the care plan thoroughly. A statement of family problems may be included.
- Be aware that this is a stressful period for family and friends as well as the resident
- Know that sometimes unexpected interactions occur
- Not offer advice or take sides
- Listen quietly and be supportive
- Remember not to repeat to either the resident or the family or friends information that has been shared with you
- Be supportive, courteous, and respectful
- Maintain eye contact and use the resident's name
- Offer physical comfort to visitors by advising them of the location of rest areas, rest rooms, and nutrition sources
- Permit family members to participate in simple caregiving activities if they desire. This gives them a sense of being needed and assisting in the resident's comfort.
- Frequently communicate with the nurse any changes in the resident's condition.

Coping Techniques to Protect Self-Esteem in Response to Grief

- Anger
- Irritability
- Crying
- Withdrawal
- Agitation
- Restlessness
- Sleep disturbance
- Weight gain
- Chronic complaining
- Muscle aches

Figure 32-8 These responses may be experienced by anyone coping with grief: resident, staff, family, or other residents.

Caregivers and the Grieving Process

The staff must deal with their feelings about death, the loss of the resident, and their own mortality at the same time that they must be providing support to the resident and the family. Staff members who have developed close relationships with residents will also experience the grieving process.

When caregivers first encounter the process of dying and death, the experience can be frightening and stressful. This is especially true if the caregiver has a close relationship with the resident or if the resident is young. The loss of a young person is especially difficult to understand and accept. With experience, the caregiver realizes that supporting and caring for the dying resident are important services.

There is no one way to prepare yourself completely for the first experience of death, but some things you can do may help:

- Discuss your feelings about life and death with colleagues in a private setting.
- Discuss your thoughts about death with a member of the clergy of your faith.
- Give yourself permission to feel the grief and sadness that accompanies the loss of a resident.
- Believe that the tasks will become easier with experience.

Religious Practices Related to the Dying Process and Death

Many residents who have a **terminal illness** gain strength and peace through the practice of their religious beliefs. Each religion has practices related to death. For example, for gravely ill Roman Catholic residents a priest will be summoned to perform **last rites**, also known as the **Sacrament of the Sick**.

> **⊘N THE JOB**
>
> You will feel grief when a resident you have cared for dies at a time when others are looking to you for support.

Residents of other religious groups may desire the spiritual support of the clergy of their own faith. Spiritual readings may provide some comfort. Be open to their needs and requests.

Figure 32-9 shows a sampling of practices related to death and dying for major religions.

Culture/Religion	Religious Belief
Adventist (Seventh Day, Church of God)	Some believe in divine healing, anointing with oil, and prayer.
American Indian	There are many different tribes, and beliefs vary with each. Some believe an owl is an omen of death. Some tribes have family members prepare the body for burial. Some tribes will not touch the dead person's belongings after death. Some tribes believe the dead are happy in the spirit world. Others believe the body is an empty shell. Some have extensive preparation of the body and visitation of the deceased. If a member of some tribes dies at home, the house is abandoned forever or may be burned.
Armenian Church	Holy Communion may be given as a form of last rites; laying-on of hands is practiced.
Baptist	Pastor, resident, and family counsel and pray. Resident may be given Communion. Some practice healing and laying-on of hands.
Black/African American	The deceased is highly respected. Health care providers usually prepare the body. Cremation is usually avoided. May have concerns about organ donation.
Black Muslim	Practices for washing the body, applying the shroud, and funeral rites are carefully prescribed.
Brethren	Anointing with oil is done for physical healing and spiritual guidance.
Buddhist Churches of America	The priest is contacted to provide Last Rites. Chanting may be done at the bedside after death.
Cambodian (Khmer)	Monks recite prayers. Family wants to be present at time of death and may want to care for the resident. Incense may be burned. Death is accepted in a quiet, passive manner. Family and monks may wish to prepare the body. A white cloth is used as a shroud, and mourners wear white.
Central American	Catholics may want a priest to administer Sacrament of the Sick. Candles may be used if oxygen is not in use in room. Family members may wish to prepare the body.

Figure 32-9 Cultural/religious beliefs affecting care at the time of death.

(continues)

Culture/Religion	Religious Belief
Chinese American	Family may prefer resident not be told of impending death, or may prefer to inform the resident themselves. May not want to talk about the terminal illness with anyone. Some believe that dying at home is bad luck. Others believe that the spirit gets lost if the resident dies in the hospital. Family members may place special cloths and amulets on the body. Some prefer to bathe their own family members after death.
Christian Scientist	A Christian Science practitioner may be called for spiritual support. Have concerns about organ donation.
Church of God	Believe in divine healing through prayer. Speaking in tongues may be used.
Church of Jesus Christ of Latter Day Saints (LDS or Mormon)	Body is dressed in white temple clothing before viewing by family members. Cremation is discouraged. Believe in baptism for others who have died and preaching to deceased.
Colombian	Catholic prayer and anointing of the sick common. Family may practice Catholic prayer at bedside. Family members may cry loudly or become hysterical. All family members may want to see the body before it is taken to the morgue. In Colombia, the deceased are usually buried within 24–36 hours. The nurse may need to inform them that in the United States the body may not be buried this quickly.
Cuban	Family may not want resident told of impending death. This varies according to Cuban culture. Family members may stay with resident 24 hours a day during terminal phase of illness.
Eastern Orthodox	Last rites are given. Anointing of the sick is performed as a form of healing with prayer. Cremation is discouraged.
Episcopal	Last Rites are available, but not mandatory. May practice prayer, Communion, and confession.
Ethiopian	Friends are told of death before family so they can be present when family is informed. Female family members are never told first. Great displays of feelings are encouraged at death. They may cry loudly and hysterically. Women may tear their clothing and beat their chests. Men may cry out loud. Some families may want to say goodbye to the deceased before the body is removed from the room.
Filipino	Head of family is informed away from resident's room. Catholic priest is called to deliver Sacrament of the Sick. DNR decisions may be made by the entire family. Religious objects may be placed around the resident. Family may pray at the bedside when resident is dying. After death, they may cry loudly and hysterically. Family may wish to wash the body. Death is considered a very spiritual event. All family members may say goodbye before body is removed from the room.
Friends (Quaker)	Do not believe in life after death (spiritual afterlife).
Greek Orthodox	The priest should be called while the resident is still conscious. Practice Last Rites and administration of Communion. Believe that life should be preserved until terminated by God.
Gypsy	In general, discussion of death is avoided in this culture. Eldest in authority is informed of death first. A priest may be present for body purification. Family may want the window open at the time of death and afterward so the spirit can leave the room. May ask for special personal items in room at the time of death. An older female relative may remain at the window to keep spirits out of room. The moment of death and the resident's last words are very significant. The body after death may represent a source of spiritual danger to the family. Family may want body embalmed immediately after death to remove blood. They may sit with the body around the clock after death, and will eat and drink at this location.
Haitian	Elaborate rituals after death. When death is imminent, family will cry hysterically and uncontrollably. Family members may bring religious symbols and medallions. They have a deep respect for the dead. Family members may wish to wash the body and participate in postmortem care.
Hindu	Specially prescribed rites. Priest may tie a thread around wrist or neck and place water in mouth. The family washes and dresses the body, and only certain persons may touch the dead. May prefer cremation to burial.
Hmong	Important to wear fine traditional Hmong clothing at the time of death. Family may put amulets on body, which should not be removed. The family usually prepares the body at the funeral home. The body cannot be buried with hard objects, buttons, or zippers against the body.

Figure 32-9 (Continued)

Culture/Religion	Religious Belief
Iranian	Death is seen as the beginning of a spiritual relationship with God, not the end of life. Family may wish to be present at all times when resident is dying, and may cry and pray at bedside. Families may wish to wash the body.
Islam (Muslim)	Begging forgiveness and confession of sins must be done in presence of family members before death. There are five steps to preparing the body for burial. The first step involves washing of the body by a Muslim of the same gender. May offer special prayers at bedside to ease pain and suffering. Some have spiritual leader give resident holy water to drink prior to death to purify body. After death, arms and legs are straightened and the toes tied together with a bandage. May be opposed to autopsy.
Japanese	Resident and family may be aware of impending death, but will not speak about it. Family may wish to remain at bedside during terminal stage of illness. Cleanliness and dignity of the body are very important.
Jehovah's Witness	Practice baptism and Communion. May be opposed to autopsy.
Judaism (Orthodox and Conservative)	Jews believe in the sanctity of life. Medical care is generally expected, and there are no medication restrictions. Most surgical procedures are permitted, but body parts that have been removed are traditionally saved for later burial. For most Jews, medical treatment cannot be stopped once it has been started, but members are not required to use extraordinary measures to prolong life. May be opposed to prolonging life if resident has irreversible brain damage. However, active euthanasia is forbidden. Traditional Jews use a burial society to care for the body after death. Society members may or may not be members of the deceased's congregation. They usually prefer no autopsy, but this is permitted if legally required. Embalming is generally discouraged. The resident is buried as soon after death as possible. Cremation is discouraged. For traditional Jews, mourning begins with a seven-day period called shiva, in which men do not shave, and family and close friends do not read the newspaper or watch television. Mourning extends over a year. Jewish practices and beliefs can be very different from family to family. Asking the resident or family members about their practices is probably best. Asking is not offensive, and shows that you care about and respect the resident's and family's wishes.
Korean	Chanting, incense, and praying may be used. Family crying and mourning may be extreme. Family may want to spend time alone with the resident after death. Some may wish to wash the body.
Lutheran	Practice prayer. Last Rites optional; the resident may request anointing of the sick.
Methodist	May request donation of body or body parts to medical science.
Mexican American	Entire family may be obligated to visit the sick and dying. Pregnant women may be prohibited from visiting. Spiritual items may be important. May want to die at home because of the fear that the spirit will get lost in the hospital. Crying loudly and wailing is culturally accepted and a sign of respect. A Catholic priest is called for the Sacrament of the Sick. A family member may wish to assist with postmortem care. Family will want time alone with the body before it is removed from the room.
Orthodox Presbyterian	Scripture reading and prayer. Full forgiveness is granted for any illness connected with a sin.
Puerto Rican	If death is imminent, family may stay around the clock. Some believe that all immediate family members must be present at the time of death. Believe that the body must be treated with great respect.
Roman Catholic	Prayer and the rite for anointing of the sick are desired. Resident or family may request anointing if prognosis is poor.
Russian	Family may not want the resident to know of a terminal diagnosis. Depending on religion, family may wish to wash the body and dress it in special clothes.
Russian Orthodox	Practice prayer, Communion, and Last Rites by priest. Many wear a cross necklace, which should not be removed if at all possible. After death the arms are crossed, and fingers set in the form of a cross. Clothing must be a natural fiber so the body changes to ashes sooner. May be opposed to autopsy, embalming, or cremation.
Samoan	Resident and family prefer to be told of terminal diagnosis as early as possible. Family would prefer to care for resident at home, if possible. Family members usually prefer to prepare the body.
Sikh	Believe that the soul remains alive after death. Family washes the body and dresses deceased member in new clothing.
Unitarian Universalist	Cremation may be preferred to burial.

Figure 32-9 (Continued)

Culture/Religion	Religious Belief
Vietnamese	DNR decisions are made by entire family. For Catholic families, religious items are kept close to resident. For Buddhist families, incense is burned. Families prefer time alone with the deceased before body is moved. The body is highly respected, and the family may prefer to wash it. Some may prefer the body left as it is.
West Indian	When death is near, close family and friends wish to remain at the bedside to pray. Family members may wish to view the body exactly as the resident was at the time of death. Most wish to be alone with the deceased.

Figure 32-9 (Continued)

Nursing Assistant Responsibilities

You have a special opportunity to be of service to the resident with a terminal diagnosis and to his or her family. Because of your day-to-day contact, you are in a position to provide the emotional and physical support needed. Make an effort to build and maintain a trusting relationship with each resident. Make sure the resident feels secure and knows you will not abandon him or her. Watch carefully for verbal and nonverbal clues as to what the resident feels and needs. Use your own special touch and listening skills to comfort the resident.

You can help the dying resident by:

- Making frequent contact with the resident
- Increasing contact as death approaches
- Keeping the resident comfortable and clean
- Changing resident's position every 2 hours
- Providing proper mouth care
- Using moistened applicators on the lips and inside the mouth
- Meeting basic physical needs
- Monitoring vital signs carefully
- Keeping the room quiet but well lit

You can help the family by:

- Giving proper care to the resident
- Treating the resident with respect and ensuring the resident's dignity
- Listening quietly to their concerns
- Providing privacy

? EXERCISE 32-2

COMPLETION
Select the correct terms from the following list to complete each statement.

accept	living will
care	dying
common	punishment
death	resuscitation
dignity	Sacrament of the Sick
hospice care	terminal
life	

1. A universal experience shared by all is _____.
2. Caring for dying residents is a(an) _____ experience in a long-term care facility.
3. The dying person should be able to keep his or her _____.
4. All people do not _____ the concept of death in the same way.
5. Death is part of the natural _____ cycle.
6. A life-ending process is called _____.
7. Efforts to revive a resident whose heart has stopped is called _____.
8. One way to help family members feel useful is to allow them to participate in resident _____.

SIGNS OF APPROACHING DEATH

Approaching death is signaled by a slowing of body functions and a loss of control. Signs and symptoms include:

- The body seems to relax and the jaw drops.
- Breathing becomes labored.
- Control of bowels and bladder or both may be lost (incontinence).
- Circulation slows.
- Blood pressure drops.
- Extremities become colder.
- Profuse perspiration is common.
- Respirations become labored (dyspnea) or temporarily cease (apnea).
- Periods of dyspnea followed by apnea, known as Cheyne-Stokes respirations, may occur.
- The pulse becomes more rapid and weaker.
- The skin pales and **mottling** (discoloration) may occur.
- The eyes do not respond to light.
- Hearing is the last sense to be lost. Do not assume that the resident can no longer hear. You must be careful in what you say. Always remember to treat the dying person with dignity and respect. This also holds true for handling the body after death.

Continue to talk to the resident in a normal tone even if the resident is **comatose** (unconscious).

Gradually, breathing becomes more labored and then stops. If the nurse is away from the bedside, note the time that breathing ceases and inform the nurse when the vital signs are absent. If the resident's family is present at the time of death, they will be asked to step outside while the nurse examines the resident and then calls the physician. Under no circumstances is the nursing assistant to inform the family that death has occurred. This is the responsibility of the nurse or physician.

Provide a comfortable, private area for the family and stay with them unless they prefer to be alone. It is appropriate to let the family know how much the resident meant to you, so do not be embarrassed if you feel like crying. Do, however, try to control your emotions because the family members will need your support.

POSTMORTEM CARE

The care given immediately after death is called **postmortem care**. The changes in the resident's body after death are listed in Figure 32-10. Make sure the resident is positioned naturally, with limbs straightened.

Postmortem signs include:
● Gradual cooling of body temperature
● Loss of circulation
● Body discoloration with pressure
● Evacuation of bowel or bladder or both
● Rigor mortis (stiffening of muscles and joints) beginning with head and neck and progressing downward

Figure 32-10 Postmortem signs.

This is important because **rigor mortis** (stiffening of the body muscles) will occur some hours after death. Return dentures to the mouth if they were normally worn. Make sure the linen is clean. Family members may want to spend a little time with the body. Stay with them, if requested, but provide privacy otherwise.

After the death of a resident, your behavior should be dignified and restrained. Death in the facility is upsetting to other residents. Residents are informed of the deaths of other residents. Some will experience feelings of the loss of a friend; others will be reminded that their own lives are limited. Some residents withdraw and others may openly grieve. Let the residents know that you understand their feelings and that such feelings are natural. Be willing to listen. Be patient if a resident seems irritable or angry. Report the resident's reactions to the nurse so the care plan will reflect the proper staff response.

As residents grieve for their deceased friend, they may want to recall their relationship. Be supportive as they express their feelings of grief (Figure 32-11).

Some facilities hold memorial services for deceased residents. Members of the family, residents, and staff are invited to celebrate the life of the resident. The services help to bring closure.

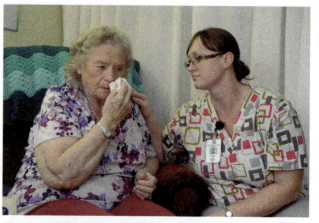

Figure 32-11 Remember that residents often form close friendships. When one dies, you must be prepared to offer comfort to those who remain.

PROCEDURE 32-98
Giving Postmortem Care

1. Carry out each beginning procedure action.

2. Assemble equipment:

   - Disposable gloves
   - Shroud or morgue pack (Figure 32-12)
   - Basin and warm water
   - Washcloth and towels
   - Linens and underpads as needed
   - Swabs for oral care

3. Put on disposable gloves.

4. Remove all appliances, drainage tubing and containers, and used articles if instructed to do so according to agency policy.

NOTE: All drainage tubes remain in the body if an autopsy is to be performed.

5. Work quickly and quietly; maintain an attitude of respect.

6. Elevate the head of the bed 30 degrees. Position the body on the back, with head and shoulders elevated on a pillow.

   - Close the eyes by gently pulling the eyelids down and holding shut for a few seconds (Figure 32-13).
   - Remove watch and all jewelry except wedding band, according to facility policy.
   - Provide mouth care using moistened oral care swabs or sponges.
   - Insert artificial eye, if appropriate.
   - Close mouth. Place a rolled washcloth under the chin to keep the mouth closed, if necessary.
   - Bathe the body, straighten arms and legs and groom hair.
   - Replace soiled linens.
   - Place disposable pads under the resident because urine and stool continue to seep from the body when the sphincters relax.
   - Apply clean dressings, if needed.
   - Put a gown on the body and replace top linens.
   - Attach identification tags according to facility policy.
   - Remove gloves and discard appropriately.
   - Wash hands.

7. Allow the family privacy when viewing the body:

   - Make sure the room is neat, remove any unnecessary equipment.
   - Adjust the lights to a subdued level.
   - Place chairs nearby for family members.

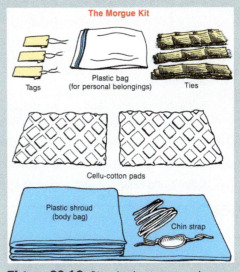

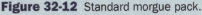

Figure 32-12 Standard morgue pack.

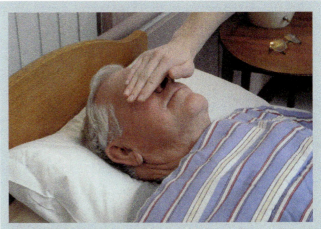

Figure 32-13 Gently close the resident's eyes.

(continues)

PROCEDURE 32-98
Giving Postmortem Care (Continued)

8. Collect all belongings and place them in a bag:

   - Per agency policy, if appropriate, clean the resident's dentures and insert in the resident's mouth or place them in a labeled denture cup to be sent to the funeral home with the body.

   - Complete and sign inventory list according to facility policy.

   - Personal items are given to the family. However, if no family members are present, follow agency policy.

9. After the family leaves:

   - Wash your hands and put the shroud (paper, plastic, or cloth) on the body according to agency policy. Wear gloves if your hands will be soiled with body fluids.

   - Close the door until representatives from the funeral home arrive to transport the body.

   - Notify the nurse when the representatives arrive and assist with moving the body, if necessary.

   - Strip and clean the unit according to facility policy.

? EXERCISE 32-3

1. Five actions the nursing assistant can take to help the dying resident and family include:

   a. _____

   _____

   b. _____

   _____

   c. _____

   _____

   d. _____

   _____

   e. _____

   _____

2. Seven nursing assistant actions that can be taken to assist the dying resident include:

   a. _____

   _____

   b. _____

   _____

   c. _____

   _____

(continues)

? EXERCISE 32-3 (Continued)

d. _____
_____

e. _____
_____

f. _____
_____

g. _____
_____

3. Briefly describe nursing assistant actions that will help the other residents after a death in the facility.
_____
_____
_____
_____
_____
_____

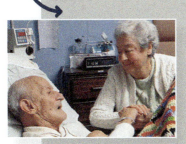

LESSON SYNTHESIS: Putting It All Together

You have just completed this lesson. Now go back and review the Clinical Focus. Try to see how the Clinical Focus relates to the concepts presented in the lesson. Then answer the following questions.

1. Why do you think Mr. Sperling is behaving the way he is?

2. How do you think the marital history of Mr. and Mrs. Sperling might affect their emotional response to this terminal condition and death?

3. How could the nursing assistant be supportive?

4. What special sacrament would be appropriate when Mr. Sperling is dying?

32 REVIEW

A. Match each term (items a–e) with the proper definition.

 a. comatose

 b. mottling

 c. moribund

 d. postmortem

 e. Sacrament of the Sick

1. _____   discoloration

2. _____   dying

3. _____   Last Rites

4. _____   unconscious

5. _____   after death

B. Provide brief answers for each of the following.

6. List five signs of approaching death.

7. List the five stages of grieving.

8. List six ways the nursing assistant can help the dying resident.

C. Answer each statement true (T) or false (F).

9. T F Death is a natural part of the life cycle.

10. T F Everyone responds to the thought of death in the same way.

11. T F A terminal illness is curable.

12. T F Given time, residents can move steadily forward through each stage of grieving.

13. T F Rigor mortis develops immediately after death.

D. Select the one best answer for each of the following.

14. Signs of approaching death include

 (A) blood pressure rises

 (B) circulation speeds up

 (C) extremities become warmer

 (D) breathing becomes labored

15. When a resident is dying,

 (A) other residents are not affected

 (B) staff members are not upset

 (C) family members are not concerned

 (D) other residents may be deeply affected

16. The Sacrament of the Sick is administered to

 (A) Buddhist residents

 (B) Jewish residents

 (C) Roman Catholic residents

 (D) residents who are members of the Church of Christ

17. After death of a resident who belongs to the Christian Scientist faith

 (A) the body will be anointed with oil

 (B) there may be concerns about organ donation

 (C) the Bible is read

 (D) the body will be dressed in new clothing

18. When a resident is comatose, he

 (A) may be able to see

 (B) may be able to hear

 (C) cannot hear

 (D) is able to speak

19. Signs of death are:

 (A) Loss of consciousness and coma

 (B) Increased body temperature and profuse perspiration

 (C) Absence of pulse, respirations, and blood pressure

 (D) Fixed and unequal pupils of the eyes

20. Rigor mortis refers to:

 (A) Loss of circulation

 (B) Body discoloration and mottling

 (C) Loss of control of bowel and bladder

 (D) Stiffening of body muscles

E. Clinical experience

21. Juan is working in the hospice unit of a long-term care facility. Mrs. Sophen, who has metastatic pancreatic cancer, is one of his residents.

    a. How would Mrs. Sophen's prognosis be described?

    b. What word best describes the kind of care Mrs. Sophen is receiving?

    c. What is the focus of this care?

    d. Who, besides Juan, provides this care?

    e. Where else might this care be given?

22. Liza is caring for Mr. Simms, who has been comatose for 12 hours. His breathing has just ceased. The nurse is away from the bedside.

    a. What action should Liza take?

    b. Should Liza inform the family members who are in the waiting room?

    c. When the family returns to the resident's room, what should Liza do to offer them support?

    d. Mr. Simms was a resident in the facility for 18 months. Liza liked him and feels very sad about his death. Is it appropriate for her to let the family know that she will also miss him very much?

LESSON 33
CARING FOR THE PERSON IN SUBACUTE CARE

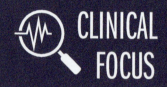 **CLINICAL FOCUS**

Think about the care that is required by residents in subacute units as you study this lesson.

OBJECTIVES

After studying this lesson, you should be able to:

- Define vocabulary words and terms.
- Describe the purpose of subacute care.
- List the differences between acute care, subacute care, and long-term care.
- Describe the responsibilities of the nursing assistant when caring for residents receiving the special treatments discussed in this lesson.
- Demonstrate the following:

  Procedure 33-99   Taking Blood Pressure with an Electronic Blood Pressure Apparatus

  Procedure 33-100   Using a Pulse Oximeter

  Procedure 33-101   Changing a Gown on a Resident with a Peripheral Intravenous Line in Place

VOCABULARY

alopecia (al-oh-PEE-shee-ah)

anorexia (an-oh-RECK-see-ah)

central venous (CV) catheter (SEN-tral VEE-nus KATH-eh-ter)

chemotherapy (kee-moh-THER-ah-pee)

dialysis (dye-AL-ih-sis)

enteral feedings (EN-ter-al FEED-ings)

epidural catheter (ep-ih-DOO-ral KATH-eh-ter)

fistula (FIS-tyou-lah)

graft (graft)

hemodialysis (he-moh-dye-AL-ih-sis)

hyperalimentation (high-per-al-ih-men-TAY-shun)

intravenous (IV) therapy (in-trah-VEE-nus THER-ah-pee)

narcotic (nar-KAH-tick)

CASE STUDY

Steven Goldstein has been a nursing assistant for several years. He has just been hired to work in a subacute care unit of a long-term care facility. Steven will need to participate in additional inservice education to fulfill the requirements of his new job. He is looking forward to the challenge of learning and acquiring new skills.

oncology (ong-KOL-oh-jee)
patient-controlled analgesia (PCA) (PAY-shent kon-TROLD an-al-JEE-see-ah)
peripheral intravenous central catheter (PICC) (per-IH-fer-al in-trah-VEE-nus SEN-tral KATH-eh-ter)
peritoneal dialysis (per-ih-toh-NEE-aldye-AL-ih-sis)
piggyback (PIG-ee-bak)
pulse oximetry (puls ox-IM-ih-tree)
radiation therapy (ray-dee-AY-shun THER-ah-pee)

sleep apnea (sleep ap-NEE-a)
subacute care (sub-ah-KYOUT kair)
total parenteral nutrition (TPN) (TOH-tal pah-REN-ter-al new-TRIH-shun)
tracheostomy (tray-kee-OS-toh-mee)
transcutaneous electrical nerve stimulation (TENS) (trans-kyou-TAN-ee-us ee-LEK-trih-kal nerv stim-you-LAY-shun)
transitional care (tran-ZIH-shun-al kair)

DESCRIPTION OF SUBACUTE CARE

Subacute care is a type of "step-down" care given to persons who have been acutely ill. These individuals are out of the acute phase of illness but still need monitoring and ongoing treatment and services. Subacute care is sometimes called transitional care. The purpose of subacute care is to provide the care a person needs but at a lower cost than care given in an acute care facility (hospital). Subacute care units may be located in a section of a long-term care facility, in a hospital, or in a free-standing unit. Most residents in subacute care units are there for several weeks or longer. Residents with terminal illness or with acquired immune deficiency syndrome (AIDS) may be there for a longer time. Residents who can be discharged may go to:

- Their own home
- A long-term care facility
- An assisted living facility
- A group home

On a subacute care unit, there are:

- Residents with clinically complex care needs
- Highly trained nurses and nursing assistants
- More medications and frequent treatments than on a regular skilled unit
- More frequent physician's visits
- More sophisticated types of equipment

Types of Care Provided in a Subacute Care Unit

Most subacute care units provide specialized care in one or two areas. Some examples are:

- Rehabilitation—all therapies are provided and the resident participates in rehabilitation for up to 5 hours a day, 6 or 7 days a week
- Peritoneal dialysis—a method of ridding the body of wastes for a person who has kidney failure

- Ventilator weaning and tracheostomy care—for persons who have been unable to breathe without the help of a ventilator
- Cardiac monitoring—for persons who have had a myocardial infarction or acute heart failure
- Pain management and control—for persons who have acute or chronic pain
- Oncology—the care of persons with cancer who are receiving treatments such as chemotherapy or radiation
- Wound management—for persons with severe stage 3 or stage 4 pressure ulcers, ulcers related to peripheral vascular disease, or burns
- Specialized care—for persons who have suffered brain damage resulting from trauma or stroke
- AIDS—for persons in the terminal stages of AIDS who need 24-hour-a-day care
- Hospice care—for persons in the terminal stages of any disease
- Postoperative care (care given to individuals who have had surgery) for persons who have other complicating conditions—for example, a person who has had repair of a hip fracture and who also has chronic obstructive pulmonary disease or diabetes
- Infusion therapy for persons needing intravenous fluids, medications, or nutrition
- Pre- and post-transplant care for persons waiting for an organ transplant or during the period of stabilization after transplantation

Types of subacute care are listed in Table 33-1.

If you work on a subacute care unit you will participate in special inservice training to meet the needs of the residents in your care. A nursing assistant on a subacute unit will be expected to:

- Work closely with registered nurses who are specialists in critical care or in a specific area of nursing such as rehabilitation or wound care
- Have extensive knowledge of the types of residents cared for on the subacute care unit

Type of Subacute Facility	Description	Typical Medical Problems of Patients Admitted	Goals of Care	Average Length of Patient's Stay
Transitional subacute unit	• A less expensive setting than the acute care hospital • Provides 24-hour-a-day RN coverage • RNs in this unit have special acute care education, experience, and certifications • Rehabilitation therapies are available 7 days a week • Respiratory therapy is available 24 hours a day • A registered dietitian is regularly available	• Severe words of stage 3 or 4 pressure ulcers • Strokes • Patients who have had open heart surgery, heart attack, acute congestive heart failure, or other heart conditions • Patients with tracheostomy who require respiratory management • Cancer, including chemotherapy and radiation therapy • Patients who require intensive rehabilitation programs • Medically complex patients with diabetes, digestive problems, or renal disorders	• Manage care and therapy in a less expensive setting than the acute care hospital • Discharge patient to home, an assisted living facility, or a skilled nursing facility	5–40 days
General medical/ surgical subacute unit	• Care for patients with complex medical care and monitoring needs, rehabilitation therapy, nursing assessment and intervention • RN coverage is provided 24 hours a day • RNs working in this unit have special acute care education, experience, and certifications • Rehabilitation therapies are available 7 days a week • Respiratory therapy is available 24 hours a day • A registered dietitian is regularly available	• Patients requiring long-term IV therapy for infection, nutrition, or other medical problems without other significant complications • Patients with stable medical problems, including cardiac, digestive, renal, or diabetes • Patients who have had strokes that require 1–3 hours of therapy (PT, OT, and/or speech) daily • Patients with neurologic or orthopedic conditions requiring 1–3 hours of therapy each day • Patients with HIV disease/AIDS	• Manage care and therapy in a less expensive setting than an acute care hospital in a cost-effective manner • Discharge patient to home, an assisted living facility, or a skilled nursing facility	7–21 days

Table 33-1 Types of Subacute Care Units

(continues)

Type of Subacute Facility	Description	Typical Medical Problems of Patients Admitted	Goals of Care	Average Length of Patient's Stay
Chronic subacute unit	• Care for patients with little hope of recovery or return to functional independence • RN on duty at least 8 hours a day • If an RN is not on duty, an LPN or LVN is in charge • Restorative nursing care is provided for comfort and to prevent deformities, maintain self-esteem • A registered dietitian is regularly available • Physical, occupational, speech, and respiratory therapies are available	• Patients who are dependent on ventilators for breathing • Long-term comatose patients • Patients with progressive neurologic conditions • Patients requiring restorative care from nursing staff with guidance, teaching, or assistance from therapy personnel	• Provide care in the most cost-effective manner, considering medical problems and needs	60–90 days
Long-term transitional subacute unit	• Care for medically complex residents and those who depend on an acute ventilator • Many different types of physician specialists must be available to care for patients in this type of unit • Unit director is a highly skilled, educated, and qualified RN with acute care experience • Residents require a high degree of RN intervention because of their acute medical problems • Respiratory therapists usually provide daily services • A registered dietitian is available, if needed	• Acute ventilator-dependent patients who require complex daily care and management of respiratory problems • Medically complex residents with at least two medical or surgical diagnoses, requiring special medical services and daily RN assessment and intervention	• Manage care and therapy in a less expensive setting than an acute care hospital • Discharge resident to home, an assisted living facility, or a skilled nursing facility	More than 25 days

Table 33-1 (Continued)

Type of Subacute Facility	Description	Typical Medical Problems of Patients Admitted	Goals of Care	Average Length of Patient's Stay
Specialized subacute unit	• Care of specialized groups of patients, such as pediatric patients • Many different types of physicians and other specialists must be available to care for patients in this unit • Unit director is a highly skilled, educated, and qualified RN with experience in the unit specialty • Patients often require a high degree of RN intervention because of their acute medical problems	• Medically complex patients grouped together according to need or medical diagnosis	• Manage care and therapy in a less expensive setting than an acute care hospital • Discharge patient to home, an assisted living facility, or a skilled nursing facility	Varies with the type of unit; commonly 60–90 days
Specialized subacute unit	• RN staffing determined by the speciality nature of the unit; most provide RN services 24 hours a day • Patients require daily RN assessment and intervention • Respiratory therapists usually provide daily services • Rehabilitation therapies are available 7 days a week • A registered dietitian is available, if needed			

Table 33-1 (Continued)

• Care for residents receiving complicated treatments
• Have excellent observational skills because of the complex conditions of the residents on the unit
• Be a member of an interdisciplinary health care team that includes highly trained professionals in areas like physical therapy, occupational therapy, speech therapy, respiratory therapy, and social services

It is important that the staff on a subacute care unit be able to provide for the resident's emotional well-being. Many of the residents on the unit will be able to return to their homes. For them, this is a time for rejoicing and for making plans for the future. Some of the residents, however, will have an uncertain future. For example:

• Will the resident receiving dialysis receive a kidney transplant in time?
• Will the cancer be cured in the resident receiving radiation or chemotherapy?
• Will the resident on the ventilator be able to be weaned off the ventilator or will it be a life-long need?
• Will the resident receiving rehabilitation gain enough independence to be able to go home?

? EXERCISE 33-1

TRUE OR FALSE
Indicate whether the following statements are true (T) or false (F).

1. T F Most subacute care units provide specialized care in one or two areas.
2. T F On a subacute care unit, staff are more highly trained as patient needs are more complex.
3. T F There is only one type of subacute care.
4. T F Subacute care is given only in the hospital.
5. T F The length of time a resident is in a subacute care unit is 1 to 2 days.
6. T F Physicians visit more often in a subacute unit than in a long-term care unit.
7. T F Fewer medications are usually given to residents in subacute units.
8. T F Ventilator weaning is carried out in subacute care units.
9. T F Peritoneal dialysis is used to remove wastes from the body.
10. T F Hospice care is provided in the subacute care unit.

SPECIAL PROCEDURES PROVIDED IN THE SUBACUTE CARE UNIT

You may care for residents who are receiving special treatments because of their health problems. These treatments may require the use of equipment that is unfamiliar to you. As a nursing assistant you will not be expected to be responsible for these procedures. However, you will be providing the same personal care and procedures that you would with any residents. In addition you will need to know what observations to make for these residents.

CARE OF THE SURGICAL PATIENT

It is possible that you may care for a resident who was admitted or readmitted to the facility shortly after surgery. Be sure you know what nursing care is expected. You may find that:

- Vital signs are taken more frequently and utilizing electronic monitors (Figure 33-1)
- The resident has devices connected to drainage tubes
- Intravenous feedings are running

  When caring for a resident who has had surgery:

- Encourage the resident to breathe deeply, cough, and move in bed. The position should be changed every 2 hours.
- Turn the resident's head to one side and support if vomiting. Have an emesis basin ready, as well as tissues and a wet cloth.

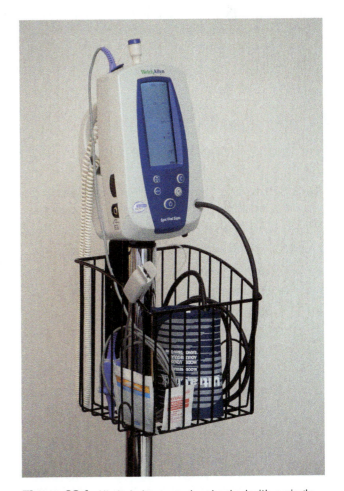

Figure 33-1 All vital signs may be checked with a single instrument.

- Report any signs of drainage from the operative area.
- Report complaints of pain promptly.

⚠ GUIDELINES FOR ... ELECTRONIC BLOOD PRESSURE MONITORING

RESIDENT SELECTION

- This procedure can be done on residents of all ages and sizes, but appropriately sized cuffs must be used.
- At least one blood pressure reading should be taken using the auscultation method before an electronic blood pressure device is used. The auscultation reading is needed as a baseline with which to compare the values from the electronic device.

The procedure is contraindicated in residents with:

- Extreme hypertension or hypotension
- Very rapid heart rates
- Excessive body movement or tremors
- Irregular heart rhythms or atrial dysrhythmias

Residents for whom electronic blood pressure monitoring is not acceptable should be known to all caregivers and identified on the care plan or Kardex. If in doubt, check with the nurse for instructions for residents with very high blood pressure or rapid or irregular heart (pulse) rates.

Do not place a cuff on an arm that has:

- Edema
- Paralysis
- Site of an intravenous (IV) infusion
- A pulse oximeter on it
- The site of a dialysis access device
- A fracture
- A burn
- The same side as a recent mastectomy or other surgical procedure site

APPLICATION OF THE CUFF

- Select the proper size cuff. The width should be equal to 40% of the arm circumference.
- The upper arm is the preferred location for the monitoring cuff, but the forearm or ankle also may be used. However, using alternate sites may result in inaccurate blood pressure readings. Check with the nurses; these sites should be used for blood pressure monitoring only when use of the upper arm site is not possible (see Procedure 33-99).

PROCEDURE 33-99
Taking Blood Pressure with an Electronic Blood Pressure Apparatus

NOTE: This procedure is generic and applies principles used for common types of electronic blood pressure monitoring devices. Follow the instructions for the specific device you are using. The operating instructions are slightly different for each type of machine. Your instructor will inform you if the directions for the equipment you are using differs from those listed here.

1. Carry out beginning procedure actions.
2. Assemble equipment:
   - Electronic blood pressure device
   - Assortment of cuffs and tubes
3. Bring the electronic blood pressure unit to the bedside. Place it near the resident and plug into a source of electricity.
4. Locate the on/off switch and turn on the machine.
5. Select the appropriate cuff for the machine and size for the resident's extremity.
6. Remove restrictive clothing.
7. Squeeze excess air out of the cuff.
8. Connect the cuff to the connector hose.
9. Wrap the cuff snugly around the resident's extremity, verifying that only one finger can fit between the cuff and the resident's skin. Make sure the "artery" arrow marked on the outside of the cuff is correctly placed over the brachial artery.
10. Verify that the connector hose between the cuff and the machine is not kinked.

(continues)

PROCEDURE 33-99
Taking Blood Pressure with an Electronic Blood Pressure Apparatus (Continued)

11. Set the frequency control for automatic or manual.
12. Press the start button.
13. If the cuff will take periodic, automatic measurement, set the designated frequency of the blood pressure measurements.
14. Set upper and lower alarm limits for systolic, diastolic, and mean blood pressure readings.
15. Remove the cuff at least every 2 hours and use alternate sites, if possible. Evaluate the skin for redness and irritation. Report abnormalities to the nurse.
16. Carry out procedure completion actions.

PULSE OXIMETRY

Pulse oximetry is routinely used on subacute units to determine the amount of oxygen in the arterial blood (Figure 33-2). The method is simple, painless, and relatively inexpensive. When the pulse oximeter is in place, it continuously measures the amount of oxygen in the resident's hemoglobin that is carried by the red blood cells to all the other cells of the body. The pulse oximeter can sense critical changes in the oxygen levels in the body, and early corrective treatment can be started before the skin color changes. Before the pulse oximeter is applied, check the resident's oxygen if it is being used. Document the liter flow. (Refer to Procedure 33-100.)

The pulse oximeter is applied to the resident's skin. Several different sensors are available. These can be clipped on or adhered to the finger (Figure 33-3A), toe, earlobe, bridge of the nose (Figure 33-3B), or forehead. The finger and toe sensors work best on dark-skinned clients. Poor circulation interferes with the use of the pulse oximeter.

The probe has two light-emitting diodes (LEDs). One is red, the other is infrared. The sensor (photodetector) then measures the absorption of light as it passes through the tissues. This measure shows the amount of oxygen in the resident's arterial blood (Figure 33-3C). The pulse oximeter converts this to a percentage, which can be viewed on a digital display. The physician will order the minimum level of oxygen saturation for the resident. The nurse will inform you of this level for each resident. A measurement of 95% to 100% is considered normal. Readings below 90% suggest complications. When the reading reaches 85%, there may not be enough oxygen for the tissues. Readings below 70% are life threatening. The pulse oximeter is not used for persons with known or suspected carbon monoxide poisoning.

The pulse oximeter has an alarm, which is usually preset by the manufacturer to normal limits. Make sure the alarm is in the "on" position, and is set as ordered. Never turn the alarm off. (Refer to Procedure 33-100.)

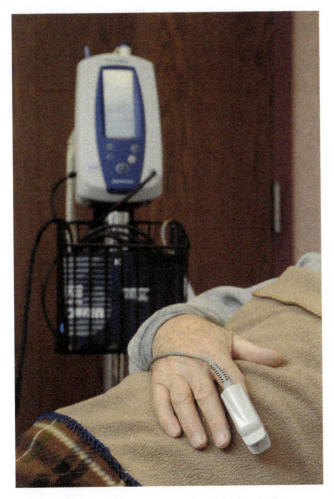

Figure 33-2 Pulse oximetry monitors the level of oxygen in arterial blood as a percentage on the display.

PROCEDURE 33-100
Using a Pulse Oximeter

1. Carry out each beginning procedure action.

2. Assemble equipment:
   - Pulse oximeter unit
   - Sensor appropriate to the site
   - Tape, if needed, to secure the sensor

3. Note the presence of fingernail polish or acrylic nails (if finger site is to be used to attach sensor) and make sure that the hand is not directly under a light source:
   - Remove fingernail polish according to facility policy (an opaque coating on the nail can decrease light transmission).
   - Acrylic nails (without polish) do not affect the accuracy of the sensor.
   - Make sure the sensor is not directly under a bedside lamp, which may affect the accuracy of the sensor.

4. Select and apply the sensor. If the sensor has position markings, align them opposite each other to ensure an accurate reading.

5. Fasten the sensor securely, or the reading will not be accurate. Make sure the sensor is not wrapped so tight with tape that it restricts blood flow.

6. Attach the sensor to the resident cable on the pulse oximeter.

7. Turn on the unit. You will hear a beep with each pulse beat. Adjust the volume as desired. Some units also have light bars, indicating the strength of the pulse. Note the percentage of oxygen saturation. Inform the nurse and document according to facility policy.

8. Monitor the resident's pulse rate, if the unit provides this reading. Compare the resident's actual pulse to make sure the unit is picking up each beat. Inform the nurse and document according to facility policy.

9. Monitor the resident's respirations and general appearance. Inform nurse and document according to facility policy. If the resident's general condition changes at any time, notify the nurse.

10. Carry out procedure completion actions.

Monitoring the Resident

You must monitor the resident regularly when a pulse oximeter is being used. Reporting to the nurse is part of your procedure completion actions. Report the resident's initial pulse oximeter reading and vital signs to

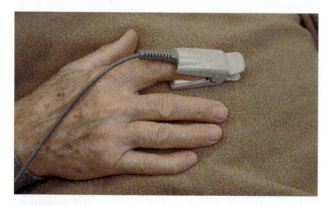

Figure 33-3A The finger-clip sensor should be rotated at least every 2 hours.

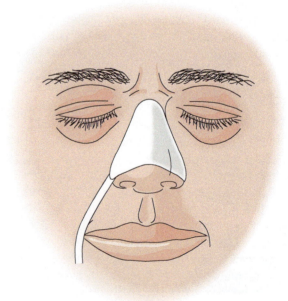

Figure 33-3B The nasal sensor.

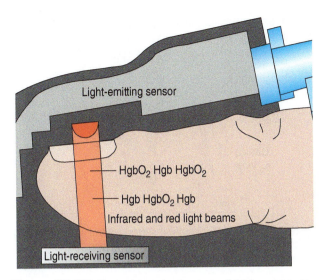

Figure 33-3C The pulse oximeter uses light to measure the amount of oxygen in the arterial blood.

the nurse; this provides important baseline information for the nurse. If these values are abnormal, the nurse will further assess the resident and provide care based on the abnormal values.

If the resident's vital signs or appearance change significantly from the baseline values, promptly notify the nurse. Immediately notify the nurse if the resident's pulse oximeter readings are less than the level ordered by the physician. Each time that you are in the room, monitor the resident's oxygen delivery system. Make sure that the liter flow rate is at the level prescribed by the physician.

Rotate the position of the finger sensor at least once every 4 hours. The spring-clip sensor should be moved every 2 hours. Rotating the location of the sensor reduces the risk of skin breakdown and complications related to pressure. If adhesive tape is used to secure the sensor, observe the skin for any signs of tape allergy, and if present, notify the nurse. Reapply sensor with hypoallergenic tape or with a spring-clip sensor.

INTRAVENOUS THERAPY

Intravenous (IV) therapy refers to medication or solutions administered directly into a vein. Standard intravenous therapy is given into a peripheral vein (a large vein in the arm). This is called an IV. The IV may consist of a single bag of solution connected to a simple tubing with a needle or small catheter on the end. Sometimes an additional small bag of fluid is attached to tubing that is connected to the main (primary) tubing. This is called a **piggyback**. This small bag contains medication such as an antibiotic that is given intermittently into the vein (Figure 33-4).

The nurse is responsible for the intravenous infusion and will immobilize the IV insertion site to prevent

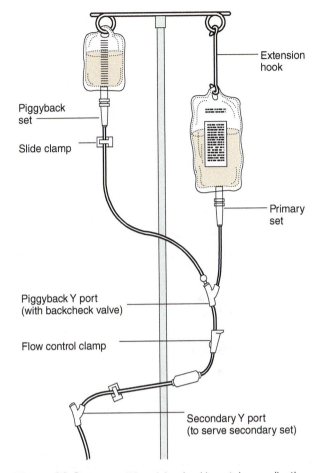

Figure 33-4 The small bag (piggyback) contains medication that is given over a short period of time.

the IV needle or cannula from moving and becoming dislodged from the vein (Figure 33-5). However, it is your responsibility to monitor the IV site and tubing each time you are in the room. Refer to Guidelines for Caring for Residents with Intravenous Lines.

Central Venous Insertion

Intravenous therapy can also be administered through a **central venous (CV) catheter**. A special catheter is inserted into a vein near the resident's collar bone (see Figure 33-7). The catheter tip ends in or near the heart chamber. CV therapy is used to administer medications or to provide total parenteral nutrition.

Peripheral Intravenous Central Catheter Line

A **peripheral intravenous central catheter** or **PICC** line consists of a catheter that is inserted into a peripheral vein and threaded upward through the vein to the jugular or subclavian vein. It is used to administer medications or to provide total parenteral nutrition (Figure 33-6).

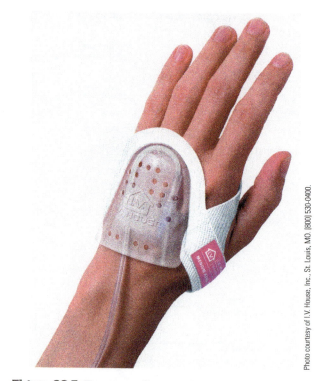

Figure 33-5 The nurse will secure the IV insertion site with a transparent dressing or device to prevent movement. Look through the transparent material to check the skin for signs of infiltration.

Insertion: Basilic vein (peripheral)
Termination: Superior vena cava

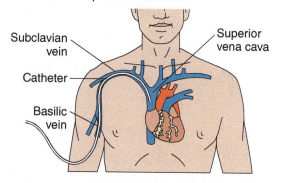

Figure 33-6 The peripherally inserted central catheter (PICC) is usually inserted into the upper arm. The long catheter is threaded into the superior vena cava of the heart.

Total Parenteral Nutrition

Total parenteral nutrition (TPN) is also called **hyperalimentation**. TPN is given to a resident whose bowels need complete rest. All required nutrients (carbohydrates, proteins, and fats) are given directly into the vein so the bowels do not have to work to digest food. Residents receiving TPN may need to be weighed daily or every other day. This should be done at the same time

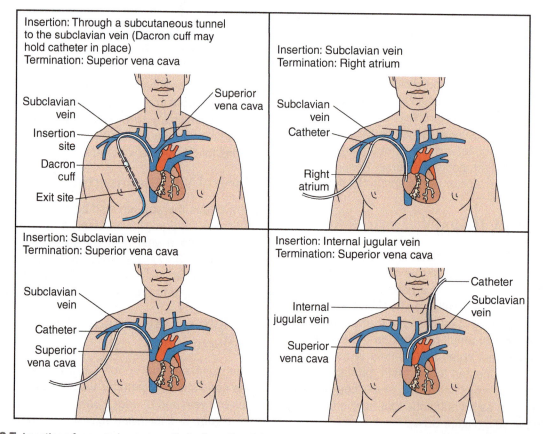

Figure 33-7 Locations for central venous catheter insertion. Infection is a high risk with a central catheter. Sterile technique is used to care for the insertion site.

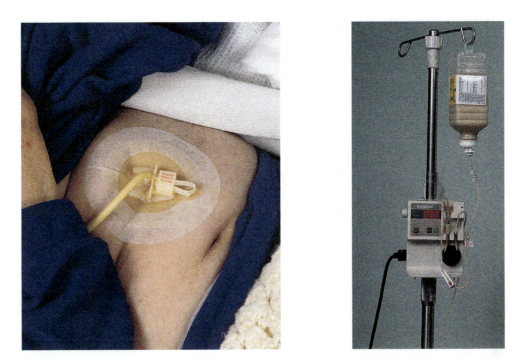

Figure 33-8 Nourishment may be given through a tube inserted into the resident's stomach.

of day with the resident wearing the same type of clothing. The resident may be gradually changed to **enteral feedings**. With an enteral feeding, liquid nourishment is administered through a tube inserted into the resident's stomach (Figure 33-8). TPN feedings bypass the organs of the digestive system, allowing them to rest and heal. The RN will care for the insertion site. Be sure the tubing is not obstructed or kinked. Be very careful when moving or caring for residents with TPN to avoid dislodging the tubing. Many health care facilities keep a special clamp, called a Kelly clamp (Figure 33-9) at the bedside of residents with lines in the subclavian vein. Serious complications occur if the tubing breaks or becomes dislodged. The Kelly is used to clamp the tubing close to the resident's body if the line breaks or is accidentally pulled loose. If air is

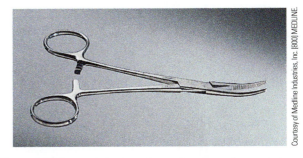

Courtesy of Medline Industries, Inc. [800] MEDLINE.

Figure 33-9 The Kelly clamp is used to clamp the central catheter close to the body in case of breakage.

allowed to enter the line, it could be fatal. The Kelly should be readily available and visible at all times. Avoid storing it in a drawer or removing it from the room.

⚠ GUIDELINES FOR … CARING FOR RESIDENTS WITH INTRAVENOUS LINES

1. Make sure the solution is dripping. Notify the nurse if the drip chamber is full.

2. Avoid pulling or twisting the tubing. Make sure the resident does not lie on the tubing. Do not adjust clamps on tubing.

3. Handle the arm carefully; notify the nurse if you:
   - Observe for signs of swelling, redness, or warmth.
   - Note any signs of moisture that may indicate the tubing is leaking.

4. Always keep IV solution above the needle insertion site.

5. Report to the nurse immediately:
   - Signs of dyspnea, cyanosis, chest pain, or back pain
   - If the alarm sounds on an IV pump
   - Redness, swelling, or complaints of pain or burning at the needle insertion site
   - Wetness or moisture at the insertion site or where the tubing connects to the IV catheter

(continues)

⚠ GUIDELINES FOR ... CARING FOR RESIDENTS WITH INTRAVENOUS LINES (Continued)

- If the solution in the IV bag or bottle is empty or low. The container should never run dry.
- If the IV is not dripping, seems to be dripping too fast, or the drip changer is completely full
- If the needle becomes dislodged
- If the tubing pulls apart from the needle
- If the solution appears to be leaking

6. When caring for residents with any type of IV therapy, never:
   - Change the drip rate
   - Disconnect any tubing

- Manipulate the needle or tubing: If the tubing or needle accidentally separate, put firm pressure on the needle insertion site with a gloved hand and call for the RN immediately.
- Remove, change, or manipulate any dressing over the site
- Adjust the clamps on the tubing
- Take a blood pressure on the arm with an IV infusion
- Turn off an alarm on an IV pump or other infusion equipment

? EXERCISE 33-2

1. Name four observations related to the resident receiving intravenous fluids that must be reported immediately to the nurse.

   a. _____
   _____

   b. _____
   _____

   c. _____
   _____

   d. _____
   _____

2. State four actions that a nursing assistant should never perform when caring for a resident with an intravenous line.

   a. Never _____
   b. Never _____
   c. Never _____
   d. Never _____

You may be required to assist the nurse with sterile dressing changes over the IV infusion site. When caring for residents with a CV catheter, immediately notify the nurse if:

- You see blood in the IV tubing
- The resident has an elevated temperature or experiences chills
- You observe swelling or redness around the collarbone or near the infusion site
- The resident complains of pain in the neck or chest
- The resident becomes short of breath, or develops elevated blood pressure or edema
- The catheter is broken or cracked
- The alarm sounds on the IV infusion pump

PAIN MANAGEMENT PROCEDURES

Pain management may be the major reason why some residents are admitted to a subacute unit. Other residents may be undergoing pain management related to other conditions such as recent surgery or pain related to cancer. Both drug and nondrug treatments can be successful in helping to prevent and control pain. Various types of relaxation and positioning techniques are frequently used for pain management.

Patient-Controlled Analgesia

Patient-controlled analgesia (PCA) is used for acute, chronic, or postoperative pain. *Analgesia* means pain relief. A device is inserted into the resident's vein. It is connected to a solution that contains a narcotic. A **narcotic** is a drug such as morphine that is used for pain relief. The dosage is controlled by equipment that has been preset. The patient or the nurse pushes the PCA button at times of discomfort.

Report to the nurse if you note any change in the resident's:

- Level of consciousness
- Rate and pattern of respirations
- Pupil size
- Skin color

Other complications of this therapy that you should report to nurse are:

- Nausea and/or vomiting
- Difficulty urinating or inability to urinate
- Excessive drowsiness
- Confusion
- Itching
- Preset pump alarm sounds

Constipation is a common side effect of narcotic medications. The resident must be carefully monitored to avoid serious problems. Encourage the resident to drink liquids, eat the fiber foods on the meal tray, and be as active as possible as determined by the plan of care. Accurately monitor and document the resident's bowel activity. Report any verbal complaints from the resident or signs of constipation to the nurse.

Pain Management with an Epidural Catheter

An **epidural catheter** is implanted beneath the resident's skin. It is inserted near the spinal cord at the first lumbar (L1) space (Figure 33-10). A local anesthetic is administered either intermittently or continuously through the catheter. The resident may have leg numbness and weakness for the first 24 hours after the catheter is inserted. Report to the nurse at once if:

- Catheter becomes dislodged from the insertion site
- You note changes in respiration rate and pattern
- Resident complains of itching
- Resident vomits or complains of nausea

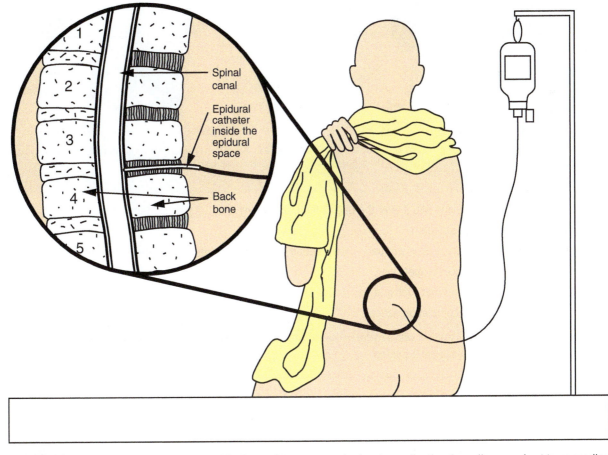

Spinal canal

Epidural catheter inside the epidural space

Back bone

Figure 33-10 The epidural catheter is used for intermittent or constant pain medication (usually on a short-term medication delivery).

PROCEDURE 33-101
Changing a Gown on a Resident with a Peripheral Intravenous Line in Place

NOTE: This procedure is to be used only when the IV is not run through an electronic pump. When a pump is used, the resident may wear a gown that snaps at the shoulder. In this case, the gown can be removed without touching the IV bag or tubing. If the resident is wearing a non snap gown, call the nurse if the gown is to be changed. Never disconnect the tubing from the pump.

1. Carry out each beginning procedure action.
2. Assemble equipment:
   - Clean gown
3. Make sure windows and door are closed to prevent chilling the resident.
4. Remove gown from the arm without the IV and bring gown across resident's chest to other arm.
5. Place clean gown over resident's chest to avoid exposure.
6. On the arm with the IV, gather material of gown in one hand so there is no pull or pressure on the line, and slowly draw gown over tip of fingers (Figure 33-11).
7. With free hand, lift IV free of standard and slip gown over bag of fluid (Figure 33-12), removing gown from resident's body. Never allow the bag of fluid to be lower than the resident's arm.

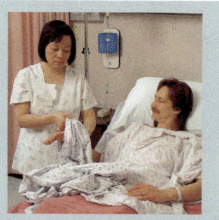

Figure 33-11 Gather material of gown in one hand so there is no pull or pressure on the line. Slowly draw the gown over tips of fingers.

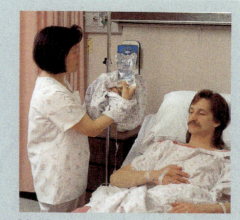

Figure 33-12 With free hand, lift IV free of stand and slip gown over bag of fluid.

8. Take sleeve of clean gown and slip it over the bag of fluid, the tubing, and up the resident's arm.
9. Replace bag of fluid on IV standard.
10. Remove soiled gown and place at end of bed. Finish putting clean gown on resident's other arm. Secure neck ties.
11. Place soiled gown in laundry hamper.
12. Make sure IV is dripping and that tubing is not kinked or twisted.
13. Carry out each procedure completion action.

NOTE: If you are changing a gown for a resident with a centrally inserted line, you will not need to lower the fluid container. Change the gown in the usual manner, taking care not to manipulate the tubing.

Transcutaneous Electrical Nerve Stimulation

Transcutaneous electrical nerve stimulation (TENS) is a drug-free method of pain relief. Mild, harmless electrical current stimulates nerve fibers to block the transmission of pain to the brain. Electrodes are taped to the resident's skin. The location of the electrodes depends on the areas related to the pain. The electrodes are attached to wires that are attached to a control box. The intensity of the stimulation is set on the control box by the nurse.

CARING FOR RESIDENTS WITH TRACHEOSTOMIES

You may care for a resident with a tracheostomy. A tracheostomy is a tube that is inserted into a surgical opening in the resident's trachea (windpipe). A tracheostomy is performed when the resident is unable to breathe in air through the nose. The tube allows the resident to "breathe" as air goes directly into the trachea and then into the lungs. A person who is on a ventilator for a long time will have a tracheostomy that is connected to the ventilator. The resident may have secretions coming from the chest and through the tube. The nurse will need to use suction to remove the secretions.

The tube may be made of plastic or metal. Tracheostomy tubes consist of an inner removable tube called a cannula and an outer tube called a neckplate that is held in place with neck ties. The neckplate rests between the clavicles (breastbones). There is a slot on each side. Tracheostomy ties are inserted here to secure the tube in place (Figure 33-13). Residents with tracheostomies can usually take a bath or shower but must keep the water away from the opening. Avoid using powders, sprays, or shaving cream around the tube. When you care for a resident with a tracheostomy, observe for:

- Changes in respiratory rate, depth, quality
- Cyanosis
- Changes in mental status such as confusion, restlessness, or irritability that indicate the resident is not getting enough oxygen

Report to the nurse immediately if the:

- Tube becomes dislodged from the opening or blocked
- Resident is having trouble breathing
- Resident needs suctioning

Be sure you know how the resident communicates. The incision in the trachea will interfere with the resident's ability to talk.

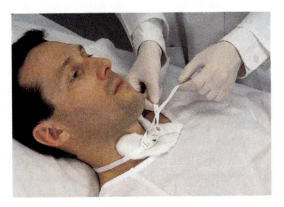

Figure 33-13 Ties hold the tracheostomy tube in place.

CARING FOR THE RESIDENT WITH SLEEP APNEA

Sleep apnea is a common but potentially serious sleep disorder. The resident experiences one or more pauses or shallow breathing patterns while asleep. It is often accompanies by loud snoring. The person who has sleep apnea frequently complains that they feel tired even though they may have slept through the night. Most people who have sleep apnea are unaware of the condition except when a family member or a bed partner complains of the snoring.

There are two main types of sleep apnea, obstructive sleep apnea (OSA) and central obstructive sleep apnea. (OSA), the latter of which is the most common and will be the main focus of our discussion. The airway collapses or becomes blocked during sleep; this causes the pauses or shallow breathing pattern. Central sleep apnea (CSA) occurs when the brain fails to send the proper stimuli to the muscles that control breathing.

Signs and symptoms of both types of sleep apnea overlap. These include:

- Loud snoring (less typical with CSA)
- Abrupt awakening with shortness of breath
- Observed episodes of breathing cessation
- Difficulty staying asleep
- Awakening with a dry mouth
- Excessive daytime sleepiness
- Morning headaches

When the muscles in the back of the throat relax, the airway narrows and closes as the person takes in a breath. Breathing stops for a few moments, but this closure is sufficient to lower the level of oxygen in the blood. When the oxygen level is lowered, the person is roused from sleep to reopen the airway. This happens so quickly, the person does not remember it occurring. The person may gasp for air or make a snorting sound. It is possible that this pattern of breathing may repeat itself many times in an hour. An overnight sleep study frequently is recommended before starting treatment.

Risk factors include:

- Excess weight
- Hypertension
- Narrowed airway
- Older males (over age 65)
- Family history
- Smoking (increased irritation to the airway)
- Alcohol, sedatives, or tranquilizers (relax throat muscles)

One of the most popular treatment modalities for sleep apnea is the use of positive airway pressure.

continuous positive airway pressure (CPAP) and bi-level positive airway pressure (BIPAP) may be used. The CPAP machine is ideally used whenever the person is sleeping (during naps or at night). This machine increases the air pressure in the throat to prevent it from collapsing when the person takes a breath. Several types of machines are available:

- Prongs that fit in the nose
- Mask that covers the face
- Mask that covers the nose only, nasal continuous airway pressure (NCPAP), the most common type. (See Figure 33-14.)

Some residents may use a BIPAP machine. This type of machine provides two different pressures. A higher pressure used during inspiration and a lower pressure during expiration. This type of machine is used for persons who have difficulty expiring against pressure. Have the nurse instruct you in applying the mask or prongs and in the use of the machines.

Even though CPAP is a safe and painless treatment, it must be used long-term. Some residents may experience side effects. If you note any of the following in residents who use this therapy, notify the nurse.

- Facial skin irritation or skin allergies
- Dry mouth
- Nasal congestion, sneezing, runny nose, or nosebleeds
- Stomach bloating or discomfort
- Noisy machine
- Failure to keep the mask in place

CARING FOR THE RESIDENT RECEIVING DIALYSIS TREATMENTS

Dialysis is a process by which the blood is cleansed of liquid wastes artificially when the kidneys are unable to remove the wastes. This procedure is needed when a person has kidney failure. Without dialysis the person would die as the waste products accumulated in the bloodstream. Dialysis is usually considered a temporary treatment that will continue until a suitable kidney is found for a kidney transplant. The two types of dialysis are hemodialysis and peritoneal dialysis.

Hemodialysis

During **hemodialysis** treatment the resident's blood is circulated outside of the body into an artificial kidney machine (Figure 33-15). In the dialysis machine, the blood is cleansed with a liquid substance called dialysate and then returned to the resident's body. Most persons needing hemodialysis treatments are treated in a dialysis center. However, you may care for residents in the subacute unit who go as outpatients to the dialysis center for their treatments. Dialysis is usually done three to four times a week. Each treatment takes several hours. To do dialysis, a connection must be made between the resident's circulatory system and the artificial kidney machine. Minor surgery is done to create either a fistula or a graft or shunt. The **fistula** (Figure 33-16A) is created when a vein is attached to an artery either in an arm or leg. When a **graft** is used (Figure 33-16B), synthetic material is inserted to form a connection between an artery and a vein. Two needles are inserted for treatment with either the fistula or graft. The needles are connected to tubes that go to and from the artificial kidney machine. As a nursing assistant, you are not expected to care for the fistula or graft. You need to be aware that the resident will:

- Have fluid restrictions
- Have dietary restrictions for calories, sodium, protein, potassium, calcium, and phosphorus
- Need all fluid intake and output measured and recorded

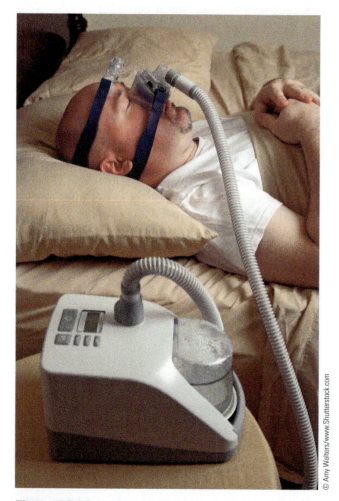

© Amy Walters/www.Shutterstock.com

Figure 33-14 A CPAP machine being used to treat sleep apnea.

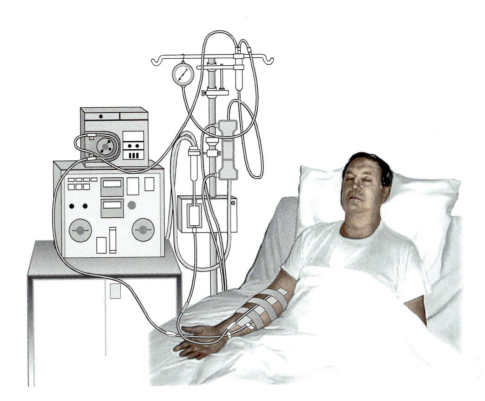

Figure 33-15 Dialysis removes wastes and impurities from the resident's blood. Blood leaves the body through an artery, is filtered by the machine, then returns through a vein.

A.V. Fistula

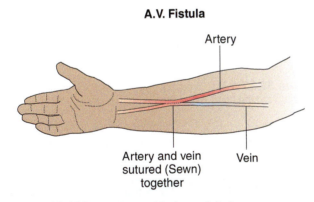

Artery

Artery and vein sutured (Sewn) together   Vein

Figure 33-16A Fistula used for hemodialysis.

Graft

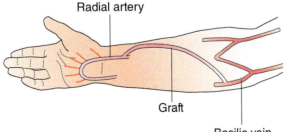

Radial artery

Graft

Basilic vein

Figure 33-16B Graft or shunt used for hemodialysis.

- Need to be weighed regularly at the same time of day and with the same type of clothing; if in a wheelchair, same chair, cushions, and foot pedals.
- Need to be monitored and have blood pressure taken frequently after dialysis. Remember that blood pressure should not be taken in the arm used for dialysis.

Report to the nurse if the resident has:

- Swelling (edema) of the hands or feet
- Changes in vital signs (blood pressure, temperature, pulse, or respirations)
- A change in weight
- A change in intake and output measurements
- Shortness of breath
- Complaints of pain at the site of the fistula or graft

Following hemodialysis, the resident may complain of weakness. Observe the resident, especially when ambulating. He or she may have periods of dizziness and faintness. Monitor vital signs frequently as prescribed after the procedure.

Peritoneal Dialysis

Peritoneal dialysis is also a process of cleansing the blood. In peritoneal dialysis, the process takes place within the resident's body in the peritoneal (abdominal) cavity, rather than outside the body in a machine (Figure 33-17). During dialysis the dialysate is introduced into the abdominal cavity, allowed to stay in for some time, and then drained out. As blood flows through the vessels in the peritoneum, waste products are filtered and excess fluids are removed. The nurse instills the dialysate through a catheter that is surgically implanted through the wall of the abdomen into the abdominal cavity. This is done using sterile technique.

Nursing assistants are not expected to administer peritoneal dialysis. You may be responsible for monitoring the resident's vital signs every 10 to 15 minutes for the first 1 to 2 hours after a treatment and then every 2 to 4 hours. Notify the nurse if there are any changes in vital signs.

Other signs and symptoms that are to be reported to the nurse include:

- Returned dialysate that appears bloody or has blood clots in the solution
- Complaints of abdominal pain
- Wet or soiled abdominal dressing
- Fluid leaks around the catheter insertion site
- Disconnected tubing or catheter
- Dialysate solution that appears to be running very slowly or not at all
- Drainage container that is almost full
- Resident is weak or unsteady
- Resident has low blood pressure or complains of dizziness
- Resident is short of breath or complains of difficulty breathing

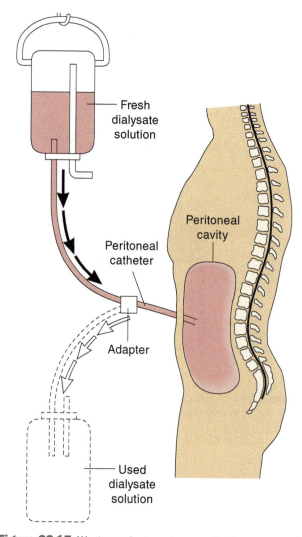

Figure 33-17 Waste products and excess fluid are removed as the dialysate flows out of the peritoneal cavity.

Labels: Fresh dialysate solution; Peritoneal cavity; Peritoneal catheter; Adapter; Used dialysate solution

---

? **EXERCISE 33-3**

CLINICAL SITUATION

Read the following situations about residents in subacute care and complete the statements.

1. Mrs. Kraft is 87 years of age and has suffered from failing kidneys for 3 years. She is on hemodialysis three times weekly. Mrs. Kraft:

    a. Will have a special site in her _____ where the dialysis needles are inserted.
       (arm) (neck)

    b. Will have fluids _____
       (forced) (restricted)

    c. Will need to be _____ regularly.
       (measured) (weighed)

    d. Should be carefully monitored for _____
       (mood) (intake/output)

INCENTIVE SPIROMETRY

An incentive spirometer is used by residents to improve lung function and keep lungs clear when coughing and deep breathing are ineffective or inadequate. The incentive spirometer measures the amount of air taken in with each inspiration. It is especially useful following surgical procedures and for residents who may have prolonged periods of bed rest, or following trauma to the ribs.

When using the incentive spirometer the person is instructed to sit up as straight as possible, to put the mouthpiece into the mouth and to seal the lips around it as tightly as possible. Then the person is instructed to breathe as deeply as possible to raise the ball in the chamber to the goal level as instructed. The breath is held for as long as possible or for at least 5 seconds. The ball will drop in the chamber. The person should rest for a few seconds and then repeat the process. The incentive spirometer can be used as many as 10 times per hour but, in any event is used many times during the day, per physician orders. Pulse oximetry, discussed earlier in this lesson, is used to assess the level of oxygenation achieved. The resident should also be instructed to increase the intake of fluids to help thin secretions in the lungs.

ONCOLOGY TREATMENTS

Oncology is the care and treatment of those with cancer. Cancer may be treated with surgery, radiation, chemotherapy, or a combination of any of these.

Radiation Therapy

Residents receiving radiation therapy in the long-term care facility will be transported to a special cancer treatment center or to a hospital to receive the therapy as an outpatient. Radiation therapy is the use of high-energy radiation to kill cancer cells. It is considered a local therapy because it kills only the cancer cells in the area being treated. Residents receiving radiation may complain of the following side effects that should be reported to the nurse:

- Nausea, vomiting
- Fatigue
- Diarrhea
- Skin redness, irritation, peeling
- Change in ability to taste
- Irritation of mucous membranes
- Cough
- Shortness of breath

When caring for residents receiving radiation therapy:

- Do not remove markings made on the skin for treatment purposes.
- Do not use any heat or cold treatments on the area being treated.
- Wash the area only with tepid water and a soft washcloth. Do not apply any soaps, powders, deodorants, perfumes, makeup, lotions, or skin preparations to the area.
- Instruct resident to avoid wearing tight clothing over area.

Protecting Yourself from Radiation Exposure

Residents who have radiation therapy, such as that previously described, are not "radioactive" (do not give off radiation). However, some residents are treated with a radiation source that is implanted in the body for a short period of time. When this radiation source is inside the resident's body, the radiation penetrates throughout the body. If you care for residents who have radiation implants, you will be taught special precautions to reduce

---

? EXERCISE 33-4

MATCHING
Match the term on the right with the definition on the left.

Definition
1. _____ used to measure the amount of oxygen in arterial blood
2. _____ a drug used for pain relief
3. _____ nondrug method of pain relief
4. _____ liquid nourishment administered through a tube inserted into the resident's stomach
5. _____ total parenteral nutrition
6. _____ special catheter inserted into the subclavian artery or right atrium
7. _____ method of ridding the body of wastes for a person with kidney failure

Term
a. hyperalimentation
b. pulse oximetry
c. narcotic
d. hemodialysis

e. TENS
f. enteral feeding
g. central venous catheter

your risk of radiation exposure. These residents will stay in bed while an implant is in place in the body. A list of special precautions will be placed on the resident's chart or in the Kardex. In general, the precautions relate to:

- *Time* spent in the resident's room
  - Stay no longer than necessary.
  - Special care plans are developed.
  - Inform the nurse if you are pregnant, or suspect that you are pregnant. (You will not be assigned to care for the resident.)
- *Distance* you are from the source of radiation
  - Stand at least 3 feet away from the resident unless giving direct care.
  - Never touch an implant if it becomes dislodged (notify the nurse).
- *Shielding* (use of lead aprons and the like for extra protection) when close contact with the resident is required
  - Find out if special precautions are needed for handling soiled lines, tissues, dressings, food trays, bedpans, and body fluids.

Chemotherapy

Chemotherapy is the use of drugs to kill cancer cells within the body. The drugs may be given by mouth (orally), through the vein (IV), or in the muscle (intramuscular [IM]). The nurse or physician administers the drugs. Because the drugs that are given target the rapidly regenerating cancer cells, they also affect all other cells in the body that quickly regenerate. The cells in the gastrointestinal tract, the blood cells (red and white blood cells), the hair and nails all will become affected by the action of the drugs. For these reasons, the residents may complain of nausea and vomiting, **anorexia** (loss of appetite), and soreness in the mouth. In addition, these residents are prone to infection because the white blood cells that help to fight infection are killed. They may also be short of breath because there are not enough red blood cells to carry hemoglobin and oxygen through the bloodstream. Some residents will develop bleeding gums or bleed more heavily from wounds because the platelets that help with blood clotting are destroyed as well. Modern treatment techniques and advanced medication therapy can help to minimize some of these symptoms. Hair loss (**alopecia**) will occur, but it is usually temporary. The hair usually comes back after the treatments are completed. Some persons prefer to wear a wig, a hat, or scarf during this time. Respect the resident's wishes regarding personal appearance and support the resident during the period when the side effects of the drugs are most intense.

? EXERCISE 33-5

1. Mr. Ornstein, 81 years of age, has a diagnosis of cancer of the colon. He has had the tumor removed but is now receiving radiation therapy. Mr. Ornstein:

   a. Will probably experience periods of _____.

   　　　　　　　　　　　　　　　　(high energy) (fatigue)

   b. Should be instructed to avoid wearing _____ clothing over the area of radiation.

   　　　　　　　　　　　　　　(loose) (tight)

   c. Should wash the area using _____ water.

   　　　　　　　　　　　　　　　　　(hot) (tepid)

   d. Should _____ the skin markings made for treatment.

   　　　(remove) (avoid removing)

2. Mrs. Santoz has cancer of the ovaries. It is too far advanced for surgery. She is receiving chemotherapy. Mrs. Santoz:

   a. Will receive her medication from the _____.

   　　　　　　　　　　　　　(nurse) (nursing assistant)

   b. Will probably experience _____ appetite.

   　　　　　　　　　(increased) (decreased)

   c. May _____ some of her hair.

   　　　(grow) (lose)

? EXERCISE 33-6

COMPLETION
Select the correct term(s) from the following list to complete each statement.

alarm	nasal cannula	stomach
bowel	oxygen	tracheostomy
chemotherapy	peripheral	III
finger	sleep apnea	IV

1. A person who has been unable to breathe without the help of a ventilator will require _____ care.

2. Cancer patients in subacute care may be receiving treatment with _____ or radiation.

3. Most people who have _____ _____ are unaware of the condition except when a family member complains of loud snoring.

4. Wound management is given for residents who have stage _____ or stage _____ pressure ulcers.

5. Never turn off the _____ on the pulse oximeter.

6. The most common way oxygen is administered to residents in subacute care units is with _____.

7. Pulse oximetry is used to monitor the level of _____ in the arterial blood.

8. In pulse oximetry the photodetector is usually placed over the _____.

9. Standard intravenous therapy is given into a _____ vein.

10. Total parenteral nutrition is given when the _____ needs complete rest.

11. Enteral feedings are given through a tube inserted into the resident's _____.

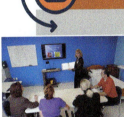

LESSON SYNTHESIS: Putting It All Together

You have just completed this lesson. Now go back and review the Clinical Focus. Try to see how the Clinical Focus relates to the concepts presented in this lesson. Then answer the following questions.

1. Consider the different types of care that subacute units provide. If Steven works in a unit with residents receiving dialysis, what should he know about kidney function and kidney disease?

2. Using the knowledge presented in earlier lessons in this text, what differences would you expect between acute care, subacute care, and long-term care?

3. What challenges would you expect to accept if you work in a subacute care unit?

4. How would you prepare yourself for meeting these challenges?

33 REVIEW

A. Select the one best answer for each of the following.

1. Subacute care is given to persons who
   (A) have been acutely ill
   (B) have had a long, progressive illness
   (C) require only custodial care
   (D) require intensive care

2. The purpose of subacute care is to
   (A) increase the population of long-term care facilities
   (B) discharge patients from the hospital as quickly as possible
   (C) provide the care a person needs at a lower cost
   (D) provide preoperative care

3. Examples of the type of persons treated in subacute care include all of the following *except* those
   (A) requiring dialysis
   (B) being held for observation
   (C) receiving wound care
   (D) requiring high levels of rehabilitation

4. A nursing assistant working in subacute care would need to
   (A) learn how to start intravenous feedings
   (B) have excellent observational skills
   (C) learn how to administer chemotherapy
   (D) instruct residents in pain management techniques

5. If you accept a position in a subacute care unit, you will not be required to learn
   (A) why hyperalimentation is given
   (B) your responsibilities for residents receiving dialysis
   (C) more about the rehabilitation process
   (D) advanced burn care

6. The procedure to measure the level of oxygen in arterial blood is called
   (A) hemodialysis
   (B) pulse oximetry
   (C) total parenteral nutrition
   (D) intravenous therapy

7. A central venous catheter is inserted into
   (A) a vein in the resident's arm
   (B) an artery in the resident's arm
   (C) the jugular or subclavian vein
   (D) the epidural space

8. Total parenteral nutrition (TPN) is used for residents
   (A) who need to lose weight
   (B) who are unconscious
   (C) who refuse to eat
   (D) whose bowel needs complete rest

9. The nursing assistant's responsibility for caring for residents with intravenous feedings is to
   (A) insert the needle into the vein
   (B) add medication to the bag of fluid when it is due
   (C) observe for complications
   (D) change the drip rate if it is going too fast or too slow

10. Patient-controlled analgesia is used for all of the following, *except*
    (A) to allow the patient to receive as much medication as he or she wants at any time
    (B) for administering narcotics for pain
    (C) to allow the resident to receive the medication when he or she needs it
    (D) for acute, chronic, or postoperative pain

11. An epidural catheter is used for
    (A) pain management
    (B) administering nutrition
    (C) emptying the bladder
    (D) intravenous feedings

12. When caring for residents with tracheostomies, you should
    (A) not allow the resident to take a bath or shower
    (B) observe for changes in respiratory rate, depth, and quality

(C) maintain the resident on a liquid diet

(D) be responsible for changing the tracheostomy tube

13. Dialysis is a procedure for

(A) cleansing the blood of liquid wastes

(B) relieving postoperative pain

(C) administering oxygen

(D) giving total parenteral nutrition

14. A resident on dialysis will have all of the following, except

(A) fluid restrictions

(B) dietary restrictions

(C) frequent weights taken

(D) unchanged blood pressure

15. When caring for residents on dialysis, you should report

(A) edema of the hands and feet

(B) stable vital signs

(C) muscle aches

(D) no change in weight

16. Oncology is the care and treatment of residents with

(A) severe wounds

(B) kidney failure

(C) cancer

(D) terminal illness

17. When caring for residents receiving radiation therapy, you should

(A) remove the markings made on the skin for treatment purposes

(B) apply cold treatments to the area

(C) avoid applying soaps, powders, lotions, deodorants, or other substances to the treated area

(D) wrap the treatment area with an elastic bandage

18. A person with sleep apnea may manifest all *but one* of the following signs and symptoms:

(A) Loud snoring

(B) Excessive daytime sleepiness

(C) Waking with a dry mouth

(D) Evening headaches

19. Risk factors associated with sleep apnea include all *but one* of the following:

(A) Hypotension

(B) Obesity

(C) Family history

(D) Man over age 65

B. Fill in the blanks by selecting the correct word or phrase from the list.

dialysis	pulse oximetry
enteral	transcutaneous
hyperalimentation	electrical nerve
long-term narcotic	stimulation
piggyback	transitional care

20. Subacute care is also called _____.

21. A procedure for removing liquid wastes from the blood is called _____.

22. _____ is used for measuring the oxygen level in arterial blood.

23. A _____ refers to a small bag of fluid containing intravenous medication that is connected with a tube to the primary tubing.

24. Total parenteral nutrition (TPN) is also called _____.

25. A feeding administered through a tube into the resident's stomach is called an _____ feeding.

26. A _____ is a potent drug used for pain relief.

27. The use of electrical current to treat pain is done with a procedure called _____.

28. Continuous positive airway pressure (CPAP) treatments are _____ therapy.

LESSON 34
CARING FOR THE PERSON IN THE HOME SETTING

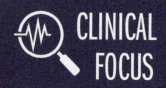 **CLINICAL FOCUS**

Think about the role of the nursing assistant in providing care in the home setting as you study this lesson.

OBJECTIVES

After studying this lesson, you should be able to:

- Define vocabulary words and terms.
- State the benefits of working in home health care.
- Name the members of the home health care team.
- List 8 to 10 important characteristics of the home health nursing assistant.
- Describe the duties of the home health nursing assistant.
- Identify how to maintain a safe, clean, and comfortable home environment.
- Describe why time management is an important characteristic for the home health nursing assistant.
- List at least 8 to 10 ways to protect your personal safety while working in the home environment.
- Describe the home health nursing assistant's responsibilities for record keeping, documentation, and reporting.

VOCABULARY

client care records (KLI-ent kair RE-kords)
home health nursing assistant (home health NUR-sing ah-SIS-tant)

intermittent care (INTER-mi-tent kair)
time and travel records (TI-m and TRA-vl RE-kords)

CASE STUDY

Emily Hancock has been a certified nursing assistant for several years. She has recently decided to work in the home setting. She is looking forward to the challenges of using her skills in caring for clients in their own home environment.

INTRODUCTION

Health care has been provided for persons in their own homes for centuries. However, it was not until the mid-twentieth century in the United States that the trend changed to move the care from the person's home into community health care facilities (namely hospitals). Now the pendulum is swinging in the opposite direction, with hospitals being used predominately for more acutely ill persons. As discussed in previous lessons, increasing numbers of persons are being cared for in various types of long-term care facilities, as well as in day care and home settings.

Over the years the rules for nursing practice have become more strict. Initially there were few legal restrictions placed on persons who provided care in a client's home. Laws now specifically state the actions an RN can and cannot perform in any setting. Anyone who practices nursing without a license can be held liable.

Home care has become a preferred option for a number of persons. Factors that are important in promoting the interest and increase in the use of home care services include:

- High cost of hospital care; home care is usually less expensive
- Early discharge from the hospital because the diagnosis-related groups (DRGs) limit the length of a hospital stay based on the client's diagnosis
- Growing population of persons with chronic illness
- Personal preference to remain in the home setting to receive personalized care
- Increasing acceptance of staying at home to die with dignity

The Omnibus Budget Reconciliation Act (OBRA), in addition to developing the national standards for care in long-term care facilities, has also set standards for care that are received in the home. The Client's Rights in Home Care are displayed in Figure 34-1. Periodically review these client rights to ensure that you are following these guidelines when you are giving care in the home.

BENEFITS OF HOME HEALTH CARE

For the Client

There are a number of benefits of home care for the client and the family:

- The client remains a member of the family unit.
- Care is provided in a familiar setting.

Client's Rights in Home Care

The persons receiving home health care services or their families possess basic rights and responsibilities. These include:

The right to:

1. be treated with dignity, consideration, and respect
2. have their property treated with respect
3. receive a timely response from the agency to requests for service
4. be fully informed on admission of the care and treatment that will be provided, how much it will cost, and how payment will be handled
5. know in advance if you will be responsible for any payment
6. be informed in advance of any changes in your care
7. receive care from professionally trained personnel, to know their names and responsibilities
8. participate in planning care
9. refuse treatment and to be told the consequences of your action
10. expect confidentiality of all information
11. be informed of anticipated termination of service
12. be referred elsewhere if you are denied services solely based on your inability to pay
13. know how to make a complaint or recommend a change in agency policies and services

The responsibility to:

1. remain under a doctor's care while receiving services
2. provide the agency with a complete health history
3. provide the agency all requested insurance and financial information
4. sign the required consents and releases for insurance billing
5. participate in your care by asking questions, expressing concerns, stating if you do not understand
6. provide a safe home environment in which care is given
7. cooperate with your doctor, the staff, and other caregivers
8. accept responsibility for any refusal of treatment
9. abide by agency policies which restrict duties our staff may perform
10. advise agency administration of any dissatisfaction or problems with your care

Figure 34-1 The client's rights in home care.

- The client has more control over daily activities (e.g., time to get up and go to bed, when and what to eat, leisure activities, visitors).
- Continuity of care is personalized to individual needs.
- Risk of infections is minimized. (The client is not exposed to the more serious infections found in a health care facility.)
- Care is usually less expensive than that provided in other settings.

1. List at least four benefits of home care for the client and family.

    a. _____

    b. _____

    c. _____

    d. _____

2. Benefits for the home health nursing assistant include:

    a. _____

    b. _____

    c. _____

    d. _____

    e. _____

For the Home Health Nursing Assistant

Each setting for providing care for those in need is unique. There are advantages to working in each type of setting. Advantages to providing care in the home setting are:

- Satisfaction for giving care to one client at a time in his or her own setting
- Opportunity to work with the same person over a period of time (Figure 34-2)
- Varied assignments
- The chance to work as a member of a team, but with greater independence
- The prospect of working part-time, if desired

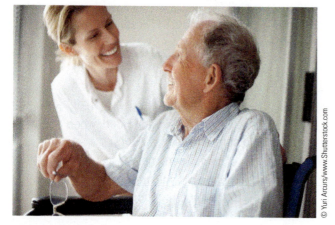

Figure 34-2 Caring for the same client over a period of time provides great satisfaction.

THE HOME HEALTH CARE TEAM

A number of persons from a variety of disciplines make up the team that provides care in the home setting:

- Client—the person who needs care
- Family members—may be alternate caregivers, may live in the client's home, and may or may not be supportive of the client
- Case manager—assesses the overall needs of the client and determines which services should be provided; may be the RN or social worker
- Registered nurse—also may be the case manager; coordinates care in the home: performs assessment, initiates plan of care, and evaluates effectiveness of care; teaches and supervises health care nursing assistants
- Licensed practical nurse—provides direct care, such as giving medications and treatments
- Health care nursing assistant—provides for direct client care (Figure 34-3) and for client's safety and comfort; observes and reports client changes; documents observations and care given
- Physician—writes orders and acts as a consultant
- Other health care personnel who may be involved in care:
  - Physical therapist
  - Registered dietitian
  - Occupational or speech therapist
  - Social worker
  - Respiratory therapist

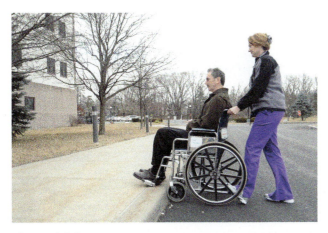

Figure 34-3 Equipment may be purchased, rented, or borrowed from other organizations or agencies.

CHARACTERISTICS OF THE HOME HEALTH NURSING ASSISTANT

The home health nursing assistant needs special preparation and knowledge to apply the information learned in a basic nursing assistant course in order to care for a client in the home setting. As a home health nursing assistant, you need to:

- Possess strong clinical skills.
- Be dependable.
- Have excellent observational skills, being able to recognize and report unusual or abnormal signs and symptoms.
- Be willing and able to follow instructions and pay attention to details, carrying out procedures as taught.
- Be self-directed and motivated, knowing the duties and carrying them out without being told.
- Be mature and self-disciplined, carrying out tasks without wasting time (texting on your phone, drinking coffee).
- Be organized and have good time management skills, yet be flexible enough to work around the client's schedule (not your own).
- Have a strong sense of honesty. You may be handling the client's money and belongings. Keep all receipts from purchases as well as an accurate record of all money spent.
- Be creative and adaptable. Equipment may not be readily available; you may have to improvise. For example, an ice bag can be made from a household zippered bag filled with ice and covered with a towel.
- Be accepting of the client and family. Remember that you are a guest in the client's home. Clients will be of all ethnic backgrounds and socioeconomic levels.
- Have good interpersonal skills and work well with others. You are a member of a team that includes the client and family.
- Be punctual and have dependable transportation.
- Have good personal hygiene.
- Know your own limitations and when to ask for help.

HOME HEALTH NURSING ASSISTANT DUTIES

The duties of the home health nursing assistant are planned around the needs and routine of the client and the family. Duties will likely include:

- Providing a safe environment at all times
- Assisting with activities of daily living (ADLs); skills may need to be adapted to home setting (Figure 34-4)
- Providing comfort measures such as positioning and special mouth care
- Performing range-of-motion exercises and other special treatments
- Monitoring the client, such as checking and documenting vital signs (Figure 34-5)
- Changing linens and making the bed
- Doing light housekeeping

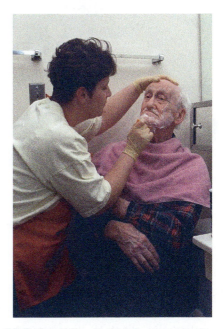

Figure 34-4 The skills you have learned may be adapted for care in the home.

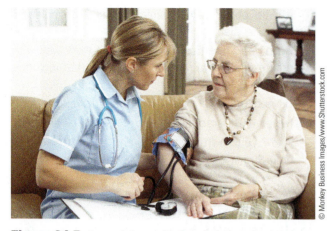

Figure 34-5 Accurately monitoring vital signs is an important responsibility.

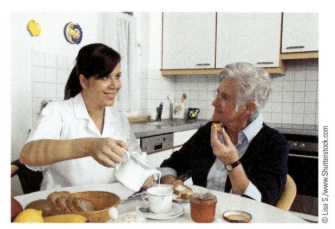

Figure 34-7 Help prepare meals for the client.

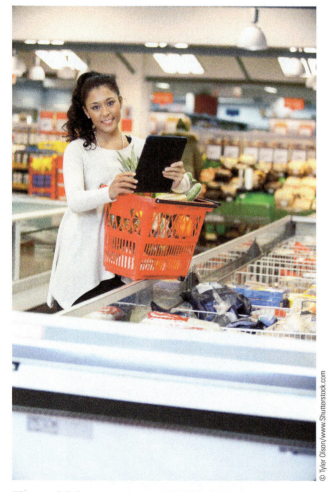

Figure 34-6 Your duties may include shopping for groceries. Prepare a list before leaving for the store.

- Shopping for meals (Figure 34-6)
- Preparing meals for the client (Figure 34-7)
- Laundering the client's personal items and bed linens
- Transporting the client to appointments as per agency protocol (Figure 34-8)

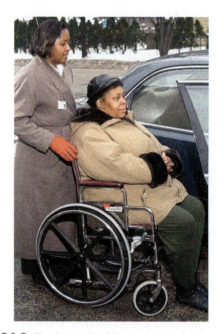

Figure 34-8 The home health nursing assistant may be responsible for transporting clients to clinic appointments and therapy.

- Reminding the client to take prescribed medications or monitoring client's self-administration of medications
- Caring for medical equipment and supplies (cleaning and disinfecting equipment and supplies used for the client)

The home health nursing assistant is *not* expected to:

- Do heavy housework such as washing windows, moving heavy furniture, or doing yard or garden work
- Make decisions about the purchase of food, unless the client is unable and the family or case manager instructs you to do so

- Become involved in the family affairs, disputes, or decisions (do not take sides)
- Handle the client's money, unless specific directions are provided by the agency (keep all receipts)

ADAPTATIONS FOR THE HOME SETTING

All of the equipment, especially disposable items, may not be available to you in the home. Sometimes the family will rent or purchase equipment, such as hospital-type beds or bedside commodes. The client may own a wheelchair or walker. No matter how many adaptations you make to adjust to the client's setting, you *cannot* adapt the principles of standard precautions. You must frequently wash your hands. If contact with blood and body fluids is likely, use personal protective equipment as you would in any health care setting and clean up any spill using the proper protocol.

If a hospital bed is not available, it is possible to raise a standard bed on wooden or cement blocks to a safe working height. Care should be taken so that the blocks are secure, the bed cannot fall, and the client will not be injured. If the bed is not raised, take care to use good body mechanics when working around the bed (e.g., when bathing the client or making the bed) so that you are not injured. You may need to kneel or squat when working around the bed.

Figure 34-9 shows ways to make equipment using readily available materials. Additional types of adaptations that may be required in the home setting include:

- Using a bed tray in place of an overbed table for eating and other activities
- Making a draw sheet from a folded twin size sheet
- Enclosing a portion of a plastic tablecloth or shower curtain to make an incontinence pad
- Using several pillows to maintain a sitting position, if the head of the bed cannot be raised
- Cutting and padding a cardboard box to make a backrest
- Hanging a shoe bag under the mattress to provide compartments for personal items within easy reach for the client
- Taping a paper bag to the mattress to collect soiled tissues and other small trash (The entire bag can be disposed of and replaced with a clean bag when necessary.)
- Using a pillowcase or a plastic bag on the back of the chair to collect linen

TIME MANAGEMENT

The home health nursing assistant is responsible for planning and completing the assigned care within a designated time period. You may be caring for one client for an entire shift or several clients during the course of a shift. It is your responsibility to be at each client's home at the specified time. In order to make the best use of your time:

- Be prepared. Have everything you need for your assignments for the day before you leave home (e.g., watch with a second hand, gloves, waterless hand cleaner, stethoscope, blood pressure cuff).
- Organize your time and supplies before you begin your care. Have a work plan in mind (e.g., prioritize the activities: bathing, shampoo, laundry, food preparation).
- Discuss essential information with the client and family; avoid distractions and lengthy conversations.
- Call your next client if you are running late.
- Determine with the client and his or her family if it is appropriate for you to read or watch television while the client naps during your shift. Make sure all of your duties are performed before spending time on personal matters.
- Do not sleep if you are caring for a client on the night shift, even if the family gives you permission to do so.

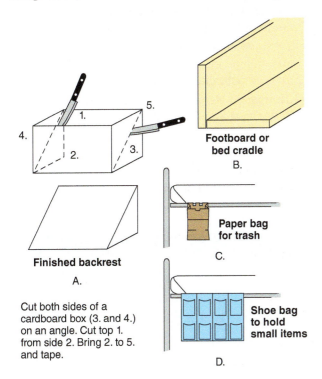

Finished backrest

A.

Cut both sides of a cardboard box (3. and 4.) on an angle. Cut top 1. from side 2. Bring 2. to 5. and tape.

Footboard or bed cradle

B.

Paper bag for trash

C.

Shoe bag to hold small items

D.

Figure 34-9 Make equipment using readily available materials.

SAFETY IN THE HOME

Personal Safety

Safety is always a concern for health care workers in the home. Always be aware of people and conditions around you. If you believe that conditions are unsafe, immediately notify your employer and/or 911, depending upon the circumstances. Every day, thousands of health care workers make home visits and there are few incidents of violence. However, trust your own instincts. If something does not seem right, then perhaps it is not. You should be "streetwise."

Ways of protecting your personal safety include:

- Know where you are going, map out your route in advance, and take the most logical route.
- Notify your employer of the time you will arrive.
- Lock your purse or valuables in the trunk of your car when you begin the day. Use a "fanny pack" or pockets to carry essential items, such as a driver's license and pens. Do not wear jewelry. Men carry your wallet in a front pocket.
- Wear clothing that identifies you as a health care worker, such as scrubs or a lab coat (according to agency policy). Always wear your name tag.
- Use car safety measures. Keep the gas tank full. Keep windows up and doors locked at all times. Park in well-lighted areas. Avoid parking on deserted streets or in vacant lots. Do not hitchhike or pick up hitchhikers.
- Most agencies will provide or reimburse the use of a cell phone. Keep the phone with you at all times.
- Attend classes on self-defense and personal safety. (Some employers make classes available as part of continuing education.)
- If an emergency arises, stay calm. Give the robber what he wants (money or keys). Be alert and always note the person's height, build, and any important characteristics such as tattoos or scars.

If the request is for your wallet or keys, throw them as far from you as possible and run the opposite direction.

- Lock the door after you enter the client's home.

Safety in the Home

The Centers for Disease Control and Prevention (CDC) report that each year a fall occurs for one of every three adults. Falls may lead to potentially serious conditions such as fractures and head trauma; complications may lead to death. According to the National Safety Council, falls are the leading cause of injury-related deaths in persons over the age of 73 and the second leading cause in people age 60 to 72 years.

With the aging population increasing, the number of persons who become injured will also increase. As a nursing assistant in the home setting, you can play an important role by helping to prevent injuries.

The RN will assess the home setting and the client before your first visit. However, it is your responsibility to check for possible safety hazards at each visit and to report any concerns to the nurse or the primary caregiver in the home. When you are working in the home, you should assess for:

- Polished, waxed floors that may be slippery
- Scatter rugs with no nonskid backing
- Unstable or broken furniture
- Clutter on the floor or stairs
- Poor lighting, especially in halls and on stairs; failure to use night-lights
- Electrical cords that may cause the client to trip and fall or electrical cords that may be under rugs—a potential fire hazard
- Overloaded electric outlets—potential fire hazards when using an electric lift device
- Liquid spills anywhere, but especially on kitchen or bathroom floors
- Loose or broken handrails or treads on stair steps, both indoors and outdoors

? EXERCISE 34-2

1. Name at least five ways to protect yourself while on the job as a home health nursing assistant:

   a. _____

   b. _____

   c. _____

   d. _____

   e. _____

- Lack of smoke detectors or fire extinguisher
- Medications or chemicals (cleaning supplies) stored inappropriately or in an unsafe manner
- Faulty ambulatory aids and equipment: worn straps on braces; worn rubber tips on canes, walkers, or crutches; frayed electric cords on electric lifts and other equipment
- Thermostat on hot water set at too high a temperature (should be no more than 120°F); inadequately marked hot and cold water faucets

It is not your job to completely reorganize the home but to ensure that the home environment is safe. Any situations that you feel are unsafe should be discussed with the RN. If you think there may be ways to make the environment safer, also discuss these ideas with the RN. For example, the client may need:

- Grab bars and nonskid strips installed or a bath bench in the bathtub (Figure 34-10)
- A raised toilet seat; grab bars next to toilet
- A commode to use if the bathroom is not easily accessible
- An over-the-bed trapeze to assist with mobility while in bed
- A mechanical lift for use in transfers out of bed

Many of these items are readily available from durable equipment providers. Payment is usually possible through Medicare or insurance companies if this equipment is essential to the care of the client. However, the nurse must have the physician write an order before the equipment is purchased.

Sometimes the home must be modified to meet the needs of the client. For example, a ramp may need to be installed. Do not attempt to arrange for or make any modifications; contact the RN. It may be possible for the occupational therapist to visit the client and family and make suggestions for needed renovations or modifications.

A list of emergency telephone numbers should be kept by the telephone. This may save time during an emergency. Be sure to keep a listing of the client's current medications as well as the telephone numbers for the:

- Agency
- Supervising nurse/case manager
- Physician
- Family member
- Poison control center
- Emergency 911 or the numbers for the police, fire department, hospital, and ambulance (Figure 34-11)

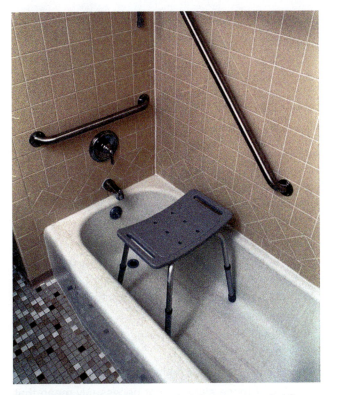

Figure 34-10 Bath bench or chair is recommended for the unsteady client. Grab bars and nonskid strips in the tub to prevent falls.

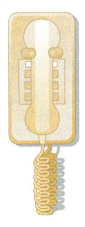

EMERGENCY NUMBERS

DOCTOR............636-9010
FIRE DEPT.........632-4000
POLICE.............636-1001
AGENCY............963-4520
DAUGHTER.........632-1698
POISON
CONTROL..........632-5000
MEDICATIONS TAKE BY CLIENT

Simvastatin 80 mg qd

Etodolac 400 mg tid

Atenolol 50 mg qd

Ranitidine HCL 150 mg
   2 tablets qd

or EMERGENCY 911
(if in use in immediate area)

Figure 34-11 Important phone numbers and medications taken by the client should be in large print and posted next to the telephone, this may save precious moments at the time of an emergency.

? EXERCISE 34-3

1. List at least five things in the home setting that may increase risk for client falls.

    a. _____

    b. _____

    c. _____

    d. _____

    e. _____

Know whether the person:

- Wears medical alert devices (bracelet or necklace)
- Has advance directives: out-of-hospital codes, papers, or a living will
- Stores important medical information in a special place that may be needed in an emergency (sometimes the IPOLST is on the refrigerator door)

Safe Administration of Medication

As a nursing assistant, you are not responsible for administering medications in the home setting. You are not legally authorized to give any drugs, even over-the-counter medications. The physician prescribes the medications, but you need to supervise the client as he or she self-administers the medications. You may need to assist the client with opening the container and ensure the medications are taken at the correct time. Sometimes medications are placed in a container that holds a week's supply. It is the responsibility of the family member or the RN to fill the container with the correct medications. This makes it easy for you to assess that the client has taken the appropriate medications. The client's family should provide a list of all current medications and dosages. Medications should be stored in a safe area (Figure 34-12). The top shelves of a closed cabinet may be a good choice, especially if the client is disoriented.

It is the home health nursing assistant's responsibility to carry out any monitoring actions that must be performed before giving a drug. Sometimes it is necessary to take a pulse, blood pressure, or blood sugar measurement before the client takes medication; as well as to remind the client to take the medications at the appropriate time.

Elder Abuse

You have been looking at various aspects of safety that impact you and the home situation. Protecting the client is an important aspect of your job as well. Sometimes the client is a victim of self-abuse or abuse by family members. The home health nursing assistant

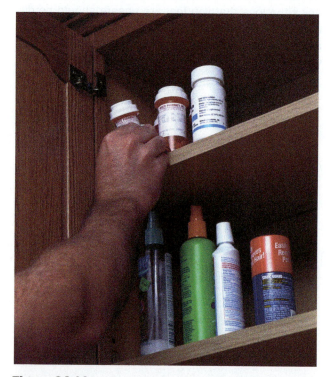

Figure 34-12 Keep medications and other potentially dangerous substances (cleaning supplies) in cabinets on a high shelf.

must look for signs that may indicate possible abuse and has a *responsibility* to report to the RN any signs of suspected abuse, such as:

- Signs of neglect such as poor hygiene
- Verbal statements made by the client that reflect abuse or neglect
- Unexplained injuries (bruises, fractures, wounds)
- Changes in personality
- A disabled person's unwillingness to accept help with ADLs
- Signs of unusual drowsiness or weakness

Any of these signs do not necessarily mean that abuse has occurred. However, there may be a need for further investigation by the RN.

? EXERCISE 34-4

1. List at least three things that may indicate possible abuse of a home care client:

a. _____

b. _____

c. _____

The reporting of elder abuse is mandated by the laws of individual states rather than by the federal legislation. Health care professionals, as well as personnel who work in long-term care facilities and mental health professionals, are among the group who are mandated, or required by law, to report any suspected elder abuse. In addition, to mandated reporters, some states have a requirement that anyone who knows of suspected elder abuse must report this to the appropriate authorities. This type of reporter is referred to as a permissive reporter and may include bank tellers, attorneys, neighbors, or anyone who suspects abuse. Because each state individually defines what constitutes elder abuse, reports should be made to the local Adult Protective Services (APS) or any local agency on aging.

HOME MANAGEMENT

Combining Client Care and Housekeeping Tasks

Care of the client is most important. However, the housekeeping tasks are not to be ignored. It is important to plan the activities of the day before beginning. The order in which the tasks are completed is frequently not important, although the day's activities should be planned around the needs of the client. You may want to clean the bathroom, for example, after you complete the client's bath and toileting activities.

Housekeeping Tasks

Some of the tasks described herein may be part of the assignment for the home nursing assistant. Always incorporate principles of standard precautions as you go about your duties.

Cleaning the Client's Room

An orderly environment can help raise a person's spirits and help prevent infection. Ask permission before rearranging the client's possessions.

- Pick up any trash; don't allow clutter to accumulate.
- Keep the client's room tidy.

- Dust the room daily.
- Clean and put away equipment after use.
- Prepare and store food properly.
- Put clean clothes away.
- Line wastebaskets with a plastic bag; empty regularly.

Cleaning the Kitchen

The kitchen is an area that requires special attention because it can be the main source of infection. Always work from the clean areas to the dirty areas.

- Clean up after each meal; do not allow dishes or trash to accumulate.
- Store leftover food appropriately.
- Wash dishes by hand or in the dishwasher, as instructed.
- Wash pots and pans by hand in hot, soapy water.
- Clean the countertops, stove, microwave oven, and sink.
- Dispose of trash.
- Sweep the floor after each meal.
- Wash the floor weekly, or as needed.

Cleaning the Bathroom

Daily thorough and careful cleaning of the bathroom is essential because this room is a major source of infection. Use the cleaning products that the family prefers and wear utility gloves to:

- Clean inside and outside the sink, wiping faucets and countertops
- Clean the tub and shower after use
- Mop the floor
- Replace towels and washcloths with clean ones
- Clean the toilet

Laundry

Your daily tasks may include laundering the client's clothes and bed linens.

- Ask for instructions before using the washing machine (or any appliance).

- Wear gloves and disposable gown when sorting clothes and loading the washing machine if contact with blood or other body fluids is likely.
- Check clothes for stains, pretreat with stain remover, and wash light colors separately from dark colors.
- Hang drip-dry clothes, as instructed; dry others in the dryer at the correct temperature.
- Remove clothes from the dryer promptly; fold them, and put them away.
- Make sure the clothing hamper is clean and ready for reuse.

Food Selection and Preparation

Work with a family member or the client to plan menus in advance. Make out weekly menu plans that meet the client's nutritional needs as well as food preferences. Take into consideration the cultural and ethnic background of the client, as well as any religious prohibitions. If it is not possible to consult with the family, keep these additional guidelines in mind:

- Spend according to the client's budget.
- Buy only what you need; large quantities are not a bargain if they will be thrown in the trash (Figure 34-13).
- Look for quality bargains.
- Keep a list and all receipts for purchases.

Using your weekly menus as a guide, prepare foods in such a way that the client's dietary needs are met. In addition:

- Wash your hands at least 10 to 15 seconds before handling food.
- Wash your hands well after handling fresh meats and poultry.
- Wash fruits and vegetables thoroughly before use.

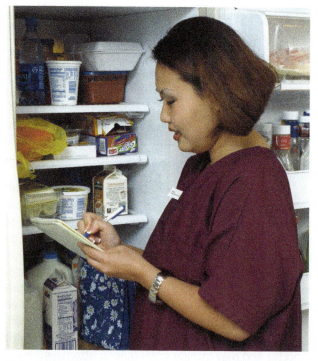

Figure 34-13 A nursing assistant is checking the refrigerator for needed groceries.

- Store dairy products and meats in the refrigerator; freeze meats that will be used later in the week.
- Thaw frozen meats in the refrigerator, not on the counter at room temperature.
- Wash the lids of cans before opening; do not use if the cans are bulging.
- Check the expiration dates on foods before preparation.
- Cook foods at proper temperature.
- Keep hot foods hot and cold foods cold.
- Store leftover foods as soon as possible.

? EXERCISE 34-5

You will be preparing food to meet client's dietary needs. Using the list below, complete the following statements regarding safe food handling for the caregiver.

after	fruits	room
before	refrigerator	vegetables
expiration		

1. Wash hands _____ handling food.
2. Always wash hands _____ handling meat.
3. Wash _____ and _____ before use.
4. Thaw frozen meat in the _____ and not at _____ temperature.
5. Check _____ dates.

COMMUNICATION AND DOCUMENTATION

Family Interactions

Some family members may reside in the home with the client and are present while you provide care. You may see them each time you visit the client. Other family members may be at work while you are in the home and some may live many miles away. Family members may telephone while you are in the home seeking information about the client's condition. It is preferable to have the client speak directly with the family member. If this is not possible, be objective in your comments. Be honest; if you do not know the answer to the question, say so and do not give false information. Refer all medical questions to the physician or RN.

When you are in the client's home you are a guest. Be sensitive to cultural and ethnic values and beliefs of the client and family. Tact and courtesy are important characteristics to use when communicating with family members. Make sure you have the client's permission to share information with the family members. If you sense there is a problem, discuss the situation with your supervisor.

Make sure that you complete all your assigned tasks for your shift. Do not leave your work to be completed by the family members.

Reporting

Each time you visit the client, it is your responsibility to assess the client and report your activities as well as any new problems that may arise. Communicate with the RN regarding any problems associated with:

- Mobility, getting in or out of bed
- Eating or swallowing
- Urinary or bowel incontinence or using the toilet
- Bathing or dressing
- Safety issues
- Marked changes in vital signs, acute illness, injuries

Your agency will have protocols for handling these problems. The nurse also will need to visit and reassess the client to alter the plan of care, if indicated. It is always better to report something immediately rather than risking the chance of endangering the client, the agency, or yourself.

Client Care Records

Documenting observations of the client and the care that you have given is an essential part of your job. These **client care records** become a permanent part of the client's chart. All documentation must be complete, accurate, and up to date. Many home health agencies are now using electronic charting, by means of a variety of devices. Computers (laptop, handheld, or tablets) as well as Smartphones may be equipped with the appropriate software. Point of care charting in this manner is paperless. After the data is entered into the computer, it can then be transmitted via numerous modalities; sometimes using secure telephone or email lines. In addition to automated visit notes, a system of this type can help to keep time sheets, mileage records, and help in billing for services.

If the agency is utilizing paper records, use a blue or black ink pen to complete your records per agency protocol. If you make an error on the record, cross through the entry with a single line; mark "error" and initial that entry (as per agency policy) and proceed with the correct documentation. Do not use Wite-Out® or leave any blank spaces. If the client is using Medicare benefits or insurance to cover the cost of care, the auditors for the agencies will check the records to see that the tasks assigned are actually what is done in the home. If the records are inaccurate or falsified, the agency may not be paid for the services. *If it is not charted, it is considered not to have been done.*

You will be recording:

- Care given: bath, position change, range-of-motion exercises
- Client's response to care given
- Household tasks assigned by the nurse
- Observations:
  - Vital signs
  - Changes in client's health status
  - Condition of the skin
  - Intake: food and fluid
  - Appetite
  - Incidents: falls or other injury
  - Mental status: orientation, alertness, mood, behavior

The agency will provide the appropriate forms and the guidelines for documentation. Figures 34-14 and 34-15 are examples of the types of forms to be completed by the home care nursing assistant. In some agencies, you submit your documentation at the end of the week. However, you may be required to keep some records by the month for such things as monitoring of blood sugar or blood pressure.

Time and Travel Records

Time and travel records indicate how you spent your time caring for the client (Figure 34-16). Your careful record keeping includes:

- Time of arrival at the home
- Time of departure
- Length of time required for specific duties

RIVERVIEW HOME HEALTH SERVICE
8987 Walkman Ave
Parkhurst, Nebraska
Client Care Plan / Progress Notes

HOME HEALTH ASSISTANT YOLANDA BROWN, CNA
CLIENT NAME NICHOLAS FRENCH SOC. SECURITY # 123-45-678
ADDRESS: 529 ANYWHERE AVE. PARKHURST, NEBRASKA

	ACTIVITY
0800	Arrived, Determined needs, planned activities Client seemed fatigued "Slept poorly". On nasal O_2 2.5L
0830	Circumoral pallor noted. Vital signs checked. Dyspneic on exertion.
0900	Put laundry into washing machine. Started breakfast. Client ate 1 sl. toast, 8 oz oatbran cereal / milk 6oz orange juice
0930	Prepared equipment for A.M. care – complete bath, shave and denture care.
1000	Asst to commode, soft brown formed stool.
1030	Made comfortable in easy chair. Reading newspaper. Nasal O_2 Cleaned kitchen including refrigerator
1100	Linen changed – dusted and dust mopped bedroom. Vacuumed living room.
1130	Prepared lunch.
1200	Client ate 1/2 chicken sandwich, 8 oz. tea, chocolate pudding, 8 oz. tomato soup.
1230	Client returned to bed for nap
1300	Cleaned lunch dishes and prepared salad, jello for evening meal
1330	Put washed laundry into dryer.
1400	Cleaned bathroom, washed kitchen floor Put bed linen into washer.
1430	Made out shopping list for A.M.
1500	Client awake. Assisted into living room. Watching T.V. Ordered O_2 tank replacement.
1530	Folded and put clean laundry away. Put washed linens in dryer.
1600	Client seems more rested. Color improved. Resp. easier. Notified supervisor of client's progress.
1630	Left client's home @ 3^{25} P.M.

Y. Brown CNA

VITAL SIGNS	T	P	R	B/P
	97^4	92	26	108/64
INTAKE				
OUTPUT				

SUP. SIGNATURE ____________

Figure 34-14 Client care record—narrative type.

? EXERCISE 34-6

TRUE OR FALSE

Indicate if the following statements are true (T) or false (F).

1. T F If a family member wants information about the client it is best for them to speak directly to the client.
2. T F It is important for the nursing assistant to be objective in comments.
3. T F If you do not know an answer to a question, answer it to the best of your ability.
4. T F Refer all questions to whatever nurse assistant is on duty after you.
5. T F If you are not able to get all your tasks done, the family can do them later.
6. T F Your documentation is a permanent part of the client's chart.
7. T F If you make an error while documenting, use Wite-Out® to fix it.
8. T F It is okay to wait until the end of your shift to document.
9. T F Time and travel records are part of your documentation.
10. T F If you handle clients' money, it is their responsibility to save receipts and record money spent.
11. T F It is important to work around your schedule instead of the client's.
12. T F It is important to avoid wasting time by doing non-work-related tasks (making phone calls, drinking coffee).
13. T F A benefit of home health care is that the home health nursing assistant does not have to worry about being on time.

HOME HEALTH AIDE RECORD

85-1008

Home Health   *Client Information Is Confidential / Call RN if change in condition.*

CLIENT: _____

First Visit of Week, HHA to view instruction sheet and transfer instruction ✔ to box left of task.
Last Visit of Week, HHA to submit completed form to office.

✔		Date	Sun. __/__/__	Mon. __/__/__	Tues. __/__/__	Wed. __/__/__	Thurs. __/__/__	Fri. __/__/__	Sat. __/__/__
✔	Safety Precautions								
	Bath								
	Grooming								
	Dressing								
	Mobility								
	Transfer								
	ROM								
	Splints/Braces								
	Toileted								
	Catheter								
	TPR								
	BP								
	Weight								
	Other as per Instruction Sheet (list)								
	Housekeeping								
	Meals								
	Time In: (List time and a.m. or p.m.)								
	Time Out: (List time and a.m. or p.m.)								
	HHA Initials: (Initials and Signature Below)								

Initials	Signature and Title	Initials	Signature and Title
		Reviewed by:	

Figure 34-15 Client care record—checklist type.

RIVERVIEW HOME HEALTH SERVICE
8987 Walkman Ave
Parkhurst, Nebraska
Time and Travel Log

CARE GIVER
NAME ___Siadto, Laura CNA___ TITLE ___Home Health Assistant___ EMPT. NO. _62718_ DATE _Aug. 29_

CLIENT NAME/ADDRESS (Last, first)	SERVICE PROVIDED	VISIT CODE	NON BILL CODE	TIME IN	TIME OUT	CLIENT CONTACT TIME	ODOMETER READING	MILES
Volheim, Eleonore	Bedbath, Shampoo	4		8¹⁵	9⁰⁵	50 min	From: 45,061 To: 45,068	7 miles
Jaronello, Sharri		1		9³⁰	9⁴⁵	15 min	From: 45,068 To: 45,083	15 miles
Doyle, Kindra	Enema, bedbath, amb	4		10¹⁰	11³⁰	1 hr. 20 min.	From: 45,083 To: 46,001	18 miles
Hammond, Rachel	Ass't c̄ colostomy cath care, bath, ROM	4		11⁵⁰	1²⁰	1 hr. 30 min.	From: 46,001 To: 46,017	16 miles
Minzey, Aimee		2		1³⁰	1³⁵	—	From: 46,017 To: 46,025	8 miles
Galloway, Rosa		5		1⁵⁰	2⁰⁰	10 min	From: 46,025 To: 46,028	3 miles
							From: To:	

Total Visits ___6___   Total Mileage ___67___   Parking Fees ___—___

Visit Code
1 IE Initial Eval & Rx   4 HC Home Care
2 FV Follow Up Visit   5 Hospital/Hospice
3 DV Discharge Visit   6 MC Maternal/Child

Supervising Nurse: _Bruce Davenport R.N._

Nonbill Code
1. Refused Care
2. Patient Not Home
3. Non-Bill
4. Expired
5. Delivered Supplies

Figure 34-16 A sample time/travel record.

- Travel time if caring for more than one client
- Mileage or transportation costs

Accurate record keeping is essential. Update the record as you complete each assignment; do not wait until the end of your shift. Some agencies require the signature of the client or family member to verify that your travel and time information is correct.

LESSON SYNTHESIS: Putting It All Together

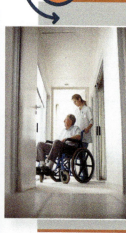

You have just completed this lesson. Now go back and review the Clinical Focus at the beginning of the lesson. Try to see how the Clinical Focus relates to the concepts presented in the lesson. Then answer the following questions.

1. What benefits will Emily derive from working as a nursing assistant in the home setting?

2. How did Emily's experience working in a long-term care facility help her prepare for caring for clients in the home?

3. What challenges might you expect if you work in a home health care setting?

4. How would you prepare yourself to meet these challenges?

34   REVIEW

A. Select the one best answer for each of the following.

1. The person who receives care in the home setting is referred to as the

    (A) patient

    (B) resident

    (C) recipient

    (D) client

2. The home health nursing assistant must adapt to all of the following, except

    (A) visiting multiple clients on the same day

    (B) doing laundry for the family members of the client

    (C) working in a variety of home settings

    (D) making and adjusting your plan for client care

3. Which one of the following is a form of client abuse?

    (A) Preparing special diets according to instruction

    (B) Observing skin integrity during the bath

    (C) Buying a soda for yourself when you shop with the client's money

    (D) Reporting that the client's blood pressure reading is lower than usual

4. Home care services are increasing because

    (A) families can provide care

    (B) more services are available to the client

    (C) there are not enough hospitals

    (D) people prefer to be at home

5. Time and travel records should *not* include

    (A) mental status of the client

    (B) time of arrival in the home

    (C) travel time

    (D) mileage or transportation costs

6. Which of the following problems does not require further assessment by the RN?

    (A) Incontinence

    (B) Inability to get out of bed

    (C) Dislike of the food you prepared

    (D) Inability to swallow

7. When preparing food for the client, it is best to avoid

    (A) washing fruits and vegetables

    (B) refrigerating leftovers as soon as possible

    (C) checking expiration dates on food

    (D) thawing frozen meat on the counter

8. Which one of the following is *not* a safety problem?

    (A) Storing medications on a high shelf

    (B) Overloaded electrical outlets

    (C) Clutter on the stairs

    (D) Highly polished wood floors

9. All of the following are desirable characteristics of the home health nursing assistant, except

    (A) honesty and dependability

    (B) need for close supervision

    (C) having dependable transportation

    (D) being self-directed

10. As a home health nursing assistant, you will *not* be expected to

    (A) wash windows

    (B) read to the client

    (C) make out a weekly menu

    (D) remind the client to take medications

B. Answer each statement true (T) or false (F).

11. T F The home health nursing assistant may be responsible for nursing care and housekeeping tasks.

12. T F Documentation is an important responsibility of the home health nursing assistant.

13. T F If you make an error in your charting, you may erase it.

14. T F The bathroom is one of the most dangerous rooms in the house.

15. T F If you work the night shift and the family gives permission, you may sleep while the client sleeps.

16. T F The home health nursing assistant must know when to ask for help with a client.

17. T F In the home, you may need to use equipment that is different from that in a long-term care facility.

18. T F You must administer the client's medication while you are in the home.

19. T F Family members are not members of the home health care team.

20. T F When the client has a problem with a family member, the nursing assistant may side with the client.

C. Complete the following statements in the space provided.

21. The home health nursing assistant may be responsible for nursing care and for _____ _____ .

22. In some home health agencies, the case manager may be _____ .

23. Keep a list of the client's medications

_____ .

D. Short answer. Briefly answer the statements in the space provided.

24. List five potential hazards in the home that may present problems for an older client.

_____

_____

_____

25. List three activities the home health nursing assistant may perform in addition to nursing care.

_____

_____

_____

Employment

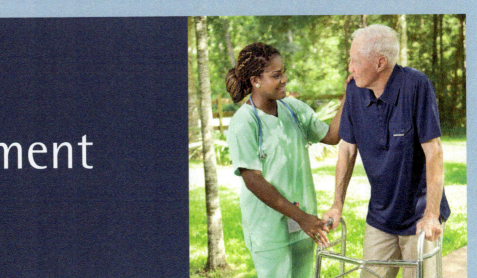

LESSON 35   Seeking Employment

10

LESSON 35
SEEKING EMPLOYMENT

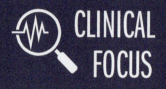 **CLINICAL FOCUS**

Think of the process involved in successfully seeking employment as you study this lesson.

OBJECTIVES

After studying this lesson, you should be able to:

• Define vocabulary words and terms.

• List objectives to be met in obtaining and maintaining employment.

• Describe a process for self-evaluation.

• List sources of nursing assistant employment.

• Explain how to prepare for a successful interview.

• Prepare a résumé and letter of resignation.

VOCABULARY

cross-training (kros-TRAYN-ing)
interview (IN-ter-vue)
networking (NET-werk-ing)

references (REF-er-en-ses)
résumé (REH-zoo-may)

CASE STUDY

Ruby Stepp has just completed a program that has prepared her to work in a long-term care facility. She has passed all tests. Ruby is now ready to enter a field of service and personal satisfaction as she seeks her first full employment.

CONGRATULATIONS ARE IN ORDER

You have done it! You have passed the certification tests and have proven your ability in the clinical area. You are now certified and are ready to make your contribution to the care of residents in a long-term care facility.

You will now begin the search for available positions and prepare yourself to apply for them. You can do several things to make the search easier and more productive.

STEP I — SELF-APPRAISAL

The first step is a self-appraisal—an honest look at your own strengths and limitations (Figure 35-1). You can do this by making a list.

On one side of a sheet of paper, list all the things you have to offer an employer. Be as specific as you can about personal as well as educational assets or strengths. For example, write statements about:

- Your sense of responsibility—Are you a punctual person?
- Your nursing assistant skills—How well trained and prepared are you?
- Your attitude—Are you caring and patient?
- Your personal appearance—Are you clean and neat at all times?

These are important characteristics in a successful nursing assistant.

On the other side of the paper, list any restrictions to your employment. Write statements about:

- Your availability for work—Are there hours when you cannot work (e.g., when you must be home to care for children)?
- Preferred location of work—Do you have to work within a specific area because you rely on public transportation?
- Resident's levels of care and your ability to work with them—What types of residents have you cared for?

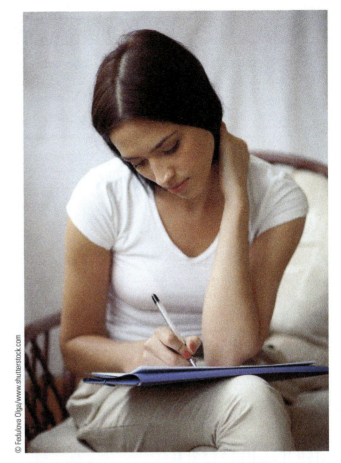

Figure 35-1 Nursing assistant listing strengths and limitations.

- Personal responsibilities you may have—Do you have any responsibilities that may interfere with the performance of a job?

Think of ways to manage your responsibilities so they will not interfere with your employability. For example, if you have an older parent living with you and must be home to prepare meals, is there a neighbor or other family member who could prepare meals on the days or hours that you work?

Put the list away and then review it in a day or two. There may be items you will want to add or revise.

? EXERCISE 35-1

COMPLETION

Complete the following statements by writing in the correct words.

1. The four steps in carrying out self-appraisal are:

   a. _____

   b. _____

   c. _____

   d. _____

(continues)

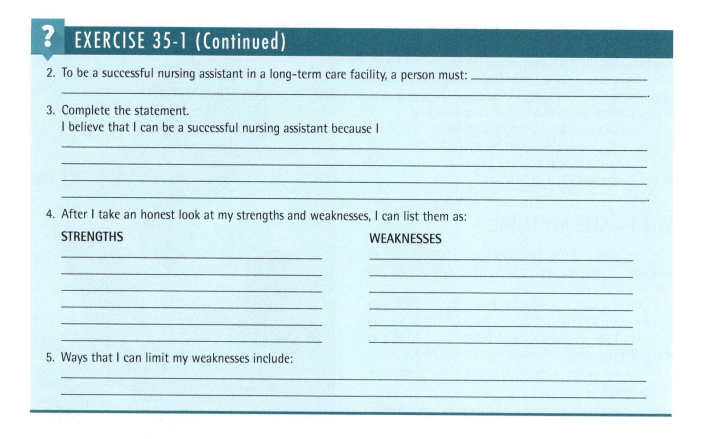

? EXERCISE 35-1 (Continued)

2. To be a successful nursing assistant in a long-term care facility, a person must: _____
_____.

3. Complete the statement.
I believe that I can be a successful nursing assistant because I
_____
_____
_____
_____.

4. After I take an honest look at my strengths and weaknesses, I can list them as:

STRENGTHS   WEAKNESSES

_____   _____
_____   _____
_____   _____
_____   _____
_____   _____
_____   _____

5. Ways that I can limit my weaknesses include:
_____
_____

STEP II—JOB SEARCH

You have listed your strengths and limitations. Now it is time to search for job possibilities. Where do you look?

- Start with the Internet
  - The Internet may be helpful to search and apply for jobs. Use a job search site such as *www.carebuilder.com*, *www.monster.com*, or *indeed.com* or go to the facility website to check job listings. If you do not have a computer, one may be available at the public library or Career Center of the Department of Labor (DOL) office in your area. In some states the use of a computer, fax machine, and copier may be available to those doing a job search through the DOL.
- Investigate the facility where you had your clinical experience. Nursing administrators often will invite nursing assistants who have trained in their facility to join the staff on completion of training. There are advantages to this policy. For one thing, you have already spent time in the facility so less time is needed to orient you as a new employee. Also, the staff has had time to evaluate you while observing you during your training period.

- **Networking** is a valuable technique that can reveal opportunities (Figure 35-2). Let friends and colleagues know that you are looking for employment. Jobs are often located on the recommendation of a network of friends. Making connections and learning of opportunities through people one meets is called networking. Networking means

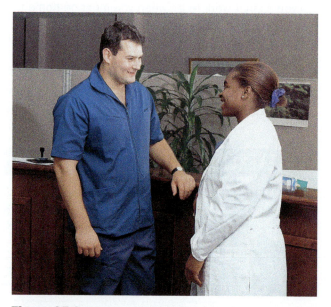

Figure 35-2 Friends, classmates, and colleagues are valuable sources of information about potential jobs.

contact the staffing agency when they need workers, including nursing assistants.

The agency then sends workers to the facilities. The worker is free to accept the assignment or not. The worker's salary is usually higher than those of facility-employed workers because no benefits are included. The agency takes a percentage of the worker's salary for the placement service. Agency employment offers flexibility in hours, variety of experience, and higher income, but requires constant adjustment to the routines of different facilities.

Nurse Aide Registry

All 50 states and the District of Columbia maintain a database of all persons who meet the federal requirements to provide care to residents of skilled nursing facilities. After you have completed your training and have successfully passed the written and skills text and there are no findings of abuse, neglect, or misappropriation of funds in your record, your name is added to the registry. This process enables prospective employers to check the status of the person applying for the job during the interview process. It is the responsibility of the registry to inform the staff of these facilities of persons who are ineligible to work in a long-term care facility. The registry also maintains an up-to-date work history on the nursing assistant.

If you move to another state and seek employment, be sure to contact the state registries in the state where you are certified as well as the state to which you are moving in order to transfer your eligibility. Since your status is maintained in that database, the information can be transferred to the state in which you are seeking employment. If you have not worked as a caregiver for pay in the previous 24 months, you will be told that you must re-train and re-test in order to again be eligible to work.

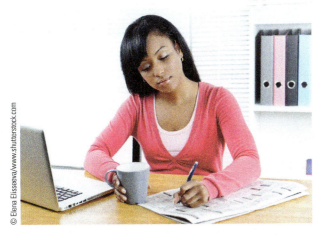

Figure 35-3 Classified ads are a good place to start your job search.

gathering a group of people with similar needs and interests to learn about:
- Working conditions
- Job openings
- Special ways of carrying out your responsibilities

Utilize job placement counselors at your school or college.
- Use the newspapers
  - The classified advertisements are your best bet here (Figure 35-3). Circle those that list positions located within your desired work area and that have openings for the shift you need to work.
  - Look in the telephone book for facilities in your area and visit the facilities.
  - List names, numbers, and addresses. Follow up and contact them.

Staffing Agency

Some health care facilities will use a private staffing agency to fill positions. The long-term care facility will

? EXERCISE 35-2

1. The aide may find out about job opportunities by:
_____
_____
_____
_____

2. What advantage is there in making applications to the clinical facility associated with your training?
_____
_____
_____
_____

(continues)

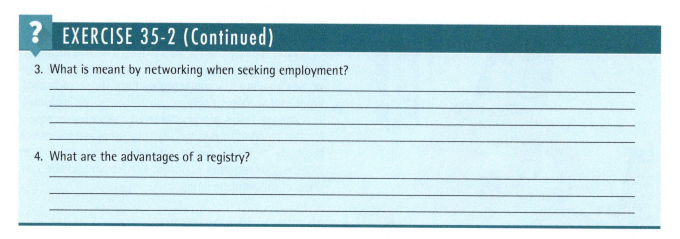

? EXERCISE 35-2 (Continued)

3. What is meant by networking when seeking employment?

_____
_____
_____
_____

4. What are the advantages of a registry?

_____
_____
_____

STEP III—THE RÉSUMÉ

A **résumé** is a summary of your education and prior work experience. The résumé should be neatly prepared, preferably typed. It is helpful to a prospective employer to have the résumé before and after your interview is held.

When an employer interviews many applicants, it is sometimes difficult to remember all the information given during a particular conversation. A note on your résumé by the interviewer can make all the difference between being hired and not being hired.

The résumé should include:

- Your name, address, telephone number, and email address
- Your educational background. List your most recent education first, giving dates and a brief summary of the content.
- Your work history, especially if it shows successful experience in the same or related areas as the position for which you are applying. Include your work history over the past 5 years. List your most recent experience first. Include the name and address of the employer, dates of employment, and job duties. Employers will look at length of employment for each job listed. Remaining in the same position for at least 2 years is typically viewed more favorably.
- Other experiences you have had can be valuable. Jobs in which you have shown initiative, reliability,

and trustworthiness are a plus and should be included. If you have not had paid employment, indicate how you spent your time. Worthwhile endeavors that might be included are:
  - Taking care of children
  - Finishing school
  - Doing volunteer work for your church or community
- List three references (people who know you and can comment on your character and abilities). *Note:* You must get permission from your references before using their names.
- Include some personal information, such as hobbies, certifications, and other interests. It is not necessary to include your:
  - Ethnic origin
  - Religion
  - Age
  - Marital status
  - Awards or certifications

Note: Some people feel that to include personal information such as height, weight, sex, marital status, or religious affiliation is an invasion of privacy. Some of this information may be discussed in the interview, but it is not necessary to include it on your résumé.

Make several copies of your résumé. Always keep the original so that you can make more copies if necessary. Put a copy in your own file. Carry a copy of your résumé whenever you seek employment. It is a ready reference as you fill out forms.

? EXERCISE 35-3

1. What five basic areas of information should be included in the résumé?

a. _____
b. _____
c. _____
d. _____
e. _____

STEP IV — REFERENCES

References are people who know you and who are willing to comment, either in writing or over the telephone, about you and your abilities. The references need to know you well enough to make an honest evaluation, but they should not be part of your family. Always get permission to use their names before listing references in your résumé. This is a matter of courtesy and ethics.

You may want to refresh the memory of your references about dates of employment or experiences that you have listed in your résumé. When listing these references be sure to include:

- Names
- Accurate titles
- Addresses
- Telephone numbers

STEP V — TAKING THE STEP

You have made your assessment of your strengths, limitations, and needs. You have searched the market for opportunities and prepared your résumé. Now you must apply for a job:

- Select three facilities that you are most interested in.
- Call and ask for the Director of Nursing or Personnel Department (Figure 35-4).
- If you are responding to advertisements in the newspaper, follow the printed instructions about the person to contact and if your résumé must be mailed or personally delivered to the facility.

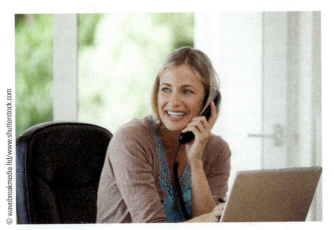

Figure 35-4 Call for an appointment to schedule an interview.

- Ask if there are any openings for a nursing assistant. If yes, ask what application procedure is to be followed.

The person in charge of hiring may ask you some questions about your education and experience, so be prepared to answer in a positive manner. He or she may set up an appointment for an interview. This is a specific time to meet and discuss your possible employment. Before you call, it is helpful if you know when you will be available and how you would reach the facility to keep the appointment.

Before hanging up:

- Obtain the name of the person to whom you are speaking.
- Thank this person by name.

STEP VI — THE INTERVIEW (PUTTING YOUR BEST FOOT FORWARD)

Before the Interview

You must sell yourself during the interview. Prepare carefully for the interview by:

- Planning what you will wear:
  - Do not overdress but avoid distracting or revealing clothing.
  - Be sure your clothes are neat and clean.
  - Polish your shoes.
  - Check you clothing for loose or lost buttons and stains; repair hems if necessary.
- Being sure to use deodorant.
- Making sure your hair is neat and clean.
- Making sure a beard or mustache is trimmed.
- Avoiding the use of heavy makeup or strong perfume or aftershave.
- Avoiding dangling or excessive jewelry.
- If possible, check to determine the dress code for the facility regarding highly colored or multi-colored hair, body piercings, tattoos, and head-dresses. Remember the first impression is an important one.

Next, make a list of information you want to share with the interviewer (Figure 35-5). You will of course share your background and answer questions the interviewer will ask. The interviewer will want proof of citizenship. Many facilities require drug testing, physical examination, and a criminal background check. Information from the certified nursing assistant registry of each state in which you were previously employed will be gathered. Be honest.

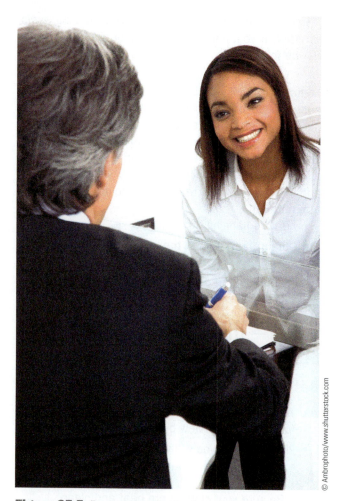

Figure 35-5 Be prepared for the interview. Know what you want to learn and what you want to share with the interviewer.

You will be asked to complete an employment application. Be sure you have a copy of your résumé for reference. Also have with you your nursing aide certificate, CPR card, proof of continuing education, and some form of identification such as your driver's license.

Think about the questions you will be asked during the interview as well as those you want to ask. Make a list of those questions and tentative answers; preparing responses to potential questions in advance helps minimize nervousness.

Typical questions may include:

- Why do you want to work in this facility?
- Why are you leaving your present employment, or why did you leave your last position?
- What are your career goals?
- What do you feel are your strongest skills?

- What are your weakest skills and how have you tried to improve them?
- How well would your coworkers and supervisors feel you related to them?
- How do you feel about people who need much care and are often demanding?
- How do you set priorities?

    In turn, you will want to learn the following:

- Starting salary
- Schedule of raises
- Fringe benefits
  - Health benefits
  - Retirement
  - Tuition reimbursement
  - Availability of credit union
  - Holiday pay or overtime
- Hours of work, including weekend schedule
- Responsibilities (ask for a job description)
- Uniform regulations
- When are job evaluations performed? Who will evaluate me?
- What type of employee orientation program is offered?
- What are the drug testing policies for the facility?
- Opportunities for growth (inservice, education, and orientation)

Interview

To make sure your interview is a success:

- Be on time for your interview, early enough to complete the employment application.
- Turn off your cell phone or leave it in the car.
- Offer a firm handshake.
- Stand until you are invited to sit.
- Be careful of body language; remember you are "selling" yourself.
- Make good eye contact with the interviewer; be open.
- Let the interviewer lead the questioning.
- Listen carefully to the interviewer's question. If you do not understand the question, ask for clarification. Your answers should reflect your positive attributes.
- Answer all questions honestly and frankly, but avoid negative comments about others.

❓ EXERCISE 35-4

INTERVIEW

1. Prepare for the interview by paying attention to your appearance. This includes:

_____
_____
_____
_____
_____
_____

2. What typical questions should you be prepared to answer during the interview?

_____
_____
_____
_____
_____
_____
_____
_____

3. Seven items of information you will wish to learn during an interview include:

a. _____
b. _____
c. _____
d. _____
e. _____
f. _____
g. _____

4. Your proper behavior during the interview includes:

_____
_____
_____
_____

5. After an interview, you should:

_____

- Emphasize your reasons for wanting to be part of the staff.
- Use the list you prepared as a guide for your questions about the job, salary, benefits, and so on (refer to section on preparing for the interview).
- Thank the interviewer(s) at the end of the interview, whether you are hired or not.
- Leave a copy of your résumé, if you have not already done so. If an opening occurs in the near future, your file is available and you will be remembered.

AFTER THE INTERVIEW

- Congratulate yourself if you are hired.
- Do not be discouraged if you are not hired. Think through the interview. Consider changes that you may want to make in your answers for future interviews.
- Send a short thank-you note to the person who interviewed you. Thank the person for giving you the opportunity to be interviewed for the job (Figure 35-6).

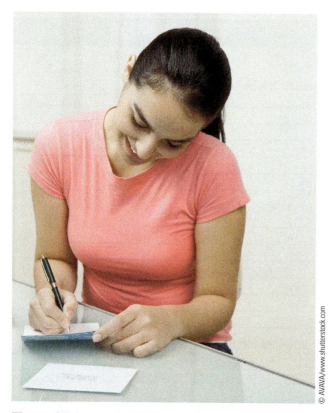

Figure 35-6 Send a thank-you note after the interview. It is considerate and helps the interviewer remember you.

Job hunting is not easy. It is emotionally stressful and can be physically exhausting. Keep trying and you will find a position to challenge you. Good luck!

KEEPING THE JOB

Getting the job was only the beginning; now you must keep it. You can secure your position if you:

- Arrive on time and always in proper uniform (Figure 35-7).

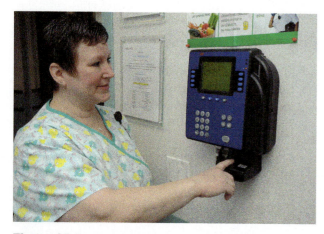

Figure 35-7 Secure your new job by being prompt.

- Perform your work as taught, and be flexible about change.
- Follow the rules of ethical and legal conduct.
- Maintain an open positive attitude; be ready to learn and grow. *Remember:* Learning is a lifelong challenge.

GROWING

You will continue to grow if you take advantage of each new experience and the opportunities you find.

- Watch experienced staff members and learn by their example.
- Do not be afraid to ask questions at the appropriate times.
- Use the nursing and medical literature that is available to learn more about the conditions of the residents (Figure 35-8).
- Participate in the care plan conferences with an open mind so that each can become a learning experience for you.
- Listen to your periodic evaluation with an open mind and follow the suggestions for improvement.

Investigate ways of advancing your education, such as:

- A general education course offered at the high school or college in your area.
- Courses in communication, listening, English, and psychology. These can be helpful in your career.
- **Cross-training** courses to increase your skills in related work. For example, you may be trained to draw blood or perform specific respiratory care procedures. Such a program may be available in your facility, at a local community college or vocational school, or in an acute care hospital.

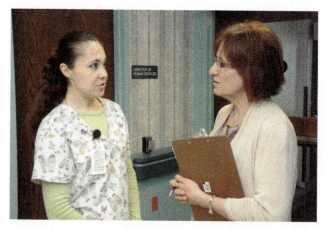

Figure 35-8 Take every opportunity you can to increase your knowledge.

- Courses offered for continuing education credit for nurses. These are sometimes available, without credit and at a reduced price, for non-licensed persons.
- Courses offered by hospitals or public health facilities on subjects of general public interest, such as hypertension, weight control, and diabetes.
- Selecting books at the library about aging and the aging process.
- Programs that can prepare you for professional development as a licensed practical nurse or registered nurse.
- Learning about advanced positions in your own facility for which you may be qualified now or could study to qualify for at a later time.

Inservice Education

All staff members are expected to participate in inservice education programs. This is called *staff development*. Some of the programs will be attended by all members of the interdisciplinary team. Other programs may be presented for nursing assistants only (Figure 35-9). OBRA requires that all nursing assistants participate in a minimum of 12 hours of inservice education each year. At these programs, you will learn:

- New or revised state and federal regulations
- New facility policies
- New procedures for resident care
- Use of new equipment
- Care of residents with unusual diagnoses or unique problems
- Issues in health care

The more you learn, the better you can care for residents and the more you will enjoy your work.

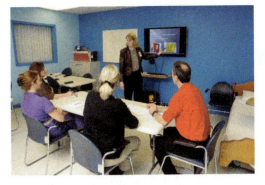

Figure 35-9 Inservice education helps the staff grow in their understanding of residents and resident's needs.

RESIGNING

The time may come when you find it necessary to leave your current job. To do this properly, check your facility policy before making your resignation plans. Then give notice as early as possible and submit a letter of resignation. Appropriate notice is usually equal to the time of a pay period, or 2 weeks on the average.

Your letter of resignation should include:

- The date
- A salutation to the Director of Nursing
- A brief explanation of your reasons for leaving. *Note*: Even if you feel upset by something that happened, make your reasons positive in nature.
- The date your resignation is to be effective
- A thank-you for the opportunity to have worked and learned as an employee of the facility
- Your signature

Remember that if you do not work as a nursing assistant for one 8-hour shift in 24 months, you must recertify before you can be reemployed.

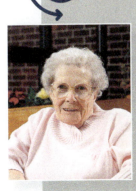

LESSON SYNTHESIS: Putting It All Together

You have just completed this lesson. Now go back and review the Clinical Focus. Try to see how the Clinical Focus relates to the concepts presented in the lesson. Then answer the following questions.

1. Why is honest self-appraisal the first step a nursing assistant must take when seeking employment?

2. Why should a reference be someone who is unrelated to the applicant?

3. Why is it important to dress "appropriately" for an interview?

4. Why is it important to be truthful during the initial interview about any limitations or restrictions related to employment?

35 REVIEW

A. Match each term (items a–d) with the proper definition.

a. interview   c. references

b. networking   d. résumé

1. _____ gathering a group of people with similar needs and interests to learn about work-related opportunities

2. _____ specific time to meet and discuss possible employment

3. _____ summary of education and work experiences

4. _____ people who know you and are willing to comment about you and your abilities

B. Answer each statement true (T) or false (F).

5. T F The first step in preparing to find a job is to call for an interview.

6. T F A positive attitude is important in a person who is seeking a job.

7. T F Personal appearance is important in making a first impression on a prospective employer.

8. T F After giving a person's name as a reference, you should always obtain permission from that person.

9. T F During the interview you should learn about the responsibilities of the job.

10. T F Thank the interviewer whether you are hired or not.

11. T F Being prompt to an interview indicates interest.

12. T F Before the interview, you should make a list of the information you want to share with the interviewer and the information you want from the interviewer.

13. T F During the interview, avoid eye contact with the interviewer.

C. Provide brief answers for each of the following:

14. List two factors that may limit the location where you can work.

15. Name three places to start looking for job opportunities.

D. Select the one best answer for each of the following.

16. When completing a résumé, include your

(A) ethnic origin

(B) religion

(C) educational background

(D) marital status

17. A person listed as a reference should be able to comment on your

(A) character and abilities

(B) age and marital status

(C) religion and ethnic origin

(D) height and weight

18. When listing a reference, be sure to include the person's

(A) place of employment

(B) ethnic origin

(C) marital status

(D) accurate telephone number

19. You can grow in your career if you

(A) never ask questions

(B) attend related educational courses

(C) do not attend care plan conferences

(D) read books on flower arranging

20. During the interview you will want to learn about all of the following, except

(A) salary

(B) benefits

(C) hours of work

(D) public transportation schedule

21. If you have not had paid employment recently, you should:

(A) give a detailed explanation of your hobbies

(B) list worthwhile endeavors

(C) list your least recent experience first

(D) make up something and hope the employer will not check

E. Clinical experience

22. Sarah has been employed by her facility for a year. She enjoys her work and the people she works with but she would like to be more challenged. What actions can she take to help her meet her needs?

23. Tilly has just received her evaluation. Her supervisor suggested several ways she can improve her performance. Tilly is upset by the evaluation and complains about her supervisor to her friend during lunch. What do you think of Tilly's response? Is it a productive response? How would you respond?

24. Charlie is going to his first inservice education meeting. What kinds of information might he learn? How many hours of inservice education must Charlie have each year?

25. Marie is a single mother with two small children. She is thinking of working through the registry in her town. Why might this be a good plan for her?

GLOSSARY

A

abandonment leaving or walking from the premises before another worker has been designated to care for your residents

abbreviation the shortened form of a word or phrase

abdominal area the area of the trunk between the thorax and pelvis

abdominopelvic cavity the body cavity extending between the diaphragm and the floor of the pelvis

abduction movement away from the midline or center

abscess localized collection of pus in any body part that is usually caused by bacterial contamination

abuse willful injury or mistreatment

accelerated increased motion, as in pulse or respiration

acceptance favorable reception; final stage of the grief process

accuracy completing assignments carefully, without mistakes

acetone a colorless liquid produced in the body during digestion of fats; found in the blood and urine of persons with diabetes

acquired immune deficiency syndrome a progressively fatal disease that is spread by contact with blood and body fluid

active assistive range of motion carrying out of specific exercises by the resident with some help from the care provider; exercises are designed to move each joint through its range of motion

active range of motion a resident carries out exercises without help; all joints are moved through their full range of motion

activities of daily living (ADL) the activities necessary for the resident to fulfill basic human needs

acupressure therapy that uses pressure at specific points to treat illness or relieve pain

acupuncture therapy from Chinese medicine that uses insertion of small needles in specific areas of the skin to treat illness or relieve pain

adaptive behavior the degree to which a person meets standards of personal independence and social responsibility appropriate for the person's age and culture

adaptive device ordinary items that are modified or changed in some way so that the equipment can be used by individuals with specific disabilities

adduction movement toward midline or center

adjunctive (complementary) therapy a treatment that goes with and supplements primary medical care

ADLs activities of daily living

administrator one who manages a facility

adrenal glands glands, located on top of the kidneys, that produce hormones

adrenaline epinephrine—hormone produced by adrenal glands

advance directive a document signed when the individual is still in good health, indicating the person's wishes regarding the type of care he or she wishes to receive when the person is unable to communicate; two forms: living will and durable power of attorney

advocate one who speaks and acts on behalf of another

age-related macular degeneration the leading cause of blindness in persons over 50 years of age

agitation an increase in physical activity, usually accompanied by anger and irritation

aiding and abetting not reporting dishonest acts that are observed

AIDS acquired immune deficiency syndrome; a progressively fatal disease caused by the HIV virus that is spread by contact with blood and body fluids

airborne precautions techniques to prevent transmission of airborne organisms

akinesia abnormal absence or slowing of muscular activity

alignment proper position

allergen a substance that causes sensitivity or allergic reactions

alopecia hair loss

alternative therapy a regimen or treatment that is used instead of conventional health practices

alveoli (sing. alveolus) tiny air sacs that make up the bulk of the lungs

Alzheimer's disease a disorder of the brain that involves thinking, memory, and judgment; a form of dementia

ambulate/ambulation to walk; to move from one place to another

amenorrhea abnormal cessation or absence of the menses

amputation removal of a limb or other body appendage

amulet protective charm

anastomosis a surgical connection made between two body structures (such as blood vessels) that are not normally joined

anatomic position standing erect, facing the observer, feet flat on the floor, arms extended, palms forward

anatomy the study of the structure of the human body

anemia the deficiency of red blood cells in the blood

aneurysm a sac formed by dilation of the wall of a blood vessel (usually an artery) and filled with blood; a weak spot in an arterial wall

anger a feeling of hostility or rage

angina pectoris acute pain in the chest caused by interference with the supply of oxygen to the heart

ankle-foot orthosis an assistive device that provides medial lateral support for an unstable ankle

anorexia loss of appetite

anoxia lack of oxygen

antecedent a cause that goes before an action

anterior in anatomy, in front of the coronal or ventral plane

antibiotic a medication to fight infection caused by bacteria

antibody a protein formed in the body in response to a specific foreign agent (antigen); may be beneficial or harmful

antidepressant a medication effective against depressive illness

antigen a foreign or pathogenic substance that enters the body and stimulates the production of antibodies

antihypertensive a medication effective against hypertension (high blood pressure)

antioxidant a substance that inhibits oxidation and cellular damage from free radicals

anuria the absence of secretions of urine by the kidneys

anus the outlet of the rectum lying in the fold between the buttocks from which waste products are eliminated

aorta the great artery arising from the left ventricle of the heart

apathy indifference; lack of emotion

apex the pointed end of a cone-shaped structure, such as the heart

aphasia language impairment; loss of ability to communicate through speech or writing

apical pertaining to the apex of a structure such as the heart

apical pulse pulse rate taken by placing a stethoscope over the tip of the heart

apical/radial pulse a comparison of the apical pulse rate and the radial pulse rate

apnea a period of no respirations

approach steps to be taken to reach a goal

aromatherapy an inhalation treatment using oils and scent to relieve pain and promote relaxation

arteriosclerosis a general term meaning a narrowing of the blood vessels, which can result in subsequent tissue hypoxia; degeneration and hardening of the walls of the arteries and sometimes of the valves of the heart

artery a vessel through which the oxygenated blood passes from the heart to various parts of the body

arthritis joint inflammation

articulation the point where two bones meet; the ability to speak or write clearly

artificial nutrition ways other than eating to provide nutrition for a resident

ascites fluid accumulation in the abdomen

asepsis without infection or pathogenic microorganisms

Asepto syringe a plastic syringe with a bulb; used to perform moist treatments

aspiration drawing foreign material (food, fluid, or other materials) into the respiratory tract

assault a violent act; an unlawful threat or attempt to harm another physically

assessment the act of evaluating

assignment a designated list of duties

assistive device equipment used to help a person be more effective in his or her physical activity

asthma a chronic respiratory disease characterized by bronchospasms and excessive mucus production

ataxic cerebral palsy a form of cerebral palsy in which the principal disturbance is a lack of balance and coordination

atherosclerosis a degenerative process involving the lining of arteries, in which the lumen eventually narrows and closes

athetoid cerebral palsy a form of cerebral palsy characterized by involuntary, slow, incessant movements of the parts of the body that are affected

atrium (pl. *atria***)** one of the upper heart chambers

atrophy shrinking or wasting away of tissues

attitude the state of mind that is indicative of feelings or opinions

audiogram hearing test

audiologist a physician specializing in hearing problems

auditory nerve the nerve carrying sound from the ear to the brain

aura a peculiar sensation preceding the onset of a convulsion or seizure

aural pertaining to the ear

autoclave a sterilizing machine

autoimmune antibodies against components of one's own body

automatic external defibrillator a nonintrusive device that restores the heartbeat and rhythm by means of electric shock

autonomic dysreflexia a syndrome that may occur in persons who have had an injury to the spinal cord below the level of T-5 or T-6 that cause the portion of the nervous system that is intact to send out signals causing constriction of the blood vessels that result in increased blood pressure and decreased pulse rate

axilla the armpit

Ayurveda an Eastern Indian system of medicine that uses body types (doshas) as the basis for prevention, diagnosis, and cure of disease

B

bacteremia the presence of bacteria in the blood

bargaining attempting to make a "deal" to influence the final outcome of a situation

battery an unlawful attack or touching of another person without consent

behavior modification an approach that is based on rewarding positive behaviors and initiating corrective action for negative behaviors

benign prostatic hypertrophy non-cancerous enlargement of the prostate gland

bile a secretion of the liver needed to prepare fats for digestion

biofeedback therapy that trains the user to gain voluntary mental control over normally involuntary bodily responses

biohazard contaminated with blood or body fluids and having the potential to transmit disease

bladder a membranous sac containing fluid, such as the urinary bladder

blood pressure pressure of blood exerted against the arterial walls

body alignment correct body position

body language nonverbal communication signaled by behavior, facial expressions, body stance, or gestures

body mechanics the correct use of the muscles of the body to move or lift heavy objects

body work hands-on therapies that involve manipulation, massage, and realignment of the body

bowel intestine

Bowman's capsule the tubule surrounding the glomerulus of the nephron in the kidney

bradycardia unusually slow heartbeat

Braille a system of raised dots representing letters A through Z and numbers 0 through 9 that allows sight-impaired residents to "read" through the sense of touch

brain stem the part of the brain that includes the medulla oblongata, diencephalon, pons, and midbrain

bridging a technique used to reduce pressure on ischemic areas by use of pillows and pads

bronchi (sing. bronchus) tubes that connect the lung to the trachea in the lungs

bronchioles one of the finer subdivisions or branches of the bronchial tree

bronchitis inflammation of the bronchi

burnout loss of enthusiasm and interest in an activity

bursa (pl. *bursae***)** a small synovial-filled sac located around a joint that helps reduce friction

bursitis inflammation of a bursa

C

calculi (sing. calculus) stones or concretions

calorie-restricted diet a diet that limits the intake of calories

cancer a malignant tumor; malignancy

cannula a small tube that may be inserted into a cavity to allow the passage of fluid

capillary hair-like blood vessel; the link between arterioles and venules

carbohydrates material used by the body to produce heat and energy

carbon dioxide gas that is a waste product in cellular metabolism

cardiac arrest sudden heart stoppage

cardiac cycle all the events (mechanical and electrical) that occur between one cardiac contraction and the next

cardiac muscle special tissue making up the muscular wall of the heart

cardiogram a record of cardiac pulsation produced by cardiograph

cardiopulmonary resuscitation (CPR) emergency medical procedure undertaken to restart and sustain heart and respiratory functions

cardiovascular pertaining to the heart and blood vessels

care plan a plan developed by the interdisciplinary health care team that describes the goals and approaches that all team members are to use in caring for the resident

care plan conference a meeting of team members to plan resident care

caries dental cavities, tooth decay

carrier a person who harbors infectious organisms that can be transmitted to others but who shows no sign of illness personally

cartilage a type of connective tissue

cast a rigid covering to keep a joint or other body part immobile

cataract opacity of the lens, resulting in loss of vision

catastrophic reaction the severe and unpredictable violent behavior of a person with dementia

catheter a tube for evacuating or injecting fluids

caustic burning, corrosive, or destructive to living tissue

cavity an enclosed area; space within the body that contains the organs

cell the basic unit in the organization of living substance

cellulose a basic substance of all plant foods, which can supply the body with roughage

Celsius a scale for measuring temperature in which the boiling point of water is 100°

centimeter one-hundredth of a meter

central nervous system (CNS) the brain and spinal cord

central venous (CV) catheter a small tube placed in a major vein, such as the subclavian vein

central venous pressure (CVP) the measurement of blood pressure in the large central veins

cerebellum the part of the brain responsible for balance and muscle coordination

cerebral pertaining to the brain

cerebral palsy a motor disorder that results in the inability to control body movement

cerebrospinal fluid a watery, clear fluid that surrounds the brain and spinal cord

cerebrovascular accident (CVA) caused by a sudden disruption in blood to the brain; may be caused by breakage of a small blood vessel or a blood clot; may cause motor or cognitive deficits; also called brain attack or stroke

cerebrum the largest and main portion of the brain that's responsible for sensory interpretation and voluntary muscle activity

certification the official recognition of successful completion of education, learning, and testing; also, an inspection process for facilities that accept federal funds as payment for health care

character (of pulse) the rhythm and volume of pulse

chart the record of medical information concerning a resident

cheeking storing food in one side of the mouth

chemical restraint drugs used for staff convenience to influence or control a resident's behavior

chemotherapy treatment with drugs or chemicals

Cheyne-Stokes respiration periods of apnea alternating with periods of hyperpnea

CHF see congestive heart failure

Chinese medicine an ancient form of medicine and therapies based on a universal energy or vital life force that flows through the body

chiropractic a system of therapy that uses manipulation and adjustment of bodily structures, particularly the spinal column, to relieve pain and promote health and healing

chlamydia a type of sexually transmitted infection

choroid the vascular layer, or coat, of the eye; contains the iris

chronic persisting over a long period

chronic bronchitis a condition, such as emphysema, in which there is excessive mucus secretion in the bronchi

chronic disease a condition that continues over a long period; incurable but treatable

chronic obstructive pulmonary disease (COPD) any condition, such as emphysema, that causes interference with normal respirations over a prolonged period

circadian daily biorhythmic functions and cycle

clear liquid diet a diet in which all nutrients must be in the form of liquid that is clear

clergy ministers, priests, rabbis; religious leaders

client a resident; a person receiving care

client care records the documentation of care provided in the home setting

climacteric menopause; the combined phenomena accompanying the cessation of the reproductive function in the female or diminution of testicular activity in the male

clitoris a small, cylindrical mass of erotic tissue; part of the external female reproductive organs analogous to the penis in the male

CNS central nervous system

code blue an emergency signal given when a resident is in danger of dying so that lifesaving techniques can be used

cognitive impairment a term used to describe intellectual impairment; any form of dementia

colon large intestine

colostomy a surgically established opening between the colon and the surface of the abdomen to allow elimination of feces

comatose unconscious; in a coma

combining form the part of a word that may be arranged in different ways to form new words

comminuted fracture a fracture in which the bone is broken or crushed into small pieces

commode a portable toilet

communal pertaining to something that is shared with others

communicable capable of being transferred from one person to another directly or indirectly, such as infectious disease

communicate to make known

communication the exchange of information

community services special services provided outside of the facility

compassion fatigue a form of burnout that can affect persons in the health care profession

compensation in psychology, the act of seeking a substitute for something unacceptable or unattainable

compliance obedience; following directions; doing what one is supposed to do

compound fracture a fracture in which the broken bone protrudes through the skin

concentration an increase in strength by evaporation

condom a rubber sheath used to cover the penis that is used for urinary drainage for an incontinent male

confidential keeping what is said or written to oneself; private; non-sharing

congestive heart failure (CHF) a chronic inability of the heart to maintain an adequate output of blood from one or both ventricles, resulting in an inadequate blood supply to the body tissues and retention of fluid

conjunctiva mucous membrane that covers the eye and lines the eyelids

connective tissue special body tissue that holds other tissues together and provides support for organs and other structures of the body

connective tissue cell a cell that produces connective tissue

constipation difficulty in defecating; passage of hard, dry stool from the rectum

constricting making narrower or smaller

constriction a narrowed or compressed area

consultant one who offers professional advice

contact precautions practices used to prevent the spread of pathogens by direct or indirect contact

contagious communicable or easily spread

contaminated unclean; impure; soiled with germs

continent able to control elimination of feces and urine

contract an agreement between two or more people, especially one that is written; to shorten, to decrease in size

contracture the permanent shortening or contraction of a muscle because of spasm or paralysis

convulsion an involuntary muscle spasm

COPD chronic obstructive pulmonary disease, for example, pulmonary emphysema and chronic bronchitis

cornea the clear (transparent) anterior covering of the eye through which light passes

coronary artery a major blood vessel of the heart that nourishes the heart muscle with fresh blood

coronary occlusion closing off or blockage of a coronary artery

corporal punishment the use of painful treatment to correct behavior

cortex the outer covering or portions of an organ

cortisone the hormone produced by the adrenal cortex

Cowper's glands two small glands located beside the male urethra and below the prostate gland, which secrete a fluid into the semen

CPR cardiopulmonary resuscitation

cross-training instruction in different skills across (health care) areas

cubic centimeter (cc) in health care, equivalent to 1 milliliter (1 mL)

cultural heritage an individual's beliefs, customs, and language

culture and sensitivity a laboratory test to determine the type of microorganism causing a disease and the specific drugs that can be used to treat the disease

cutaneous relating to the skin

cutaneous membrane skin

cuticle the area around the base of a fingernail or toenail

CVA cerebrovascular accident

CVP central venous pressure

cyanosis bluish skin discoloration of the nails, skin, and lips from lack of oxygen

cyanotic pertaining to blueness most commonly observed as a result of lack of oxygen

cystocele bladder hernia

cystoscopy a procedure using a cystoscope for visualization of the urinary bladder, ureter, and kidney

D

day care center a place where senior citizens may go for various services

debilitating weakening

debridement the removal of foreign matter or necrotic tissue from a wound

decline deterioration or negative change in a resident's condition or abilities

deconditioned a state in which tissues and organs become weakened from lack of use

decubiti (sing. decubitus) pressure sores; bedsores; decubitus ulcers

defamation of character making false or damaging statements about another person that harm that person's reputation

defecation a bowel movement that expels feces

defense mechanism a psychological reaction or technique for protection against a stressful environmental situation or anxiety

defibrillation the artificial restoration of the heartbeat and heart rhythm by means of electric shock

deficiencies incomplete, inadequate, lack of important elements of care; areas of noncompliance with relevant standards

dehydration excessive loss of fluid from the body

delegation passing on of orders or responsibilities

delirium a mental condition marked by confusion and excitement; may be due to varied causes (fever, anxiety, shock, drug overdose)

delusion a false belief

demanding behavior unreasonable requests for service, special meals, or special treatment

dementia progressive mental deterioration caused by organic brain disease

dendrite the branch of a neuron conducting impulses toward the cell body

denial an unconscious defense mechanism, refusing to recognize something as the truth

dental hygienist a person licensed and specially trained to perform oral hygiene, including cleaning of teeth

dentist a person licensed and specially trained to practice dentistry and/or dental surgery

dentures false teeth

deoxygenated to have lost oxygen

dependability trustworthiness; reliability

depressant something (e.g., a drug) that decreases body function

depression feelings of sadness and despair

dermal ulcer a skin lesion; a term that includes: pressure ulcers (decubiti), arterial or venous ulcers, and diabetic ulcers

dermis the layer of skin beneath the epithelium

deteriorate to progressively break down or disorganize

developmental disability a severe, chronic disorder apparent before age 22, caused by mental and/or physical impairment

developmental tasks in psychology, normal steps in personality development

diabetes mellitus a disorder of carbohydrate, fat, and protein metabolism

diabetic coma a loss of consciousness caused by lack of treatment for or unregulated diabetes mellitus

diabetic ketoacidosis (DKA) inadequately controlled diabetes mellitus

diabetic retinopathy damage to the eye and vision that may be the result of diabetes mellitus

diagnosis determination of the specific disease or condition causing a patient's symptoms

diagnostic-related group (DRG) the method used to determine the number of hospital days allowed for a specific illness

dialysis a treatment given when kidneys fail to remove accumulated wastes from the blood

diaphoresis profuse sweating

diaphragm the dome-shaped muscle that divides the ventral cavity into a thorax and an abdominopelvic cavity

diarrhea the passage of multiple, watery stools

diastole the period during which the heart muscle relaxes and the chamber fills with blood

diastolic pertains to the relaxation phase of the cardiac cycle

diathermy treatment with heat

diet the food and drink necessary for body nourishment

dietetics the science of regulation of the diet for therapeutic purposes

dietitian (or dietician) a person specially trained in the field of nutrition and the science of dietetics (diets)

digestion the process of converting food into a form that can be used by the body

dilating enlarging

diplegia a movement disturbance that primarily affects the legs

dirty contaminated with microbes

disability persistent physical or mental defect or handicap

discharge planner the social worker who arranges for care after discharge from a facility and helps the resident make the transition from the long-term care facility to the community

discharge planning a cooperative procedure that involves all members of the interdisciplinary health care team

disinfection the process of destroying pathogenic organisms or agents on articles or surfaces

dislocation a bone or joint displaced from its normal alignment with another

disorientation the loss of recognition of person, time, place, or location

displacement an unconscious defense mechanism in which an emotion such as anger is directed at an inappropriate person or object

distal farthest away from a central point, such as point of attachment of muscles

distended stretched or enlarged

diuretics drugs that increase urine output

diverticuli(a) (sing. diverticulum) small blind pouches that form in the lining and wall of the colon

diverticulitis inflammation of diverticula

diverticulosis presence of many diverticula

DNR See do not resuscitate order

document the process of recording observations and data about a resident's condition

documentation substantiating statements

do not resuscitate (DNR) order physician order indicating that the resident is not to be revived when cardiac and respiratory arrest occur

dorsal posterior or back

dorsal cavity the posterior body cavity consisting of the cranium and vertebral canal

draw sheet a sheet placed horizontally under the resident and extending from above the shoulder to below the hips

DRG diagnosis-related group

drip chamber part of the equipment used to administer parenteral fluids

droplet precautions the practices used to prevent the spread of microbes transmitted by droplets in the air produced by laughing, talking, singing, sneezing, or coughing

dry sterile dressing (DSD) a sterile dressing that is applied dry to a wound

duodenum the first part of the small intestine

durable power of attorney a document that permits a person to delegate to someone else the power to make any health care decisions that the person is unable to make

dyspepsia indigestion

dysphagia difficulty in swallowing

dyspnea difficult or labored breathing

dysuria painful urination

E

ECG See electrocardiogram

edema excessive accumulation of fluid in the tissues

ejaculation forcible, sudden expulsion of semen from the penis

ejaculatory duct the part of the male reproductive tract extending from the seminal vesicles to the urethra

electrocardiogram (ECG or EKG) a recording of the electrical activity of the heart

electroencephalogram (EEG) graphic recording of the electrical activity of the brain

electrolytes compounds that play an essential role in body function

elimination excretion; discharge from the body of indigestible materials and of waste products of body metabolism

embolus a blood clot that moves through the vascular system

emergency an unexpected occurrence that requires immediate action

Emergency Medical Services (EMS) services provided by specially trained people at the scene of the emergency and in the ambulance

emesis vomitus or vomiting

emotional lability easily upset; emotionally unstable

empathy the ability to understand how someone else feels

emphysema chronic obstructive pulmonary disease in which the alveolar walls are destroyed

empowerment power or authority

EMS Emergency Medical Services

Encephalopathy malfunction of the brain caused by toxic materials such as ammonia that are not broken down by the liver

endocrine gland the gland that secretes hormonal substances directly into the bloodstream; ductless gland

endometrium the lining of the uterus

endotracheal within the trachea

endotracheal tube a tube placed in the trachea to assist respiration

enema the introduction of liquid into the lower bowel or the rectum to be returned or retained

enteral feedings feedings that bypasses the mouth and goes directly into the intestinal tract

enteric pertaining to the alimentary canal; intestinal

environment surroundings

environmental services the department and workers responsible for maintaining clean and comfortable surroundings for residents and staff

enzymes organic catalysts produced by living cells but capable of acting independently of the cells producing them

epidermis the top layer of skin

epididymis an elongated, cordlike structure along the posterior border of the testes, in the ducts of which the sperm is stored

epidural catheter a tube inserted into the spinal area for delivery of medication

epilepsy a noninfectious disorder of the brain manifested by episodes of motor and sensory dysfunction, which may or may not be accompanied by convulsions and unconsciousness

epithelial cell cell that produces and forms epithelial tissue

epithelial tissue tissue that forms the skin and parts of the secreting glands and that lines the body cavities; specialized in its ability to absorb, secrete, excrete, and protect

equilibrium sense of balance

ergonomics adapting the workplace and the job to the workers' needs

erythrocytes red blood cells

esophagus a tube extending from the pharynx (back of throat) to the stomach

estrogen a hormone produced by the ovaries

ethical code rules governing the right and wrong of professional behavior

ethics the study of standards of conduct or moral judgment

ethnicity special groups of persons within a culture who share certain characteristics such as customs, language, and national origin

evaluation judgment; critical review of a situation or condition; determination of how the resident's plan of care is working

exacerbation a period of increased severity of symptoms

excreta excretions, such as feces, urine, and perspiration

expectorant a medication to aid in expectoration (spitting up phlegm)

expectorate to spit

Health Maintenance Organization (HMO) an insurer that provides a range of services on a group basis, a network of physicians and other healthcare providers. All care must be approved by the HMO to be eligible for coverage

holistic applying to the whole; seeing a person as a complete, integrated entity with many aspects; it also can be used to describe the exclusive use of alternative treatments

home health nursing assistant a person who performs personal and nursing care skills, such as bathing the client, under the supervision of a registered nurse

home health services help provided at a person's home after an acute hospitalization and during chronic illness

homeopathy therapy based on the theory that a person can be cured of disease by giving small amounts of agents that cause disease

homeostasis a state of balance or equilibrium

hormone a secretion of the endocrine gland; chemical messengers that originate in the endocrine glands of the body

hospice a special facility or arrangement to provide care of terminally ill persons

hot-line number a toll-free number residents may use to reach authorities outside the facility to register complaints

hot soak a treatment in which a part of the body, such as a hand, is placed in warm water as a method of applying heat

human immunodeficiency virus (HIV) the microorganism that causes HIV disease, which may progress to AIDS

Huntington's disease a progressive degenerative disease of the brain that results in uncontrolled movements and mental deterioration

hydrotherapy a treatment that uses water for healing purposes

hygiene a system of principles or rules designed for the promotion of health

hyperalimentation parenteral nutrition; nutrition delivered directly into the bloodstream

hyperbilirubinemia the presence of bilirubin in the blood stream

hyperglycemia excessive level of blood sugar

hypertension high blood pressure

hyperthyroidism a condition in which the thyroid gland is enlarged and over-produces thyroid hormones

hypertrophy an increase in size of an organ or structure, which does not involve tumor formation

hypoglycemia abnormally low level of sugar in the blood

hypotension low blood pressure

hypothermia greatly reduced core body temperature

hypothyroidism deficient functioning of the thyroid gland

hypoxia lack of adequate oxygen supply

hysterectomy surgical removal of the uterus

I

IADL's *See* (IADL's)

I&O *See* intake and output

ice bag a type of cold treatment

IDDM *See* insulin-dependent diabetes mellitus

ileostomy a surgically made opening in the ileum through the abdominal wall

ileum the lower three-fifths of the small intestine, lying between the jejunum and cecum

illusion a mental impression derived from misinterpretation of an actual sensory stimulus

IM *See* intramuscular

immunity the ability of the body to fight off disease caused by microbes; the state of being protected from disease

immunization the process of making a person more resistant to infectious agents

immunosuppression the failure of the body to begin an immune response when exposed to an antigen

impaction the condition of being tightly wedged or stuck (as feces in the bowel)

impairment disability

implementation to put into action; process of carrying out a plan

impotence lack of physical strength or weakness; inability to perform sexually

incident something of consequence that happens unexpectedly; an event that might result in harm to a resident

incontinence the inability to predict and control elimination of body wastes

incontinent unable to control elimination

indwelling catheter a small tube that remains in the patient's bladder to provide continuous drainage of urine (Foley catheter)

infarction death of tissue

infection the invasion and multiplication of any organism and the damage this causes in the body

inferior below another part

inferior vena cava the large vein that returns blood to the right atrium of the heart

inflammation a localized protective reaction of the body due to injury, characterized by heat, redness, swelling, and pain

inflammatory response tissue reaction to injury, whether direct or referred

influenza an acute, contagious respiratory viral disease spread by droplets

informed consent permission given by one who fully understands all the facts relating to what is going to happen

infusion introduction of a solution into a vein by gravity such as an intravenous infusion (IV)

inguinal hernia a condition in which intestines push through the abdominal wall in the groin area

inhibition that which restrains an action, emotion, or thought

insertion distal point of attachment of skeletal muscle

inspiration the drawing of air into the lungs (inhalation)

instrumental activities of daily living (IADL) higher-level tasks performed by adults, such as money management and driving

insulin the hormone secreted by the islets of Langerhans in the pancreas that regulates glucose metabolism

insulin-dependent diabetes mellitus (IDDM) a condition in which the person must rely on insulin injections as part of the therapy

insulin shock hypoglycemia (a decrease in blood sugar), accompanied by anxiety, excitement, perspiration, delirium, or coma

intake and output (I&O) measurement of all fluids the resident ingests and excretes in a 24-hour period

integrity a personality trait consisting of sincerity and honesty

integumentary system the body system consisting of the skin, its various layers, and its accessory structures (hair, nails, and skin glands)

intellectual disability a condition diagnosed before the age of 18 that includes below-average intellectual function, and a lack of skills needed for everyday living

intelligence quotient (IQ) the ability to solve problems, to adapt to the demands of the environment, and to understand abstract relationships appropriate to one's age

intention tremor trembling of hands that increases with efforts to control trembling

intercostals between the ribs

intercourse interchange or communication between individuals; an alternate term for sexual relations

interdisciplinary health care team a group of health care providers in different specialties who act together to plan and implement the plan of care for each resident

intermittent care care that is given at periodic intervals

intermittent positive pressure breathing (IPPB) a technique in which a machine is used to deliver air or oxygen and medication under pressure to a person's lungs; a technique for assisting breathing

interpersonal relationships how people interact with each other

intervention actions that influence the eventual outcome of a situation

interventricular septum the dividing portion between the ventricles of the heart

interview a formal meeting with a prospective employer to assess the qualifications of an applicant and provide information about available jobs

intramuscular (IM) within muscles

intravenous (IV) therapy an intravenous infusion of fluids, nutrition, or medication injected by means of a sterile needle and tubing directly into a vein

invasion of privacy revealing information of a personal nature regarding a resident

involuntary muscle a type of muscle forming the walls of organs; also known as visceral or smooth muscle

involuntary seclusion being kept apart from others against one's will

IPPB intermittent positive pressure breathing

IQ intelligence quotient

iris the colored portion of eye

ischemia deficient blood supply to body tissues

islets of Langerhans special cells in the pancreas that produce insulin

isolation a place where a resident with easily transmitted diseases is separated from others

isolation technique special procedures carried out to prevent the spread of infectious organisms from an infected person

J

jaundice yellowing of the skin

JCAHO See Joint Commission for Accreditation of Healthcare Organizations

jejunum the portion of the small intestine between the duodenum and the ileum

job description the duties and responsibilities involved in a position

joint the point of articulation between bones

Joint Commission for Accreditation of Healthcare Organizations an organization that inspects and accredits health care agencies to ensure the agency meets high quality standards

K

Kardex a type of file in which nursing care plans are kept

keratosis roughened, scaly, wartlike lesion

ketones products from fat metabolism

ketosis abnormal levels of ketones in the blood; a complication of diabetes mellitus

kidney dialysis See hemodialysis

kidney glandular organ that secretes urine

kilogram 1,000 grams; 2.2 pounds

kyphosis extreme dorsal curvature of the spine in the thoracic area (hunchback)

L

labia majora two large, hair-covered, liplike structures that are part of the vulva of the female

labia minora two hairless liplike structures found beneath the labia majora of the female

laceration an injury or wound made by tearing or cutting of the flesh

lactose a form of sugar found in milk

larynx the voice box

last rites a special service of confession and blessing practiced by clergy for Catholic residents when gravely ill; also called Sacrament of the Sick

lateral to the side; away from the midline

lateral position side-lying position

laxative medicine to relieve constipation

legal guardian one who has the legal authority to make decisions and act on behalf of another

lens the portion of the eye that bends light rays

lentigines elevated yellow or brown spots or patches that occur on exposed skin; "liver spots"

lesion abnormal change in tissue formation

leukemia a malignant disease of the blood-forming organs, characterized by abnormal proliferation and distortion of the leukocytes in the blood and bone marrow

leukocytes white blood cells

Lhermitte's sign seen in multiple sclerosis; a feeling of tingling and pain (like an electric shock) in the spinal column when the neck is flexed

libel any oral or written defamatory statement

libido sex drive

licensed practical nurse (LPN) a person licensed by the state who provides direct care under the supervision of a registered nurse; in some states LPNs are called licensed vocational nurses or LVNs

licensure permission to operate or practice from a state agency that regulates a business or profession

ligaments bands of fibrous tissue that hold joints together

light therapy a treatment regimen that uses controlled light to influence and regulate bodily processes

lipase a fat-splitting enzyme produced by the pancreas

lipodystrophy any disturbance in fat metabolism

living will a document describing the wishes of a terminally ill resident relating to health care

long-term care facility health care institution that provides care for residents with chronic diseases and personal care needs

lower extremities pertains to the legs and feet

low-fat diet a diet in which the amount of fat has been reduced

low-sodium diet a diet that limits the amount of sodium chloride, a mineral salt

LPN licensed practical nurse

lumen a channel (opening) within a tube-like organ

LVN a licensed vocational nurse. See licensed practical nurse

lymph fluid found in lymphatic vessels

lymph node a mass of lymphatic tissue along lymph vessels; mainly acts as a filter

M

magnetic resonance imaging (MRI) a procedure using computer and magnetic fields to visualize inner body organs

magnetic therapy the use of magnets in treatments to relieve pain and promote healing

malignancy cancerous

malpractice negligence or unethical conduct that results in harm, injury, or loss to a resident

manipulative behavior actions designed to control the responses of others

mastication the act of chewing food with the teeth in preparation for swallowing

masturbation sexually stimulating oneself

maturity the state of full development, physically, mentally, and psychologically

MDS *See* Minimum Data Set

meatus an opening or channel

mechanical lift a device used to transfer residents who are unable to bear weight or are very heavy

mechanical soft diet a diet in which the foods are specially prepared to make them easier to chew

medial close to the midline of a body or structure

mediastinum the space between the lungs

Medicaid the federal- and state-funded program that pays for medical costs for those whose income falls below a certain level

medical asepsis procedures followed to prevent the spread of infection

medical chart a legally binding record of pertinent information relating to the resident, the resident's progress, and care

medical terminology specialized words, phrases, and abbreviations used in the field of medicine

Medicare the federal program that assists the disabled and those over 65 years of age with hospital, long-term, and/or home health care

medulla the internal portion of a gland; also refers to the lowest part of the brain stem, where the vital centers for respiratory, cardiac, and vasomotor control are located

membrane a thin lining or covering of cells

memo a brief written or electronic communication

meninges the three-layered serous membrane covering the brain and spinal cord

menopause the period when ovaries stop functioning and menstruation ceases; female climacteric

menstruation the periodic shedding of the endometrium

mental abuse making verbal threats to hurt, punish, or humiliate a resident

mental retardation former clinical term for "intellectual disability," which was changed by Rosa's Law in 2010, because the term has become widely used in today's society to degrade and insult people with intellectual disabilities; *see* intellectual disability

mercury a toxic silvery metal that is liquid at room temperature; was frequently used in clinical thermometers and is now banned

metabolism the sum total of the physical and chemical processes and reactions taking place in the body

metastasis the spreading of cancer to other body parts or locations

meter the metric distance measurement equaling 39.371 inches

methicillin-resistant *Staphylococcus aureus* (MRSA) a common infectious microbe that is resistant to the effect of most antibiotics

metric system a system of weights and measurements based on the meter and having all units based on some power of 10

microbe a tiny organism that can only be seen with a microscope; some may cause disease

micturition urination

midplane an imaginary line that divides the body evenly into a right side and left side

milliliter (mL) a measurement of capacity—volume of 1 g of water at standard temperature and pressure; the same as one cubic centimeter (cc)

mineral an inorganic chemical compound found in nature; many minerals are important in building body tissues and regulating body fluids

Minimum Data Set (MDS 3.0) an assessment completed for all residents admitted to a skilled care facility; the basis for the care plan

mite a tiny, often parasitic organism that cannot be seen with the naked eye

mitered corner a bedmaking technique in which the top sheet is tucked in at the front of the bed, forming a 45° angle with the perpendicular edge of the mattress

mitosis the division of the cytoplasm and nucleus in the cell

mixed incontinence simultaneously experiencing two types of incontinence such as stress and urge incontinence; this type most often occurs in women

mL milliliter

mobility the ability to move or to be moved easily from place to place

mobility skills a person's ability to move easily from place to place

morbidity the state of being diseased; conditions inducing disease

mortality rate the proportion of deaths to population

motor nerve the nerve that carries messages to muscles from the brain

mottling discoloration of skin or irregular areas

MRI magnetic resonance imaging

MRSA methicillin resistant *Staphylococcus aureus*

MSDS Material Safety Data Sheets

mucolytic destroying or dissolving mucus

mucous pertaining to or resembling mucus; also, secreting mucus

mucous membrane special tissues that secrete a sticky substance called mucus; these membranes line body cavities that open to the outside

mucus the secretion of mucous membranes; thick, sticky fluid

multiple sclerosis (MS) a chronic disease of the central nervous system that causes degeneration to the covering of the nerve fibers and interferes with the conduction of nerve impulses

muscle the tissue composed of contractile (contracts and relaxes) fibers or cells

muscle cell cells characterized by their ability to contract and relax and to bring about movement

muscle tissue the tissue that forms the body wall and organs and is specialized for movement

myasthenia gravis (MG) a disease characterized by muscular weakness caused by inadequate neurotransmitters

myocardial infarction an area of dead heart tissue caused by lack of blood flow

myocardial ischemia the lack of blood flow to the heart muscle

myocardium heart muscle

myth a commonly accepted belief that is untrue

N

narcosis a stuporous state produced by drugs

narcotic a drug that relieves pain and may induce sleep

nasogastric (NG) tube a soft rubber or plastic tube that is inserted through a nostril and into the stomach that can be used for feeding or for medical procedures

naturopathic medicine a medical system based on wellness, emphasizing prevention and self-care

necrosis tissue death

neglect the failure to provide services to residents to prevent physical harm or mental anguish

negligence the failure to give care that is reasonably expected under the circumstances that results in unintended injury to the resident

nephron a microscopic kidney unit that produces the urine; made up of the glomerulus, Bowman's capsule, and the convoluted tubules

nerves bundles of nerve processes (axons and dendrites) that are held together by connective tissue

nerve cell a cell that carries electrical messages to and from different parts of the body

nerve impulses electrical waves that transmits messages

nervous tissue highly specialized tissue capable of conducting a nerve impulse

networking a line of communications among individuals with a common interest or goal

neurons cells of the nervous system

neurotransmitter a chemical compound that transmits a nervous impulse across cells at a synapse

NG tube nasogastric tube

NIDDM *See* non–insulin-dependent diabetes mellitus

NIOSH-approved respirator a type of personal protective equipment for breathing that is approved by the National Institute for Occupational Safety and Health

nitroglycerin a vasodilator drug used mainly to relieve pain for angina pectoris

no-code (DNR) (do not resuscitate) an order not to resuscitate (revive) a resident

nocturia excessive urination at night

non–insulin-dependent diabetes mellitus (NIDDM) relative insulin deficiency or resistance to insulin action; controlled by diet, exercise, and oral medication; insulin may not be needed

nonverbal communication sending messages without the use of words, such as facial expressions or gestures

non-weight bearing no weight to be borne by hip(s)/leg(s); unable to stand or walk on one or both legs

nosocomial infection older term used to refer to an infection that occurs while the resident is in a health care facility; now called "Healthcare Acquired Infection (HAI)"

nurse's notes a section of a resident's medical record that contains documentation of medications, observations, and procedures given by nurses

nurses' station the area on a resident unit where medical records and care plans are kept

nursing assistant a nurse's aide or orderly

nursing diagnosis a nursing statement of a patient problem and its probable cause

nursing process a four-step process for determining resident care: assessment, nursing diagnosis, planning, implementation, and evaluation

nutrient food that supplies heat and energy, builds and repairs body tissue, and regulates body functions

nutrition the process by which the body uses food for growth and repair and to maintain health

nystagmus involuntary and jerky repetitive movements of the eyes

O

obesity the condition of being overweight

objective observation observations made by seeing, hearing, feeling, touching, and smelling

OBRA *See Omnibus Budget Reconciliation Act of 1987;* a law that set many standards for the health care industry, including education, licensure, certification, and regulation of nursing assistants

observation something that is noticed

occult hidden blood; blood that cannot be seen by the naked eye

occupational exposure coming into contact with a hazard (infectious or chemical) while carrying out assignments

Occupational Safety and Health Administration (OSHA) the federal government agency responsible for developing and enforcing health and job safety standards to protect employees

occupational therapist a person licensed to provide rehabilitative services to evaluate and treat persons with physical injury or illness, psychosocial problems, or developmental disabilities

occupied bedmaking making of the bed while the resident is in the bed

oil gland a sebaceous gland that is found in the skin and secretes an oily substance into the follicles

olfactory pertaining to the sense of smell

oliguria scant urine

ombudsman a public official designated to investigate complaints objectively and act as an advocate

Omnibus Budget Reconciliation Act legislation that regulates the education and certification of nursing assistants in the long-term care industry

oncology the study of neoplasms or tumors (cancer)

open reduction/internal fixation a surgical method of stabilizing fractures

ophthalmologist a physician who specializes in the treatment of defects and diseases of the eye

opportunistic infection an infection that results from a defective immune system that cannot defend the body against pathogens that are commonly found in the environment

optic nerve the nerve carrying messages from the eye to the brain

optometrist a health care provider who specializes in measuring visual acuity

oral pertaining to the mouth

oral hygiene care of the mouth and teeth

orally through the mouth

organ any part of the body that carries out a specific function or functions, such as the heart

origin proximal point of attachment to skeletal muscle

orthopnea a condition in which there is difficulty breathing, except when sitting upright

orthopneic position a resident must sit, supported, in an upright position, while leaning slightly forward, to relieve respiratory distress

orthosis a device used to maintain the position of an extremity

orthostatic hypotension a fall in blood pressure when a person assumes an upright position from a reclining position

orthotic device a device, such as a brace or splint, that restores or improves function and prevents deformity

OSHA Occupational Safety and Health Administration

osteoarthritis a degenerative joint disease caused by disintegration of the cartilage that covers the ends of the bones

osteoporosis the most common metabolic disease of bone in the United States; characterized by a decrease in the mass of bony tissue; more commonly affects women past middle age but also affects men; may lead to fractures with minimal or no trauma

ostomy a suffix/word ending that means to create a new opening, as colostomy

output the measured amount of fluid excreted in a given period

ovaries endocrine glands located in the female pelvis; female gonads

overflow incontinence form of incontinence when bladder cannot fully emptied; the bladder becomes over-distended and causes small, frequent voiding

oviduct; fallopian tube the part of the female reproductive tract that carries ova from the ovaries to the uterus

ovulation a discharge of an egg from the ovary

ovum (pl. ova) the female egg

oxygen gas essential to cellular metabolism and life

oxygen mask a cuplike appliance attached to an oxygen source that is placed over a resident's nose and mouth to deliver oxygen

oxygenated carrying oxygen

P

pacemaker an artificial device placed in the body to regulate heartbeat

pacing repeatedly walking back and forth

PAINAD scale a scale that has been specifically developed to rate pain in a person with advanced dementia

palliative relieving symptoms but not curing disease

pallor less color than normal of the skin

pancreas a gland located behind the stomach that secretes several enzymes necessary for digestion, plus insulin and glycogen

papilloma a benign tumor of the skin or mucus membrane, also referred to as a wart or polyp

paralysis loss or impairment of the ability to move parts of the body

paranoia a state in which one has delusions of persecution and/or grandeur

paraplegia paralysis of both legs

parathormone a hormone produced by the parathyroid glands; important in managing the level of body calcium and phosphorus in the blood

parathyroid glands several small glands located on the posterior thyroid gland that produce the hormone parathormone

Parkinson's disease a neurological disease due to deficiency of dopamine; characterized by stiffness of muscles and tremors; occurs later in life

paroxysmal abrupt in onset and termination

partial weight bearing limited amount of weight can be borne on one or both legs

passive range of motion movement of the resident's joints by the caregiver

pathogen a microorganism or other agent capable of producing a disease

pathology changes caused by disease

patient a person who needs care; usually in a hospital

patient-controlled analgesia (PCA) a device used by a patient (resident) to control pain medication; administration is through an intravenous site

pelvic cavity that portion of the ventral cavity shaped like a basin surrounded by the pelvic bones

pelvis the lower portion of the trunk of the body; a basin-shaped area bounded by the hip bones, the sacrum, and the coccyx

penis the male organ of copulation

pension retirement income or fund

perceptual deficit an inability to reason, to think systematically, to make judgments, or to use common items

perceptual process the interpretation of information

pericardial pertaining to the pericardium (the sac enclosing the heart)

pericardium the membrane that surrounds the heart

perineal care specific cleaning of the genital and rectal areas

perineum in the male, the area between the anus and scrotum; in the female, the area between the anus and vagina

peripheral pertaining to the outside or outer part

peripheral intravenous central catheter (PICC) a small tube inserted into a vein in the arm and threaded through to a larger vein, such as the superior vena cava

peripheral nervous system (PNS) nerves that carry messages to and from the brain and spinal cord

peripheral vascular disease a disease resulting from decreased blood supply to and from the extremities

peristalsis a progressive, wavelike movement that occurs involuntarily in hollow tubes of the body, especially in the alimentary canal and the urinary tract; moves food and waste products through the gastrointestinal tract and urine through the ureters

peritoneal cavity that portion of the abdominopelvic cavity that is enclosed within the membranous peritoneum

peritoneal dialysis the process of cleansing the blood of waste products; a sterile fluid (dialysate) is introduced into the peritoneal cavity where it remains for a period of time; waste products from the body enter the fluid, which is then drained from the body

peritoneum a delicate serous membrane that lines the abdominal pelvic cavity and covers the organs

perseveration the constant repetition of an action such as finger tapping or lip licking

personal inventory a list of a resident's personal belongings

personal protective equipment (PPE) equipment such as waterproof masks, gowns, gloves, and goggles that protects the caregiver against the transmission of infectious organisms

personality the sum of the behavior, attitudes, and character traits of an individual

petit mal seizure a type of epilepsy attack, generally short in nature; "absence attack"

pet therapy providing animals to bring pleasure to severely impaired residents

phalange any bone of a finger or toe

phantom pain pain that seems to exist in a body part that has been removed, such as an amputated limb

pharynx the muscular and membranous tube between the mouth and the esophagus; throat

phlebitis inflammation of a vein

phlebotomy incision of a vein for the purpose of withdrawing blood

phlegm thick mucus found in the throat or respiratory tract

physical abuse any physical contact that intentionally causes pain or discomfort

physical needs needs that include maintaining hygiene and cleanliness and maintaining nutrition and fluid intake

physical restraint a device used to inhibit body movement; also prevents personal access to the body

physical therapist a licensed professional who provides services to persons to help them regain function and prevent disability following disease, injury, or loss of a body part

physician a licensed medical doctor

physiology the science that deals with the functioning of living organisms

PICC peripheral intravenous central catheter

piggyback a small bag of fluid that is attached to the main intravenous tubing to allow intermittent administration of medication

piles hemorrhoids

pineal gland a small gland found deep in the brain, it secretes serotonin and melatonin to help regulate sleep-wake cycles; and to delay puberty until an appropriate age

pitting edema a condition in which the tissue remains indented when pressure is applied to an edematous area

pituitary gland the gland located in the brain that serves a variety of functions, including regulation of the gonads, thyroid, adrenal cortex, and other endocrine glands; "master gland"

plane an imaginary line used to describe the relationship of one body part to another

plaque an irregular patch or flat lesion that forms on an artery lining in atherosclerosis; also, a gummy, decay-causing substance that grows around the base and the roots of the teeth

plasma liquid portion of blood

platelet thrombocyte; involved in the blood-clotting mechanism

pleura the membranes that surround the lungs

pleural pertaining to the pleura

pneumonia inflammation of the tissues of the lungs

PNS peripheral nervous system

podiatrist a physician specializing in foot problems

point of attachment areas where arms and legs are attached to the torso

policy book a book that outlines the rules governing the facility and explains what will be done for the residents

Physician Orders for Life Sustaining Treatment (POLST) standardized medical order form that identifies the type of life-sustaining treatments to be performed on the seriously ill resident

polydipsia excessive thirst

polyphagia excessive ingestion of food

polyuria excessive excretion of urine

pore opening of one of the ducts leading from the sweat glands to the surface of the skin

position sense the ability to tell how one's extremities are positioned without looking at them

posterior back or dorsal

postmortem after death

postmortem care care of the body after death

postural drainage positioning a patient to encourage drainage from the respiratory tract

postural hypotension a fall in blood pressure when a person assumes an upright position from a reclining position

postural support pads, pillows, or rolls used to help residents remain in proper alignment

potassium an element essential to the body; an electrolyte

potency power; especially the ability of the male to perform coitus

potentially infectious material material that might possibly cause infection

power of attorney for health care a legal document that authorizes someone other than the resident to carry out the health care wishes of the resident when the resident is unable to do so

PPE personal protective equipment

Preferred Provider Organization or Participating Provider Organization (PPO) managed care organization of medical doctors, hospitals, and health care providers who have agreed with an insurer to provide services at a reduced cost

prefix a term placed before a word that changes or modifies the meaning of the word

prepuce foreskin; a fold of skin covering the glans penis

presbycusis progressive loss of hearing due to normal aging

presbyopia impaired vision as a result of the aging process (farsightedness)

pressure ulcer ulcerations that form as the result of ischemia of tissues due to pressure; also called dermal ulcers or decubitus ulcers

procedure the steps taken to accomplish a particular task; a course or plan of action

procedure book a reference for procedures

professionalism a knowledgeable, compassionate, responsible manner of delivering health care

progesterone the hormone produced by the ovaries

prognosis the probable outcome of a disease or injury

progressive mobilization a process used to increase a resident's mobility skills

projection an unconscious defense mechanism in which an individual sees his or her own defects as belonging to another

prolapse the falling down or downward displacement of a body part or organ

prone a position in which the resident is lying on the abdomen; also, turning the forearm so the palm is facing downward

prostatectomy removal of all or part of the prostate gland

prostate gland the gland of male reproductive system that surrounds the neck of the urinary bladder and the beginning of the urethra

prosthesis an artificial substitute for a missing body part, such as a denture, hand, or leg

protein the basic material of every body cell; an essential nutrient to build and repair tissue

protocol a plan of treatment; a particular stated or standard method or procedure

protraction to be brought forward

proximal closest to the point of attachment

pruritus itching

psychiatrist (gero) a physician who specializes in the study, treatment, and prevention of mental disorders of the elderly

psychologist licensed mental health professional who is trained in methods of analysis, counseling, and research but may not prescribe medications for clients

psychosocial relating social conditions to mental health

psychotic completely out of touch with reality

puberty the condition or period of becoming capable of sexual reproduction

pubic pertaining to the pubis or pubic bone, which forms the center bone of the front of the pelvis

pulmonary artery the blood vessel that carries deoxygenated blood from the right ventricle to the lung

pulmonary emphysema a chronic lung disorder in which the terminal bronchioles become plugged with mucus and lung elasticity is lost

pulmonary veins four large veins that return blood from the lungs to the left atrium of the heart

pulse a wave of pressure exerted against the walls of the arteries in response to ventricular contraction that can be felt on the outside surface of the body

pulse deficit the difference between contractions of the heart and pulse expansions of the radial artery

pulse oximetry a procedure used to determine oxygen levels in the bloodstream

pulse pressure the difference between the systolic and diastolic pressure

pulse rate number per minute of impulses transmitted to the arteries by contraction of the left ventricle

pupil the opening in the center of the iris of the eye that regulates light entering the eye

PVD peripheral vascular disease

pylorus the narrow, tapered end of the stomach opening into the duodenum

pyorrhea periodontitis; loosening of the teeth caused by gum disease

Q

quadrant one of four imaginary sections of the surface of the abdomen

quadriplegia paralysis of all four limbs

quality assurance program (QA) measurement of care provided to residents; an internal review done by facility staff to identify problems and find solutions for improvement

R

race classification of people by shared physical characteristics such as skin color, facial features, hair texture, and bone structure

RACE acronym for a series of activities to take during a fire: r = remove all residents, a = activate alarm, c = contain, e = extinguish/evacuate

radial artery a blood vessel carrying oxygenated blood, located on the lateral anterior wrist at the base of the thumb; most often used to determine pulse rate

radiation therapy treatment of cancer using high-energy radiation

rales an abnormal respiratory sound heard in auscultation of the chest

range of motion (ROM) exercises a series of exercises specifically designed to move each joint through its full range

rapport a relationship of understanding and trust between two people

rationalization an unconscious defense mechanism in which one devises a logical, self-satisfying, but incorrect explanation for one's behavior or feelings

reality orientation techniques used to help residents remain oriented to the environment, to time, and to themselves

receptor a peripheral nerve ending; specialized for response to a particular type of stimuli

recovery position a modified lateral position used for persons who are recovering from certain emergencies, such as unconsciousness

rectocele protrusion of part of the rectum into the vagina

rectum the lower part of large intestine, about 5 inches long, between the sigmoid flexure and the anal canal

references in a résumé, statements about abilities and characteristics; persons who give such statements

reflex involuntary response to a stimulus

registered nurse (RN) a person who has completed a 2- to 4-year program in a nursing school and is licensed by the state to assess, to plan for, to implement, and to evaluate the nursing care needs of residents

regular diet a routine or balanced diet; sometimes called a house diet

regularity routinely eliminating waste products from the body

regurgitate swallowing air and expelling it in a controlled manner for speech, or the backflow of food from the stomach to the mouth

regurgitating "throwing up" undigested food from the stomach

regurgitation the backward flow of fluids in the body

rehabilitation the restoring of physical or mental abilities following an accident or illness

rehabilitation aide a specially trained nursing assistant who helps residents regain lost skills or teaches new skills; works under the direction of an occupational or physical therapist

reiki a Japanese term meaning universal energy; it is also a energy medicine, similar to the Chinese *chi,* but focuses on positive energy rather than disharmony within the body

reminiscing recalling past events

remission a period of decreased severity of symptoms in chronic disease, or when symptoms subside

renal calculi kidney stones

renal pelvis the portion of the kidney that collects the urine and directs it into the ureter

reprisal retaliation

resident a person who receives care in a long-term care facility

resident care plan a nursing plan of care for a resident in a long-term care facility

Resident Council a group of residents who meet regularly; the councils give residents a method for communication with each other and with staff

resident unit a room occupied by a resident and his or her personal possessions; may be shared by other residents

residual limb a portion of a limb left after part has been removed

respiration the process of taking oxygen into the body and expelling carbon dioxide

respiratory arrest cessation of breathing

restoration basic nursing care designed to maintain or improve the resident's function and to assist the resident to return to self-care

restorative care describing care in which the interdisciplinary health care team assists the resident to reach the highest level of function

restraints physical, manual, or mechanical devices that are attached or adjacent to the resident's body that the resident cannot easily remove; these are used, when necessary, to protect the resident or other residents

résumé a short account of one's career and qualifications

resuscitation restoration to life of one who has cardiac and respiratory arrest

retention the inability to excrete urine that has been produced

retina the innermost or third layer of the eye, which receives images

retinopathy noninflammatory disease of the retina

retirement period after leaving employment

retraction to be brought backward

retroperitoneal space the area of the anterior cavity behind the peritoneum; in it are the kidneys, aorta, and inferior vena cava

Reye's syndrome a rare but deadly disease that affects all organs but is most harmful to the brain and liver, which affects predominately children through young adults who have had a viral infection and been treated with aspirin-containing products

rheumatoid arthritis an autoimmune response that results in inflammation of the joints

rhinitis inflammation of the mucous membranes of the nose

rhythm regular action or motion

ribs the 24 long, flat bones forming the wall of the thorax

rigor mortis a stiffening of the body 2 to 4 hours after death

RN registered nurse

RO reality orientation

ROM range of motion exercises

rotation the act of turning about the axis of the center of a body, as rotation of a joint

rubra unusual redness or flushing of skin

rupture the bursting of a part

S

Sacrament of the Sick given by a clergyman to a Catholic person who is terminally ill (dying); also called last rites

Safety Data Sheets (SDS) information sheets on chemicals used in a facility that list the health hazards, safe use, and emergency procedures for chemical exposure

safety device? a device that in some way restricts the activity of a resident to protect that resident or others

saliva a digestive secretion produced by the salivary glands and found in the mouth

sclera the white of the eye

scrotum a saclike pouch that holds the male gonads

sedative medication that has a calming effect; used to control nervousness, irritability, and excitement

seizure a convulsion; a condition characterized by involuntary shaking and jerking of the body

self-care (functional) deficit an inability to perform activities of daily living

Self-Determination Act a federal law passed in 1990 stating that competent adults have the right to be adequately informed about their medical conditions and the options of treatment available to them, and then to make their own decision as to their degree of participation

self-esteem? an opinion about oneself

self range of motion exercises done by the resident

seminal vesicles pouch-like sacs found in the male, located on the posterior wall of the bladder, that produce the bulk of the seminal fluid

semiprone position a modified prone position in which body is supported on pillows to relieve pressure on most of the bony prominences

semisupine position lying partially on the back and side; tilt position

senescent growing old

senescent changes normal aging changes

senile affected with the infirmities of age

senile keratosis? roughened, scaly, slightly elevated wartlike lesions, believed to be related to sun damage in fair-skinned individuals

senile lentigines yellow or brown spots that occur on exposed skin surfaces

senior a person over the age of 65

senior citizen center a place where seniors can meet for social and other activities

sensitive showing awareness or understanding of the feelings of others

sensitivity the state of acute or abnormal responsiveness to stimuli; the ability to recognize needs that are expressed or not expressed

sensory deprivation the lack of stimulation to the sense of vision, hearing, smell, taste, or touch

sensory nerve nerve that carries messages—about pain, temperature change, changes in body position, taste, touch, sound, and sight—toward the brain for interpretation

sensory-perceptual changes? an inability to recognize and use common objects such as eating utensils, combs, or pencils

sensory stimulation activities that increase the resident's awareness of his or her surroundings

sensual pertaining to the senses or sensation

sensuality the quality or state of being sensual

sepsis infection

septicemia an infection in the bloodstream

septum a wall or partition dividing a body cavity or space

seropositive producing a positive reaction to serologic tests (e.g., HIV positive)

serous membrane? a special tissue that secretes a serous fluid; covers organs and lines cavities that do not open to the outside

serum the clear liquid portion of the blood remaining after removal of the solid components and blood-clotting elements

sexual abuse using physical or verbal threats to force a resident to perform any sexual act; tormenting or teasing a resident with sexual gestures or words

sexuality the attitude of a person in relation to sex and sexual behavior

sharps needles, razors, or any sharp or cutting items

shearing force of skin over bone when the skin remains at the point of contact but the bone moves, causing skin damage; slides toward the lower gradient while the skin remains at its point of contact; the tissues between become ischemic

sheath covering

shift report information regarding resident status given to on-coming shift from those going off duty

sign? an observation apparent to an examiner or viewer

signing using hands and facial expression to communicate without speaking words

simple fracture a fracture that does not produce an open wound in the skin

sitz bath a bath providing moist heat to the genitals or anal area

skeletal muscle muscle tissue that is attached to the bone and provides voluntary movement

skilled nursing facility a long-term care facility

skin the external covering of the body

skin tear shallow injuries in which the epidermis is torn or ripped

slander? a false and damaging oral statement that injures the reputation of another person

sleep apnea stopping of breathing during sleep

SLIDE board a smooth, waxed board used for a sitting transfer, such as bed to wheelchair

sling a support used for an upper limb

smooth muscle a type of tissue that forms the walls of organs—involuntary or visceral

social worker a person licensed by the state to assess and provide services for non-medical and psychosocial needs of the residents

society a group of people who have common interests

spastic cerebral palsy a form of cerebral palsy in which the muscles are tense, contracted, and resistant to movement

spasticity? a condition of rigidity or spasm of muscle

spatial-perceptual deficit difficulty in distinguishing between left and right, up and down

specimen a sample of body secretion, excretion, or tissue used for diagnosis or determination of condition

speech-language pathologist a person trained and educated to diagnose and treat swallowing problems and speech and language disorders

sperm the male reproductive cell

sphincter a circular muscle that constricts a passage or closes a natural orifice; when relaxed, it allows passage of materials

sphygmomanometer an instrument for determining arterial pressure; blood pressure gauge

spinal column backbone or vertebral column

spiritual healing? treatment through prayer and invocation of supernatural forces to achieve healing and unity with a higher power

spirituality the state of being spiritual-minded or religious

splint a rigid device applied to maintain a body part in a specific position

spouse a marriage partner; gender neutral; husband or wife

sprain an injury to a ligament caused by sudden overstretching

sputum expectorated matter, composed of saliva and mucus from the lungs and throat

square corner a bedmaking technique in which the top sheet is tucked in at the bottom of the bed by forming a line parallel to the perpendicular edge of the mattress

Standard Precautions infection control practices used to prevent the spread of infection to health care workers and others

status? condition or state of health

stent a mesh device used to keep the artery open

stereotype a characteristic assigned to entire groups of people; rigid, biased ideas about people as a group

sterile free from microorganisms; incapable of reproducing sexually

sterilization a process that removes infectious agents from surfaces and equipment; a process that renders an individual incapable of reproduction

steroids a group name for certain compounds that include progesterone, the adrenocortical and gonadal hormones, bile acid, and sterols such as cholesterol

stethoscope an instrument used in auscultation to make audible the sounds produced in the body

stimulant an agent that produces stimulation or elicits a response

stoma? an artificial, mouthlike opening

stool another name for feces

strain excessive stretching of a muscle resulting in pain and swelling of the muscle

strengths activities that an individual can perform

stress feelings that cause a person to be anxious about his or her well-being

stress incontinence the inability to prevent small amounts of urine to escape when coughing, sneezing, laughing or lifting

stroke a cerebrovascular accident or brain attack; damage to the blood vessels of the brain

stump the distal end of a limb remaining after amputation

subacute care? care provided to persons who are not critically ill but have complex care needs

subcutaneous beneath the layers of the skin

subcutaneous tissue tissue that attaches the skin to the muscles

subjective observation observation based on reports of the resident (symptom)

subluxation incomplete dislocation of a joint

suffix a term added to the end of a word that changes or modifies the meaning of the word

sundowning increased confusion and restlessness in late afternoon, evening, or night

superior toward the head; upward

superior vena cava? the large blood vessel that drains the blood from the upper part of the body into the right atrium of the heart

supine lying in a face-up position on the back, or turning the forearm so the palm is facing upward

supportive care providing comfort measures

support services services not directly involved in resident care, for example, building and ground maintenance, housekeeping, kitchen work, administration duties

suppository a semisolid medication inserted in the rectum or vagina where it dissolves

suppression consciously refusing to acknowledge unacceptable feelings and thoughts

suprapubic situated, occurring or performed from above the pubis

survey a review and evaluation to make sure the long-term care facility maintains acceptable standards of practice and quality of care

surveyor? a representative of a private or governmental agency who reviews facility policies, procedures, and practices for quality care

sweat gland glands found in the skin that produce perspiration

symbol a mark or character that represents some quality, relationship, or word

sympathy feeling of pity or sorrow for another's situation or condition

symptom a subjective observation; indication of disease or disorder reported by the person but cannot be seen by others, such as pain

synapse the space between the axon of one cell and the dendrites of others

syncope faint; sudden loss of consciousness or strength

syndrome a group of signs and symptoms that may cause illness but are not a specific cause

synovial membrane? a special membrane that lines movable joint cavities

synovium joint lining

syphilis a sexually transmitted disease that may cause lesions in almost all tissues of the body and seriously affect the nervous system; a person may be asymptomatic for years

system a group of organs organized to carry out a specific body function or functions, such as the respiratory system

systole contraction, or period of contraction, of cardiac muscle

systolic applies to the contraction phase of the cardiac cycle

T

tachycardia an unusually rapid heartbeat

tachypnea respiratory pattern of rapid, shallow respirations

tact sensitive mental perception

tactile? pertaining to touch

tai chi an ancient Chinese form of meditative movement practiced through a series of exercises and breathing techniques; thought to improve the life energy flow

talisman engraved stone, ring, or other object used to ward off evil

task segmentation breaking down a complex task into a series of single steps

TED hose support hose for legs

temporal artery an artery located in the forehead and temple; assessed to measure temporal artery temperature

tendon a fibrous band of connective tissue that attaches skeletal muscle to bone

TENS See transcutaneous electrical nerve stimulation

terminal final, life-ending stage

terminal condition an illness, injury, or condition that will result in death

terminal illness a condition for which there is no cure

testes? male sex glands (gonads) found in the scrotum that produce sperm and the hormone testosterone

testicles testes

testosterone male sex hormone produced by the testes

theft taking that which does not belong to you; stealing

therapeutic pertaining to results obtained from treatment; a healing agent

therapeutic diet a planned intake of food and fluid to treat a specific disease condition

therapeutic recreational specialist a person trained and educated to use physical recreation as a rehabilitation therapy

therapy a treatment designated to eliminate disease or other bodily disorder

thermometer an instrument used to determine temperature

thoracic pertaining to the chest

thoracic cavity chest cavity

thorax the chest; the part of the body between the neck and the abdomen, encased by the shoulder girdle, ribs, and diaphragm

thrombocyte a blood platelet that is formed in the bone marrow and is important in blood clotting

thrombophlebitis development of thrombi (clots) as the result of inflammation of the lining of the veins

thrombus (pl. thrombi) blood clot

thyroid gland an endocrine gland located in the anterior neck in front of and on either side of the trachea that produces hormones thyrocalcitonin and thyroxine

thyroxine the hormone of the thyroid gland that contains iodine

TIA See transient ischemic attack

time and travel records records kept of the time spent with clients and the distance between client locations

tipping giving money as a reward or thanks for service rendered; not connected to salary

tissue a group of similar cells and fibers forming a particular structure; a piece of paper used for cleansing (e.g., toilet tissue, facial tissue)

toe pleat a bedmaking technique in which an extra fold of the top sheet is made at the foot of the bed to provide extra room for the resident's feet

withdrawal the retreat from reality or from social contact that is associated with severe depression and other psychiatric disorders

withhold? an order to refrain from serving a resident certain foods or fluids or all food

womb another term for the female uterus

word combination a joining or merging of different parts or qualities in which the component elements are individually distinct?

word root a word form whose basic meaning can be used in forming new words by combining it with prefixes and suffixes

work practice controls specific procedures to prevent the spread of infection

Y

yeast one type of fungus

yoga a system to promote union between the mind and body; includes a combination of breath control, postures, relaxation, and meditation

INDEX

Note: Page numbers followed by f or t represent figures or tables respectively.